Healing Traditions

Healing Traditions

The Mental Health of Aboriginal Peoples in Canada

Edited by Laurence J. Kirmayer and Gail Guthrie Valaskakis

UBCPress · Vancouver · Toronto

16 15 14 13 12 11 10 09   5 4 3 2 1

Printed in Canada on acid-free paper

Library and Archives Canada Cataloguing in Publication

    Healing traditions : the mental health of Aboriginal peoples in Canada / edited by Laurence J. Kirmayer and Gail Guthrie Valaskakis.

Includes bibliographical references and index.
ISBN 978-0-7748-1523-9

    1. Native peoples – Mental health – Canada. 2. Native peoples – Mental health services – Canada. I. Kirmayer, Laurence J., 1952- II. Valaskakis, Gail Guthrie

RC451.5.I5H44 2008   362.2'08997071   C2008-906205-1

Canadä

UBC Press gratefully acknowledges the financial support for our publishing program of the Government of Canada through the Book Publishing Industry Development Program (BPIDP), and of the Canada Council for the Arts, and the British Columbia Arts Council.

This book has been published with the help of a grant from the Canadian Federation for the Humanities and Social Sciences, through the Aid to Scholarly Publications Programme, using funds provided by the Social Sciences and Humanities Research Council of Canada.

UBC Press
The University of British Columbia
2029 West Mall
Vancouver, BC V6T 1Z2
604-822-5959 / Fax: 604-822-6083
www.ubcpress.ca

Contents

Illustrations

Figures

Table

Foreword

GEORGES HENRY ERASMUS

When one considers the material consequences of Canada's century-long policy of state-sponsored, forcible assimilation, a simple fact emerges: for generations, opportunities to live well *as an Aboriginal person* have been actively frustrated. Successive governments, committed to the notion that Aboriginal cultures belong only to the past, have made no provision for the well-being of these cultures in the present and future. In the arrangement of Canada's social affairs, only the assimilated Indian has been offered even the prospect of wellness. For those who resisted or refused the benefits of assimilation, government policies assured a life of certain indignity. That is the essence of life in the colony: assimilate and be like us or suffer the consequences.

But to go on blaming government for our problems is, as we know, to stop short of solutions. Canada has responsibilities, articulated in treaties and in other formal agreements with Aboriginal people. Canada furthermore has a role to play in the present work of healing and reconciliation. However, our healing and well-being are and ought to be our own responsibility. What Wilfred Pelletier wrote of freedom is true also of wellness: "It is not something government can give you. Government does not have it, you have it, and when you realize this you exercise it responsibly" (*No foreign land* 1973, 149-50). The task of securing our well-being and that of our children is the ultimate task of our cultures. As noted in one of the contributions to this volume, "culture is treatment, and all healing is spiritual."

For many years now, Aboriginal people have been on a healing journey. We began to address the conditions of our communities even before the demise of the government-managed Indian residential schools. Focusing on addictions and a renewed commitment to traditional Aboriginal teachings, the healing movement in its early days embraced a holistic view of individual and community wellness. Perhaps the most dramatic example of community healing to date has been Alkali Lake (Esketemc First Nation), in British Columbia. The return of this society from a state of near-universal addiction became the subject of a video, *The Honour of All: The Story of Alkali Lake*. The case of Alkali Lake, which achieved a 95% rate of sobriety, demonstrates hope and potential when even one dedicated person is committed to the goal of community wellness.

Fortunately for us, there are today thousands of committed Aboriginal people across Canada and indeed across the world. Their strength and resilience is a source of much-needed encouragement. Every year many more rise, take the first uncertain steps, and add to a growing momentum that we hope will carry us forward.

Since 1998 the Aboriginal Healing Foundation has encouraged and supported community-based healing initiatives that address the intergenerational legacy of physical and sexual abuses suffered in Canada's Indian residential school system. We know today that the residential schools have contributed to unresolved historical trauma and that the healing of this trauma is critical to our ability to address other pressing social concerns. And so, like the authors, the Aboriginal Healing Foundation looks forward to a time when Aboriginal people have addressed the effects of unresolved trauma in meaningful terms, have broken the cycle of abuse, and have enhanced their capacity as individuals, families, communities, and nations to sustain both their well-being and the well-being of future generations.

This collection challenges many common assumptions, as it should. The terrain of mental health is broad, varied, and incompletely seen from any one vista. In the following pages, mental health is considered from a variety of critical perspectives that subject even the notions of mental illness and Aboriginal healing to constructive analysis. What these writings bear in common is a commitment to the principle that we as Aboriginal people must take possession of our wellness. This principle includes the freedom to critique, to debate, and, one hopes, to arrive at a constructive consensus of the definitions of healing.

This collection will contribute to just such a discussion.

Masi.

Preface

This is the first book dedicated to bringing together research and reflection on the mental health of Aboriginal peoples in Canada from a wide range of perspectives, with contributions from psychiatry, psychology, anthropology, women's studies, sociology, and education. This is not a handbook of practice but a resource for thinking critically about current issues in the mental health of indigenous peoples. Thus there is an emphasis on cultural analysis of the concepts, values, and assumptions that shape mental health theory and practice and on the nature of Aboriginal identity and experience. Understanding the multiple meanings of Aboriginal identity requires an appreciation of history and contemporary and political realities. This book examines some of these contexts and cultures – and traces their implications for mental health. Although the focus is necessarily on social suffering and affliction, we have tried to strike a balance between looking unflinchingly at the problems faced by Aboriginal peoples and recognizing their equally evident well-being, resilience, and renewal. We believe this approach will be useful for a wide range of readers in Aboriginal communities as well as in the general population, including health professionals, community workers, planners and administrators, social scientists, researchers, educators, and students.

Our title, *Healing Traditions,* has several potential meanings. First, it refers to recovering and applying traditional methods of healing. Aboriginal peoples had a wide range of methods of healing that served to integrate the community and provide individuals with systems of meaning to make sense of suffering. These traditions were displaced and actively suppressed by successive generations of Euro-Canadian missionaries, governments, and professionals. Restoring these traditions, therefore, makes available a great variety of potentially effective forms of healing that may fit especially well with the values or ethos of contemporary Aboriginal peoples.

More broadly, the recovery of traditional healing involves ceremonies and practices that engage not just individuals but also families and communities in ways that can promote solidarity, social support, and collective transformation. Many indigenous ways of understanding the person include an ecocentric sense of self that contrasts with the individualism that underwrites most contemporary mental health theory and practice. For most Aboriginal peoples, traditional subsistence activities (e.g., hunting, fishing, trapping) were deeply integrated with spiritual beliefs as well as with family and community relationships. Returning to the land to take part in these activities may then have healing value for both troubled individuals and whole communities.

Traditional healing is also healing through tradition. The recovery of tradition itself may be healing, both at individual and collective levels. Efforts to restore linguistic, religious, and communal practices can be understood as fundamental acts of healing. Retrieving and transmitting the knowledge associated with healing practices reaffirms core cultural values and maintains the historical continuity of Aboriginal cultures.

Finally, traditions themselves need to be reconfigured to meet the challenges of the contemporary world. The effort to reassert cultural traditions results in individuals and communities taking political action to claim their place in the larger world, at the levels of regional, national, and global society, and this too may have positive effects on health. Establishing legal claims to traditional lands and self-government may also be viewed as crucial elements of reasserting the autonomy that was central to traditional culture, even when the forms of social life, community, and governance necessarily reflect contemporary political structures.

Notions of mental health and illness cover a broad territory that includes well-being, everyday problems in living associated with bodily symptoms of stress and anxiety, mild depression, and seasonal fluctuations in mood and energy, as well as more severe psychiatric disorders, such as major depression, bipolar disorder, schizophrenia, and other psychotic disorders. There are several reasons for collecting such a diverse group of conditions under the broad term "mental health": they all involve processes of behaviour and experience related to mental or psychological functions; there are overlapping causes, symptoms, and, in some instances, similar treatments that work to ameliorate many of these conditions, promoting health, resilience, and recovery; and finally, these all fall under the domain of the "psy" professions in contemporary health care – psychiatry, psychology, social work, family therapy, and so on.

Concepts of mental illness and psychiatric disorder focus on problems and pathology. The clinical professions are committed to trying to understand and help those who are obviously ill, suffering, and disabled by offering specific forms of therapy, marshalling appropriate resources, and engaging in social advocacy. At the same time, we recognize that mental afflictions are part of the human condition: we all have difficulties at times, and we are all striving for better functioning, greater well-being, and positive life attitudes and experiences. Recognition of the universal importance of mental well-being suggests that we focus not only on mental illness but also on mental health. A focus on health, well-being, and resilience draws attention to what works, to what can be learned from those who are healthy despite adversity – those who find creative solutions to life's challenges.

The term "mental health" is therefore both less stigmatizing and more positive than mental illness, which is likely why it is preferred by many individuals and organizations.

There is the risk, however, that in focusing on the positive, on solutions, and on the milder end of the spectrum, we ignore those who are carrying the heaviest burden of illness, whose behaviour and experience may be more out of the ordinary, strange, and disturbing, and who may be blamed, stigmatized, and scapegoated. We therefore think it is crucial to retain this broad and flexible use of the term "mental health," which encompasses the whole range of human problems, in an effort to reduce the stigma attached to mental illness and to signal a commitment to address all forms of suffering.

Although psychology and psychiatry tend to focus on the individual, many of the problems people face involve interactions with others – in couples, families, communities, or wider social networks, including governments and global economic systems. As the contributors to this volume emphasize, what is distinctive about Aboriginal mental health is the shared history and social predicament that has made many communities vulnerable to a range of social problems that, in turn, increase the risk of emotional suffering. The challenge for mental health theory and practice is to develop perspectives that are deeply informed by an understanding of this social and cultural history and current political and economic contexts.

The book is divided into four sections: an introduction to the mental health of indigenous peoples; origins and representations of social suffering; transformations of identity and community that contribute to resilience; and traditional healing and mental health services. However, all of the contributors discuss issues that span these divisions, so the book is structured more like a spiral that returns to core questions again and again in ways that can enlarge our understanding. The cross-cutting themes make it possible to pursue many paths through the book, to follow discussions of the impact of colonialism, sedentarization, and forced assimilation; the importance of land for indigenous identity and an ecocentric self; the notions of space and place as part of the cultural matrix of identity and experience; the processes of healing; and the importance of spirituality as a counterbalance to the competitiveness and materialism intrinsic to urban industrialized societies and consumer capitalism.

In the introductory chapter, Laurence Kirmayer, Caroline Tait, and Cori Simpson outline some of the historical background and current context needed to understand what is distinctive about the mental health of Aboriginal peoples. The diverse indigenous cultures of North America developed many unique ways of life and rich cultural traditions reflecting the ecological contexts in which they lived. These were radically challenged and transformed by European colonization and the policies of forced assimilation adopted by governments. Although it is difficult to prove a direct causal link, it is likely that the collective trauma, disorientation, loss, and grief caused by these short-sighted and often self-serving policies are major determinants of the mental health problems faced by many Aboriginal communities and populations across Canada.

In the second chapter, Mason Durie, Helen Milroy, and Ernest Hunter note the similarities in experiences of Anglo-settler colonialism in Australia, Canada, New Zealand, and the United States. Their discussion of Aboriginal and Torres Strait Islander Australians and of Mäori New Zealanders provides an illuminating set of comparisons to the situation in Canada. Despite the parallel history, there are important differences between the countries in demography, culture, and politics. The high proportion of indigenous people in the population of New Zealand has contributed to a new era of bicultural national identity that bodes well for the health of Mäori. In Australia the more fragmented and marginalized Aboriginal population has continued to struggle with devastating social problems and, until recently, a lack of basic recognition and restitution from government.

In his contribution, anthropologist James Waldram critiques the ways that the notion of Aboriginality itself has been constructed and construed in mental health research. He identifies four main approaches in quantitative research that define Aboriginal identity in terms of blood quantum, legal status or self-identification, geographic region or culture area, and individual cultural orientation or acculturation. Each approach raises problems because it overgeneralizes, essentializes, and stereotypes identity in terms of sets of traits or qualities that do not characterize any single individual.

Psychologists Grace Iarocci, Rhoda Root, and Jacob Burack provide an overview of developmental approaches to understanding social competence and mental health among Aboriginal youth. They discuss integrative developmental models that include the interactions of individuals, families, and communities with culture, social context, and the ecological environment. They review research on resilience among inner-city youth and ethnic minority groups as well as the much smaller quantity of research on Aboriginal children and youth. These studies make it clear that resilience is not a single global trait or fixed characteristic of individuals but an ongoing process of adaptation based on diverse processes of growth and transformation. Individuals may show strength and resilience in one domain while having difficulties in other areas. Iarocci and her co-authors draw out the broad implications of a developmental perspective for mental health promotion and future research.

The contributions to the second section look more closely at the predicaments of particular communities, major historical changes, and specific types of mental health problems to trace the origins of the social suffering experienced by many Aboriginal communities. At the same time, they look at the prevalent social representations of these problems. The ways that Aboriginal peoples and communities are represented in popular mass media, as well as in academic writing and government reports, can play an important role in improving or aggravating their predicaments.

Colin Samson describes the Innu predicament in terms of the metaphor of the double-bind. In Gregory Bateson's formulation, the double-bind is a no-win situation in which one is faced with inescapable contradictions and is prohibited from leaving the situation or talking explicitly about the paradox. Samson describes the profound social changes brought by sedentarization and forced relocation for the Inuit. Mental health professionals tend to emphasize individual agency and culpability and do not see the sociopolitical and historical "big picture," so they end up blaming individuals for social suffering, pointing to unhealthy parents, corrupt leaders and undersupervised and misguided children. Governments also tend to downplay or ignore the historical context because it allows them to sidestep their own responsibility. As a result of ignoring this larger context, even well-intentioned interventions tend to aggravate existing problems.

Jo-Anne Fiske explores another form of silencing and marginalization: the refusal to see the oppressive effects of the residential school system mandated by the Canadian government, which carried out a regime of forced assimilation for almost one hundred years. Fiske shows how the residential school was divided into gendered places: the outdoor fields where boys laboured and the indoor workshops where girls learned domestic skills. This symbolic organization of space was motivated by another powerful and pervasive dichotomy between the domestic and the wild, or between modern civilization and primitive savagery. The residential school as a whole was viewed as a domestic space, which served effectively to hide its political functions of containment, assimilation, and elimination of indigenous peoples through the education of their children. This elision of colonial history persists today and causes some to doubt on the claims of survivors of residential schools that they have suffered violent cultural oppression as well as physical and sexual abuse. Their claims of abuse are viewed as incredible – or at least, hard to credit – because they challenge the underlying assumption that a benevolent nation and church bestowed the gifts of civilization on backward peoples.

Dara Culhane describes the situation of urban Aboriginal women in Vancouver who are struggling with drug addiction, HIV infection, homelessness, and loss. Her interviews with these women reveal how their predicaments emerge from a cascade of events that reflect their poverty, marginalization, and disempowerment as Aboriginal women. Although the women themselves emphasize their own bad choices in life, it is clear that they have been choosing from the limited range of options created by bureaucratic systems and the exclusionary practices that affect Aboriginal people in both rural and urban society. Despite the harshness and desperation of their lives, the women emerge as struggling for a moral stance and presence in others' lives.

Drawing from his fieldwork in a Cree community in Manitoba, Ronald Niezen focuses on the phenomenon of suicide clusters. He details the historical changes faced by this community, including residential schools and the social impact of hydroelectric development, mining, and other forms of large-scale resource extraction. Like Samson, he notes the "inherently contradictory efforts to impart autonomy and self-sufficiency through the imposition of alien values." The fact that suicides have tended to occur in clusters in some Aboriginal communities may tell us something important about the dynamics of suicide and other forms of self-destructive behaviour. Suicidal youth may be those who suffer estrangement from family and community, resulting in a lack of connection across the generations, and fall back on a small subgroup of similarly suffering and disaffected youths who reinforce each other's risky behaviour, impulsivity, and desperation, limiting their ability to imagine life-affirming alternatives or ways out of their shared quandary.

Caroline Tait examines recent concerns about an "epidemic" of fetal alcohol syndrome (FAS) among Aboriginal peoples. The pre-existing association of Aboriginal people with alcohol and drug abuse, coupled with new evidence about the potential effects of maternal substance use on the developing fetus, has led many to assume that problems related to fetal alcohol exposure are endemic in Aboriginal populations. However, this assumption has occurred in the absence of actual clinical diagnosis. Once FAS was identified as a potential problem, resources were made available to support intervention. This has encouraged communities to self-label in ways that fit the funding priorities. Tait points to the risk that, in this case, individuals and communities are accepting a label that implies permanent disability, and this may ultimately undermine collective aspirations for autonomy.

The third section continues the discussion of the impacts on mental health of the history of internal colonialism, sedentarization, and forced assimilation, but the emphasis shifts to consider notions of resilience – that is, what processes account for the fact that many individuals and communities have done well despite historical and contemporary adversities.

Michael Chandler and Christopher Lalonde present their influential work on the social correlates of suicide in Aboriginal communities. This research was originally inspired by Chandler's work on the development of adolescent identity and sense of personal self-continuity, but they have extended this to a community-psychology approach that seeks correlations between health outcomes and social factors at the level of region, band, or community. Although most of their work to date has focused on suicide, more recently they have begun to examine outcomes like the frequency of accidents or school completion. Their developmental theory frames this in terms of individual and cultural continuity, yet continuity is not simply about preserving the past but equally about forging strong commitments to the future. They end with a plea for more effective knowledge transfer and suggest that encouraging communities to share their knowledge "laterally" with other communities may avoid some of the problems associated with the culture of experts, which tends to reproduce the colonial hierarchies of dominance and the devaluing of indigenous knowledge.

Reflecting on his work with the Cree of Mistissini over three decades, Adrian Tanner describes the social suffering brought about by sedentarization. However, he emphasizes the ways that the community has responded to this predicament by political engagement and by developing new healing practices. Individuals within Cree communities are exploring traditions that include pan-Indian spirituality, Pentecostalism, and Cree animism to create the diverse strands of what Tanner calls "the healing movement," which involves annual gatherings and other collective activities aimed at cultural renewal and collective solidarity. Of course, there are significant differences of opinion over the right direction, and the community must contend with new tensions and conflicts between groups following divergent paths. Nevertheless, the active engagement with these healing activities constitutes a source and expression of vitality in the community.

In her chapter, Naomi Adelson also addresses the varieties of religion, tradition, and healing in Cree communities in Quebec. She reviews some of the history of Christian missionizing among the Cree, which led the community to make the religion its own. Based on interviews with church Elders, she provides a different point of view on the dilemmas posed by the new Native spirituality, which is rooted in pan-Indianism or in the recuperation of specifically Cree traditions. These dilemmas take on a particular dynamic in the light of generational differences, particularly given the experiences of youth with new levels of mobility and their connections to a global network.

The Inuit in Canada's North have faced one of the most rapid and dramatic changes in way of life of any people. In a chapter based on ethnographic fieldwork and clinical experience in Nunavik, Laurence Kirmayer, Christopher Fletcher, and Robert Watt describe Inuit concepts of mental health and illness. Contemporary understandings of mental health problems draw from popular psychology, Christian religious ideas, and more specifically Inuit notions of both spirituality and an ecocentric self. The person is seen as intimately connected to the land through diet, activities, and values. Mental health and healing can be powerfully influenced by eating country food, hunting, and camping on the land. These indigenous notions of an environmental, or land-based, psychology offer an important complement to current models of the person in mental health.

Inuit mental health and well-being are also the topic of the chapter by Michael Kral and Lori Idlout, who discuss the transformations of identity and community in Nunavut. The creation of Nunavut itself, as a political entity, has been an important milestone, affording the Inuit a greater measure of authority in their own land. Despite this political advance and government programs promoting "healthy communities," many settlements have continued to suffer high rates of suicide, domestic violence, and other social problems. Some Inuit communities have done well, and Kral and Idlout explore possible reasons for these regional differences. They discuss the factors that may contribute to a sense of collective agency and *nunalingni silatuningit,* or community wisdom.

The last section considers issues of treatment intervention, illness prevention, and health promotion with discussions of Aboriginal healing and the provision of mental health services.

Rod McCormick outlines contemporary approaches to psychological counselling grounded in Aboriginal values and perspectives. These approaches start with the recognition that substance use and related mental health problems are not only symptoms of individuals' distress but also efforts to cope with untenable social situations brought on by a history of collective oppression.

Gregory Brass presents an ethnographic study of healing and identity in a residential therapeutic program for a diverse group of Aboriginal men in the correctional system. The treatment program used a generic construction of Aboriginal identity, emphasizing pan-Indian spirituality, combined with standard methods of counselling and psychotherapy, to create hybrid forms of group and individual therapy. This hybrid Aboriginal identity and therapeutic practice was meaningful to many clients, who differed from one another in cultural, linguistic, and personal backgrounds. However, some participants found the pan-Indian symbolism or the psychological idioms strange and uncomfortable.

At present, more than half of all Aboriginal people live in cities. Mary Ellen Macdonald examines the predicament of urban Aboriginal residents in the Montreal region seeking mental health services. Most Aboriginal people in the city are expected to make use of mainstream services, where there is virtually no attention to issues of Aboriginal identity and culture. Community organizations like the Native Friendship Centre provide some counselling and support but are not well integrated with other resources. Unlike Toronto, Winnipeg, and some other cities in Canada, Montreal has no specialized clinics or services for most Aboriginal people. However, Macdonald's interviews with members of the Aboriginal community in Montreal reveal caution and ambivalence about the potential to develop ethnospecific services, with many expressing concerns about confidentiality, stigma, and further marginalization.

Cornelia Wieman describes the unique mental health services developed at the Six Nations reserve in Ontario. The community is large enough to sustain its own comprehensive mental health clinic with psychiatric nurses, social workers, psychologists, and several part-time psychiatrists. The aim is to provide quality mental health care that is respectful of local values and traditions. Their links to the community give practitioners inside knowledge and understanding of how to mobilize social networks and supports to enhance care. At the same time, conflicts over jurisdiction and funding force staff to engage in constant struggles in order to ensure a secure future for the service.

Writing from his perspective as a Native American clinical psychologist, educator, and researcher, Joseph Gone discusses the perils of academia and professional education. Education provides credentials needed to achieve a social status and to command the power and resources to effect change. At the same time, education involves acquiring a set of identities, practices, values, and ways of knowing that belong to the "whiteman." Psychotherapies provide languages of selfhood rooted in Euro-American culture that have particular moral and political implications – some of which may be at odds with indigenous values. Gone suggests, therefore, that Aboriginal communities should be more cautious in adopting the latest popular psychological theory or treatment fad. Although some indigenous scholars have been deeply suspicious of the value system inherent in science, Gone makes the provocative argument that "scientific knowing is *probably all that recommends psychology as a profession*." The epistemology of science allows a kind of systematic inquiry and verification that goes beyond commonsense knowledge, and this approach should be claimed and used by indigenous scholars and practitioners.

In the concluding chapter, Kirmayer, Brass, and Gail Guthrie Valaskakis examine some of the implications of the many forms of healing and diverse interpretations of tradition presented throughout this volume. Healing is a universal human experience built out of symbols, metaphors, and actions that are grounded in specific traditions. Recuperating these traditions is, thus, a way to restore cultural riches that belong to a people and that, through them, are of significance to all of humanity. "Tradition" is a term of veneration, linking contemporary knowledge and identity to a valorized past. But all living traditions undergo constant renovation and reinvention. To recognize the ways forward for Aboriginal peoples in Canada, we need to understand this process of inventing the present by simultaneously respecting the past and imagining the future.

This book has had a long gestation, and many people have contributed to bringing it to completion. At various stages in its development, the co-ordinators of our Québec Aboriginal Mental Health Research Team and the National Network for Aboriginal Mental Health Research have done background research and managed the logistics. Deepest thanks to Gregory Brass, Aimee Ebersold, Shannon Dow, Tara Holton, Cori Simpson, Caroline Tait, and Marsha Vicaire. Dianne Goudreau generously contributed her editorial expertise and Robert Lewis ably copy-edited the final manuscript. Kay Berckmans and Antonella Clerici provided administrative and secretarial support and facilitated the meetings and conferences that led to this publication. Darcy Cullen of UBC Press shepherded the manuscript through the editorial and production process with tact and creativity.

This book has been published with the help of grants from the Aboriginal Healing Foundation and the Canadian Federation of the Humanities and Social Sciences, through the Aid to Scholarly Publications Programme, using funds provided by the Social Sciences and Humanities Research Council of Canada. Preparation of this volume was also supported by grants from the Canadian Institutes of Health Research (CIHR), the Institute of Aboriginal Peoples' Health, and the Institute for Neurosciences, Mental Health and Addictions. We thank Jeff Reading and Remi Quirion for their vision in fostering the National Network for Aboriginal Mental Health Research. The Aboriginal Healing Foundation supported Gail Guthrie Valaskakis' co-leadership of the Network and participation in this book project. The Department of Psychiatry and the Lady Davis Institute for Research of the Sir Mortimer B. Davis – Jewish General Hospital in Montreal have supported our work in Aboriginal mental health since its inception.

The National Network for Aboriginal Mental Health Research, founded with a grant from the CIHR Institute of Aboriginal Peoples' Health, is a vehicle for training and fostering collaborative, community-based research that can contribute to improving the mental health of Aboriginal peoples. This volume is one fruit of this ongoing collaboration. This book has many Aboriginal voices, but there are still too few involved in the fields of mental health research and practice. It is our hope that these essays will inspire others to take up the challenge of rethinking mental health and healing from diverse perspectives.

Laurence J. Kirmayer
Gail Guthrie Valaskakis
2007

With great sadness, I note the untimely death of my friend and colleague Gail Guthrie Valaskakis. Her creative vision, wise counsel, and steadfast commitment made the National Network for Aboriginal Mental Health Research a reality. Although she was not able to see this book in print, it stands as a testament to her belief in the value of socially relevant research and collaboration among researchers from diverse disciplines and backgrounds as a means to further the health and well-being of indigenous peoples in Canada and throughout the world.

Laurence J. Kirmayer
2008

PART 1
The Mental Health of Indigenous Peoples

1

The Mental Health of Aboriginal Peoples in Canada: Transformations of Identity and Community

LAURENCE J. KIRMAYER, CAROLINE L. TAIT, AND CORI SIMPSON

Around the world, indigenous peoples have experienced colonization, cultural oppression, forced assimilation, and absorption into a global economy with little regard for their autonomy or well-being. These profound transformations have been linked to high rates of depression, alcoholism, violence, and suicide in many communities, with the most dramatic impact on youth (Waldram, Herring, and Young 2006; Warry 1998). Despite these challenges, many communities have done well, enjoying high levels of health and well-being and continuing to transmit their cultural knowledge, language, and traditions to the next generation. This book brings together scholars, researchers, and clinicians from a range of backgrounds and perspectives to consider some key issues in the mental health of Aboriginal peoples, particularly in Canada.

In this introductory chapter, we provide an overview of the social and historical context that underpins current mental health disparities found among Aboriginal peoples of Canada. We first outline the profound changes in the material, social, and political conditions of life for Aboriginal peoples brought about by European colonization. Although it is not easy to prove causality when describing the unfolding of large-scale historical events, it seems clear that intensive interactions with colonizers and settlers as well as with the economic, bureaucratic, and technocratic institutions of Canadian society have been major determinants of the social distress experienced by Aboriginal communities today. We then review the clinical information available on the type and prevalence of mental health problems in Aboriginal populations. Next, we consider some of the ongoing transformations of individual and collective identity as well as the forms of community that have persisted despite adversity and that hold the seeds of resilience and renewal for Aboriginal peoples. The concluding section explores some implications of an emphasis on identity and community for mental health services and health promotion.

Aboriginal Peoples in Canada

According to the 2006 census, 1.17 million people self-identify as Aboriginal in Canada, representing 3.8% of the total population (Statistics Canada 2008). First Nations constitute

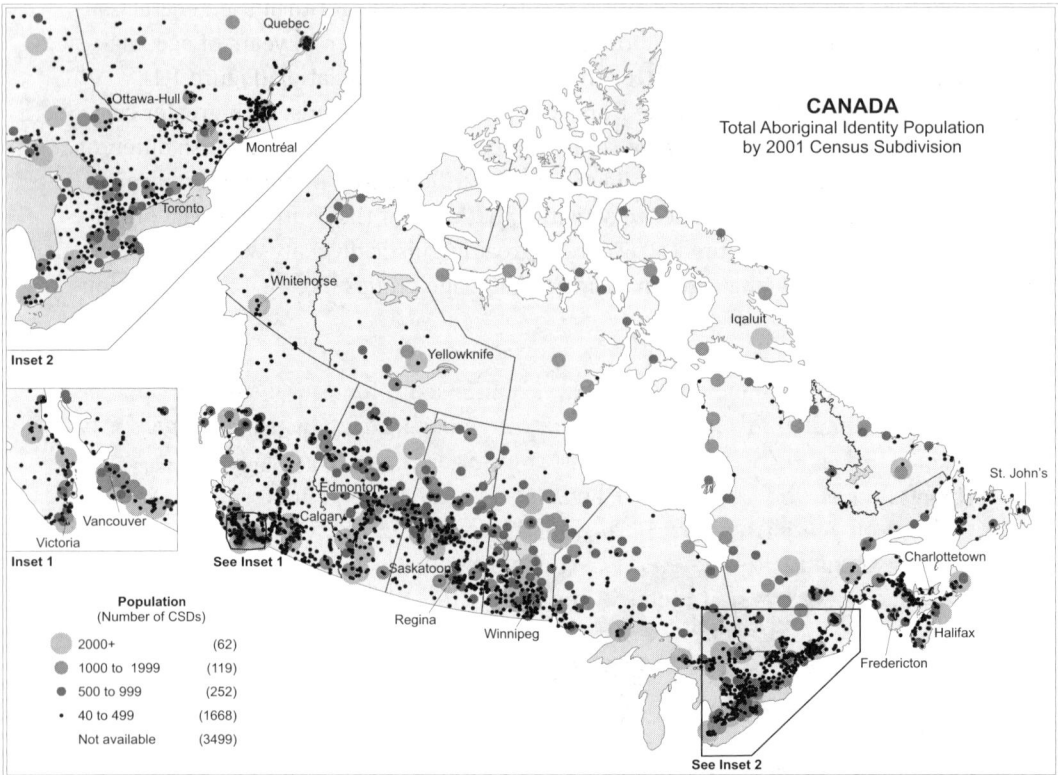

FIGURE 1.1 Geographic distribution of the Aboriginal population in Canada. Total Aboriginal population in Canada by census division, 2001. *Source:* Statistics Canada, 2001.

about 60% of the Aboriginal population, Métis 33%, and Inuit 4%.[1] First Nations are administratively divided into status and nonstatus Indians under the federal Indian Act (Imai 2003). In 2006, 698,025 people identified themselves as First Nations, of whom 564,870, or 81%, were registered as status Indians. The 2006 census estimated the Inuit population at 50,485, and there were 389,785 Métis. The nonurban population is distributed across many small communities that include 615 First Nations bands and 2,284 reserves and 52 Inuit communities (Frideres 2004; Government of Canada 2006; Statistics Canada 2008). More than half (54%) of Aboriginal people live in urban centres. About 60% of First Nations people live off-reserve, 3.4% of them in urban areas. Almost 70% of Métis live in urban areas. Fully 80% of Aboriginal persons live in Ontario and western Canada, with the greatest concentrations in the North and on the Prairies (Statistics Canada 2008). Most Inuit live in small settlements in the northern regions of Canada, mainly Nunavut (50%), Nunavik (northern Quebec) (19%), Nunatsiavut (northern Labrador) (4%), and the Inuvialuit region of the Northwest Territories (6%); about 17% of Inuit live in urban areas across Canada.

LAURENCE J. KIRMAYER, CAROLINE L. TAIT, AND CORI SIMPSON

Demographically, the Aboriginal population is substantially younger than the general Canadian population: almost half of the Aboriginal population is under 24 years of age, making the mean age 27, compared to 40 for the non-Aboriginal population (Figure 1.1).

Indigenous people in Canada come from very diverse backgrounds, with greater cultural and linguistic differences between some groups than those that distinguish different European cultures. Broad culture areas have been described based on the importance of local ecology for traditional subsistence activities that were at the centre of social organization and cultural values (Figure 1.2). There is great linguistic diversity within this population, with more than 55 languages in 11 major language groups (Figure 1.3). In addition

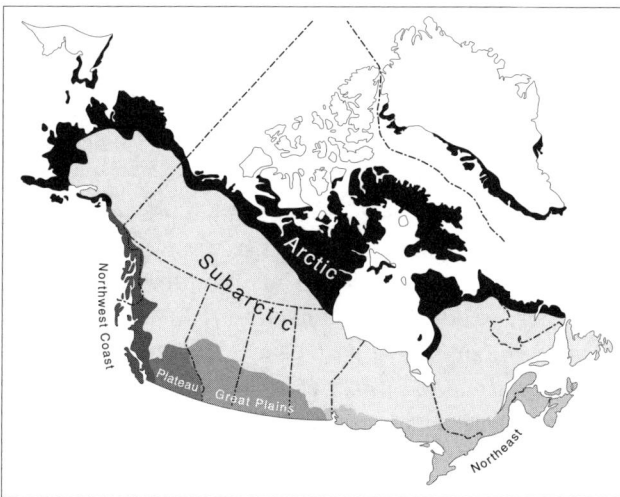

FIGURE 1.2   Cultural-ecological regions. *Source:* Natural Resources Canada.

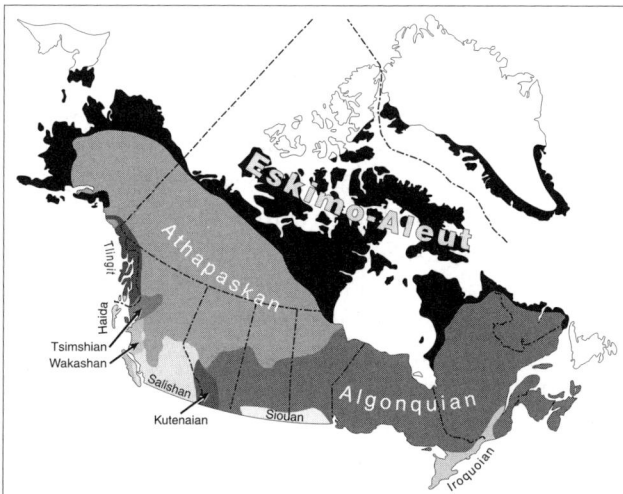

FIGURE 1.3   Language groups. *Source:* Natural Resources Canada.

to the social, cultural, and environmental differences between groups, there is an enormous diversity of values, lifestyles, and perspectives within any community or urban Aboriginal population. This diversity makes lumping groups together under generic terms like "Aboriginal" or "indigenous" misleading (see Waldram, Chapter 3). Nevertheless, although First Nations, Métis, and Inuit each have a unique historical relationship with European colonization and Canadian governments, they do share a common social, economic, and political predicament that is the legacy of colonization. This shared predicament has motivated efforts to forge common political fronts (i.e., the Assembly of First Nations and the Métis National Council) and, to some degree, a collective identity across diverse groups (e.g., the National Aboriginal Health Organization, the Native Women's Association of Canada, and Quebec Native Women). Globally, there are also striking parallels in the histories of indigenous peoples around the world, suggesting that although biological, social, cultural, and political factors vary, there are common processes at work (Durie et al., Chapter 2; Kunitz 1994; Stephens et al. 2005).

Although there have been improvements in recent years, there continues to be a significant gap in life expectancy between Aboriginal peoples and the general Canadian population. According to Health Canada, in 2001 the average life expectancy for First Nations men was 70.4 years, compared to 77.1 for the general population; the corresponding figures for women were 75.5 versus 82.2.[2] Among Inuit, the figures for 1999 revealed an even greater disparity, with life expectancies of 67.7 for men and 70.2 for women. Aboriginal peoples suffer from a wide range of health problems at much higher rates than other Canadians (MacMillan et al. 1996; Waldram, Herring, and Young 2006). They have 6 to 7 times greater incidence of tuberculosis, are 4 to 5 times more likely to be diabetic, 3 times more likely to have heart disease and hypertension, and 2 times as likely to report a long-term disability. Injuries and poisonings are the main cause of potential years of life lost; Aboriginal peoples have 1.5 times the national mortality rate and 6.5 times the national rate of death by injuries and poisonings. The potential years of life lost before age 75 due to accidents or health problems is about 50% higher in geographic regions with a high proportion of Aboriginal residents (Allard, Wilkins, and Berthelot 2004). Almost 40% of these years lost are due to injuries, mainly suicide and motor vehicle accidents. The regions with the highest levels of premature years lost and lowest expectancies of living free of disabilities are characterized by being remote and rural and by having the sparsest population, high levels of unemployment, low educational attainment, and low household income. Social problems are also common. In a recent survey, fully 39% of Aboriginal adults reported that family violence is a problem in their community, 25% reported sexual abuse, and 15% reported rape (Health Canada 2002). The incarceration rates of Aboriginal adults are 5 to 6 times higher than the national average, and Aboriginal people account for fully 18.5% of the federal prison population (Brzozowski, Taylor-Butts, and Johnson 2006).

These health disparities and social problems are paralleled by elevated rates of mental health problems in some communities (Petawabano et al. 1994; Waldram et al. 2006). Age-standardized suicide rates of Aboriginal youth are 3 to 6 times that of the general population (Kirmayer et al. 2007). In 2001 survey rates of emotional distress reported were about 13% among First Nations individuals living off-reserve, compared to 8% in the general population (Government of Canada 2006, 164). The rates may be higher on some reserves. Although these problems affect individuals, both their high prevalence and the great variability across communities underscore the need for a social perspective if we are to understand the sources of illness and suffering as well as resilience and healing.

Social Origins of Distress

Despite creation stories rooted in a timeless past and notions of cultural continuity, traditional Aboriginal societies in North America were not static over their 15,000 years or more of migration and development throughout the Americas, nor were they entirely free of disease or social problems (Ray 1996). However, a dramatically accelerated process of cultural change began in the sixteenth century through interactions with European outsiders, which included those on fishing expeditions, explorers, itinerant traders whose ships put in for provisions, missionaries, fur traders, and colonists. In addition, there were encounters with Mesoamerican and Caribbean Natives who accompanied European expeditions (Trigger and Swagerty 1996).

The origins of the elevated rates of mental and social distress found in many Aboriginal populations are not hard to discern. Aboriginal peoples in Canada have faced cultural oppression and social marginalization through the actions of European colonizers and their institutions since the earliest periods of contact. Culture contact brought with it many forms of depredation. Economic, political, and religious institutions of the European settlers all contributed to the displacement and oppression of indigenous people.

Early missionary activities focused on saving heathen souls through religious conversion. In many cases, this involved suppression or subversion of indigenous spiritual beliefs and practices that were integral to subsistence activities and to the structure of families and communities. Although Aboriginal peoples engaged in trade to further their own interests, early trade and military alliances with Europeans were generally arranged without regard for Aboriginal cultural values or relationships. With colonization, these sporadic encounters took on a new scale and intensity, resulting in escalating levels of violence against Aboriginal peoples – violence driven by fear and avarice and justified by ideologies that viewed the indigenous peoples of the Americas as "savages" and that declared the entire continent *terra nullius,* "no man's land," a land unclaimed and free for the taking.

The history of the European colonization of North America is a harrowing tale of decimation of the indigenous population by infectious disease, warfare, and active suppression of culture and identity, an undertaking that was tantamount to genocide (Stannard 1992; Thornton 1987). Despite the escalating levels of violence toward indigenous peoples, the greatest killers were new diseases brought by the colonizers, including smallpox, measles, influenza, bubonic plague, diphtheria, typhus, cholera, scarlet fever, trachoma, whooping cough, chicken pox, and tropical malaria. Estimates of the indigenous population of North America prior to the arrival of Europeans range upward from about 7 million.[3] Close to 90% of these people died as a result of the direct and indirect effects of culture contact. For example, the population of northern Iroquoian peoples is estimated to have dropped from about 110,000 in the early seventeenth century to about 8,000 by 1850 (Trigger and Swagerty 1996).

Colonization did not end with the creation of new nation-states. Over the past century, Canadian and American government policies have continued the process of destruction of indigenous cultures and ways of life through forced sedenterization, creation of reserves, relocation to remote regions, residential schools, chronic underfunding and poor resourcing of essential services such as health care and education, and bureaucratic control (Miller 2000; Neu and Therrien 2003; Richardson 1993). For example, the crowded, poor-quality housing in most Aboriginal settlements increased the risk of transmission of contagious diseases, including tuberculosis, which necessitated prolonged hospitalizations, further subverting the integrity of families and communities (Grygier 1994). Increasing reliance on European foodstuffs contributed to the growing dependence of indigenous peoples on European market economies. The negative health and social effects of this shift in diet and lifestyle are evident today, with problems of obesity and diabetes now endemic in many Aboriginal communities (Waldram et al. 2006).

Although the process of sedentarization began with the response of indigenous peoples to the presence of fur traders and missionaries, it took new form with the systematic efforts of the government to police, educate, and provide health care for remote populations. The location of virtually every Aboriginal settlement was chosen by government or mercantile interests rather than by the Aboriginal peoples themselves (Dickason 2002). In some cases, this resulted in arbitrary groupings of individuals or families with no history of living together in such proximity. Groups of people were essentially forced to improvise new ways of life and social structures. In many cases, Aboriginal peoples were relegated to undesirable parcels of land out of the way of the settlers' expanding cities and farms. When new land was needed for the settlers, Aboriginal communities were pushed still farther to the margins. Other forced relocations took place for more complicated political reasons. The disastrous "experiment" of relocating Inuit from Nunavik to the far North to protect Canadian sovereignty was a late chapter in this process of forced culture change that revealed the government's lack of awareness of basic cultural and ecological realities crucial to survival (Marcus 1992; Royal Commission on Aboriginal Peoples 1994; Tester and Kulchyski 1994).

These policies served the economic, social, and political interests of the dominant non-Aboriginal society and were supported by both explicit and subtler forms of racism and discrimination. Active attempts to suppress and eradicate indigenous cultures were rationalized by images and arguments that portrayed Aboriginal people as "primitive," "savage," and uncivilized (Titley 1986). This discounting of Aboriginal peoples' ways of life justified legislation that prohibited traditional religious and cultural practices like

LAURENCE J. KIRMAYER, CAROLINE L. TAIT, AND CORI SIMPSON

the Potlatch or Sun Dance (Hoxie 1996). Aboriginal peoples were viewed as incapable of understanding and participating in democratic government, thereby motivating efforts to "civilize" and assimilate them into mainstream Canadian society.

Aboriginal children, particularly First Nations children, became the central target for assimilation strategies through their forced attendance at residential schools and out-of-community adoption into non-Aboriginal families. These efforts were part of an orchestrated plan of forced assimilation that emerged at roughly the same time in Canada, Australia, and New Zealand in accordance with British colonial policy (Armitage 1995).

The Canadian government informally recognized indigenous communities of Canada as peoples or nations, but they were viewed as uncivilized and hence unable to exercise rights as citizens in a democratic polity. The Bagot Commission Report (1844) argued that reserves in Canada were operating in a "half-civilized state" and that in order to progress toward civilization, Aboriginal peoples needed to be imbued with the principles of industry and knowledge through formal education. This report began a shift in Indian policy in Canada away from the principle of protection and toward active assimilation. This shift was reinforced by the Davin Report (1879), which recommended a policy of "aggressive civilization." Aboriginal adults and Elders were described by this second report as having "the helpless mind of a child." To be integrated into the emerging nation, therefore, Aboriginal children had to be separated from their parents and "civilized" through a program of education that would make them talk, think, and act like mature British Canadians.

From 1879 to 1973 the Canadian government mandated church-run boarding schools to provide education for Aboriginal children (Miller 1996). Following the recommendations of the Davin Report, residential education for Aboriginal children in Canada was modelled after the system of boarding schools for Native American children in the United States (Miller 1996; Milloy 1999). Although portrayed as places of education and enlightenment, most of the residential schools in fact functioned as "total institutions" (Goffman 1961) or "carceral spaces" (Foucault 1977) – enclosed places of confinement with a highly regimented social order apart from everyday life. The schools were located in isolated areas, and the children were allowed little or no contact with their families and communities. There was a regime of strict discipline and constant surveillance of every aspect of their lives, and cultural expression through language, dress, food, and beliefs was vigorously suppressed.

Over the span of 100 years, about 100,000 Aboriginal children, mainly First Nations, were taken from their homes and subjected to an institutional regime that fiercely denigrated and suppressed their heritage. At their height, there were 80 residential schools operating across Canada, with a peak enrolment in 1953 of over 11,000 students.[4] Although some families welcomed the opportunity for formal education of their children, others desperately tried to avoid sending their children to the schools (Johnston 1988). The extent of the physical, emotional, and sexual abuse perpetrated in many of the residential schools has only recently been acknowledged (Haig-Brown 1988; Knockwood and Thomas 1992; Lomawaima 1993; Milloy 1999). Beyond the impact on children of abrupt separation from their families, multiple losses, deprivation, and frank brutality, the residential school system denied Aboriginal communities the basic human right to transmit their traditions and maintain their cultural identity (Chrisjohn, Young, and Maraun 1997).

Intensive surveillance and control of the lives of Aboriginal peoples in Canada went far beyond the residential school system. Assimilation of Aboriginal peoples was the explicit motivation for the removal of Aboriginal children to residential schools. Aboriginal parents were not necessarily seen as "unacceptable" parents, only as incapable of educating their children and passing on "proper" European values (Fournier and Crey 1997; Johnston 1983). Beginning in the 1960s, the federal government effectively handed over the responsibility for Aboriginal health, welfare, and educational services to the provinces, despite remaining financially responsible for status Indians. Provincial child and welfare services focused on the prevention of "child neglect," which emphasized the moral attributes of individual parents, especially mothers, and on enforcing and improving care of children within the family (Swift 1995). In the case of Aboriginal families, "neglect" was mainly linked to endemic poverty and other social problems, which were dealt with under what social workers referred to as "the need for adequate care." However, improving care within the family was not given priority, and provincial child-welfare policies did not include preventive family counselling services, as they did in the case of non-Aboriginal families. Since there were no family reunification services for Aboriginal families, social workers usually chose adoption or long-term foster care for the Aboriginal children they took into care, resulting in Aboriginal children experiencing much longer periods of foster care than their non-Aboriginal counterparts (MacDonald 1995).

Beginning in the 1960s, as a result of heightened surveillance and concerns about child welfare, large numbers of Aboriginal children were taken from their families and communities and placed in foster care. By the end of that decade, between 30% and 40% of the children who were legal wards of the state were Aboriginal – in stark contrast to the rate of 1% in 1959 (Fournier and Crey 1997). By the 1970s about one in four status Indians could expect to be separated from his or her parents; rough estimates on the rates of nonstatus and Métis children apprehended from their families show that one in three could expect to spend his or her childhood as a legal ward of the state. Eventually, many of these children were adopted into non-Aboriginal families in Canada and the United States. Termed the "Sixties Scoop," this practice lasted almost three decades – and statistics indicate that there is still an overrepresentation of Aboriginal children in the care of non-Aboriginal institutions and foster families (Gough et al. 2005).

The large-scale removal of Aboriginal children from their families, communities, and cultural contexts through the residential school system and the "Sixties Scoop" had damaging consequences for individuals, families, and whole communities. Much like former residential school students, who often returned to their communities in a culturally "betwixt and between" state, Aboriginal children relegated to the care of the state or non-Aboriginal families have experienced problems of identity and self-esteem growing up at the margins of two worlds. Physical and sexual abuse, emotional neglect, internalized racism, language loss, substance abuse, and suicide are common in their stories (Fournier and Crey 1997; York 1990).

The intense governmental surveillance and bureaucratic control of the lives of Aboriginal peoples in Canada was mandated and institutionalized by federal Indian policy (Neu and Therrien 2003). Some of these policies were well intentioned, but most were motivated by a condescending, paternalistic attitude that failed to recognize either the autonomy of Aboriginal peoples or the richness and resources of their cultures and communities (Titley 1986).

The Indian Act (1876) was the most comprehensive piece of federal legislation directed toward the management of Aboriginal peoples in Canada. Although established over a century ago, this document continues to play an integral role in the lives and juridical identities of Aboriginal peoples. The Indian Act defines First Nations people as wards of the Crown, subjects for whom the state has a responsibility to provide care (Imai 2003). The broad application of the Act has included prohibiting participation in cultural activities such as the Potlatch and the Sun Dance, restricting movement by means of the pass system, creating social categories of identity such as "status" and "nonstatus Indians," and exempting status Indians from taxation (Tobias 1976; Miller 1990).

The Indian Act has been the focus of great conflict and contestation in many First Nations communities, which have been forced to reconcile local notions of membership, citizenship, political participation, and structure with imposed legal sanctions and controls (Lawrence 2004; Sissons 2005; Valaskakis 2005). For example, until quite recently, the patrilineal descent recognized by the Indian Act resulted in the removal of Indian status from many First Nations women (and their children) who married non-First Nations men.

Acknowledging the colonial nature of the Indian Act and its negative consequences in communities across Canada, government officials have made some efforts to replace the Indian Act with a more modern document defining a more contemporary arrangement. In 1969 the federal government produced its "White Paper," which asserted that existing Indian policies were discriminatory and argued that removing special status by abolishing the Indian Act would end this discrimination. However, the liberal philosophy behind the White Paper did not address some of the most basic values, concerns, and aspirations of Aboriginal people (Turner 2006, 29ff): it did not consider the legacy of colonialism and other institutions of forced assimilation that created a persistent pattern of inequalities and marginalization; it did not acknowledge indigenous rights as a unique form of group rights, not merely another instance of ethnocultural minority rights in the framework of Canadian multiculturalism; it failed to recognize the contested legitimacy of the initial formation of the Canadian state, in which Aboriginal peoples were incorporated into the new state with loss of land, power, and autonomy; and most critical for the process of creating a viable political arrangement, the White Paper was produced without the participation of Aboriginal peoples themselves. Far from being perceived as a positive step toward political equality, the "ex cathedra" manner in which the White Paper was produced, its paternalism, and its lack of recognition of the autonomy of Aboriginal peoples created a sense of betrayal that has made leaders wary of subsequent efforts at reform (Turner 2006). In 2001 the Liberal government proposed the First Nations Governance Act (FNGA), which also met with considerable opposition since there was great concern that this legislation would disempower First Nations peoples and communities. The proposal was dropped, and debate continues on ways to rework the formal relationship between the government and Aboriginal peoples.

The Indian Act confers official status only on some First Nations individuals. Other Aboriginal peoples, including nonstatus Indians and Métis, have no official status. This has significant consequences for their relationship with government institutions. Along with nonstatus Indians, the Métis were denied access to programs such as the Non-Insured Health Benefits Program (which provides free medical services to status Indians and Inuit who are not covered by provincial health-insurance plans). Programs provided by the federal government to status First Nations and Inuit under the umbrella of the Medical Services Branch – more recently renamed the First Nations and Inuit Health Branch (FNIHB) – such as health centres, federal alcohol- and drug-abuse programs, initiatives for at-risk children, and a healthy-babies program, are not available to Métis and nonstatus First Nations, many of whom live in communities adjacent to the First Nation reserves that are served by these programs. Despite facing the same social and health problems, none of the provincial or territorial governments has yet to offer parallel programming for Métis and nonstatus First Nations (Chartrand 2006, 23).

The history of urbanization in Canada is also the history of the displacement and marginalization of Aboriginal peoples. The sites upon which many Canadian cities are built were traditional meeting places used by indigenous peoples as gathering spots or settlement areas (Newhouse and Peters 2003, 6). Prior to the mid-1990s, a variety of policies ensured Aboriginal peoples were excluded from urban centres. These policies reinforced an image that Aboriginal culture and identity are incompatible with urban residence. Urban migration has therefore often been interpreted as a decision by Aboriginal people to leave their rural communities *and* cultures in order to assimilate into mainstream society. Of course, there is no reason why an Aboriginal person cannot maintain and develop a distinctive identity and community in urban settings. By the 1980s, however, the focus of concern over Aboriginal urbanization had shifted from questions of cultural adaptation to the impact of poverty. By extension, the presence of indigenous people in cities came to be viewed as detrimental to the moral and physical conditions of both Aboriginal peoples and the urban community, providing another rationale for the further removal of indigenous people from city areas.

Over the past 50 years the percentage of indigenous people living in Canadian cities has risen to approximately 56% of the total Aboriginal population (Siggner 2003, 16). The most urbanized groups are nonstatus Indians and Métis, with 73% and 66%, respectively, living in urban areas (Norris and Clatworthy 2003, 51). It remains relatively easy for Aboriginal people to move back and forth between rural or reserve communities and the city.[5] Although indigenous peoples face some of the same challenges as other migrants,

LAURENCE J. KIRMAYER, CAROLINE L. TAIT, AND CORI SIMPSON

many indigenous people are travelling within their traditional territories and expect that their indigenous rights and identities should make a difference to the ways that they are able to live their lives in urban areas (Norris and Clatworthy 2003, 6).

"Residential instability," which is marked by frequent migration back and forth from cities as well as by high mobility within cities, may diminish the well-being of urban Aboriginal populations (Norris and Clatworthy 2003). High mobility may weaken social cohesion in communities and neighbourhoods where large concentrations of indigenous people live. Residential instability is associated with family instability and with a high proportion of female lone-parent families with low incomes that may experience high rates of crime and victimization. High mobility also makes it more difficult to deliver services such as schooling and housing to this population, and it destabilizes organizations such as Friendship Centres that provide health, employment, and education outreach and social services (Norris and Clatworthy 2003, 69-70). As a consequence, individuals and families living in these areas exhibit greater social problems (e.g., poorer education attainment, divorce, crime, suicide), which in turn leads to even greater levels of social disintegration. Therefore, a major challenge for indigenous peoples living in cities is to maintain social cohesion through collective activities and community strategies that reinforce indigenous cultural identity and develop urban institutions that reflect indigenous values.

To the organized efforts to assimilate, regulate, or destroy Aboriginal cultures are added the corrosive effects of poverty and economic marginalization. In 1991 the average income for Aboriginal people was about 60% of that of non-Aboriginal Canadians. Despite efforts at income assistance and community development, this gap had widened over the decades since 1980, and it has continued to grow (Frideres 2004). In the 1996 census 43.4% of Aboriginal people lived below the poverty line; in 2001 the figure was 55.9%. The effects of poverty are seen in many ways, including the poor living conditions on many reserves and in many remote settlements. A government survey in 2001 found that two-thirds of Aboriginal reserves had water supplies that were at risk for contamination.[6] In the 2001 Aboriginal Peoples Survey, 34% of Inuit living in the North, 19% of Aboriginal people in rural areas, and 16% of those in urban areas reported that there were times in the year when their drinking water was contaminated. Aboriginal people are much more likely than the non-Aboriginal population to live in crowded housing. The 2006 census found that 31% of Inuit lived in crowded conditions, compared to 15% of First Nations people (26% of those living on reserves), and 3% of the non-Aboriginal Canadian population (Statistics Canada 2008). Aboriginal people are also much more likely than non-Aboriginal people to have a home in need of major repairs.

Of course, the current notions of poverty are the creation of the social order in which Aboriginal peoples are embedded, one that has economically marginalized traditional subsistence activities while creating demands for new goods. The presence of mass media even in remote communities makes the values of consumer capitalism salient and creates feelings of relative deprivation and lack where none existed before. Even those who seek solidarity in traditional forms of community and ways of life find themselves enclosed and defined by a global economy that treats "culture" and "tradition" as commodities or useful adjectives in advertising campaigns (Krupat 1996).

These realities of globalization, together with the legacy of internal colonialism, contribute to the continuing political marginalization of Aboriginal peoples. Some groups, however, have been able to exploit the logic of mass media and the market to further their efforts to regain local control and stewardship of their land and people. For example, the Cree of northern Quebec have successfully fought against hydroelectric development in their territory through publicity aimed at influencing public opinion in the United States and abroad (Salisbury 1986). They have appealed to a global audience through moral arguments and suasion to achieve an influence beyond their local political or economic power. These manifest successes in challenging the Quebec provincial government, achieved on a global stage, likely have had a positive effect on the sense of efficacy and mental health of many Cree. This example illustrates the extent to which efforts at revitalization of communities and collective identities must be understood not only in terms of local politics or of the agendas of provincial and federal governments but also in terms of the forces of globalization that reach into even the most remote communities in contemporary Aboriginal Canada.

Mental Health Consequences of Cultural Suppression and Forced Assimilation

The terms "mental health" and "mental illness" cover a broad domain that encompasses personal growth and well-being, everyday problems in living, such common mental disorders as anxiety and depression, and severe mental disorders like schizophrenia or manic-depressive illness. Many social problems, including interpersonal violence, child abuse, alcohol and drug abuse/dependence, gambling, and antisocial behaviour, are also prominent mental health concerns because of their causes and consequences.

Qualitative ethnographic and epidemiological studies have documented high levels of mental health problems in some Canadian Aboriginal communities (Kirmayer 1994; Government of Canada 2006; Royal Commission on Aboriginal Peoples 1996; Waldram 1997a; Waldram et al. 2006). However, there are many gaps in knowledge and a great need for further systematic research to identify the prevalence, causes, and effective responses to specific mental health problems as well as the factors that contribute to health and well-being in many communities.

Epidemiological Studies of Mental Health

Older studies of mental health problems used symptom checklists or clinical impressions of individuals' overall level of distress and impairment without distinguishing different types of problems. Contemporary psychiatric epidemiology uses structured interviews administered by clinicians or trained lay interviewers to elicit reports of the specific symptoms, behaviours, and experiences. This information can then be used to make diagnoses following the diagnostic criteria of the World Health Organization (1992) or the American Psychiatric Association (2000). This gives a more detailed picture of the prevalence and co-occurrence of specific types of disorders, which may require different types of treatment intervention and have very different courses and outcomes. Psychiatric epidemiology faces many challenges in cross-cultural application because of differences in how people experience and express distress (Kleinman 1987; Kirmayer 1989; van Ommeren 2003). Generally, the way to address these limitations is to begin with careful qualitative ethnographic work in order to understand local models of illness and idioms of distress (Manson, Shore, and Bloom 1985; Canino, Lewis-Fernandez, and Bravo 1997; de Jong and van Ommeren 2002; Beals et al. 2003; Waldram 2006). This understanding of local cultural knowledge and practice can then be used to revise interviews, questionnaires, and criteria in order to ensure that they make sense and capture the relevant dimensions of illness experience.

Most estimates of the prevalence of psychiatric disorders in Aboriginal populations are based on clinic- or service-utilization records. Case reviews based on psychiatric consultation in Aboriginal communities indicate high rates of depressive disorders in some communities (e.g., Abbey et al. 1993; Armstrong 1993). However, since many people never come for treatment, service-utilization studies are usually at best only a low-end estimate of the true prevalence of distress in the community and may not give an accurate profile of problems in the community.

The few community surveys of prevalence rates among North American Aboriginal peoples indicate rates of psychiatric disorders that vary widely from levels less than the general population to levels twice those of neighbouring non-Aboriginal communities. This variation likely reflects both methodological difficulties in accurately assessing mental health across cultures and real differences among populations and communities that may provide important clues to the social origins of distress.

In the United States, Kinzie and colleagues conducted a 1988 follow-up study of a Northwest Coast village originally studied by Shore and colleagues in 1969 (Shore et al. 1973). In all, 31.4% of subjects met criteria for a current psychiatric diagnosis (Kinzie et al. 1992; Boehnlein et al. 1993). A marked sex difference was observed, with nearly 46% of men being affected, compared to only 18.4% of women. The presence of a psychiatric disorder was not related to age, marital status, or educational level, but men were much more likely to be affected (46%, compared to 18.4% of women). The surveys in both 1969 and 1988 found a very high rate of alcohol-related problems, with a lifetime rate of alcohol dependence of almost 57%, and an abuse rate of about 21%. Similar or still higher rates have been reported in other American Indian populations (Kunitz et al. 1999a).

More recently, Beals and colleagues have published results from the first large-scale epidemiological surveys of rural Indian reservations in the United States, conducted as part of the American Indian Services Utilization, Psychiatric Epidemiology, Risk and

Protective Factors Project (AI-SUPERPFP). The project involved surveys of a total of 3,084 members of two Tribes living on or near their home reservations in the Southwest and on the Northern Plains. These community surveys, conducted from 1997 to 2000, found that the overall rate of psychiatric disorders in the two Tribes was roughly comparable to that of the general population, but the rates of specific diagnoses differed (Beals et al. 2005a; Beals et al. 2005c). Compared to the general population, alcohol dependence and post-traumatic stress disorder were more frequent in the American Indian communities (Spicer et al. 2003).

Major depressive disorder was actually substantially less frequent in the American Indian samples (the 12-month prevalence was 3.8% for men and 7.9% for women) than in the general US population (6.1% for men and 11.0% for women) (Beals et al. 2005a). The researchers found this hard to reconcile with the prevalence of social problems and evident distress in the community, and they reasoned that this low rate might reflect methodological difficulties with the version of the Composite International Diagnostic Interview (CIDI) used in these studies. The CIDI asks individuals about the two cardinal symptoms of major depression: depressed mood and anhedonia (loss of interest or ability to take pleasure in ordinary activities). The interview has a "skip-out" so that if respondents have not had either of these two key symptoms, they are not asked about other symptoms of depression. As a result, individuals who have other culturally mediated or inflected ways of expressing depression may not be identified by the survey (Kirmayer and Jarvis 2005). In the AI-SUPERPFP surveys, Northern Plains Tribal members were much less likely to report either depressed mood or anhedonia than the Southwest Tribe or the general population (Beals et al. 2005b; Beals et al. 2005c). The authors speculated that this might be due to local cultural attitudes that regard admitting to feelings of depression as a sign of weakness; it may also reflect specific cultural idioms of distress that lead individuals to express depressed mood in terms of loneliness, boredom, or anger (O'Nell 1996 and 2004; Jervis et al. 2003).

To diagnose a discrete episode of depression, the CIDI also asks respondents to indicate whether their symptoms co-occurred during a two-week period. This proved difficult for survey participants from both Tribal groups. To salvage the data from this survey, the authors tried an alternative method of scoring, relaxing the criteria for co-occurrence of symptoms. With these modified criteria, the rates of depression were higher than those in the general population, but it is difficult to know how to interpret these results.

Rates of exposure to potentially traumatic events were very high in these communities, up to 67% for males and 70% for females (Manson et al. 2005). This compares to levels previously reported in the general population in the United States of 61% for males and 51% for females. The rates for women in particular were very elevated, reflecting increased levels of sexual and domestic violence.

Data pertaining to Aboriginal children's mental health are limited, but there is clear evidence of high rates of problems, including suicide and substance abuse among adolescents in many communities (Beiser and Attneave 1982; Gotowiec and Beiser 1994; Beals et al. 1997). The Flower of Two Soils Re-Interview Study followed up on 109 of 251 Northern Plains adolescents (aged 11 to 18) who had taken part as children in the earlier study (Beiser et al. 1993; Sack et al. 1994). Fully 43% of the respondents received a diagnosis of at least one DSM-III-R disorder, with the most frequent diagnoses being disruptive behaviour disorders, 22% (including conduct disorder, 9.5%); substance use disorders, 18.4% (including alcohol dependence, 9.2%); anxiety disorders, 17.4%; affective disorders, 9.3% (including major depression, 6.5%); and posttraumatic stress disorder, 5%. Rates of comorbidity were very high, with almost half of those with behaviour or affective disorders meeting criteria for a substance-use disorder. Almost two-thirds of respondents reported having experienced a traumatic event; the most frequent events were car accidents and death or suicide. There is evidence that rates of conduct disorder are increasing in some American Indian communities in the United States owing to increasingly high levels of family breakdown (Kunitz et al. 1999a). Conduct disorder before age 15 is a risk factor for adult alcohol abuse in this population (Kunitz et al. 1999b).

Surveys using symptom measures suggest high rates of common mental disorders, with as many as 25% of individuals in some communities suffering from current depression, but the lack of specific diagnostic measures makes it difficult to judge the reliability of these estimates (Haggarty et al. 2000). The 1997 First Nations and Inuit Regional Health Surveys, conducted across Canada, found elevated rates of depression (18%) and problems with alcohol (27%) (First Nations Information Governance Committee 2007).[7] The 2002 Regional Health Survey found that 30% of First Nations individuals had experienced a period of two weeks or more in the previous year when they were sad, blue, or depressed, a cardinal symptom of depression. Data from the Canadian Community Health Survey in 2001, which used the CIDI, indicate that 12% of First Nations people living on-reserve had an episode of major depression, compared to 7% of the general population.

Surveys undertaken by the Province of Quebec among the Cree in 1991 (Clarkson et al. 1992) and among the Inuit in 1992 (Boyer et al. 1994) and 2006 (Kirmayer, Paul, and Rochette 2007) used brief measures of generalized emotional distress, specific questions about suicidal ideation and attempts, and a few questions about people with chronic mental illness within the family. Again, these methods give only a very crude estimate of the level of distress in the population and provide little information about specific disorders or service needs.

Suicide is one of the most dramatic indicators of distress in the Aboriginal populations. In many communities, First Nations, Inuit, and Métis have elevated rates of suicide, particularly among youth; however, rates are in fact highly variable (Kirmayer 1994; Kirmayer et al. 2007). In Quebec, for example, the Inuit, Attikamekw, and several other nations have very high rates of suicide, while the Cree have a rate comparable to that of the general population of the province (Petawabano et al. 1994). This variation has much to teach us about the community-level factors that affect suicide risk.

Compared to the general population, a smaller proportion of Aboriginal people consume alcohol (79% versus 66%, respectively) (First Nations Information Governance Committee

2007). However, the rate of problem drinking is higher in the Aboriginal population, with 16% of First Nations individuals reporting heavy drinking on a weekly basis, compared to 6.2% in the general population. The Northwest Territories Health Promotion Survey found that 33% of the territories' Aboriginal persons were considered heavy drinkers, compared to 16.7% in the non-Aboriginal population (Northwest Territories Bureau of Statistics 1996). In the same survey, use of cannabis was also greater for Aboriginal persons (27.3%) than for non-Aboriginal persons (10.8%). The survey also asked about the history of solvent use and found that the percentage of Aboriginal people who had used solvents was particularly high (19.0%), compared to 1.7% among non-Aboriginal people.

A survey of drug use in Manitoba assessed Aboriginal (Indian and Métis residents off-reserve) and non-Aboriginal adolescents over four consecutive years from 1990 to 1993 (Gfellner and Hundleby 1995). The Aboriginal groups had consistently higher rates of use of marijuana, nonmedical tranquilizers, nonmedical barbiturates, LSD, PCP, other hallucinogens, and crack. For both LSD and marijuana, the average rate of use for Aboriginal adolescents was over 3 times higher than the corresponding non-Aboriginal rate. In the same survey, glue sniffing was more frequent among the Aboriginal group than among the non-Aboriginal groups.

Inhalant use (e.g., gas, glue, solvents) is an increasing problem among young people worldwide but is much more common in some Aboriginal communities than in the general population (Howard et al. 1999; Neumark, Delva, and Anthony 1998; Weir 2001). In a survey of Inuit youth in one community in Quebec, 21% reported having used solvents at one time, and 5% had used them within the past month (Kirmayer, Malus, and Boothroyd 1996). Individuals who had used solvents were 8 times more likely to have made a suicide attempt. The 2004 Nunavik Health Survey found that 5.9% of respondents had used solvents in the previous 12 months; for those 15 to 19 years of age, the rate was 13.5% (Muckle et al. 2007).

Qualitative Ethnographic Research

Whereas epidemiological research identifies the magnitude and distribution of mental health and social problems of Aboriginal peoples in Canada, qualitative studies implicate the collective exposures of Aboriginal peoples to forced assimilation policies as prime causes of poor health and social outcomes. The policies of forced assimilation have had profound effects on Aboriginal peoples at every level of experience, from individual identity and mental health to the structure and integrity of families, communities, bands, and nations.

Narratives and life histories suggest that the residential school experience has had enduring psychological, social, and economic effects on survivors (Haig-Brown 1988; Milloy 1999; York 1990). Of course, the links between events and outcomes made by individuals in their narratives do not prove causality, but they give a clear picture of how suffering is understood and can identify plausible connections for more systematic study. Transgenerational effects of the residential schools identified through such qualitative research include the structural effects of disrupting families and communities; the transmission of explicit models and ideologies of parenting based on experiences in punitive institutional settings; patterns of emotional responding that reflect the lack of warmth and intimacy in childhood; repetition of physical and sexual abuse; loss of knowledge, language, and tradition; systematic devaluing of Aboriginal identity; and, paradoxically, essentializing Aboriginal identity by treating it as something intrinsic to the person and thus static and incapable of change. These studies point to a loss of individual and collective self-esteem, to individual and collective disempowerment, and, in some instances, to the destruction of communities.

The legacy of the policies of forced assimilation is also seen in the current relationship of Aboriginal peoples with the larger Canadian society. Images of the "savage" and stereotypes of the "drunken Indian" continue to recur in popular media. Racism is still widespread, if sometimes subtle, and beyond active discrimination there is a continuing lack of historical awareness of the experience of Aboriginal peoples with colonization and the enduring impact on their well-being and social options. Governmental, bureaucratic, and professional tutelage and control continue to undermine Aboriginal efforts at self-direction.

The impact of local control on mental health has been strikingly illustrated in the studies by Michael Chandler and Chris Lalonde (1998; see also Chapter 10; Chandler et al. 2003) that compare the rates of completed suicide in 80 bands in British Columbia. There was wide variation in rates, with some communities exhibiting no suicides, while others suffered very high rates. Each community was scored on seven measures of what was termed "cultural continuity": self-government, involvement in land claims, band control of education, health services, cultural facilities, police services, and fire services. The rate of suicide was strongly correlated with the level of these factors. Communities with all seven factors had no suicides, while those with none of the factors had extremely high suicide rates. Of course, it is possible that some of these factors are markers for healthy communities and that the link to suicide is through other co-varying but unmeasured factors, including collective self-efficacy and self-esteem, better infrastructure or community organization, and more job opportunities or active roles for youth. Labelling these factors as "cultural continuity" is also questionable, as the involvement of Aboriginal people in contemporary institutions like municipal government or formal school systems can hardly be viewed as cultural traditionalism. "Local control" seems a more accurate term, and it is a factor that probably reflects cultural adaptability and pluralism rather than the maintenance of tradition. Nevertheless, this study provides compelling evidence for the impact of community-level factors and should encourage other studies of determinants of mental health that are based on careful analysis of the history, structure, and dynamics of communities.

Cultural continuity remains an interesting construct and one that is important in the light of ongoing efforts of Aboriginal peoples to recuperate and reclaim traditional knowledge and values as an explicit basis for collective identity and community cohesion. Cultural continuity can be expressed in many ways, but all depend on a notion of culture as something that is potentially enduring or continuously linked through processes of historical transformation with an identifiable past or tradition. To some extent, it is precisely this notion that has been challenged by recent critical writing on the idea of culture itself that emphasizes its constant contestation, invention, and renegotiation by members of a community in dialogue with other cultures and with global systems of knowledge and practice.

Transformations of Identity and Community

The wide variation in rates of suicide and other indices of distress across Aboriginal communities suggests the importance of considering the nature of communities and the different ways that groups have responded to the ongoing stresses of colonization, sedentarization, bureaucratic surveillance, and technocratic control. It is likely that the mediating mechanisms contributing to high levels of emotional distress and problems like depression, anxiety, substance abuse, and suicide are closely related to issues of individual identity and self-esteem (Chandler 1994; Chandler and Ball 1989; Phinney and Chavira 1992), which in turn are strongly influenced by collective processes at the level of band, community, or larger political entities (Tester and McNicoll 2004).

All cultures are in constant flux, so cultural and ethnic identity must be understood as a construction of contemporary people responding to their current situation (Niezen 2003; Roosens 1989; Sissons 2005). This is not to question the authenticity of tradition but to insist that culture be appreciated as a co-creation by people in response to current circumstances – an ongoing construction that is contested from both within and without. For Aboriginal peoples, two important arenas for this contestation and change are the relationship of individual groups to movements founded on pan-Indian political and ethnic identity and the relationship of traditional healing practices to cosmopolitan medicine and religion, including their appropriation by "New Age" practitioners.

Notions and experiences of being a Native involve cross-cutting historical, cultural, linguistic, geographic, and political dimensions (Krupat 1996; Vizenor 1999). To a large extent, they are situational, emerging out of specific encounters with others who are viewed as sharing a generalized Aboriginal heritage or a political position (Trimble and Medicine 1993). Of course, Aboriginal identity is also embodied and linked to behavioural and physical attributes (e.g., brown skin, brown eyes, black hair), but these attributes too are shaped by cultural scripts (e.g., braided hair, choice of clothing) that determine how people identify or fail to identify each other as Aboriginal.

LAURENCE J. KIRMAYER, CAROLINE L. TAIT, AND CORI SIMPSON

The very notion of Aboriginality is a social construction that serves as a "dividing practice" that both marginalizes and unites. Over centuries of colonial contact, the rapid and often violent usurping of indigenous lands – followed by more encompassing forms of neo-colonial bureaucratic control over remnant populations – has given way to a powerful notion that there exists a distinct category of peoples in the world distinguished by having been sociopolitically marginalized from nation-state populations. This discourse of Aboriginality was used originally by colonial powers when confronting the "others" whose territory they conquered (see Waldram 2004; Chapter 3). Colonial history and an-thropological writings about Native American cultures and peoples have had a powerful effect on their contemporary representations in North American society. Berkhofer (1979) discusses how the construction of stereotypical images impacted the self-image of Native Americans. Since anthropological investigations of Native Americans began in the nine-teenth century, they have become the objects of a Euro-American cultural gaze that creates an "other" and then polices its cultural identity. The resultant discourse on Ab-originality circulates within the wider society, including the media and popular culture, and creates commonly accepted social facts about ethnic identity and tradition. Recogniz-ing a practice as traditional marks it off from the everyday practices of a people or com-munity. This labelling, essentializing, and commodification of tradition are all features of modernity that pose dilemmas for the recuperation of history and the forging of identity.

The creation of an explicit ethnic identity requires that certain beliefs, practices, or characteristics be elevated to core values and claimed as shared experiences. This natur-ally tends to obscure individual variation and the constant flux of personal and social definitions of self and other. It also leads to the privileging of groups identified as being more "authentically" close to the ideal ethnic image while simultaneously marginalizing and even stigmatizing those groups or individuals who fail to embody this image.

A shared history invests ethnic identity with social value and thus contributes directly to mental health. Studies of how cultural and historical knowledge is used to construct ethnic identity and of the way that such ethnicity is then used for psychological coping, social interaction, and community organization can therefore contribute directly to Ab-original mental health (Trimble and Medicine 1993). For example, the development of a collective identity has posed particular problems for Métis, who have suffered from ambi-guity of status (Dickason 2002; Peterson and Brown 1993). Building a national identity of a "Métis nation" from social groups that have experienced prolonged suppression and fragmentation of their ethnic identity has proven to be a challenge. In this situation, the writing and dissemination of a group's history takes on special urgency (Sioui 1992). To be effective in welding a group together and advancing its interests and collective well-being, the expression of collective history and identity requires a public forum.

Inequality *within* indigenous communities receives significantly less attention than does inequality *between* indigenous and non-indigenous groups (Culhane et al. 2003). Because many indigenous peoples in Canada live as small, scattered minorities within polities where significant and powerful sectors of majority populations hold and exercise racist and exclusionary ideas and practices, the effects of internal group inequalities are largely ignored. Although divisions and debates within majority populations are taken as evidence of vibrancy and growth, similar conflicts within indigenous communities are frequently interpreted as signs of chaos, disorder, and political immaturity and thus deemed to legitimate ongoing external governance and administration. The burden of distress and despair wrought by generations of colonial oppression commonly renders relationships and social cohesion within and between indigenous communities fragile, and internal critics face tremendous challenges in their efforts to develop modes of constructive social and political criticism. However, ignoring or minimizing internal inequalities risks perpetuating injustices paid for in terms of poor health and high levels of social suffering among those who are most marginalized and exploited: women, Elders, youth, two-spirited people (i.e., gay or lesbian), and the disabled and ill. Indigenous women have been courageous in struggling with the personal and intimate legacies of colonialism within their families and communities, in placing issues of gender and class inequalities on the agenda of indigenous and other government bodies, and in working toward change for future generations (Culhane et al. 2003).

Despite concerted efforts at forced assimilation, Aboriginal cultures have persisted. Although at least 10 Aboriginal languages became extinct during the past 100 years and many others are endangered, several languages remain viable, with large enough numbers of speakers to ensure their long-term survival, including Inuktitut, Cree, and Ojibway (Norris 2007). According to the 2001 census, about 1 in 4 Aboriginal people are able to converse in an Aboriginal language, and about 18% use an Aboriginal language regularly (Statistics Canada 2003). Only 13% speak an Aboriginal language most often in the home. However, the learning of Aboriginal languages as a second language by young people is increasing (Norris 2007). Many communities are currently engaged in cultural immersion programs geared toward strengthening Aboriginal languages and identity. Aboriginal languages are official languages in the Northwest Territories and Nunavut, the latter being a vast region of Canada's North that on 1 April 1999 was recognized as a new territory with an Inuit-led government (Bennett and Rowley 2004).

Beyond the diversity of languages, there are distinctive cultural concepts of personhood and community among many Aboriginal peoples. Whereas the Euro-American notion of the person has been characterized as egocentric or individualistic, many Aboriginal peoples retain notions of the person as defined by a web of relationships that includes not only extended family, kin, and clan but, for hunters and other people living off the land, also animals, elements of the natural world, spirits, and ancestors. Aboriginal concepts of the person thus may be relational or communalistic as well as *ecocentric* (connected to the land, animals, and the environment) (Tanner, Chapter 11; Kirmayer, Fletcher, and Watt, Chapter 13; Tanner 1979) and *cosmocentric* (connecting the person to an ancestral lineage or to the spirit world) (Hultkrantz 1987). Although these forms of personhood have wide prevalence, it is important to recognize the great diversity of Aboriginal individuals,

LAURENCE J. KIRMAYER, CAROLINE L. TAIT, AND CORI SIMPSON

cultures, and communities, which is sometimes obscured by images in the popular media or by Aboriginal peoples themselves when they seek to make common cause in developing political and cultural institutions.

The literature of cross-cultural psychology makes a broad distinction between egoistic or individualistic cultures and sociocentric, communalistic, or collectivist cultures (Triandis 1995). Many Aboriginal cultures appear sociocentric in that the self is defined relationally and the well-being of the family, band, or community is given central importance; however, this occurs along with strong support for individual autonomy and independence. For peoples who lived in small groups of one or two extended families, such as the Inuit, the notion of a sociocentric or communalistic self is misleading since there was no social group larger than the family by which to define the self. Traditional notions of Inuit family relations have been extended to the new situations of large settlements (Dorais 1997).

Many Aboriginal peoples have a concept of the person that might be better identified as ecocentric, for they see other people, the land, and the animals as all being in transaction with the self and, indeed, in some sense, as constituting aspects of a relational self (Drummond 1997; Stairs 1992; Stairs and Wenzel 1992). Consequently, damage to the land, appropriation of land, and spatial restrictions all constitute direct assaults on the person (Sioui 1992). Traditional hunting practices are not just means of subsistence but also sociomoral and spiritual practices aimed at maintaining the health of person and community (Tanner 1979). For example, Inuit concepts of self include physical links with animals through the eating of "country food." In this light, the widespread destruction of the environment motivated by commercial interests must be understood as attacks on Aboriginal individuals and communities that are equivalent in seriousness to the loss of social role and status in a large-scale urban society. The result is certainly a diminution in self-esteem but also the hobbling of a distinctive form of self-efficacy that has to do with living on and through the land (Brody 1975, 2000).

Both contemporary environmentalism and New Age spirituality promote the notion that indigenous peoples practised a generic form of spirituality characterized by a harmonious, nonexploitative approach to nature based on an underlying animistic ontology (Hultkrantz 1987). This obscures the historical reality of diverse cultural traditions that have different mythologies, religious beliefs, and spiritual practices; it also ignores centuries of European contact and the assimilation of Christian forms of belief into syncretic religious practices (Vecsey 1990). In most First Nations and Inuit communities, organized religious denominations, such as the Anglican or Catholic churches, remain influential, especially among older populations, whose members were educated in the residential school system (Treat 1996). Moreover, in recent years the evangelical Christian movement, primarily the Pentecostal Church, has spread rapidly in many communities. Pan-Amerindian spiritual practices are strongly influenced by the vibrant cultures of the Northern Plains of the United States, but these traditions involve distinctive elements not shared with other, equally rich, Aboriginal traditions.

Whereas older anthropological writing conceived of cultures as closed, homogeneous, and sometimes static systems, contemporary ethnographers view cultures as local worlds that are constantly in flux. There is great variation in knowledge, practice, and attitudes among individuals within a cultural group, resulting in significant conflict, resistance, and contestation of dominant values. Local worlds are embedded in larger global systems that bring diverse peoples together through migration, mass media, and other forms of contact and exchange. As a result, most individuals have access to and participate in multiple cultures. Individuals use this multicultural background to navigate, communicate, and provide rhetorical supplies and discourses within which to locate and construct socially and psychological viable selves.

These social realities of cultural diversity, hybridization, flux, and change exist in some tension with Aboriginal claims for a pan-Indian cultural identity rooted in a timeless mythic past (Nabakov 1996). The reality is that, like all cultural identities, Aboriginality is not "in the blood" but emerges from and is sustained by forms of life that exist at the confluence of historical currents and contemporary forces (Waldram, Chapter 3). Aboriginal identity is nurtured within families and communities, but it is also imposed by the larger cultural surroundings. Aboriginal peoples are engaged in an ongoing process of re-articulating themselves in the modern world in ways that honour their ancestors, maintain links with crucial values, and creatively respond to the exigencies of a world simultaneously woven together by electronic media and riven apart by conflicts of culture and value.

Re-Articulating Tradition

In recent years a series of important events has begun to reverse the cultural marginalization and oppression endured by Canadian Aboriginal peoples. It is shocking for Euro-Canadians, who have been profoundly unaware of the social realities of Aboriginal peoples, to be reminded that it was only in 1967 that Aboriginal peoples gained the right to vote. A pivotal event in public consciousness was the Oka Crisis of 1990, in which the Mohawk communities adjoining Montreal confronted local and federal authorities to defend an ancestral burial ground, which was to be appropriated to extend a municipal golf course (York and Pindera 1991). During this crisis, Canadians witnessed overt acts of racism and violence against Aboriginal people and had to confront a complacent self-image as a nation of tolerance. This led directly to the 1991 Royal Commission on Aboriginal Peoples (RCAP). The public hearings held by the RCAP uncovered the widespread abuses of the residential school system. In 1993 the Royal Canadian Mounted Police (RCMP) – the federal police force long involved with law enforcement in remote regions, including Aboriginal settlements – established a Native Residential School Task Force to investigate residential schools from 1890 to 1984. The RCAP addressed many dimensions of Aboriginal health and produced special reports on suicide (1995) as well as volumes on the needs of urban Aboriginal peoples and on healing (1993). The RCAP Final Report included a volume titled *Breaking the silence,* which detailed the abuses in the residential school system (Royal Commission on Aboriginal Peoples 1996).

In 1998 the government responded to the RCAP report with *Gathering Strength: Canada's Aboriginal Action Plan,* which was intended to begin a process of reconciliation and renewal (Minister of Indian Affairs and Northern Development 1998). Several new Aboriginal organizations were created, including the Institute for Aboriginal Peoples Health (1 of 13 Canadian Institutes of Health Research replacing the Medical Research Council) and the National Aboriginal Health Organization.

A crucial component of *Gathering Strength* was the establishment of the Aboriginal Healing Foundation (AHF), a federally funded, Aboriginal-run, nonprofit organization created in March 1998 to support community-based healing initiatives of Aboriginal people affected by physical and sexual abuse in residential schools, including intergenerational impacts (i.e., "the Legacy"). The AHF received $350 million over 10 years to fund projects that address the legacy of the residential schools. The funded projects included healing centres and services; community services; conferences, workshops, and gatherings; cultural activities; material development; planning; research; traditional activities (e.g., programs for living on the land); and a variety of educational and training programs (Aboriginal Healing Foundation 2006).

Aboriginal people have also sought other avenues for reconciliation and reparation. An out-of-court program for dispute resolution organized by the federal government had resolved only 147 claims by July 2005, with almost 2,000 more cases awaiting hearing or adjudication.[8] As of September 2005, 12,455 tort claims had been filed and several class action suits were pending. Legal proceedings often involve retraumatization, and Aboriginal organizations continue to explore alternative dispute-resolution methods, including establishing a Truth and Reconciliation Commission similar to the process developed in post-Apartheid South Africa. Efforts at reconciliation are consonant with the values in many Aboriginal communities, which emphasize maintaining family and community ties and repairing breaches of trust by a public ritual of confession, expiation, and recommitment to the community. In 2006 a Residential Schools Settlement Agreement was reached between the federal government and the legal representatives of many school survivors, the churches involved in running the schools, the Assembly of First Nations, and other Aboriginal organizations. This $1.9 billion agreement will support a series of measures intended to contribute to a "resolution of the Indian Residential Schools legacy," including a Common Experience Payment to every former student; an alternative dispute-resolution process for dealing with claims of physical and sexual abuse endured at the schools; expanded access to mental health support programs (e.g., counselling by mental health professionals, trained Aboriginal health providers, and traditional healers); and a Truth and Reconciliation Commission, mandated to promote public education and awareness

(Brant Castellano, Archibald, and DeGagné 2008). Additional funds will pay for commemorative events and memorials as well as support the continued work of the Aboriginal Healing Foundation. The churches will also contribute resources for healing initiatives.

In an effort to respond to local problems in ways that affirm Aboriginal values and perspectives, communities have experimented with various forms of alternative dispute resolution and restorative justice, including sentencing circles for healing and reintegrating offenders who might otherwise be ostracized and dealt with entirely within the penal system (Drummond 1997; Ross 1996). Other therapeutic examples of meeting in circles include talking circles, in which people speak openly and listen to others' stories in order to begin to become aware of original hurts; sharing circles, in which a high degree of trust is established and people express painful emotions; healing circles, in which people can work through memories of painful experiences; and spiritual circles, in which people develop trust in their own experiences of spirituality as sources of comfort and guidance. The rules of these circles vary with their goals, but all have in common an emphasis on each person's commitment to change, an etiquette that honours the individual's voice and experience through respectful listening, and a process of reaffirming collective and communal solidarity.

The past century has seen the emergence of various forms of pan-Indian spirituality, in which practices associated with specific cultural groups have been widely adopted and have served both as effective healing rituals for groups and as symbols of shared identity and affiliation. The elements of this common spiritual tradition include a focus on the Creator, the symbolism of the medicine wheel, the use of the sweat lodge and traditional plant medicines, Pow-Wow costume dances, drumming, and tobacco offerings (Bucko 1998; Hall 1997; Waldram 1997b).

In parallel, increased awareness of the historical predicament of Aboriginal peoples has become a rallying point. In the United States the attention to trauma among Vietnam veterans provided a context to reconsider the collective trauma of American Indians (Manson et al. 1996). For Canadian Aboriginal peoples, the revelations of the evils of the residential schools have made the notion of individual and collective trauma salient (Haig-Brown 1988). Some Aboriginal people have made use of communal settings to tell the story of their suffering. In these accounts, individual traumas and losses may be explicitly linked to collective traumas. This serves to make sense of suffering and to valorize it as part of a larger collective struggle. At the same time, the metaphors of individual and collective trauma have both positive value and limitations. On the plus side, the metaphor of trauma draws attention to the severity, shock, and violence of the physical and psychological injuries inflicted on Aboriginal peoples. It locates the origins of problems in a shared past and thus motivates the reconstruction of historical memory and collective identity. Ideally, this history would insist on the importance of social and political events and thereby avoid "psychologizing" what are fundamentally political issues (Chrisjohn et al. 1997).

However, like any partial truth, the metaphor of trauma also has limitations and unwanted connotations (Kirmayer, Lemelson, and Barad 2007). Current trauma theory and therapy tend to focus on the psychiatric disorder of posttraumatic stress disorder and give insufficient attention to the other dimensions of experience that may be profoundly transformed by massive trauma and abrogation of human rights. These include issues of secure attachment and trust, belief in a just world, a sense of connectedness to others, and a stable personal and collective identity.

For Aboriginal peoples, historical events have exerted their noxious influences at many levels and in diverse ways, only some of which are captured by the concept of trauma. Indeed, an emphasis on the most overt and dramatic forms of aggression and abuse may make it harder to recognize more subtle, indirect, and insidious effects of residential schools and other forces of assimilation on individuals and communities. The location of the origins of trauma in past events may divert attention from the ongoing effects of a chaotic and constricted present and a murky future – which are the oppressive realities for many Aboriginal young people living in demoralized communities. Finally, an emphasis on past trauma as an explanation for current suffering ignores the pervasiveness of everyday, routinized practices of exclusion and marginalization.

Conclusion

Aboriginal peoples of North America, like indigenous populations in other parts of the world, have experienced profound disruption and alteration of their traditional ways of life through culture contact. This has involved diverse processes, including epidemics of infectious disease, systematic efforts at religious conversion, colonization with forced sedentarization, relocation and confinement to reserves, prolonged separation from family and kin in residential schools and hospitals, gradual involvement in local and global cash economies, political marginalization, and increasingly pervasive bureaucratic and technocratic control of every detail of their lives. This history has had complex effects on the structure of communities, individual and collective identity, and mental health.

Although mental health problems are reflections of ordinary human vulnerabilities and can be found in every population, the elevated rates of suicide, alcoholism, and domestic violence and the pervasive demoralization seen in many Aboriginal communities can be readily understood as both direct and indirect consequences of this history of colonization, cultural oppression, loss of autonomy, dislocations and disruptions of traditional life-ways, and disconnection from the land. Framing the suffering that has resulted from these historical conflicts in terms of mental health issues may command attention from politicians and health authorities and support ongoing efforts to obtain resources and to rebuild healthy communities. At the same time, exclusive attention to individual mental health problems may deflect attention from the larger social structural problems that persist and thus risk continuing the assault on the identity and vitality of Aboriginal peoples. Understanding the personal and collective processes of resilience that have emerged despite these adversities can play a crucial role in finding ways forward that support both individual autonomy and cultural survival and renewal.

Ongoing transformations of identity and community have led some groups to do well while others face catastrophe. In many cases, the health of the community appears to be linked to the sense of local control and cultural continuity. Recent successes in negotiating land claims and local government as well as forms of cultural renewal hold out hope for improvements in health status. Attempts to recover power and to maintain cultural tradition must contend with the political, economic, and cultural realities of consumer capitalism, technocratic control, and globalization.

Issues of equity in health and well-being for Canada's Aboriginal peoples must be central to any vision of a just society. The wounds of racism, abuse, and cultural oppression, inflicted through colonization's infernal machinery of residential schools and state control of the lives of Aboriginal people, have marked survivors, perpetrators, and bystanders as well. Redressing past wrongs, protecting human rights, and respecting the aspirations of Aboriginal peoples both as individuals and as members of distinct nations are all crucial for the health, well-being, and moral order of Canadian society as a whole.

Acknowledgments
Portions of this chapter are adapted with permission from Kirmayer and colleagues (2000, 2003). Preparation of this chapter was made possible by grants from the Fonds de la recherche en Santé du Québec and from the Institute of Aboriginal Peoples Health and the Institute of Neurosciences, Mental Health and Addiction of the the Canadian Institutes of Health Research.

Notes
1 The remaining 3% of respondents in the census either identified with more than one Aboriginal group or were registered Indians or members of a First Nation but did not identify as Aboriginal (Statistics Canada 2008, 9).
2 Treasury Board of Canada Secretariat (2005). *Canada's performance report 2005 annex 3: Indicators and additional information.* Ottawa: Treasury Board of Canada Secretariat. http://www.tbs-sct.gc.ca/report/govrev/05/ann304_e.asp (accessed 2 January 2007).
3 Including Central and South America, the indigenous population of the Americas prior to European contact was probably over 100 million.
4 Although most Métis and Inuit did not receive any formal education services, some did attend residential schools (Chartrand 2006, 21). In cases where Métis parents were given a choice about whether they would send their children to residential schools, many kept their children home, choosing to teach them the history, songs, dances, and values of their people.
5 A number of "push" and "pull" factors influence rural-urban migration patterns among indigenous peoples (Norris and Clatworthy 2003, 66). The push factors that prompt individuals to move from reserve and settlement communities include the lack of employment opportunities and resulting difficult social conditions; poor economic conditions; marriage and family formation; boredom and low quality of life; lack of housing, health facilities, and educational opportunities; and band politics. Factors pulling indigenous people back to reserve and rural communities include the inability to find employment or to otherwise

adjust to life in the city and lack of access to affordable or acceptable housing. Reserve and rural communities are also commonly viewed as providing a better quality of life than urban settings for raising children because of lower crime rates and less alcohol and drug abuse (Norris and Clatworthy 2003). Stronger social networks that include support from extended families, friends, and culturally appropriate activities and services are also important factors that pull indigenous peoples from cities.

6 Indian and Northern Affairs (2003). *Backgrounder—Water quality and First Nation communities.* Ottawa: Indian and Northern Affairs. CBC News Online (2006). *The state of drinking water on Canada's reserves.* http://www.ainc-inac.gc.ca/nr/prs/m-a2003/02304bk_e.html (accessed 2 June 2008). See also http://www.cbc.ca/slowboil (updated 20 February 2006; accessed 18 January 2007).

7 The Regional Health Surveys excluded Alberta and the northern and James Bay regions of Quebec.

8 From the website of the International Center for Transitional Justice, citing official statistics: http://www.ictj.org/en/where/region2/513.html (accessed 15 January 2007).

References

Abbey, S.E., E. Hood, L.T. Young, and S.A. Malcolmson. 1993. Psychiatric consultation in the eastern Canadian Arctic, Pt. 3, Mental health issues in Inuit women in the eastern Arctic. *Canadian Journal of Psychiatry* 38 (1): 32-35.

Aboriginal Healing Foundation. 2006. *Final report of the Aboriginal Healing Foundation.* Ottawa, ON: Aboriginal Healing Foundation.

Allard, Y.E., R. Wilkins, and J.M. Berthelot. 2004. Premature mortality in health regions with high Aboriginal populations. *Health Reports* 15 (1): 51-60.

American Psychiatric Association. 2000. *Diagnostic and statistical manual of mental disorders: DSM-IV-TR.* 4th ed. Washington, DC: American Psychiatric Publishing.

Armitage, A. 1995. *Comparing the policy of Aboriginal assimilation: Australia, Canada, and New Zealand.* Vancouver: UBC Press.

Armstrong, H. 1993. Depression in Canadian Native Indians. In P. Cappeliez and R.J. Flynn, eds., *Depression and the social environment*, 218-34. Montreal, QC, and Kingston, ON: McGill-Queen's University Press.

Beals, J., J. Piasecki, S. Nelson, M. Jones, E. Keane, P. Dauphinais, R.R. Shirt, W.H. Sack, and S.M. Manson. 1997. Psychiatric disorder among American Indian adolescents: Prevalence in Northern Plains youth. *Journal of the American Academy of Child and Adolescent Psychiatry* 36 (9): 1252-59.

–, S.M. Manson, C.M. Mitchell, and P. Spicer. 2003. Cultural specificity and comparison in psychiatric epidemiology: Walking the tightrope in American Indian research. *Culture, Medicine and Psychiatry* 27 (3): 259-89.

–, S.M. Manson, N.R. Whitesell, C.M. Mitchell, D.K. Novins, S. Simpson, and P. Spicer. 2005a. Prevalence of major depressive episode in two American Indian reservation populations: Unexpected findings with a structured interview. *American Journal of Psychiatry* 162 (9): 1713-22.

–, S.M. Manson, N.R. Whitesell, P. Spicer, D.K. Novins, and C.M. Mitchell, 2005b. Prevalence of DSM-IV disorders and attendant help-seeking in 2 American Indian reservation populations. *Archives of General Psychiatry* 62 (1): 99-108.

–, D.K. Novins, N.R. Whitesell, P. Spicer, C.M. Mitchell, and S.M. Manson. 2005c. Prevalence of mental disorders and utilization of mental health services in two American Indian reservation populations: Mental health disparities in a national context. *American Journal of Psychiatry* 162 (9): 1723-32.

Beiser, M., and C.L. Attneave. 1982. Mental disorders among Native American children: Rates and risk periods for entering treatment. *American Journal of Psychiatry* 139 (2): 193-98.

–, W. Lancee, A. Gotowiec, W. Sack, and R. Redshirt. 1993. Measuring self-perceived role competence among First Nations and non-Native children. *Canadian Journal of Psychiatry* 38 (6): 412-19.

Bennett, J., and S. Rowley, eds. 2004. *Uqalurait: An oral history of Nunavut.* Montreal, QC, and Kingston, ON: McGill-Queen's University Press.

Berkhofer, R.F. 1979. *The white man's Indian: Images of the American Indian, from Columbus to the present*. New York: Vintage.

Boehnlein, J.K., J.D. Kinzie, P.K. Leung, D. Matsunaga, R. Johnson, and J.H. Shore. 1993. The natural history of medical and psychiatric disorders in an American Indian community. *Culture, Medicine and Psychiatry* 16: 543-54.

Boyer, R., R. Dufour, M. Préville, and L. Bujold-Brown. 1994. State of mental health. In Santé Québec and M. Jetté, eds., *A health profile of the Inuit: Report of the Santé Québec Health Survey among the Inuit of Nunavik, 1992*, vol. 2, 117-44. Montreal, QC, and Kingston, ON: Ministère de la Santé et des Services sociaux, Gouvernement du Québec.

Brant Castellano, M., L. Archibald, and M. DeGagne, eds. 2008. *From truth to reconciliation: Transforming the legacy of residential schools*. Ottawa: Aboriginal Healing Foundation.

Brody, H. 1975. *The people's land: Eskimos and whites in the eastern Arctic*. Middlesex, UK: Penguin.

–. 2000. *The other side of Eden: Hunters, farmers and the shaping of the world*. Vancouver, BC: Douglas and McIntyre.

Brzozowski, J.-A., A. Taylor-Butts, and S. Johnson. 2006. *Victimization and offending among the Aboriginal population in Canada*. Ottawa: Statistics Canada, Canadian Centre for Justice Statistics.

Bucko, R.A. 1998. *The Lakota ritual of the sweat lodge: History and contemporary practice*. Lincoln, NE: University of Nebraska Press.

Canino, G., R. Lewis-Fernandez, and M. Bravo. 1997. Methodological challenges in cross-cultural mental health research. *Transcultural Psychiatry* 34 (2): 163-84.

Chandler, M.J. 1994. Self-continuity in suicidal and nonsuicidal adolescents. *New Directions in Child Development* 64: 55-70.

–, and L. Ball. 1989. Continuity and commitment: A developmental analysis of identity formation in suicidal and non-suicidal youth. In H. Bosma and S. Jackson, eds., *Coping and self-concept in adolescence*, 149-66. New York: Springer-Verlag.

–, and C.E. Lalonde. 1998. Cultural continuity as a hedge against suicide in Canada's First Nations. *Transcultural Psychiatry* 35 (2): 191-219.

–, C.E. Lalonde, B.W. Sokol, and D. Hallett. 2003. Personal persistence, identity development, and suicide: A study of Native and non-Native North American adolescents. *Monographs of the Society for Research on Child Development* 68 (2): 1-130.

Chartrand, L.N. 2006. Métis residential school participation: A literature review. In L.N. Chartrand, T.E. Logan, and J.D. Daniels, eds., *Métis history and experience and residential schools in Canada*, 5-55. Ottawa, ON: Aboriginal Healing Foundation.

Chrisjohn, R., S. Young, and M. Maraun. 1997. *The circle game: Shadows and substance in the Indian residential school experience in Canada*. Penticton, BC: Theytus Books.

Clarkson, M., C. Lavallée, G. Legaré, and M. Jetté. 1992. *Santé Québec Health Survey among the Cree of James Bay*. Quebec, QC: Ministère de la Santé et des Services sociaux, Gouvernement du Québec.

Culhane, D., C.L. Tait, J. Fiske, and M. Boscoe. 2003. Social determinants of Indigenous women's mental health. Working Paper 3. Indigenous Women, Inequality and Health: Intercommunity, Interdisciplinary and International Strategies Research and Action Development Project. Unpublished manuscript.

de Jong, J.T.V.M., and M. van Ommeren. 2002. Toward a culture-informed epidemiology: Combining qualitative and quantitative research in transcultural contexts. *Transcultural Psychiatry* 39 (4): 422-33.

Dickason, O.P. 2002. *Canada's First Nations: A history of founding peoples from earliest times*. 3rd ed. Don Mills, ON: Oxford University Press.

Dorais, L.J. 1997. *Quaqtaq: Modernity and identity in an Inuit community*. Toronto, ON: University of Toronto Press.

Drummond, S.G. 1997. *Incorporating the familiar: An investigation into legal sensibilities in Nunavik*. Montreal, QC, and Kingston, ON: McGill-Queen's University Press.

First Nations Information Governance Committee. 2007. *First Nations Regional Longitudinal Health Survey (RHS) 2002/03: Results for adults, youth and children living in First Nations communities*. Ottawa, ON: Assembly of First Nations.

Foucault, M. 1977. *Discipline and punish: The birth of the prison*. New York: Pantheon Books.

Fournier, S., and E. Crey. 1997. *Stolen from our embrace*. Vancouver, BC: Douglas and McIntyre.

Frideres, J.S. 2004. *Aboriginal peoples in Canada: Contemporary conflicts*. 7th ed. Toronto, ON: Prentice Hall Canada.

Gfellner, B.M., and J.D. Hundleby. 1995. Patterns of drug use among Native and white adolescents: 1990-1993. *Canadian Journal of Public Health* 86 (2): 95-97.

Goffman, E. 1961. *Asylums: Essays on the social situation of mental patients and other inmates*. New York: Anchor.

Gotowiec, A., and M. Beiser. 1994. Aboriginal children's mental health: Unique challenges. *Canada's Mental Health* 41 (4): 7-11.

Gough, P., N. Trocmé, I. Brown, D. Knoke, and C. Blackstock. 2005. Pathways to overrepresentation of Aboriginal children in care. CECW Information Sheet #23E. Toronto, ON: University of Toronto Press. http://www.cecw-cepb.ca/DocsEng/AboriginalChildren23Epdf.

Government of Canada. 2006. *The human face of mental health and mental illness in Canada 2006*. Ottawa, ON: Minister of Public Works and Government Services of Canada.

Grygier, P.S. 1994. *A long way from home: The tuberculosis epidemic among the Inuit*. Montreal, QC, and Kingston, ON: McGill-Queen's University Press.

Haggarty, J., Z. Cernovsky, P. Kermeen, and H. Merskey. 2000. Psychiatric disorders in an Arctic community. *Canadian Journal of Psychiatry* 45 (4): 357-62.

Haig-Brown, C. 1988. *Resistance and renewal: Surviving the Indian residential school*. Vancouver, BC: Tillacum Library.

Hall, R.L. 1997. *An archaeology of the soul: North American Indian belief and ritual*. Urbana, IL: University of Illinois Press.

Health Canada. 5 March 2002. *First Nations and Inuit Regional Health Survey*. http://www.rhs-ers.ca.

Howard, M.O., R.D. Walker, P.S. Walker, L.B. Cottler, and W.M. Compton. 1999. Inhalant use among urban American Indian youth. *Addiction* 94 (1): 83-95.

Hoxie, F.E. 1996. The reservation period, 1880-1960. In B.G. Trigger and W.E. Washburn, eds., *The Cambridge history of the Native peoples of the Americas*, vol. 1, *North America Part 2*, 183-258. New York: Cambridge University Press.

Hultkrantz, A. 1987. *Native religions of North America*. New York: Harper San Francisco.

Imai, S., ed. 2003. *The 2003 annotated Indian Act and related constitutional provisions*. Scarborough, ON: Carswell.

Jervis, L.L., P. Spicer, S.M. Manson, and AI-SUPERFRP Team. 2003. Boredom, "trouble," and the realities of postcolonial reservation life. *Ethos* 31 (1): 38-58.

Johnston, B. 1983. *Native children and the child welfare system*. Toronto, ON: Canadian Council on Social Development, in association with James Lorimer.

–. 1988. *Indian school days*. Norman, OK: University of Oklahoma Press.

Kinzie, J.D., P.K. Leung, J. Boehnlein, D. Matsunaga, R. Johnson, S. Manson, J.H. Shore, J. Heinz, and M. Williams. 1992. Psychiatric epidemiology of an Indian village: A 19-year replication study. *Journal of Nervous and Mental Disease* 180 (1): 33-39.

Kirmayer, L.J. 1989. Cultural variations in the response to psychiatric disorders and emotional distress. *Social Science and Medicine* 29 (3): 327-39.

–. 1994. Suicide among Canadian Aboriginal peoples. *Transcultural Psychiatric Research Review* 31 (1): 3-58.

–, M. Malus, and L.J. Boothroyd. 1996. Suicide attempts among Inuit youth: A community survey of prevalence and risk factors. *Acta Psychiatrica Scandinavica* 94 (1): 8-17.

–, G.M. Brass, and C.L. Tait. 2000. The mental health of Aboriginal peoples: Transformations of identity and community. *Canadian Journal of Psychiatry* 45 (7): 607-16.

–, C. Simpson, and M. Cargo. 2003. Healing traditions: Culture, community and mental health promotion with Canadian Aboriginal peoples. *Australasian Psychiatry* 11 (suppl.): 15-23.

–, and G.E. Jarvis. 2005. Depression across cultures. In D. Stein, A. Schatzberg, and D. Kupfer, eds., *Textbook of mood disorders*, 611-29. Washington, DC: American Psychiatric Publishing.

–, G.M. Brass, T.L. Holton, K. Paul, C.L. Tait, and C. Simpson. 2007. *Suicide among Aboriginal peoples in Canada*. Ottawa, ON: Aboriginal Healing Foundation.

–, K.W. Paul, and L. Rochette. 2007. *Nunavik Health Survey 2004/Qanuippitaa? How are we? Mental health, social support and community wellness*. Quebec, QC: Institute National de Santé Publique and Nunavik Regional Board of Health and Social Services.

–, R. Lemelson, and M. Barad, eds. 2007. *Understanding trauma: Biological, psychological and cultural perspectives*. New York: Cambridge University Press.

Kleinman, A. 1987. Anthropology and psychiatry: The role of culture in cross-cultural research on illness. *British Journal of Psychiatry* 151: 447-54.

Knockwood, I., and G. Thomas. 1992. *Out of the depths: The experiences of Mi'kmaw children at the Indian residential school at Shubenacadie, Nova Scotia*. 2nd ed. Lockeport, NS: Roseway.

Krupat, A. 1996. *The turn to the native: Studies in criticism and culture*. Lincoln, NE: University of Nebraska Press.

Kunitz, S.J. 1994. *Disease and social diversity*. New York: Oxford University Press.

–, K.R. Gabriel, J.E. Levy, E. Henderson, K. Lampert, J. McCloskey, and G. Quintero. 1999a. Alcohol dependence and conduct disorder among Navajo Indians. *Journal of Studies on Alcohol* 60 (2): 159-67.

–, K.R. Gabriel, J.E. Levy, E. Henderson, K. Lampert, J. McCloskey, G. Quintero, S. Russell, and A. Vince. 1999b. Risk factors for conduct disorder among Navajo men. *Social Psychiatry and Psychiatric Epidemiology* 34 (4): 180-89.

Lawrence, B. 2004. *"Real" Indians and others: Mixed-blood urban Native peoples and indigenous nationhood*. Vancouver, BC: UBC Press.

Lomawaima, K.T. 1993. Domesticity in the federal Indian schools: The power of authority over mind and body. *American Ethnologist* 20 (2): 227-40.

MacDonald, J.A. 1995. The program of the Spallumcheen Indian Band in British Columbia as a model of Indian child welfare. In B. Blake and J. Keshen, eds., *Social welfare policy in Canada*, 380-91. Toronto, ON: Copp Clarke.

MacMillan, H., A. MacMillan, D. Offord, and J. Dingle. 1996. Aboriginal health. *Canadian Medical Association Journal* 155 (11): 1569-93.

Manson, S.M., J. Beals, T.D. O'Nell, J. Piasecki, and D. Novins. 1996. Wounded spirits, ailing hearts: PTSD and related disorders among American Indians. In A.J. Marsella, M.J. Friedman, E.T. Gerrity, and R.M. Scurfield, eds., *Ethnocultural aspects of post-traumatic stress disorders: Issues, research and clinical applications*, 255-84. Washington, DC: American Psychological Association.

–, J. Beals, S.A. Klein, and C.D. Croy. 2005. Social epidemiology of trauma among 2 American Indian reservation populations. *American Journal of Public Health* 95 (5): 851-59.

–, J.H. Shore, and J.D. Bloom. 1985. The depressive experience in American Indian communities: A challenge for psychiatric theory and diagnosis. In A.M. Kleinman and B. Good, eds., *Culture and depression*, 331-68. Berkeley, CA: University of California Press.

Marcus, A.R. 1992. *Out in the cold: The legacy of Canada's Inuit relocation experiment in the High Arctic*. Copenhagen, Denmark: IWGIA.

Miller, J.R. 1990. Owen Glendower, Hotspur, and Canadian Indian policy. *Ethnohistory* 37 (4): 325-41.

–. 1996. *Shingwauk's vision: A history of Native residential schools*. Toronto, ON: University of Toronto Press.

–. 2000. *Skyscrapers hide the heavens: A history of Indian-white relations in Canada*. Toronto, ON: University of Toronto Press.

Milloy, J.S. 1999. *A national crime: The Canadian government and the residential school system, 1879 to 1986.* Winnipeg, MB: University of Manitoba Press.

Minister of Indian Affairs and Northern Development. 1998. *Gathering strength: Canada's Aboriginal action plan, a progress report.* Ottawa, ON: Minister of Indian Affairs and Northern Development.

Muckle, G., O. Boucher, D. Laflamme, S. Chevalier, and L. Rochette. (2007) *Alcohol, drug use and gambling profile.* Quebec, QC: Institute national de santé publique and Nunavik Regional Board of Health and Social Services.

Nabakov, P. 1996. Native views of history. In B.G. Trigger and W.E. Washburn, eds., *The Cambridge history of the Native peoples of the Americas,* vol. 1, *North America Part 1,* 1-59. New York: Cambridge University Press.

Neu, D.E., and R. Therrien. 2003. *Accounting for genocide: Canada's bureaucratic assault on Aboriginal people.* Black Point, NS: Fernwood/Zed Books.

Neumark, Y.D., J. Delva, and J.C. Anthony. 1998. The epidemiology of adolescent inhalant drug involvement. *Archives of Pediatrics and Adolescent Medicine* 152 (8): 781-86.

Newhouse, D.R. and E.J. Peters. 2003. Introduction. In D.R. Newhouse and E.J. Peters, eds., *Not strangers in these parts: Urban Aboriginal peoples,* 5-21. Ottawa, ON: Policy Research Initiative, Government of Canada.

Niezen, R. 2003. *The origins of indigenism: Human rights and the politics of identity.* Berkeley, CA: University of California Press.

Norris, M.J. 2007. Aboriginal languages in Canada: Emerging trends and perspectives on second language acquisition. In *Statistics Canada: Canadian social trends* (11-008), 19-27. Ottawa, ON: Ministry of Industry.

–, and S. Clatworthy. 2003. Aboriginal mobility and migration within urban Canada: Outcomes, factors and implications. In D.R. Newhouse and E.J. Peters, eds., *Not strangers in these parts: Urban Aboriginal peoples,* 51-78. Ottawa, ON: Policy Research Initiative, Government of Canada.

Northwest Territories Bureau of Statistics. 1996. *NWT Alcohol and Drug Survey: Report no. 1.* Yellowknife, NWT: Northwest Territories Bureau of Statistics.

O'Nell, T.D. 1996. *Disciplined hearts: History, identity, and depression in an American Indian community.* Berkeley, CA: University of California Press.

–. 2004. Culture and pathology: Flathead loneliness revisited. The 2001 Roger Allan Moore Lecture. *Culture, Medicine, and Psychiatry* 28 (2): 221-30.

Petawabano, B., E. Gourdeau, F. Jourdain, A. Palliser-Tulugak, and J. Cossette. 1994. *Mental health and Aboriginal people of Québec.* Montreal, QC: Gaëtan Morin Éditeur.

Peterson, J., and J.S.H. Brown, eds. 1993. *The new peoples: Being and becoming Métis in North America.* Winnipeg, MB: University of Manitoba Press.

Phinney, J.S., and V. Chavira. 1992. Ethnic identity and self-esteem: An exploratory study. *Journal of Adolescence* 15 (3): 271-81.

Ray, A.J. 1996. *I have lived here since the world began.* Toronto, ON: Lester.

Richardson, B. 1993. *People of terra nullius: Betrayal and renewal in Aboriginal Canada.* Vancouver, BC: Douglas and McIntyre.

Roosens, E.E. 1989. *Creating ethnicity: The process of ethnogenesis.* Thousand Oaks, CA: Sage.

Ross, R. 1996. *Returning to the teachings: Exploring Aboriginal justice.* Toronto, ON: Penguin.

Royal Commission on Aboriginal Peoples. 1993. *Aboriginal peoples in urban centres: Report of the National Round Table on Aboriginal Urban Issues.* Ottawa, ON: Royal Commission on Aboriginal Peoples.

–. 1994. *The High Arctic relocation: A report on the 1953-55 relocation.* Ottawa, ON: Minister of Supply and Services.

–. 1995. *Choosing life: Special report on suicide among Aboriginal people.* Ottawa, ON: Royal Commission on Aboriginal Peoples.

–. 1996. *Report of the Royal Commission on Aboriginal Peoples.* Ottawa, ON: Royal Commission on Aboriginal Peoples.

Sack, W.H., M. Beiser, G. Baker-Brown, and R. Redshirt. 1994. Depressive and suicidal symptoms in Indian school children: Findings from the Flower of Two Soils. *American Indian and Alaska Native Mental Health Research Monograph Series* 4: 81-94.

Salisbury, R.F. 1986. *A homeland for the Cree: Regional development in James Bay, 1971-1981.* Montreal, QC, and Kingston, ON: McGill-Queen's University Press.

Shore, J.H., J.D. Kinzie, J.L. Hampson, and E.M. Pattison. 1973. Psychiatric epidemiology of an Indian village. *Psychiatry* 36 (1): 70-81.

Siggner, A.J. 2003. Urban Aboriginal populations: An update using the 2001 census results. In D.R. Newhouse and E.J. Peters, eds., *Not strangers in these parts: Urban Aboriginal peoples,* 15-21. Ottawa, ON: Policy Research Initiative, Government of Canada.

Sioui, G.E. 1992. *For an Amerindian autohistory: An essay on the foundations of a social ethic.* Montreal, QC, and Kingston, ON: McGill-Queen's University Press.

Sissons, J. 2005. *First peoples: Indigenous cultures and their futures.* London: Reaktion Books.

Spicer, P., J. Beals, C.D. Croy, et al. 2003. The prevalence of DSM-III-R alcohol dependence in two American Indian populations. *Alcohol Clinical and Experimental Research* 27 (11): 1785-97.

Stairs, A. 1992. Self-image, world-image: Speculations on identity from experiences with Inuit. *Ethos* 20 (1): 116-26.

–, and G. Wenzel. 1992. "I am I and the environment": Inuit hunting, community and identity. *Journal of Indigenous Studies* 3 (2): 1-12.

Stannard, D.E. 1992. *American holocaust: The conquest of the New World.* New York: Oxford University Press.

Statistics Canada. 2003. *Aboriginal peoples of Canada: A demographic profile.* 2001 Census: Analysis Series No. 96F0030XIE2001007. Ottawa, ON: Statistics Canada.

–. 2008. *Aboriginal peoples in Canada in 2006: Inuit, Métis and First Nations, 2006 Census.* Ottawa, ON: Ministry of Industry.

Stephens, C., C. Nettleton, J. Porter, R. Willis, and S. Clark. 2005. Indigenous peoples' health – Why are they behind everyone, everywhere? *Lancet* 366 (9479): 10-13.

Swift, K. 1995. *Manufacturing "bad mothers": A critical perspective on child neglect.* Toronto, ON: University of Toronto Press.

Tanner, A. 1979. *Bringing home animals: Religious ideology and mode of production of the Mistassini Cree hunters.* New York: St. Martin's Press.

Tester, F.J., and P.K. Kulchyski. 1994. *Tammarniit (mistakes): Inuit relocation in the eastern Arctic, 1939-63.* Vancouver, BC: UBC Press.

–, and P. McNicoll. 2004. Isumagijaksaq: Mindful of the state: Social constructions of Inuit suicide. *Social Science and Medicine* 58 (12): 2625-36.

Thornton, R. 1987. *American Indian Holocaust and survival: A population history since 1492.* Norman, OK: University of Oklahoma Press.

Titley, E.B. 1986. *A narrow vision: Duncan Campbell Scott and the administration of Indian affairs in Canada.* Vancouver, BC: UBC Press.

Tobias, J.L. 1976. Protection, civilization, assimilation: An outline history of Canada's Indian policy. *Western Canadian Journal of Anthropology* 61 (2): 12-30.

Treat, J., ed. 1996. *Native and Christian: Indigenous voices on religious identity in the United States and Canada.* New York: Routledge.

Triandis, H.C. 1995. *Individualism and collectivism.* Boulder, CO: Westview Press.

Trigger, B.G., and W.R. Swagerty. 1996. Entertaining strangers: North America in the sixteenth century. In B.G. Trigger and W.E. Washburn, eds., *The Cambridge history of the Native peoples of the Americas,* vol. 1, *North America Part 1,* 325-98. New York: Cambridge University Press.

Trimble, J.E., and B. Medicine. 1993. Diversification of American Indians: Forming an indigenous perspective. In U. Kim and J.W. Berry, eds., *Indigenous psychologies: Research and experience in cultural context,* 133-51. Thousand Oaks, CA: Sage.

Turner, D.A. 2006. *This is not a peace pipe: Towards a critical indigenous philosophy*. Toronto: University of Toronto Press.

Valaskakis, G.G. 2005. *Indian country: Essays on contemporary Native culture*. Waterloo, ON: Wilfred Laurier University Press.

van Ommeren, M. 2003. Validity issues in transcultural epidemiology. *British Journal of Psychiatry* 182 (5): 376-78.

Vecsey, C., ed. 1990. *Religion in Native North America*. Moscow, ID: University of Idaho Press.

Vizenor, G. 1999. *Manifest manners: Narratives on post-Indian survivance*. Lincoln, NE: University of Nebraska Press.

Waldram, J.B. 1997a. The Aboriginal people of Canada: Colonialism and mental health. In I. Al-Issa and M. Tousignant, eds., *Ethnicity, immigration, and psychopathology,* 169-87. New York: Plenum.

–. 1997b. *The way of the pipe: Aboriginal spirituality and symbolic healing in Canadian prisons*. Peterborough, ON: Broadview Press.

–. 2004. *Revenge of the Windigo: The construction of the mind and mental health of North American Aboriginal peoples*. Toronto, ON: University of Toronto Press.

–. 2006. The view from the Hogan: Cultural epidemiology and the return to ethnography. *Transcultural Psychiatry* 43 (1): 72-85.

–, A. Herring, and T.K. Young. 2006. *Aboriginal health in Canada: Historical, cultural, and epidemiological perspectives.* 2nd ed. Toronto, ON: University of Toronto Press.

Warry, W. 1998. *Unfinished dreams: Community healing and the reality of Aboriginal self-government*. Toronto: University of Toronto Press.

Weir, E. 2001. Inhalant use and addiction in Canada. *Canadian Medical Association Journal* 164 (3): 397.

World Health Organization. 1992. *The ICD-10 classification of mental and behavioural disorders: Clinical descriptions and diagnostic guidelines*. Geneva, Switzerland: World Health Organization.

York, G. 1990. *The dispossessed: Life and death in Native Canada*. Boston: Little, Brown.

–, and L. Pindera. 1991. *People of the pines: The people and the legacy of Oka*. Toronto, ON: Little, Brown.

2

Mental Health and the Indigenous Peoples of Australia and New Zealand

MASON DURIE, HELEN MILROY, AND ERNEST HUNTER

The eminent New Zealand public health physician Robert Beaglehole recently commented that the critical question for public health practitioners "is how to build the social movement to support nascent political efforts to address the unacceptable levels of health inequalities in all societies" (2006, 260). This is as much a call to political action as it is a call to health policy and practice, and it clearly relates to the means by which disadvantaged populations worldwide are enabled to control their destinies, which, as noted by Michael Marmot, is critical to self-esteem and health: "Autonomy is closely linked with self esteem and the earning of respect. Both are basic and ... linked. Low levels of autonomy and low self esteem are likely to be related to worse health" (2003, 574).

These issues are particularly relevant to minority indigenous[1] populations dispossessed and displaced by settler colonialism, as happened in Australia, New Zealand, Canada, and the United States, which were all areas of "Anglo-settler colonialism" (Kunitz 1994). However, although there are macro-level historical commonalities among these countries, there are also unique factors that inform differences in health policy, health services, and broader health status (Anderson et al. 2006). Even though in all of these nations there are persistent health differentials between indigenous and non-indigenous populations, Australia stands out in that the health differentials are both larger (Kunitz 1994; Kunitz et al. 1994) and not improving (Fremantle et al. 2006; Lavoie 2004; Ring and Brown 2003; Ring and Firman 1998) (see Table 2.1). Politics and health, then, are inextricably intertwined, a point made forcefully by the Royal Australian and New Zealand College of Psychiatrists, which states in its *Principles and guidelines for Aboriginal and Torres Strait Islander mental health*: "Health professionals need to be aware that interventions within the arena of Indigenous health necessarily have political implications. Involvement in this area of professional practice often involves challenging government policy and community attitudes which have the potential to impact negatively on Aboriginal and Torres Strait Islander social, emotional, cultural and spiritual well-being" (1999, 1).

With this in mind, in this chapter we explore issues relevant to the mental health and to the social and emotional well-being of Aboriginal and Torres Strait Islander Australians and Mäori New Zealanders.

TABLE 2.1

Indigenous and non-indigenous health indicators in Canada, Australia, and New Zealand

	Life expectancy (years)	ASDR	IMR	Population < 15 years of age (%)
Canada (1991)				
First Nation M	66.9	12.71	12.30	34.4
Non-FN M	74.6	8.49	6.40	20.6
First Nation F	74.0	7.95		
Non-FN F	80.9	5.28		
Australia (1991-96)				
Aboriginal M	56.9	20.87	18.70	39.0
Non-Aboriginal M	75.6	8.39	6.05	21.0
Aboriginal F	61.7	16.86	17.30	
Non-Aboriginal F	81.3	5.42	4.95	
New Zealand (1991)				
Mäori M	67.2	11.89	14.10	33.1
Non-Mäori M	71.6	9.33	7.10	22.2
Mäori F	72.3	8.40		
Non-Mäori F	77.6	6.05		

Notes: ASDR: age-standardized death rate (per 100,000 population)
IMR: infant-mortality rate (per 1,000 life births)
Source: Where no numbers exist for female (F), the number for male (M) covers both genders (Derived from Lavoie 2004).

Origins

Most Indigenous Australian belief systems have held that human origins lie in the Dreamtime when geological features, animals, plants and humans were created by ancestral beings. People see themselves as an element in the creation of the landscape. For them there was no migration to Australia at all. The alternative western scientific view is that Aboriginal people must be part of the development of all humanity, ultimately originating somewhere in Africa two million years ago.

– B. ARTHUR AND F. MORPHY, EDS., *THE MACQUARIE ATLAS OF INDIGENOUS AUSTRALIA* (2005), 38

This quotation from *The Macquarie atlas of Indigenous Australia* raises the important issue of how indigenous and scientific knowledge systems interpret and explain origins. From the scientific perspective, the first peoples to arrive in northern Australia preceded the Polynesian arrival in Aotearoa (i.e., New Zealand) by at least 60,000 years (probably considerably more) and populated the continent in waves, entering across the Timor Sea to the Kimberley region and from the Island of New Guinea into Cape York. Consequently, Australia is a continent of extraordinary cultural and linguistic diversity, particularly across the north, with estimates of more than 250 languages prior to contact.[2] The most obvious difference in this population is between the Aboriginal inhabitants of mainland Australia and Torres Strait Islanders, whose ancestry is both Aboriginal and Papuan. Aboriginal peoples also comprise many groups or nations, the preferred terms being those of self-identification – Koori, Nyoongar, Murri, Palawa, Nunga, and Yolgnu, to name a few of the estimated 600 to 700 nations from which Aboriginal Australians are descended. By contrast, Mäori, the descendents of the great Polynesian navigators whose canoes reached New Zealand a thousand years before Europeans, speak a common language (although with distinct dialects) and observe similar cultural practices. However, these populations share fundamental kindredness and common worldviews as indigenous peoples. In this chapter, this critical feature of indigeneity will be addressed before considering the history and contemporary circumstances that inform not only current patterns of health and ill-health but also approaches to addressing social, emotional, and mental health needs.

Indigenous Worldviews

There are some 5,000 indigenous groups around the world with a total population of about 370 million, or around 5% of the global population spread across 70 countries (Horton 2006). They are descendents of those who inhabited a country or region at a time when people of different cultures or ethnic origins arrived. The new arrivals later became dominant through conquest, occupation, settlement, or other means (Bristow 2003). Although there is no simple definition of indigenous peoples or the attributes that underlie indigeneity – being indigenous – it is possible to identify shared characteristics that inform the "indigenous perspective."

As noted earlier, the indigenous peoples of Australasia and those of North America have a history of dispossession through Anglo-settler colonialism. The devastations that followed resulted from disruption of the critical bond with the land and the natural environment that is the key feature of indigeneity and is reflected in systems of knowledge and societal arrangements (Durie 2005a). For instance, the bond with the land is acknowledged by Mäori when they describe themselves as *tangata whenua,* or people of the land. In Aotearoa, Mäori were *kaitaiki,* or guardians of their lands. They developed complex systems of environmental management within which people learned to live in harmony with nature. Similarly, as the world's oldest continuous living culture, Aboriginal peoples viewed themselves as being part of the landscape, born of the country and intimately connected to it – everything had its place in the continuous cycle of life. This relationship is often referred to as "custodianship," or looking after the land for the sustainable benefit of the environment and humankind alike, with "Mother Earth" taking on a literal meaning, the sacred inscribed in a totemic landscape.

MASON DURIE, HELEN MILROY, AND ERNEST HUNTER

Both Māori and Aboriginal knowledge systems are based on experience and observation – learnings passed down through stories, ceremonies, and songs that explain the interrelatedness of all things. This interconnectivity includes kinship systems and kin groupings, traditional law, knowing tribe and "country," and language – the latter being a powerful marker of indigeneity. In contrast to Māori, the languages of Aboriginal and Torres Strait Islander Australians are extremely diverse (Schmidt 1994). Although traditional languages have been vulnerable in Australia in the face of colonization, the development of region-specific Creole (e.g., in the Torres Strait) and of a distinct Aboriginal English recognizable across the continent emphasizes the continuing importance of language as a signifier of indigeneity and as a vehicle for cultural continuity.

Traditional family structures are characterized by extensive kinship systems with enduring bonds of obligation and reciprocity. In such systems, relationships and responsibilities are clearly defined. From a non-indigenous perspective, this may involve a confusing abundance of subtle distinctions and ambiguous intragenerational relational equivalences – for instance, between sibling and cousin or between mother and aunt. Across generations, contiguity of physical and spiritual realms ensures that ancestry is a vital aspect of daily life, with experiences and understandings being powerfully influenced by dreams, symbols, visitations, spiritual gifts, premonitions, and messages. Time is experienced not only in its mundane diachronic (linear) sense but also synchronically – past, present, and future coexisting (Janca and Bullen 2003). This relationship to time can have very real impacts on priority setting and time management that can cause consternation and confusion when they collide with the agendas and demands of mainstream culture and organizations.

Indigenous knowledge systems also integrate worldviews, values, and experiences to generate a framework for a distinctive approach to health and well-being that emphasizes collectivity, spirituality, and balance – an ecological perspective. Balance is achieved through emphasis on well-being and collective identity rather than on individual achievement and prosperity. This focus is also reflected in traditional healing methods derived from a close association with the environment, and it remains crucial to Māori and Aboriginal healers, for whom health and well-being are inseparable. In the past the roles of these healers were not only to resolve illness arising from spiritual or cultural malaise but also to support indigenous knowledge systems to ensure a structured society with its own system of governance and law. When these roles and the stable social order they supported were overturned, the consequences were dire, including the undermining of social order and loss of indigenous methodologies.

Identity Transitions: Māori Views

Identity is a necessary prerequisite for mental health. Cultural identity depends not only on access to culture and heritage but also on opportunities for cultural expression and cultural endorsement within society's institutions. Ethnic identity has assumed increasing importance in the broad mental health field both in relationship to positive health and development and as a key determinant of successful counselling outcomes. Prior to colonization a tribal identity was the distinguishing characteristic between indigenous people. Tribal members not only had common lines of descent but were also closely attuned to their natural environment and often identified with geographic features such as rivers, mountains, and forests. Identity was to a large extent a collective experience (Durie 1998).

Although indigenous populations are not homogenous and are made up of individuals with a diverse range of attitudes, beliefs, and values, it is possible to identify at least three forms of cultural identity: a positive identity, an identity based on deficits, and a negative identity. In a study of 700 Māori households, a secure cultural identity was evident in one-third of participants and characterized by competence in Māori languages, regular contact with Māori cultural institutions and networks, and shares in Māori land (Te Hoe Nuku Roa 1997). Within the group, some identified strongly with tribal culture, while others were more aligned to a broader Māori culture where language, networks, and interests were embedded in communities of interest rather than in tribal alliances. The shift paralleled Māori transitions from a tribal society to an urban society.

Not all Māori, however, have positive cultural identities. Urbanization saw the emergence of an identity based on being poor and unsophisticated. Until the middle of the twentieth century, Māori were largely rural dwellers, but by 1976 more than 80% were living in urban settings. Thousands of young had migrated to towns and cities, leaving behind familiar landmarks, culture, and language for the prospect of higher wages, trade training, subsidized housing, and greater social mobility. Māori had been propelled into an urban industrial economy, largely as labourers and unskilled workers. As early as 1960, national social indicators pointed to a new class of urban dwellers who were poor, unhealthy, housed in substandard homes, more likely to offend, less likely to succeed at school – and Māori (Hunn 1961). Being Māori was measured more by deficits in comparison to the Pākehā middle class than by any notion of a positive Māori identity. Moreover, the stereotype was endorsed by implicit policies of assimilation.

Another pattern of identity was linked to lack of perceived power within the wider society. In response to marginalization and societal intolerance, a positive Māori identity was often crushed or reconfigured in a fatalistic light. Many Māori rejected their own cultural identity and either tried to imitate Pākehā New Zealanders or played out second-class roles as carefree, unambitious, and inoffensive labourers. Many opted to take a defiant stance by wearing a patch, a Māori identity that became synonymous with gang culture, while others took refuge in foreign cults such as Rastafarianism. A negative identity had been assumed in part as a defence against cultural alienation and in part as a reaction to perceived discrimination.

Among indigenous populations, negative identities accompanied by deculturation have been recognized as causes of mental ill-health, including alcohol misuse, suicide, aggression, and offending (Waldram 1997). More recently, indigenous peoples have come to

MASON DURIE, HELEN MILROY, AND ERNEST HUNTER

regard the establishment of a positive cultural identity as a key to better mental health and have developed a range of therapies that focus on cultural reawakening (Duran and Duran 1995; McCormick, Chapter 15).

Mäori models of counselling, for example, place emphasis on reducing alienation from Mäori culture. Cognitive skills (especially language competence) and cultural knowledge such as genealogy, custom, and tribal history are important, but identity also rests on being able to have first-hand contact with the wider Mäori world: traditional lands, customary meeting places *(marae)*, traditional sources of food, waterways, opportunities for social and work relationships with other Mäori, and a balanced relationship with family. Cultural therapists must be able to evaluate identity as it pertains to health status and then, using their own knowledge of indigenous networks and resources, make appropriate contacts (Durie 2001). Not all indigenous clients who have mental health problems have an insecure cultural identity; however, their relationships with family and other societal groups may be unsatisfactory, and they may be ignoring the consequences of their own attitudes, behaviours, and emotional reactions.

By itself, a secure and positive ethnic identity is not insurance against poor mental health, nor does it offer a passport to good health. An identity that confines human experience to a culturally safe environment reduces anxiety and enhances confidence in that environment, but it creates maladaptive coping behaviours and rigidities that are out of place in a mobile and changing world. Nonetheless, a secure cultural identity derived from ready access to indigenous cultural, social, and physical resources can provide a strong foundation for health if it also allows interaction with the other identities that must be incorporated into a psychological whole necessary to navigate tribal, urban, and global worlds.

Identity Transitions: Aboriginal Views

Indigenous peoples of Australia have undergone similar identity transitions, and the debate regarding Aboriginality has become increasingly complex and controversial. Although the right to decide one's own identity may be assumed, there are both moral and legal ramifications for individuals, communities, and programs in regard to just who is Aboriginal in Australia. Traditionally, Aboriginal identity was strongly linked to kinship system, skin group, and land. It followed a variety of societal and cultural rules for use of names, roles, and responsibilities, and it often included developmental rites of passage. However, following colonization, ascribed identity or classification was based on degree of descent and physical features with the imposition of the collective, diminutive term "Aborigine."

With restrictive racist legislation that controlled all aspects of Aboriginal people's lives, Aboriginal children were deemed to be under the "guardianship" of the state. For some families, the only way to retain custody of their children was to apply for exemption by denying their Aboriginality and adopting a "white" lifestyle. The denial of paternity by non-Indigenous Australians of their mixed-descent offspring and the widespread removal of lighter-skinned children from their families for the purposes of assimilation (the "Stolen

Generations") denied many Aboriginal people their cultural identity and heritage. It has also excluded them from access to their non-Indigenous heritage, in essence constituting a "double denial." The Stolen Generations and their descendents confront the ongoing challenge of reclaiming Indigenous identity and tracing cultural origins. Given the lack of positive Indigenous representations and the lack of role models and authority figures, a further challenge is how to facilitate children's development of healthy identities based on cultural strengths, not on disadvantage, disease burden, and discrimination.

As a result, in contemporary Australian society there is a continuum in terms of identification from denial of Aboriginality to identity rooted in identification with traditionality. Predictably, the influence on people's lives varies enormously. The current definition of indigeneity used nationally for administrative purposes, such as eligibility for special programs, is that an Aboriginal or Torres Strait Islander person is one who is of Aboriginal or Torres Strait Islander descent, who identifies as Aboriginal or Torres Strait Islander, and who is accepted as such by the community in which he or she lives or has lived. Although this is not based on degree of descent or physical features, identity as an Indigenous Australian continues to be a contested issue at the core of which is a persistent sense of "violation." As noted by Australia's first Aboriginal and Torres Strait Islander Social Justice Commissioner, Mick Dodson: "At the heart of the violation [of our rights as peoples] has been the denial of control over our identity ... Recognition of a people's fundamental rights to self-determination must include the right to self-definition, and to be free from the control and manipulation of an alien people" (1994, 5).

Health and Well-Being

From an indigenous perspective, health is a holistic concept exemplified by the commonly accepted definition adopted in Australia's National Aboriginal Health Strategy, which states that health is "not just the physical well-being of the individual but the social, emotional, and cultural well-being of the whole community. This is a whole-of-life view and it also includes the cyclical concept of life-death-life" (National Aboriginal Health Strategy Working Party 1989, x). This perspective is further expanded in relation to mental health in *"Ways forward,"* a national consultancy report on Aboriginal mental health: "The Aboriginal concept of health is holistic, encompassing mental health and physical, cultural and spiritual health. Land is central to well-being. This holistic concept does not merely refer to the 'whole body' but is in fact steeped in the harmonised inter-relations which constitute cultural well-being ... Crucially, it must be understood that when the harmony of these inter-relations is disrupted, Aboriginal ill-health will persist" (Swan and Raphael 1995, 19).

Māori concepts are similar and have been reintroduced into modern discourses on health in a model known as *Te Whare Tapa Wha,* which is based on a holistic approach to health and the recognition of spirituality as a significant contributor to good health (Durie 1998). Reconfiguring health in terms that make sense to Māori supports conceptual claims and ownership while balancing medical and professional dominance with community involvement and local leadership. Te Whare Tapa Wha invokes the image of a four-sided house, each wall representing one aspect of health. *Taha wairua* (spirituality) remains important to Mäori since it captures both the notion of a special relationship with the environment and a Mäori cultural identity. *Taha hinengaro* (mind) concerns the way people think, feel, and behave, and it recognizes that Mäori patterns of thought tend to value metaphor and allusion. *Taha tinana* (physical health) is not only about physical illness but also about fitness, mobility, and freedom from pain, while *taha whänau* (relationship) focuses on the nature of interpersonal relationships within the family and in the wider society. Increasingly, this model is being used as a framework for the development of Mäori approaches to health assessment, treatment, care, the measurement of outcomes, and the formulation of health policies.

Similar metaphors are found in Indigenous Australia. For instance, in the Torres Strait the "Tree of Life" (Hunter et al. 1999) draws on the image of a coconut palm tree with 10 elements that symbolize the structure of family and society as well as the balances of continuity and change. The 10 elements are roots (cultural foundations and heritage), trunk (intimate unions), leaves (extended family), new shoots (siblings), the first tier of leaves around new shoots (teachers), the second tier of leaves around new shoots (guardians of knowledge and culture), bunches of coconuts (individuals and people), dead leaves (old people – ancestors and lineage – reproduction, and rejuvenation), falling coconuts (offspring), and growth rings around the trunk (reproduction of history/story). Story and visual representation have been critical factors in cultural continuity and in supporting the reaffirmation of Aboriginal traditions and values (Caruana 1989).

Demographic Trends

For both Mäori and Indigenous Australians, the story and fabric of traditional societies were abruptly destabilized by the arrival of Europeans. With colonization, the social structures and tribal autonomy of traditional Mäori societies were undermined, the population falling from estimates of between 150,000 and 200,000 before European arrival to around 45,000 by 1896. By then, Mäori were thought to be close to extinction. Remarkably, in the century that followed there was a dramatic reversal. Although changes to statistical definitions of Mäori complicate population estimates, by the 2001 census 526,281, or 14%, of New Zealanders identified as Mäori, with 85% of these classed as urban dwellers. By 2051 the Mäori population will almost double to close to 1 million, or 22%, of the nation's population, with 33% of all children in the country being Mäori (Statistics New Zealand 2001).

The pattern for Aboriginal peoples in Australia is similar. A precontact population now estimated to be in excess of 1 million suffered a rapid decline. Frontier violence, including random killings and planned massacres, is documented well into the twentieth century (Reynolds 1999). Major losses resulted from introduced diseases, particularly smallpox (Campbell 2002), and were sustained by high mortality rates – especially among infants and children – associated with social adversity and state neglect. As with Mäori, there has been a subsequent dramatic population increase occasioned by improved survival, with recent census data also reflecting increasing self-identification and improved enumeration. According to the Australian Bureau of Statistics, the Aboriginal and Torres Strait Islander population in 2001 was 458,520, or 2.4% of the Australian population. Of this total, 90% claimed Aboriginal origin, 6% Torres Strait Islander origin, and 4% both Aboriginal and Torres Strait Islander origin. The population is also highly dispersed, about one-quarter living in remote or very remote areas and one-third living in major cities, with the majority of Australians of Torres Strait Islander descent now living on the Australian mainland. The Indigenous population is youthful: 40% are below the age of 15, compared to just 21% in the non-Indigenous population, and only 3% are aged 65 or older, compared to 13% of non-Indigenous Australians.

Health Determinants

As indigenous populations stabilized and began to recover through the early part of the last century, understandings of vulnerability began to shift away from theories of "constitutional inferiority" (Anderson 2002) and toward explanations that increasingly emphasize social determinants. This has been reinforced by the ecological transition from patterns of excess morbidity and mortality caused by communicable diseases to the current burden of chronic diseases associated with social transition.[3] Contemporary explanations for current indigenous health status can be grouped into four main causal categories: genetic predisposition, socioeconomic disadvantage, resource alienation, and political oppression (Durie 2003).

Genetic Factors

Possible genetic predispositions have been investigated in alcohol disorders, schizophrenia, and bipolar disorders, although as determinants of mental illness they are regarded as less significant than socioeconomic disadvantage. Even though there is no evidence for genetic contribution to the excess vulnerability of indigenous peoples to specific psychiatric disorders, there is evidence for vulnerability to the development of lifestyle-related chronic disease associated with the "epidemiological transition," such as diabetes and renal disease, which have significant effects on social and emotional well-being (Cass et al. 2002).

Socioeconomic Factors

Poor health status correlates with a range of indices of socioeconomic disadvantage that are demonstrably worse for Mäori and Indigenous Australians than for non-indigenous populations. These include poor educational outcomes and low employment rates, welfare-based income with widespread poverty, inadequate housing and community resources, and high levels of child removal and incarceration (Krieg 2006). These factors not only inform vulnerability but also compromise the availability of family and community resources that would otherwise support resilience – a process of risk amplification.

Mäori children, for example, are more likely to live in a lone-parent family, not to be immunized, to have no parent in paid work, and to live in a household in the lowest income quintile (Ministry of Social Development 2004). However, care should be exercised with explanations that rely solely on social disadvantage – "class" is not a sufficient explanation for the health disparities between indigenous and non-indigenous populations (Reid, Robson, and Jones 2000). Additional ethnicity-specific factors include discriminatory behaviour in the provision of services and access to economic opportunities, culturally inappropriate design of goods and services, and cultural differences in values and aspirations.

Similar findings have been demonstrated for Aboriginal populations. Data from the Australian 2001 National Health Survey (Trewin and Madden 2005) revealed that socioeconomic variables explain between one-third and one-half of the gap in self-assessed health status between Indigenous and other Australians. However, as with Mäori, there are other ethnicity-specific factors. For instance, the Western Australian Aboriginal Child Health Survey (Zubrick et al. 2004, 2005) demonstrated elevated risk for clinically significant emotional and behavioural disorders for Aboriginal children, compared to their non-Indigenous peers. Among associated social factors were the number of life-stress events in the prior 12 months (22% of children were living in families with seven or more life stresses), poor quality parenting, poor family functioning, being raised by a sole parent or by a nonparental caregiver, and a history of parental forcible separation (in Australia this included removal of children to residential institutions, non-Indigenous foster adoption and foster placement, and separation from families within mission and reserve dormitories).

Resource Alienation and Political Oppression Factors

The association of colonization and health has been extensively explored. Stephen Kunitz (1994) argues that loss of sovereignty along with dispossession created a climate of material and spiritual deprivation that increased susceptibility to disease and injury. Contemporary indigenous health status reflects the political legacies of the transition from colonial to postcolonial administrations, which have varied significantly across Anglo-settler colonial societies. It is noteworthy that although approaches to "empowerment" have included treaties (in Canada, New Zealand, and the United States), significant investment in bicultural education (e.g., in Hawaii and New Zealand), designated political representation (New Zealand), regional autonomy (Nunavut in Canada), and removal of indigenous affairs from the vagaries of regional and local politics (in the United States) (Hocking 2005; Waters 2005), none of these have occurred in Australia, which remains intransigently resistant to supporting real Indigenous autonomy.

Moreover, across all these indigenous peoples, the experiences of one generation are consequential for those that follow. In Australia, following the ravages of disease and displacement that occurred during the first century of European occupation, all states introduced legislation around the beginning of the twentieth century that provided for state control over almost all aspects of life and the forcible removal of children from their families (Hunter 1993). From a psychological perspective, this denied not only rights but also cultural identity, relegating Aboriginal people to a position of invisibility in society. Many of the Aboriginal children reared in the missions and institutions that continued to operate into the 1970s were further traumatized by abuse and substandard care. The fragmentation of families and the disruption of kinship systems continued following the repeal of racist legislation through continuing high rates of child removal and incarceration.

In 1967 a national referendum, which was overwhelmingly endorsed by the Australian electorate, provided for inclusion of Indigenous Australians in the national census and enabled the Commonwealth to legislate in Aboriginal affairs. This period, which is often associated with the beginnings of "citizenship" rights, initiated significant changes in policy and services. However, the gains in civil and political rights have not been matched by gains in social rights. Numerous commissions and inquiries have sought to address what has been termed "unfinished business," including the Royal Commission into Aboriginal Deaths in Custody in the late 1980s and the National Inquiry into the Separation of Aboriginal and Torres Strait Islander Children from their Families in the late 1990s, which confirmed that the governmental policies that caused devastation to Aboriginal families were indeed genocidal (Human Rights and Equal Opportunity Commission 1997). In these commissions, as in many other reports and reviews, the dimensions of historical and contemporary social injustice are made clear, the consequences are outlined, recommendations are made in profusion – and there it stops.

Health Experience

The health status of Aboriginal, Torres Strait Islander, and Mäori peoples at the time of colonization is believed to have been good (Webb 1995), better than among Europeans at the time and certainly better than among the despairing and diseased victims of English "justice" who were transported to Australia between 1788 and 1867. As noted at the outset, the situation is now dramatically changed: the Indigenous infant-mortality rate is 2.5 times that of the total population; low birth weight is 2 times as common – recent reliable data demonstrate that Indigenous perinatal mortalities have increased over the past two decades and are worse in remote areas (Fremantle et al. 2006); and the gap between Indigenous and non-Indigenous life expectancy is some 20 years. Although the rates are not identical, there are also disparities in New Zealand. Mäori life expectancy, as measured between 2000 and 2002, was lower by some 8.2 years for males and 8.7 years for females than for non-Mäori, while disability rates were higher (13.4% for Mäori males, compared to 9.9% for non-Mäori males, and 14.5% for Mäori females, compared to 9% for non-Mäori females) (Ministry of Social Development 2004). As with Aboriginal Australians, "lifestyle" conditions (which may be better construed as diseases of marginalization or oppression) are prominent: Mäori rates for diabetes are nearly 3 times higher than European rates and 2 times higher for heart disease, arthritis, hazardous drinking, and obesity.

Across Australia and New Zealand, reliable indigenous-specific mental health data are limited. However, a New Zealand study of primary health care demonstrated that although the rates of general-practice attendance did not differ between Māori and non-Māori, Māori patients, especially Māori women, had higher rates of mental disorder. Māori were at greater risk for all common mental disorders: anxiety, depression, and substance abuse. Māori also tended to exhibit greater severity of symptoms (MaGPIe Research Group 2005). Although socioeconomic status was an important contributor, social and material deprivation was not by itself able to explain the differences. Age is an important factor in terms of vulnerability. Thus, although the suicide rate in New Zealand in 2002 was only slightly higher for Māori than for non-Māori (12.6 vs. 10.1 per 100,000), the rates for Māori youth were significantly higher (31.2 vs. 13.7 per 100,000) (Ministry of Social Development 2005). The situation is similar in Australia: the suicide rate for young adult males in Queensland at the same time was approximately 4 times higher for Indigenous Queenslanders than for their non-Indigenous peers. Mental health problems are common, with later presentation, high rates of comorbidity (that is, co-existing mental health disorders and alcohol- or substance-abuse problems) and thus greater acuity, resulting in overrepresentation of Aboriginal Australians among those detained involuntarily in hospitals and forensic mental health facilities. The co-existence of physical-health and substance-abuse problems is the norm.

Clinical Implications

Although ethnicity has been recognized as a factor with significant implications for clinical diagnosis and treatment, mental health services have often struggled to accommodate indigenous worldviews and traditional healing alongside more conventional psychiatric methods. Notwithstanding difficulties in reconciling two worldviews, treatment outcomes will be improved if the whole treatment process makes sense in cultural terms. Incorporating cultural beliefs and values into treatment and healing has been a goal in many countries, including Australia and New Zealand, since the early 1980s, and at least four approaches have been used. First, there has been an increase in the utilization of traditional healing services, sometimes as an alternative to mainstream services, although more often as a supplementary activity. Second, several mainstream services have incorporated ethnic values and customary practices in treatment programs, creating a bicultural approach. Third, in respect to psychological therapies, a number of ethnicity-centred techniques have been developed either independent of other processes or alongside them. Usually, they aim to strengthen cultural identity. Fourth, development of an indigenous mental health workforce has led to indigenous health services and to a greater utilization of indigenous workers within conventional services.

Ethnic components have been added to clinical settings by increasing the number of bilingual ethnic therapists, by ensuring that clinicians are better informed about cultural values and ethnic communities, and by modifying treatment regimes, especially psychotherapy (Sue and Zane 1987). However, although there is evidence that outcomes are better when there is a match between the ethnicity and language of client and therapist, there is less proof that greater cultural knowledge by the therapist will have any beneficial effect on outcomes. Nonetheless, therapists who are culturally responsive are perceived more favourably by ethnic clients (Atkinson and Lowe 1995). It is likely that non-Native mental health workers will be confronted with clients who prefer to see a traditional healer as well as ethnic clinic staff or who may have quite different attitudes to gender-role definitions and perceptions of trustworthiness and may interpret psychological tests from a different set of understandings (Choney, Berryhill-Paapke, and Robbins 1995). Many tools for psychological assessment are culture-bound or culture-biased and may be insufficiently sensitive to capture cultural nuances. Standardization reflects predominantly white, middle-class samples whose value systems cannot be automatically applied to people of other cultural backgrounds (Suzuki and Kugler 1995).

As an alternative to indigenizing mental health services, another approach has been to establish indigenous health services that are centred on indigenous values and culture while also including conventional mental health methods. The focus is on adding clinical skills to an indigenous facility. In this approach, the emphasis is on reintegrating patients into indigenous communities and families within a context shaped by indigenous protocols. The inclusion of conventional mental health treatments in this environment can sometimes be seen as an intrusion and may be resisted by some staff, but in Australia and New Zealand there appears to have been a general acceptance that indigenous services can be more effective when modern psychiatric methods are introduced alongside psychological therapies that incorporate indigenous values and protocols (Durie 2001). Indigenous mental health services may be part of a wider set of tribal services or focused on urban communities. In either case, the arrangements for governance and management rest with indigenous organizations.

Both for mental health services where indigenous components are added on and for indigenous-centred services, disjunctions can arise between clinical and cultural approaches to healing and treatment. A tendency for the two dimensions to follow parallel rather than synergistic pathways can lead to conceptual and management misunderstanding and can aggravate patient anxiety and uncertainty. In addition, culture and psychopathology can be confused. Being sensitive to cultural influences demands being alert to the dangers of both pathologizing culture (i.e., misattributing illness to what is, in reality, a cultural process) and culturally rationalizing pathology (i.e., misconstruing pathology as some exotic cultural form). This is no easy task, for cultural elements are often secondarily incorporated into, for instance, psychotic-symptom formation. Ultimately, experience and informants are critical. Further, although the social adversity in which many Indigenous Australians and Māori live is clearly consequential for their health and well-being, it is important not to conflate disadvantage and disorder. The term "category fallacy" was coined by Arthur Kleinman (1987) to describe this process whereby the effects of unrelenting adversity are medicalized, as in simply diagnosing "dysthymia" in such circumstances rather than considering social and political analyses. Indeed, the cultural validity of diagnostic frameworks such as those presented in the *Diagnostic and statistical manual*

MASON DURIE, HELEN MILROY, AND ERNEST HUNTER

(DSM) and the *International classification of diseases* (ICD) have been challenged by medical anthropologists and cultural psychiatrists (Kleinman 1988). Ideally, the goal should be to value the meaning and significance of culture alongside social, biological, and psychological factors and to reach a comprehensive formulation that will lead to an intervention that makes sense in clinical as well as cultural terms.

However, the two perspectives – cultural and clinical – need not be incompatible. For example, instruments have been developed to better reflect indigenous perspectives. *Hua oranga* (a healthy result) is a quantifiable outcome measure for Mäori patients that assesses the outcome of a mental health intervention on the basis of gains in each of the four dimensions of health – spiritual, mental, physical, and social – and that incorporates ratings from clinician, patient, and a family member (Kingi 2002). It is consistent with Mäori worldviews and also provides a guide to clinical progress.

The clinical presentation of mental disorders, although often exhibiting common core characteristics that transcend cultures, is nonetheless closely linked to culture. Schizophrenia is a good example. As noted earlier, cultural factors can result in misattribution of psychopathology. However, they may also result in assessment difficulties of individuals who do suffer from a psychotic disorder. Because Mäori value allusive and metaphorical thinking and often depend on context rather than on the precise use of words to establish meaning, clinicians may confuse this style of communication with loosening of association, tangential thinking, or even delusions (Durie 2005b). Depression may also be overlooked if the biological symptoms are not recognized. Although unhappiness and guilt are prominent symptoms in Western cultures, somatic concerns or changes in energy levels may be more typical in other cultures. For example, in the Kimberley region of Western Australia, where Aboriginal mental health workers use a cultural and spiritual model to assess well-being, *ngarlu* is the term used to describe the place of the inner spirit, which is the stomach region (Roe 2000). When a person experiences a spiritual or emotional problem, this may be felt as discomfort in the epigastrium and hence can be easily misinterpreted.

There are many other communication styles that if not well understood can lead to unjustified conclusions. Patients may deliberately avoid eye contact (a sign in many cultures of respect), may minimize distress (to avoid overwhelming the interviewer), or may react with suspicion to overtly friendly approaches in order to reduce the risk of imposition. Sometimes a patient may lapse into total silence in the presence of older relatives, which is not necessarily a sign of withdrawal but an acceptance that others are better able to speak on behalf of family members.

Indigenous Workforce Development

Increasing indigenous participation in the health workforce is critical. Mäori make up around 14% of the total population but only 5% of the New Zealand health workforce. Aboriginal and Torres Strait Islander Australians are only half as likely as non-Indigenous people to have a postschool qualification. They are very significantly underrepresented in the health workforce, with this limited representation falling progressively among those with higher levels of professional education. Two broad strategies have been used to address underrepresentation: affirmative programs to enhance indigenous entry into the mainstream workforce; and the employment alongside mainstream health professionals of cultural or community health workers, who bring first-hand knowledge of community and a capacity to engage diffident patients. In Australia this approach has had obvious benefits but has been complicated by the failure of all jurisdictions, except the Northern Territory, to provide professional registration for Aboriginal Health Workers.

Research

Efforts to recognize indigenous worldviews in research have been boosted greatly by the establishment of indigenous health research teams, largely in university settings. Indigenous health research objectives are twofold: to increase the indigenous research capacity and to encourage the development of methodologies that reflect indigenous worldviews and intellectual traditions. Useful clinical applications have resulted. The publication *Te taura tieke,* for example, describes a three-part framework for describing health-service effectiveness developed by Mäori researchers (Cunningham 1996). It encompasses technical and clinical competence, structural and systemic responsiveness, and consumer satisfaction.

In Australia there has been an evolution from largely descriptive research undertaken by non-Indigenous researchers to consideration of the social correlates of mental health problems in Indigenous communities and, later, to defining historical, developmental, and social determinants (Hunter 2001). Research now is increasingly solution-focused action research, with the key national projects being undertaken through research collaborations between academic centres and Indigenous organizations. The definition of ethical guidelines by the National Health and Medical Research Council for research in Indigenous populations – which have shifted from prescriptive and proscriptive approaches to defining "ethical relationships" in research – has been important not only in approaches to this critical work but also in addressing the historical marginalization of Indigenous researchers and interests (National Health and Medical Research Council 2003). There is also increasing interest in defining and developing Indigenous research methodologies based on cultural practices such as storytelling and deep listening (Atkinson 2002).

Conclusion

Cultural and clinical approaches to mental health should, ideally, complement each other. However, the emergence of a distinctly indigenous mental health framework has exposed tensions resulting in confusion and fragmentation. Ensuring culturally informed and

MASON DURIE, HELEN MILROY, AND ERNEST HUNTER

effective services demands engagement and dialogue – it is not simply a matter of defin-ing protocols or producing one more CD-ROM. It will also require attitudinal change, which must be underpinned in policy. Ultimately, additional demands on mental health services will require aligning perspectives, priorities, and both cultural and clinical inputs to balance generic service delivery against targeted approaches to specific populations.

On this point, there is ongoing debate. Champions of neo-liberalism argue that mental health is colour blind and that individuals should be considered entirely on the basis of need without recourse to consideration of ethnicity or race. However, this view overlooks evidence suggesting a strong link between illness and ethnicity (Durie 2005b). Assessing and responding to need appropriately and effectively requires an understanding of the ways that such need is expressed, particularly an appreciation of cultural nuances and styles of communication, especially in psychiatry, where physical evidence (such as blood tests) is limited. Although being a competent clinician does not demand being a "cultural expert," work with indigenous patients does require reflective practice informed by respectful consideration of the cultural, social, and clinical dimensions of presentation, assessment, and intervention.

Finally, in the face of globalization and the consequent threats and opportunities confronting indigenous peoples, it is also critical to understand health as part of a wider indigenous-rights agenda both nationally and internationally. In this regard the fifth ses-sion of the United Nations Permanent Forum on Indigenous Issues has recently linked the objectives of the second decade of action for indigenous peoples with the global commit-ments of the Millennium Development Goals (Horton 2006). Although this focus may seem far removed from the clinical context, practitioners should be alert to the leverage pro-vided through convention, legislation, and policy (Barker 2002). The main objectives of the 2nd International Decade of the World's Indigenous Peoples, 2005-2015, are:

1   To promote non-discrimination and inclusion of Indigenous peoples at all levels of society, especially regarding laws, resources, policies and programmes.
2   To promote full and effective participation of Indigenous peoples in decisions that affect their lives and lands.
3   To redefine development policies to include a vision of equity for Indigenous peoples, respecting their cultural and linguistic diversity.
4   To adopt targeted policies, programmes, and budgets for Indigenous peoples, with a particular emphasis on women, children and youth.
5   To develop strong monitoring and evaluation mechanisms to meet these objectives. (Horton 2006)

The task, then, is to ensure both cultural empowerment and "fair equality of oppor-tunity" (Rawls 1999) for all Māori and Indigenous Australians (Hunter 2006). Doing so will strengthen not only these ancient cultures but also the modern nations of which they are part. These closing words by Aboriginal poet Jack Davis, of Western Australia (1988, 55), address the transnational issue of social justice for indigenous peoples:

> Big brown eyes, little dark Australian boy
> Playing with a broken toy.
> This environment his alone,
> This is where a seed is sown.
> Can this child at the age of three
> Rise above this poverty?

Notes

1 In this chapter the terms "Aboriginal" and "Indigenous" will be capitalized when referring to Aboriginal/ Indigenous Australians, with the uncapitalized term – "indigenous" – referring to such populations across nations.

2 A comprehensive interactive map of Indigenous Australia can be found on the Australian Institute of Aboriginal and Torres Strait Islander Studies website: http://www.aiatsis.gov.au/Aboriginal_studies_press/ Aboriginal_wall_map/map_page (accessed 16 June 2008).

3 "Ecological transition" is a concept emerging from the confluence of sociology and health sciences, particularly public health. It is used to explain the transition in health patterns and outcomes – at a population level referred to as the "epidemiological transition" – as an interactive process between health, physical, and social contexts (McLaren and Hawe 2005).

References

Anderson, I., S. Crengle, M. Kamaka, T.-H. Chen, N. Palofax, and L. Jackson-Pulver. 2006. Indigenous health in Australia, New Zealand, and the Pacific. *Lancet* 367 (9524): 1775-85.

Anderson, W. 2002. *The cultivation of whiteness: Science, health and racial destiny in Australia*. Melbourne, AU: Melbourne University Press.

Arthur, B., and F. Morphy, eds. 2005. *The Macquarie atlas of Indigenous Australia: Culture and society through space and time*. Sydney, AU: Macquarie.

Atkinson, D.R., and S.M. Lowe. 1995. The role of ethnicity, cultural knowledge, and conventional techniques in couseling and psychotherapy. In J.G. Ponterotto, J.M. Casas, L.A. Suzuki, and C.M. Alexander, eds., *Handbook of multicultural conseling*, 378-414. Thousand Oaks, CA: Sage.

Atkinson, J. 2002. *Trauma trails, recreating song lines: The transgenerational effects of trauma in Indigenous Australia*. Melbourne, AU: Spinifex.

Barker, B. 2002. *Getting government to listen: A guide to the international human rights system for Indigenous Australians*. Sydney: Human Rights International.

Beaglehole, R. 2006. The challenge of health inequalities. *Lancet* 367 (9510): 259-60.

Bristow, F., ed. 2003. *Health and well-being among indigenous peoples*. London: London School of Hygiene and Tropical Medicine and Health Unlimited.

Campbell, J. 2002. *Invisible invaders: Smallpox and other diseases in Aboriginal Australia, 1780-1880*. Melbourne, AU: Melbourne University Press.

Caruana, W. 1989. Introduction. In W. Caruana, ed., *Windows on the dreaming: Aboriginal paintings in the Australian National Gallery*, 9-12. Canberra, AU: Australian National Gallery and Ellsyd Press.

Cass, A., J. Cunningham, P. Snelling, Z. Wang, and W. Hoy. 2002. End-stage renal disease in Indigenous Australians: A disease of disadvantage. *Ethnicity and Disease* 12 (3): 373-78.

Choney, S.K., E. Berryhill-Paapke, and R.R. Robbins. 1995. The acculturation of American Indians: Developing frameworks for research and practice. In J.G. Ponterotto, J.M. Casas, L.A. Suzuki, and C.M. Alexander, eds., *Handbook of multicultural conseling*, 73-92. Thousand Oaks, CA: Sage.

Cunningham, C. 1996. *Te taura tieke: Measuring effective health services for Mäori*. Wellington, NZ: Ministry of Health.

Davis, J. 1988. Slum dwelling. In K. Gilbert, ed., *Inside black Australia: An anthology of Aboriginal poetry*, 55. Ringwood, AU: Penguin.

Dodson, M. 1994. The end in the beginning: Re(de)finding Aboriginality. The Wentworth Lecture. *Australian Aboriginal Studies* 1: 2-13.

Duran, E., and B. Duran. 1995. *Native American postcolonial psychology*. Albany, NY: State University of New York Press.

Durie, M. 1998. *Whaiora: Mäori health development*. Auckland, NZ: Oxford University Press.

−. 2001. *Mauri ora: The dynamics of Mäori health*. Auckland, NZ: Oxford University Press.

−. 2003. Editorial: Indigenous health. *British Medical Journal* 326 (7388): 510-11.

−. 2005a. Indigenous knowledge within a global knowledge system. *Higher Education Policy* 18: 301-12.

−. 2005b. *Nga tai matatu: Tides of Mäori endurance*. Auckland, NZ: Oxford University Press.

Fremantle, J., A. Read, N. de Klerk, D. McAullay, I. Anderson, and F. Stanley. 2006. Patterns, trends, and increasing disparities in mortality for Aboriginal and non-Aboriginal infants born in Western Australia, 1980-2001: Population database study. *Lancet* 367 (9524): 1758-66.

Hocking, B., ed. 2005. *Unfinished constitutional business? Rethinking Indigenous self-determination*. Canberra, AU: Aboriginal Studies Press.

Horton, R. 2006. Indigenous peoples: Time to act now for equity and health. *Lancet* 367 (9524): 1705-7.

Human Rights and Equal Opportunity Commission. 1997. *Bringing them home: Report of the National Inquiry into the Separation of Aboriginal and Torres Strait Islander Children from Their Families*. Canberra, AU: Australian Government Publishing Service.

Hunn, J. 1961. *Report on the Department of Mäori Affairs: Appendix to the Journal of the House of Representatives*. Wellington, NZ: Government of New Zealand.

Hunter, E. 1993. *Aboriginal health and history: Power and prejudice in remote Australia*. Melbourne, AU: Cambridge University Press.

−. 2001. A brief historical background to health research in Indigenous communities. *Aboriginal and Islander Health Worker Journal* 25 (1): 6-8.

−. 2006. *Back to Redfern: Autonomy and the 'middle E' in relation to Aboriginal health*. Discussion Paper 18. Canberra, AU: Australian Institute of Aboriginal and Torres Strait Islander Studies.

−, T. Batrouney, H. McGurk, R. Buchanan, J. Gela, and G. Soriano. 1999. *The Buai Sei Boey Wagel Project*. Canberra, AU: Office of Aboriginal and Torres Strait Islander Health.

Janca, A., and C. Bullen. 2003. The Aboriginal concept of time and its mental health implications. *Australasian Psychiatry* 11 (suppl.): S40-S44.

Kingi, T. 2002. *Hua oranga best outcomes for Mäori*. Palmerston North, NZ: Massey University.

Kleinman, A. 1987. Anthropology and psychiatry: The role of culture on cross-cultural research on illness. *British Journal of Psychiatry* 151: 447-54.

−. 1988. *Rethinking psychiatry*. New York: Free Press.

Krieg, A.S. 2006. Aboriginal incarceration: Health and social impacts. *Medical Journal of Australia* 184 (10): 534-36.

Kunitz, S.J. 1994. *Disease and social diversity: The European impact on the health of non-Europeans*. New York: Oxford University Press.

−, R. Streatfield, G. Santow, and A. De Craen. 1994. Health of populations in northern Queensland Aboriginal communities: Change and continuity. *Human Biology* 66 (5): 917-43.

Lavoie, J. 2004. Governed by contracts: The development of indigenous primary health services in Canada, Australia and New Zealand. *Journal of Aboriginal Health* 1 (1): 6-22.

MaGPIe Research Group. 2005. Mental disorders among Mäori attending their general practitioner. *Australian and New Zealand Journal of Psychiatry* 39 (5): 401-96.

Marmot, M. 2003. Self esteem and health: Autonomy, self esteem, and health are linked together. *British Medical Journal* 327 (13 September): 574-75.

McLaren, L., and P. Howe. 2005. Ecological perspectives in health research. *Journal of Epidemiology and Community Health* 59: 6-14.

Ministry of Social Development. 2004. *The social report: Te pürongo oranga tangata.* Wellington, NZ: Ministry of Social Development.

–. 2005. *The social report: Te purongo oranga tangata.* Wellington, NZ: Ministry of Social Development.

National Aboriginal Health Strategy Working Party. 1989. *A national Aboriginal health strategy.* Canberra, AU: Department of Aboriginal Affairs.

National Health and Medical Research Council. 2003. *Values and ethics: Guidelines for ethical conduct in Aboriginal and Torres Strait Islander health research.* Canberra, AU: National Health and Medical Research Council.

Rawls, J. 1999. *A theory of justice.* Rev. ed. Cambridge, MA: Belknap Press/Harvard University Press.

Reid, P., B. Robson, and C. Jones. 2000. Disparities in health: Common myths and uncommon truths. *Pacific Health Dialogue* 7 (1): 38-43.

Reynolds, H. 1999. *Why weren't we told: A personal search for the truth about our history.* Ringwood, AU: Viking.

Ring, I., and N. Brown. 2003. The health status of indigenous peoples and others. *British Medical Journal* 327 (7412): 404-5.

–, and D. Firman. 1998. Reducing Indigenous mortality in Australia: Lessons from other countries. *Medical Journal of Australia* 169: 528-33.

Roe, J. 2000. Ngarlu: A cultural and spiritual strengthening model. In P. Dudgeon, D. Garvey, and H. Pickett, eds., *Working with Indigenous Australians: A handbook for psychologists,* 395-401. Perth, AU: Curtin University Press.

Royal Australian and New Zealand College of Psychiatrists. 1999. *Ethical guideline # 11: Principles and guidelines for Aboriginal and Torres Strait Islander mental health.* Melbourne, AU: Royal Australian and New Zealand College of Psychiatrists.

Schmidt, A. 1994. Language maintenance. In D. Horton, ed., *The encyclopaedia of Aboriginal Australia,* 600-1. Canberra: Aboriginal Studies Press.

Statistics New Zealand. 2001. *New Zealand census of population and dwellings 2001: Mäori.* Wellington, NZ: Department of Statistics New Zealand – Te Tai Tatau.

Sue, Z., and N.S.W. Zane. 1987. The role of culture and cultural techniques in psychotherapy: A critique and reformulation. *American Psychologist* 42: 37-45.

Suzuki, L.A., and J.F. Kugler. 1995. Intelligence and personality asessment. In J.G. Ponterotto, J.M. Casas, L.A. Suzuki, and C.M. Alexander, eds., *Handbook of multicultural counseling,* 493-99. Thousand Oaks, CA: Sage.

Swan, P., and B. Raphael. 1995. *"Ways forward": National consultancy report on Aboriginal and Torres Strait Islander mental health.* Canberra, AU: Australian Government Publishing Service.

Te Hoe Nuku Roa. 1997. *Reports of the Manawatu-Whanganui and Gisborne Baseline Studies.* Palmerston North, NZ: Department of Mäori Studies, Massey University.

Trewin, D., and R. Madden. 2005. *The health and welfare of Australia's Aboriginal and Torres Strait Islander peoples, 2005.* Canberra, AU: Australian Bureau of Statistics and Australian Institute of Health and Welfare.

Waldram, J. 1997. *The way of the pipe: Aboriginal spirituality and symbolic healing.* Peterborough, ON: Broadview Press.

Waters, A. 2005. Indigeneity, self-determination and sovereignty. In B. Hocking, ed., *Unfinished constitutional business? Rethinking Indigenous self-determination,* 190-209. Canberra, AU: Aboriginal Studies Press.

Webb, S. 1995. *Paleopathology of Aboriginal Australians*. Melbourne, AU: Cambridge University Press.

Zubrick, S.R., D.M. Lawrence, S.R. Silburn, et al. 2004. *The Western Australian Aboriginal Child Health Survey: The health of Aboriginal children and young people*. Perth, AU: Telethon Institute for Child Health Research.

–, S.R. Silburn, D.M. Lawrence, et al. 2005. *The Western Australian Aboriginal Child Health Survey: The social and emotional well-being of Aboriginal children and young people*. Perth, AU: Curtin University of Technology and Telethon Institute for Child Health Research.

3
Culture and Aboriginality in the Study of Mental Health

JAMES B. WALDRAM

The study of Aboriginal mental health has, in many ways, been the study of culture and cultural difference. However, this does not mean that *culture* per se, or more specifically Aboriginal North American cultures,[1] have been adequately conceptualized or researched. A great deal of pioneering work in fields such as psychiatry, psychology, and anthropology has utilized North America's Aboriginal cultural arena to advance theoretical and methodological thinking on culture and mental health. Confronted with the immense cultural diversity and cultural change characteristic of Aboriginal peoples, researchers have logically employed conceptualizations of culture popular at the time of their work, and throughout the twentieth century the fields of psychiatry and psychology frequently looked to anthropology for guidance on how best to think about and research culture. It is evident, however, that while culture theory has continued to evolve, the notion of culture employed in much Aboriginal mental health research has not. The demands of a predominantly quantitative approach to mental health research have invariably resulted in the reduction of culture to the status of variable, a methodological development largely rejected by anthropology and one that, ironically, has served to lead us not closer to but further away from an understanding of the role of culture in Aboriginal mental health.

The purpose of this chapter, then, is to explore the relationship between conceptualizations of "culture" and methodological approaches in Aboriginal mental health research, particularly that undertaken from a clinical or epidemiological perspective.[2] My main concerns are with how "Aboriginality" has been understood in this research, how "Aboriginal" research subjects have been identified, and how culture has been employed as an explanation for their mental abilities and psychopathology. My central argument is that, although overt theorizing of culture has been largely absent from much Aboriginal mental health research, embedded within the research itself can be found elementary ideas about culture that are characteristic of several older, now anachronistic, anthropological schools. Methodological strategies, in turn, have been built upon these rigid, modernist notions of culture. The impact of this has been the creation and perpetuation of a fractured, reductionist, and essentialized understanding of Aboriginal culture and Aboriginality that is out of touch both with contemporary culture theory and, more important, with the contemporary cultural reality of North American Aboriginal peoples.

I will approach this investigation in several ways and provide selected examples from across the breadth of the research base that in the past and still today informs policy on Aboriginal health.[3] I will begin with a look at how Aboriginality has been constructed as a variable category for purposes of comparative research, focusing on the most common methods that researchers have employed to identify and categorize Aboriginal individuals and communities. I will then turn to a discussion of a singularly problematic category of Aboriginal individual, the "culturally marginalized," and the lessons this category provides for understanding broader views of culture within mental health research. I will conclude with some critical observations on the views of culture in general, and of Aboriginal "culture" specifically, that have guided much of the mental health research on Aboriginal peoples to date.

Conceptualizing Culture and Aboriginality

Anthropologist-psychoanalyst George Devereux once wrote that "anyone who understands [culture] may be said to possess the open-sesame" of the social sciences (1971, 23). Indeed, anthropologists have been struggling for well over a century to understand what culture is and how it should be researched, without achieving a consensus. Not surprisingly given a general skepticism toward the utility of a culture concept, the approach of most mental health researchers has been to keep the notion of culture as simple as possible. Early theoretical schools in anthropology – the cultural evolutionists, the historical particularists, and the diffusionists – implied through their work that North American Aboriginal cultures could be seen as bounded, isolated constellations of well-defined traits, that a culture could reasonably be seen, and studied, as though the whole were the sum of its parts, and that cultures were at once biological and sociological phenomena (for an overview of this history, see Darnell 2001). This was a simplistic view of culture but one that resonated with mental health researchers precisely because of the ease with which it could be operationalized. The issues of who, in fact, was "Aboriginal" for purposes of research and, indeed, of what being "Aboriginal" actually meant were not belaboured to any extent. Several methods have been employed in mental health research to identify Aboriginal research subjects, each one elegantly simple yet demonstrably flawed: (1) blood quantum; (2) legislative or self-identification criteria; (3) culture areas; and (4) cultural orientations or acculturation. In this section, I address each of these approaches to defining Aboriginality in turn.

Blood Quantum as a Measure of Aboriginality

"Blood quantum" is a sometimes confusing notion that suggests that Aboriginality is related to biological heritage – that is, the "amount" of "Indian blood" one is perceived to have relative to other kinds of blood. This in turn is related to ideas of cultural authenticity and is central to much political-rights discourse. The concept of "bloodedness" is one tenaciously persistent remnant of the evolutionary theory and social Darwinism of the late nineteenth and early twentieth centuries, and it reflects the confusion between biology and culture that pervades much Aboriginal research. Within this evolutionary framework, the so-called advanced races (such as Europeans) were seen to be at the forefront of cultural development, while the behaviour of "primitive" peoples, such as Aboriginal North Americans, was viewed as still anchored by essential biological properties: these peoples had yet to fully escape the bonds of their biology to become truly cultural individuals.

"Race" research was highly popular in the late nineteenth and early twentieth centuries, with race largely conceived of in phenotypical terms (e.g., skin colour, hair type) purporting to represent true genotypical differences among human populations (Barrett 1996; Garbarino 1983). Some of the early studies of Aboriginal cognitive functioning, for instance, were focused on the question of the relationship between intelligence and race (a common theme that still dogs us today) and especially conceptualized in terms of "blood quantum" (e.g., Fitzgerald and Ludeman 1926; Garth 1921, 1922, 1923, 1925, 1927; Garth, Smith, and Abell 1928; Terman 1916).[4] Many scholars, for instance, reflecting popular attitudes, hypothesized that the intelligence of Indians would improve proportionate to the amount of "white" blood they had. The supposed relationship between blood quantum and psychopathology was also established early, as demonstrated in the work of Dr. H.R. Hummer (1913), director of the first asylum for Indians in the United States. Hummer felt the need to describe some 66% of his patients as "full-bloods," implicitly suggesting that Indian biological heritage was somehow an important predisposing factor for mental illness.

Blood quantum measurements have also been central to much of the research on Aboriginal alcoholism. As the stereotype of the "drunken Indian" was firmly entrenched by the twentieth century (e.g., Leland 1976; Westermeyer 1974), considerable effort was expended to understand the biological basis for this alleged reaction to alcohol. Typically, however, self-declaration was the usual measure of bloodedness, not any biological measurement (e.g., Bennion and Li 1976; Weisner, Weibel-Orlando, and Long 1984), and the existence of even a little Indian blood frequently resulted in the individual being categorized as an "Indian." For example, Uecker, Boutilier, and Richardson (1980), in a study of Sioux alcoholics, defined as "Sioux" those individuals claiming to have as little as one-quarter Indian blood, in effect allowing for any problematic behaviours to be interpreted as the product of a kind of biological contamination.

In a more recent study, Garcia-Andrade, Wall, and Ehlers (1997) divided a small sample of Mission Indians into two groups according to their self-reports: those with more than 25% but less than 50% Indian blood and those with 50% or more Indian blood. An alcoholic drink was provided to some and a placebo to others, and subjective responses to the effects of alcohol as well as objective measures of blood pressure, pulse rate, plasma cortisol levels, and blood alcohol levels were taken after varying periods of time. Their research showed that those with 50% or more Indian blood reported feeling fewer effects of intoxication than those with lesser Indian blood. They thus concluded that, compatible with other studies, "groups at higher risk for alcoholism have a less intense subjective response to alcohol and that groups at lower genetic risk for alcoholism have a more intense subjective response to alcohol" (986). In other words, not only were individuals with greater Indian blood seen to be at higher risk for alcoholism because of the genetic nature of this disease, this was also conceptualized as a characteristic of the whole population, not of a specific family, as is the case with genetic explanations of alcoholism among non-Aboriginal people. Even still, there was no attempt to assess the impact of the other components of their subjects' biological heritage: the Indian blood, even if only 50%, was assumed to dominate any other biological heritage, and having even 25% Indian blood still meant one was biologically "Indian." Issues of culture – or more appropriately, individual lifestyle – were not considered.

A confusion of race and culture characterizes a great deal of Aboriginal mental health research. According to Brumann, in some instances the language of culture has supplanted that of race, even though the underlying premise of a "pseudo-genetic transmission" of traits remains throughout (1999, S1). Aboriginal blood quantum has also been viewed as a measure of Aboriginal cultural orientation. Weisner and colleagues (1984), for instance, compared the percentage of "Indian ancestry" with drinking levels and concluded that individuals with "50%" Indian ancestry drank more than individuals with both more and less Indian ancestry. They suggested that the problem was not biological but cultural, or more specifically, acculturative stress. The underlying premise, however, was that only half-Indians were engaged in problematic processes of cultural change, as though the biological "halfness" was the problem, which is still a biological argument. Hoffman, Dana, and Bolton (1985) also employed blood quantum as a measure of acculturation among the Rosebud Sioux in their efforts to determine the cultural validity of the Minnesota Multiphasic Personality Inventory (MMPI), and such use of this biological measure of cultural orientation is far from rare (see also Dana, Hornby, and Hoffman 1984).

Although the scientific language of race is heard less today, the idea of bloodedness remains and is still operative in the contemporary proxy of Tribal (United States) or First Nations (Canada) membership (Snipp 1997). Most Tribes and First Nations control their own membership and often use genealogies as a central criteria for establishing eligibility. In fact, the older notion of blood quantum was really genealogy dressed up in biological garb: blood quantum was usually determined by self-reported family history, if not by simple self-declaration. The contemporary manipulations of genealogy to establish how Aboriginal one is only thinly veils a persistent belief that being Aboriginal is as much biological as it is cultural, hence the prominence in much of the discourse of terms like "full blood," "pure blood," "mixed blood," and "half-breed." Some Aboriginal peoples have internalized these biological understandings of Aboriginality and use them frequently to challenge the claims to Aboriginality or authenticity of specific groups and individuals

(Weaver 2001). But specific American Indian Tribes and Canadian First Nations demonstrate considerable ambiguity in their definition of what constitutes a sufficient amount of Indian blood for enrolment and hence authentication as truly "Indian" (Norton and Manson 1996). Some American Indian membership codes allow for an Indian blood quantum of as little as one-sixteenth – in other words, an applicant can be an Indian if his father's father's father was an Indian. In Canada, for many decades, it was possible for females with no Aboriginal heritage whatsoever to gain Indian status through marriage. Hence researchers who uncritically accept Tribal or First Nations membership lists as de facto evidence of either biological or cultural purity do so at considerable peril. Their samples will likely contain diverse individuals, including those with little or no Aboriginal cultural orientation whatsoever (as in the case of a member adopted at birth by a non-Aboriginal family), individuals with no on-reserve experience (an increasingly common phenomenon in both Canada and the United States), and individuals whose biological heritage demonstrates little or no linkage with any Aboriginal population.

The Use of Legislative and Self-Identification Criteria

This brings me to the issue of the use of existing legislative as well as self-identification criteria for establishing Aboriginality.[5] Several Canadian studies published in the early and mid-1970s, which collectively proved extremely influential, serve as excellent examples of these approaches. The first of these, by Roy, Choudhuri, and Irvine (1970), involved the analysis of first-admission statistics (based on clinical case notes) at a Saskatchewan psychiatric hospital between 1961 and 1966 for 51 treaty Indians and 2,607 others. In Saskatchewan, as in Canada generally, federally recognized Indians, including those with treaty status, are readily identifiable because of a unique form of health card (which allows provinces to bill back to the federal government for services provided to Indians); this system is considered to be reliable for identifying these members of the Indian population (i.e., those with federal recognition). The other individuals in this study were said to represent "a wide variety of ethnic groups" (384), which could well have included Métis and nonrecognized (i.e., nonstatus) Indians as well as non-Aboriginal peoples from varying backgrounds, all clustered into one variable category. The statistical analysis revealed that the Indian admissions were much younger than others and that a significantly higher proportion of Indians than non-Indians were diagnosed with schizophrenia. In contrast, a significantly higher proportion of the non-Indians were diagnosed with organic psychosis. In an attempt to understand the situation further, the researchers undertook a comparative study of active psychiatric cases "in a large Indian community" (actually 10 Cree and Saulteaux reserves), which they compared to a neighbouring non-Indian community (some 18 primarily European rural municipalities). After six months of data collection, the researchers estimated that the non-Indian prevalence rate for active psychiatric disorders was almost half that of the Indians. Several important and revealing biases are evident in the study. For instance, although there was little difference between the two populations on the prevalence of alcoholism, they rejected this finding because it was "common knowledge" that excessive alcohol consumption was greater among the Indians (389); none of the other findings were balanced against this "common knowledge." And the higher prevalence of severe mental deficiency among the Indians was explained as "not altogether surprising"; making an odd comparison, they noted that as with Hutterites, "inbreeding" could be responsible (389). Finally, after combining the Cree and Saulteaux into one category and all the non-Indians into another, they described the two groups as "culturally different" and their research as "cross-cultural" despite never actually addressing the issue of culture.

Hendrie and Hanson (1972) undertook a comparison of psychiatric care for Indian, Métis, and other non-Aboriginal patients in a Winnipeg psychiatric hospital. They utilized what they termed a "social" definition of Aboriginal status and explicitly acknowledged the Métis as a distinct Aboriginal population. An Indian was defined as a person who self-identified as one, who was so identified by relatives, or who was registered as an Indian by the federal government; a Métis was someone who so identified or who was identified as such by relatives. Tellingly, whereas at least some examples were given of the backgrounds of those included in the non-Native category (e.g., English, Scottish, German), the Tribal or cultural affiliation of the other two groups, particularly the Indians, was not mentioned. Fritz (1976) published another Saskatchewan study involving a much larger database of patients in psychiatric treatment centres. In this study, an important attempt was also made to distinguish among the Aboriginal population in order to separately identify the Indians (i.e., those who self-identified and were registered) and the Métis (also self-identified); the latter category was problematic, however, in that it also included nonregistered Indians. And similar to the Hendrie and Hanson (1972) study, no mention was made of the specific cultural, community, or Tribal affiliation of the Indian participants. Since self-identification was partly employed in these studies to identify and distinguish Aboriginal subjects, the lack of data on specific cultural identity was likely a product of the type of questions asked of participants.

First Nations and Tribal membership lists, rosters of federally recognized Indians, and self-identification are perhaps the most common methods for determining "Aboriginality." As these studies demonstrated, however, what this means is rarely addressed, and there is a fairly explicit assumption that the difficult work of determining Aboriginality has in fact already been achieved by some legislative mechanism. Equally problematic is the assumption that individuals will accurately describe their cultural orientation in a manner relevant for research and distinct from the issue of self-identity; indeed, much research erroneously suggests quite clearly that cultural orientation and self-identity are synonymous. And, when convenient and without justification or explanation, it is even possible to ignore both legislative and self-identification criteria in order to group together, inexplicably, individuals from different Aboriginal communities or with different Tribal heritages. This lumping effect pertains also to the non-Aboriginal category so frequently used for comparative analyses; non-Aboriginal people are likewise assumed to exhibit an identical cultural orientation. Therefore, any result that compares an Aboriginal with a non-Aboriginal group should not be immediately read as demonstrative of cultural differences.

Culture Areas as Sampling Frames

Culture areas date back to the work of anthropologists such as A.L. Kroeber (1939) and Harold Driver (1969), who devised a schema dividing Aboriginal North America into discrete zones, or areas, predicated on the assumption that individuals and groups within each area would demonstrate significant cultural similarities with other individuals and groups in the same area and significant dissimilarities with those in other areas.[6] Driver (1969, 17) actually cautioned that his 17 North American culture areas were only a "convenient framework" for organizing thought on the immense cultural diversity of Aboriginal peoples and that the boundaries between areas were not rigid demarcations of cultural difference but regions in which cultures were blending. But this was not how many subsequent researchers viewed them. Being an extension of the historical-particularist school, which emphasized the reconstruction of the history of specific cultures as necessary to comprehending them (Barrett 1984), the culture-area scheme was in its heyday primarily trait-based, focusing on such topics as material culture and economic and social practices but not on intellectual or cognitive abilities or psychological functioning. At best, culture areas were an attempt to understand the precontact ecological adaptations of Aboriginal peoples through systematic categorization. Although the historical particularists were also interested in the diffusion of traits among different peoples and in how these were then adapted to fit the new context, this was done to understand historical cultural configurations, not contemporary ones. The culture-area concept inadvertently served to cement dynamic cultural groups into more or less permanent and static analytical categories. Despite agreeing that Aboriginal cultural development prior to colonization was shaped by the local ecology, subsequent advocates of the culture-area concept largely ignored how these cultures were constantly changing as a result of ecological alterations that followed the arrival of Europeans and their technology.

Notwithstanding these problems, culture areas have been used as a convenient means to organize cultural similarity and difference. Research that employs the culture-area framework explicitly assumes that all Aboriginal societies within an area are so similar as to be identical for research purposes, and it hypothesizes that those in another culture area are therefore significantly culturally different. The concept was never intended to comprehend individual cultural orientation, but in psychological and psychiatric research that is precisely what has happened. A contemporary *individual* from one culture area is assumed or hypothesized to be different from an *individual* from another culture area not so much because of personal experiences of enculturation or acculturation but because of the culture areas to which his or her ancestors were once slotted by anthropologists. Shore and colleagues (1987), for instance, utilized culture areas in a study of the usefulness of the Schedule for Affective Disorders and Schizophrenia-Lifetime Version (SADS-L) in identifying index cases of depression. They were primarily concerned with allowing for "intertribal comparisons," and to this end three American Indian reservation communities from different culture areas were selected. Specific details of the three communities were withheld to ensure anonymity and were thus designated simply as the Plains, Plateau, and Pueblo Tribes, representing three distinct culture areas. Contrary to their hypothesis, they found that there were few differences among individuals from the three culture areas, so they proposed the existence of "a core depressive syndrome" (11) unique to all Indians (itself a problematic notion). However, they also noted that the Plains group appeared to have a higher rate of "complicated depression ... a major depressive disorder superimposed upon an underlying chronic depression," possibly explainable by "unique cultural and genetic factors" (13). However, these cultural or genetic factors were not detailed, nor were the cultural orientations of the specific research participants addressed. Membership in a Tribe located within a culture area that had been delineated more than a half-century earlier was taken on face value as a valid measure of contemporary individual cultural orientation.

Another study of culture and depression looked at American Indian elderly by utilizing the Center for Epidemiological Studies Depression Scale (CES-D) (Chapleski et al. 1997; Curyto et al. 1998). The researchers explicitly acknowledged the difficulties in generalizing a unidimensional view of the disorder across Indian cultural boundaries and especially within the context of acculturation. They utilized a multigroup comparative strategy that identified three categories of individuals: urban residents, rural off-reservation residents, and those living on-reservation, each of which was viewed as a separate "cultural context." In so doing, they explicitly rejected as too simple the rural/urban or on-reservation/off-reservation dichotomies that guide much comparative work. Specific Tribal backgrounds were not provided, but they suggested that the target population lived in areas "which are representative of the major Tribal groups in the state, Potawatomi, Ojibwa, and Odawa" (Curyto et al. 1998, 27). Therefore, no analysis by Tribe was presented, and instead the researchers argued that since the vast majority of individuals came from Tribes to be found in the Woodlands culture area, "the sample offers a group of American Indians with similar biological and cultural roots" (Chapleski et al. 1997, 471). Yet they also acknowledged that there was great cultural variability and that intermarriage with non-Indians had resulted in a "polycultural" rather than monocultural or even bicultural reality.

Mental health researchers have continued to be attracted to the relative simplicity and ease of culture areas as sampling frames. Although the concept is rarely seen in anthropology these days, it has not been expunged entirely. Introductory textbooks on Aboriginal North American peoples commonly still frame their presentations through culture areas (e.g., McMillan 1995; Morrison and Wilson 1995), and anthropologist James Green (1999, 232) even suggested, problematically in my estimation, that culture areas represent conceptual distinctions that are "remembered" by contemporary American Indians who "recognize and respect" them.[7] The legacy of the culture-area concept is still evident in recent work in psychiatry and psychology. In what is perhaps the largest, long-term contemporary study of Aboriginal mental health and related psychological and sociological matters, spanning both Canada and the United States, Beiser and Gotowiec (2000) acknowledged their debt to anthropology in drawing participants from four culture areas for comparative purposes (see also Sack et al. 1994; Sack et al. 1987). Keeping with trends to simplify culture, researchers in psychiatry and psychology have often made dramatic alterations to the culture-area concept. McShane and Berry, for instance, reduced the total number of culture areas in North America to seven, "reflecting the lesser interest of psychology in particular cultural variations" (1988, 389). Such a desire to formulate culture at ever-increasing levels of generality serves only to reduce, and ultimately to eliminate, its existence. Individual cultural orientation disappears, and culture is conceptualized to exist not as contemporary lived experience but only at the level of geographically defined space, residence, group membership, or biology.

The Measurement of Cultural Orientation and Acculturation

Not all mental health research has deferred to pre-existing categorizations such as blood quantum or culture areas. In recent years, some scholars have written of the need to determine the contemporary cultural orientation of Aboriginal peoples as an essential part of the assessment and treatment process, a nod to the fact of cultural change that has dramatically reshaped Aboriginal cultures (e.g., Dillard 1983; Dinges et al. 1981; Garrett and Garrett 1994; Heinrich, Corbine, and Thomas 1990; Herring 1990; LaFromboise, Trimble, and Mohatt 1990; Renfrey 1992; Trimble and Fleming 1989; Trimble et al. 1996). With a focus on quantitative applications, most efforts have revolved around the construction of instruments and especially scales to measure individual cultural orientation despite anthropological conceptualizations of culture as shared, group phenomena.[8] Occasionally, however, there have been attempts to assess entire communities. Although the emphasis has frequently been on assessing acculturation and assimilation – in other words, degrees of non-Aboriginality – there have also been efforts to assess "Indianness," or "Aboriginality."

Attempts to measure the degree of orientation to Aboriginal or Euro-North American cultures have generally focused on the acquisition or retention of material goods and practices, the degree of experience in non-Aboriginal and Aboriginal culture, and the adoption of Euro-North American values versus the retention of Aboriginal values. Psychologists John Berry and Robert Annis (1974a, 1974b), who were pioneers in the study of acculturation, appeared to employ a diffusionist model of cultural change when they developed a simple "ownership scale" for use with James Bay Cree. With this scale they attempted to measure, quite literally, the extent to which a Cree person had "bought into" Canadian society by acquiring various items or services, including a radio, outboard motor, snowmobile, washer, freezer, bank account, and life insurance (Berry, Trimble, and Olmedo 1986).[9] What the acquisition of new technological items means is complex, however, and frequently researchers have simply assumed that such acquisition signals important cognitive cultural changes. Some of these goods (e.g., the outboard motor and snowmobile) represent items linked to economic activity, and since the Cree were (and still are in many ways) a hunting and fishing people, their purchase and integration into Cree life might have meant nothing more than the acquisition of better technology, as with the Crees' adoption of traps and rifles generations earlier. Furthermore, as their baseline, Berry and Annis used Cree society just prior to the introduction of some of these items to the North, ignoring that these people had been using other items of European technology for centuries.

In contrast to Berry and Annis, Graves (1967a; see also Graves 1967b) developed a 10-item "acculturation index" for American Indian populations in the Southwest that measured experiences, suggesting that "exposure, identification, and access are all required for change to occur" (345). Thus this scale included items such as "Respondent lived in town rather than in the countryside," "Respondent owned a TV set," and "Respondent reported a close Anglo friendship." Language was also important, however, and two items pertained to the use of English in particular. Chance and Foster (1962) and Chance (1965) utilized a similar approach and developed an "Inter-cultural contact scale" and a "Western Identification Scale" in their study of North Alaskan Eskimos. The contact scale included items such as knowledge of English, whether the person had ever been hospitalized or been employed, and his or her access to mass media. The identification scale included the preference for Western versus Eskimo foods, the preference for Western clothing, and participation in traditional activities, such as hunting for men and skin sewing for women.

Studies by Berry and Annis (1974a, 1974b), Graves (1967a, 1967b), Chance and Foster (1962), and Chance (1965) all had in common a materialist view of culture, one predicated on the idea that the acquisition of foreign material items was suggestive of a change in individuals' cultural orientation, their cognitive map of the world, and their place within it. These studies were guided by the acculturation theory predominant at the time, an offshoot of historical particularism, which emphasized a process of sharing of cultural traits (including material items) through intercultural contact and diffusion among cultures in sustained contact (Garbarino 1983; Redfield, Linton, and Herskovits 1936). The emphasis on the acquisition of material goods as central to the process of cultural change, as well as the assumption that Aboriginality existed only within the precontact context, can be challenged. Moreover, these studies failed to significantly consider other, more salient aspects of culture. Whereas the diffusionists were interested in how a particular material item was adapted to a new culture, these acculturation theorists seemed to believe that the acquisition of a new item automatically resulted in, or signified, important cultural change for the individual.

Aboriginality as an individualized cultural orientation has also been measured in a variety of ways, with an emphasis on the expression of values and commitment to certain cultural practices. Characteristically, Aboriginality has been conceptualized only as the continued existence of precontact cultural traits and has thus been understood to preclude any notion of a contemporary Aboriginality that exists as a product of cultural changes. Edwin Richardson (1981), for instance, designed an "Indian Culturalization Test" for Sioux people and even included Lakota expressions (although it was suggested that the scale probably had "reasonable content validity" for other Northern Plains Indians as well as the Sioux) (Uecker, Boutilier, and Richardson 1980, 359). This scale asked questions about dancing, craft making, religious practice (such as the Sun Dance), and even the consumption of dog meat (a traditional practice). Uecker and colleagues employed this Indian Culturalization Test in a study of the Minnesota Multiphasic Personality Inventory (MMPI). Compatible with Richardson's view that there were many universal American Indian values, the intent was to develop an Indian Culture Quotient (ICQ), which would then be employed in "determining how much *the* Indian Value System will affect scores" on various other psychological tests (359, emphasis added). The ICQ attempted to assess language utilization, values and behaviours, and attitudes, but it was conceptually flawed and suffered from a lack of methodological rigour.[10]

Westermeyer and Neider (1985) developed a 10-item "Indian Culture Scale" for use in their research among American Indian alcoholic clients in Minnesota. They used a three-point scale, and the items included language comprehension, contact with Indian family and friends, and engagement in activities deemed to be "Indian." These latter included attendance at Pow-Wows, ricing, beading, and practising "Indian" religion. Another even simpler approach was employed by Johnson and Lashley, who were interested in the idea of "cultural commitment" as it related to individual Native American college students' preferences for counsellors. Respondents were asked to select from among four statements the one that best described their level of cultural commitment, the options ranging from "Strong commitment to both Native-American and Anglo-American cultures" to "Weak commitment to both Native-American and Anglo-American cultures" (1989, 117). Using a three-point scale, individuals were also asked to rate their degree of participation in Tribal activities and degree of proficiency in the Tribal language (i.e., not at all, somewhat, or very).

Multimethod approaches to measuring Aboriginality have also been employed that often have combined materialist, acculturative, and cognitive understandings of culture. Hoffman and colleagues (1985) developed an instrument for use with Lakota people in order to test the validity of the MMPI-168. Working with 37 males and 32 females from the Rosebud Lakota Sioux reservation in South Dakota, they developed an acculturation scale after extensive examination of existing literature on the topic, the testing of a preliminary version in the community, and the use of a battery of tests to determine local norms (see Dana, Hornby, and Hoffman 1984). These were then reduced through statistical analysis to subscales tapping "five dimensions of Native American acculturation": "social behaviour, social membership, and social activities; value orientation and cultural attitudes; blood quantum; language preference and usage; and educational and occupational status" (Hoffman, Dana, and Bolton 1985, 245). Sack and colleagues (1987) also adopted a more complex approach by employing three measures also for use with Sioux people. The first simply attempted to determine the language spoken in the home. The second was a "traditionality" scale developed in consultation with a local community panel and included, for instance, the use of or preference for certain traditional Sioux items (e.g., "I pick wild berries" and "I use tobacco to give thanks"). A third scale sought the respondents' opinions on a variety of issues, such as whether an individual should remain on the reservation or move to the city. There are problems with the assumptions of traditionality upon which these techniques were built. For instance, the authors failed to explain how personal opinions relate to the issue of traditionality, and thus we fail to comprehend why, among other things, the researchers assumed that the most traditional Indian was the one who believed people should remain on the reservation.

Attempts have also been made to categorize entire communities on traditionality scales. Mohatt and Blue (1982) developed such a scale for use with Lakota people. Employing the Lakota concept of *tiospaye,* which describes a community's way of life, particularly its traditionality, the researchers worked closely with Lakota "cultural experts" to identify appropriate scale items and to score 21 Lakota communities. These experts were asked to offer their assessment of the degree to which a statement characterized a community. For instance, one scale item, "Balance," included statements about family and community relations, such as: "If conflict occurs, the persons and families involved are brought together and advised by an Elder." Another scale item, "Spiritual," which was related to spiritual and linguistic practices, asked whether "the people speak Lakota."

This was a radical approach given the individualistic nature of other research on this topic. It was seen by the authors as more compatible with how the Lakota viewed culture, and it can be seen as an improvement on instruments constructed solely by noncommunity members. However, several problems are still evident. One can certainly question the existence of cultural "experts," as opposed to individuals with domain-specific knowledge within a community. It is unclear what "cultural expert" means, who qualifies as such an expert, and who so designates such a person. The idea appears to privilege the views of a kind of aged cultural elite; although many communities cherish Elders, who often are the repositories of longstanding cultural knowledge, the existence of such knowledge per se does not necessarily reflect the actual, lived cultural experiences of community members, especially in a period of rapid cultural change. The idea also reinforces a conception of culture as tradition – something from the past – unchanging, and official doctrine. Not all individuals would either agree with the scale or, more important, fit with the overall evaluation of the traditionality of their community. In other words, this approach, like so many others, resulted in overgeneralization and gave short shrift to the notion of intracultural variability and the fact that many individuals may hold not only traditional but also global knowledge and values as well as engage in both traditional activities and those more readily identified as coming from outside the group.

More recently, in a pioneering and important study, psychologists Michael Chandler and Christopher Lalonde (see Chapter 10) attempted to demonstrate how certain activities deemed to be "evidence of efforts on the part of communities to preserve, rebuild or reconstruct their culture by wrenching its remnants out of the control of federal and provincial government agencies" might explain the lower rates of suicide in some British Columbia Indian reserve communities relative to others (1998, 208-9). Conceptualized as "cultural continuity," such factors as involvement in land claims, self-government, and control over education, police, fire, and health services were measured, and the analysis included an aggregate measure that allowed the authors to rate each community according to the number of these factors deemed present. From this, they observed that there was an inverse relationship between the number of "cultural" factors present and the suicide rate in the community. I would suggest, however, that none of these factors necessarily demonstrates continuity with a cultural past since each involved the development of very modern institutions. In my reading of their work, it is not cultural continuity per se that explains healthy communities but the *efforts,* however locally conceptualized, to wrest control over their lives from external institutions.

Although many measures of acculturation into non-Aboriginal society have focused on the acquisition of material items and intercultural experiences, many of the measures of Aboriginality have had, at their core, an assessment of knowledge, beliefs, and values – in other words, a cognitive view of culture. In particular, the focus on beliefs and values as essential ingredients of culture likely stems primarily from anthropological research in the decades of the 1960s, 1970s, and 1980s, when the generation of values lists was common (Kleinman 1996; Kluckhohn and Strodtbeck 1961). Some anthropologists today are more inclined to view values problematically, as constructed phenomena that, within singular cultures and as embodied within individuals, are inherently contradictory and context-specific (e.g., Nuckolls 1998; Shore 1996). Whereas anthropology has moved away from a concentration on values as integral to culture, psychology has not. Considerable recent work in cross-cultural psychology and psychiatry remains committed to the view that Aboriginal cultures consist of core, "traditional" values that continue to play important roles in cognitive and emotional functioning despite centuries of cultural contact and change (e.g., Brucker and Perry 1998; Dana 1993; Dillard 1983; Dillard and Manson 2000; Fisher and Harrison 1997; Herring 1989, 1992; Ho 1987, 1992; LaFromboise 1993; Trimble 1981; Trimble and Fleming 1989; Trimble and Hayes 1984). These core values are perceived as cultural remnants only, and in many analyses they are routinely contrasted with those alleged to characterize the colonizers. This betrays the problematic view that the Aboriginal and non-Aboriginal populations are homogeneous isolates with no shared cultural heritage.

Attempts to measure culture and acculturation are laudable and represent a golden opportunity to comprehend, from a research perspective, the significance of the contemporary cultural reality of Aboriginal peoples separate from sometimes overly romantic notions of traditionality that serve only to cement these peoples in a bygone era. However,

JAMES B. WALDRAM

both culture and acculturation represent multidimensional constructs that, to date, have beguiled researchers bent on constructing quantitative measures (Sue 2003; Trimble 2003). In addition to problems with operationalizing the concept of culture germane to all research approaches, the emphasis on quantification and instrumentation has, in practice, served to remove the individual from his or her cultural context. Efforts to construct "cultural formulations" that utilize the framework found within the *Diagnostic and statistical manual* (DSM-IV-TR) of the American Psychiatric Association (2000) (e.g., Fleming 1996; Manson 1996; O'Nell 1998) and efforts to employ clinical measures of culture based on "emic" understandings (e.g., Weiss 1997; Weiss et al. 2001) have ironically largely erased culture from the analysis (Waldram 2006). Berry (2003), perhaps the leading figure in the assessment of psychological acculturation, has recently reminded us that extensive ethnographic research is essential *prior* to the development or employment of a scale to measure culture, advice that has not always been heeded.

Cultural Marginality

The notion that there are two separate and distinct "cultures," the Aboriginal and the non-Aboriginal, has certainly dominated Aboriginal mental health research. There exists, however, a third kind of cultural category. Some researchers attempting to understand the contemporary cultural reality of Aboriginal peoples have, for the most part, adopted a negative, deficit approach. Eschewing studies of well-balanced Aboriginal individuals functionally integrated within either their own or the larger society, these scholars have focused on the existence of apparently cultureless individuals, those who have failed to make a successful transition from one culture to the next and who have become trapped in a culturally marginal position that leaves them "caught between two worlds" without a functioning cultural referent (French 1979, 1980, 1989, 1997; Trimble et al. 1996). These marginal individuals, it is thought, are "unable either to live the cultural heritage of their tribal group or to identify with the dominant society" and therefore "have the most difficulty in coping with social problems due to their ethnicity" (LaFromboise et al. 1990, 638), including alcohol problems, psychiatric disorders such as depression, and criminal behaviour (Choney, Berryhill-Paapke, and Robbins 1995; Kerckhoff and McCormick 1955; Locke 1992; Phillips and Inui 1986; Topper and Curtis 1987). They experience "acculturative stress," which is related to that form of cultural change that ensues when cultures meet for prolonged periods of time (e.g., Berry 1970, 1975, 1985, 1991; Berry and Annis 1974a, 1974b; Berry and Kim 1988; Berry et al. 1987; Berry et al. 1982), as well as "deculturative stress," which is "the stress of losing traditional beliefs and values" (Phillips and Inui 1986, 124).

The argument that such individuals are caught between two worlds is a fascinating example of the intrusion of an antiquated anthropological view of culture into the mental health arena. Both British and American anthropology in the first half of the twentieth century had legitimized the study of societies as though they were isolates, often focusing on easily identifiable cultural traits (e.g., material goods, values, practices) (Barrett 1984; Darnell 2001). The idea of cultural marginality requires one to accept the existence of two – and only two – singular cultural isolates that are vastly different as well as the notion that an individual can become trapped in some kind of limbo between them. Of course, cultural processes are much more fluid than these scholars would suggest, and the notion that there are two "cultures" in North America is nonsensical. Implicit is the notion that an individual can actually be without culture, having experienced cultural loss without a corresponding cultural gain. Such a trait-based view of culture is built on the assumptions that individuals have a limited capacity to cognitively absorb the stuff of culture and that such individuals have intense difficulty learning new cultural ways (e.g., Phillips and Inui 1986, 141). There seems to be little room in this formulation either for individual agency or for healthy, multicultural adaptation. Perhaps more important, the idea that marginality may be a function more of socioeconomic deprivation than of culture loss is rarely considered.[11]

Conclusion: Culture and Aboriginality

In the past few decades, culture has become more acceptable as an element of study in psychology and psychiatry, and the search for cultural "others" to test the cross-cultural applicability of accumulated psychological and psychiatric knowledge has focused, in part, on Aboriginal North America. A move away from the ethnography of the anthropologist and toward clinical-, community-, or disorder-based epidemiology has resulted in the creation and sustenance of a "cultural" variable. Over time, anthropology entered a reflective, critical phase, characterized by the notion of culture as a constructed entity, and the discipline became embroiled in debates over the veracity and validity of its own concepts, methods, and ethnographic portraits. Correspondingly, the discipline became increasingly uncomfortable with the notion of fixed cultures and boundaries (e.g., Borofsky et al. 2001; Geertz 1973; Keesing 1990). In contrast, psychology and psychiatry have largely continued to embrace the earlier, now disputed, cultural "truths," perhaps because such "truths" were most amenable to operationalization in comparative research. Many of these "truths" today can be thought of as anthropological anachronisms, versions of once accepted ideas of culture embedded in the evolutionary, historical-particularist, and structural-functionalist schools of anthropology (see Brumann 1999). These anachronisms include the following assumptions:

1   that there are discrete cultural or biological populations and that these can be delineated and bounded conceptually;
2   that biological heritage, community, nationality, and identity are synonymous with culture;

3   that culture can be accurately self-declared;
4   that cultures are internally consistent and known in the same way and to the same extent by each culture member;
5   that cultures can be aggregated into larger units, or culture areas, on the basis of trait similarities, and that these larger units can be conceptualized as essentially culturally homogeneous;
6   that an individual's capacity for culture is limited and that one can lose his or her culture and exist in a "cultureless" state.

Not surprisingly, then, in much mental health research, Aboriginal cultures have all too frequently been portrayed as simple, easily bounded units that harbour uniformly unicultural citizens. Such cultures, in Keesing's critique, are "hermetically sealed beyond the reaches of time and the world system" (1990, 53). When there has been an attempt to consider the implications of cultural change, the tendency has been to assume a breakdown of culture leading to social and psychological disintegration. Aboriginal peoples have clearly experienced the "overpathologizing bias" said to be characteristic of approaches to minority groups more generally (Good 1997, 239), in large part because of their perceived inability to function as healthy, modern cultural beings.

Culture, then, has been central to much of the research on Aboriginal mental health, research that has been guided by two distinct and dissociable assumptions: (1) that all Aboriginal peoples are essentially the same culturally (at least within "culture areas"); and (2) that when viewed as a totality, they are all uniformly culturally different from non-Aboriginal peoples. For example, research has frequently assumed that a registered or self-declared Indian *is* culturally different in meaningful ways from a non-Indian person or that an individual of the subarctic culture area *is* culturally different from one of the Plains culture area. Researchers have rarely explored these as empirical questions and have uniformly avoided an examination of Aboriginal cultures in a contemporary context. When differences between populations have been found in some clinical dimension – for instance, the rate for a particular disorder – the argument that this must be due to cultural differences has frequently prevailed. We need to pay more attention to Joseph Trimble's caution that cross-cultural research has frequently operated with the "tacit belief that the host people are in fact culturally different" in the absence of empirical evidence to this effect. Most such research, he has argued, attempts "to isolate sets of discriminating variables that serve to differentiate one cultural group from another" (1975, 304). In other words, researchers discursively and/or empirically create cultural difference where none may meaningfully exist and then use that "difference" to explain patterns of psychopathology.

Much clinical, community-based, and epidemiological research has required the operationalization of culture as a variable (or as a set of variables), and the problem with this is clearly articulated in the continued utilization of culture-area models as sampling frames and of broad biological, cultural, Tribal, or legal affiliations and so-called traditional values as cultural markers – as though these have been intrinsically meaningful in the late twentieth and early twenty-first centuries.[12] These are certainly convenient conceptual tools, and they have a long scientific history to support them, but as representations of *culture* they are woefully inadequate. Self-declaration is equally problematic since a cultural declaration may represent a declaration of historical heritage or a wish more than a reality – that is, a pining for a "culture" that one does not have much experience with, that may not even exist, or that may be little more than a romanticized simulation (Vizenor 1994; Waldram 1997). This seems as common among Aboriginal North Americans as it is among individuals elsewhere whose ancestors have experienced colonization or among those who have emigrated and then developed nostalgia for a lost country. Heritage is of immense importance to individuals everywhere, and it often plays a central role in our multifaceted constructions of identity. But understanding the multiple meanings of Aboriginal identity for mental health research requires a concrete, context-specific understanding of the contemporary cultural reality of Aboriginal peoples. I am not suggesting that there are no cultural issues with respect to Aboriginal mental health but rather that deferring to cultural explanations has been too readily employed at the expense of other possible explanations.

Part of a comprehension of this contemporary cultural reality, I would argue, is the need to consider the view of anthropologist Bradd Shore that "any powerful theory of cultural knowledge must clarify not just the power of culture to explain ... but also the limits of culture as an explanatory device" (1996, 315). This view is seconded by psychologist John Christopher, who has cautioned against taking culture "too seriously" by seeing Aboriginal culture as "wholly native, indigenous, and in need of protection from cultural imperialism" (1998, 4). In attempting to bring Aboriginal culture into mental health research, many have erroneously assumed that culture can meaningfully explain all aspects of problematic or distressed human behaviour and further that Aboriginal peoples in particular are first and foremost collective cultural beings, with everything explainable in terms of a shared traditional culture of longstanding. Less evident in the Aboriginal mental health research is an understanding of the implications of socioeconomic status, especially economic marginalization, for mental health. An essentialist interpretation is unavoidable: whereas the behaviour of non-Aboriginals is interpreted primarily in terms of class and socioeconomics, as though they have no culture, the behaviour of Aboriginals is too frequently explained as though it is *only* a manifestation of culture or, worse still, of biology.

Studies of Aboriginal mental health, especially those that employ a comparative and/ or epidemiological perspective, do so utilizing conceptualizations of culture that are at odds with current developments in anthropological theory. Fields such as psychology and psychiatry have eschewed the apparent navel-gazing of their anthropological colleagues in favour of a results-oriented program (Greenfield 2000). A "cultural critique" (Kirmayer, Brass, and Tait 2000, 613) of Aboriginal mental health pushes us in the direction of what Alarcón (2001), Bibeau (1997), and Kirmayer and Minas (2000) all refer to as a "creolizing" cultural psychiatry, one that recognizes the apparent cultural changes wrought by processes of globalization. For Aboriginal North Americans, globalization commenced more than 500 years ago, significant cultural changes have ensued, and cultural boundaries, if they ever existed, have become blurred, even erased. A creolizing psychiatry eschews the notion of fixed cultural boundaries, viewing cultures instead as "pastiche" (Keesing 1990, 57) or "melange" (Hermans and Kempen 1998, 1113).

This does not mean that researchers, especially anthropologists, should abandon an attempt to better theorize and operationalize culture or to develop a concrete understanding of contemporary cultural realities and lived cultural experiences of Aboriginal peoples. As culture remains central to our comprehension of human behaviour, it is incumbent upon us to make such an effort. However, the contemporary cultural orientation and distinctiveness of specific Aboriginal individuals and communities should be a matter for sound empirical investigation, not an a priori research assumption. At present, the meaning of Aboriginality, as a construct of both identity and culture, for an understanding of contemporary mental health issues remains unclear. Perhaps once we are better able to understand it, we will better comprehend not only observed patterns of psychopathology and associated suffering but also mechanisms through which many Aboriginal peoples have achieved and maintained a healthy state in a culturally complex and challenging world. This is possibly the most important new direction for Aboriginal mental health research.

Notes

1 In this chapter, I examine notions of culture and Aboriginality for North America, not just Canada. Most of the important research that I discuss has had as its focus American Indians and Alaskan Natives, yet this research has had a profound effect on Aboriginal mental health scholarship in Canada. I will use terms appropriate to the context being discussed; hence the appearance of "Indian," "Aboriginal," "Tribe," and "First Nation."

2 Due to space limitations, I will not examine the issues of theory and method in ethnographic approaches to Aboriginal mental health. A critical examination of such research can be found in Waldram (2004).

3 A more substantive analysis of the topic of culture and Aboriginal mental health is available from my book *Revenge of the Windigo: The construction of the mind and mental health of North American Aboriginal peoples* (Waldram 2004).

4 An excellent source on nineteenth-century science and Aboriginal North Americans that speaks to this and the related issue of blood quantum is Bieder (1986) (see also Gould 1996).

5 More recently, there seems to have been increasing interest in using postal codes as markers of Aboriginality, assuming an Aboriginal or cultural uniformity within communities known to be Indian reserves or predominantly Métis communities. The problems that I discuss in this section also apply to this approach.

6 Some of the most enduring "culture areas" were the arctic, subarctic (western and eastern), Plains, Plateau, Eastern Woodlands, and Southwest.

7 I find this argument hard to accept. Contemporary Aboriginal people are certainly aware of the history of co-operation with or animosity toward neighbouring Tribal groups, such as between the Dene and Cree in northern Saskatchewan and between the Plains Cree and Blackfoot in Alberta. Such co-operation or

conflict, it seems to me, was based not on a recognition and respect of culture areas but on more prag-matic issues such as economic competition and the need for alliances.

8 Attempts to measure cultural orientation or acculturation for other groups have also been made. Inkeles and Smith (1974) have dealt with this issue cross-nationally; Doob (1967) for Africa; Dawson (1969) and De Lacy (1970) for indigenous Australians; and Cuellar, Harris, and Jasso (1980), Olmedo, Martinez, and Martinez (1978), and Olmedo and Padilla (1978) for Mexican Americans. Berry and colleagues (1986) provide a good introduction to the issues involved.

9 Other items included in their list are curious and reflect the problems inherent in the imposition of exter-nal cultural referents: most Cree communities at the time of Berrys and Annis' work did not have running water, making the purchase of washers a questionable measure of acculturation, and there were no banks or life insurance agents.

10 Particularly noteworthy was the lack of mutual exclusivity in response categories, which betrayed a funda-mental lack of knowledge of the specific cultural practices for which researchers were testing. For instance, subjects were requested to select the most applicable response from among three options: (1) I believe in bad medicine; (2) Bad medicine scares me; (3) Bad medicine is evil. All three are interrelated components of the belief in bad medicine, however, and it is not clear how one of these choices could somehow indi-cate greater Indian orientation in comparison to the others.

11 For another critique of "deculturation," see Del Pilar (2004).

12 Further, in research where the individual is requested to designate his or her culture, choices offered often include cultural as well as legal and geographical designations, a confusing array presented to the respondent without a corresponding explanation of their meaning. In Canada, for instance, surveys often ask respondents to declare themselves to be "registered Indians," "treaty Indians," "Métis," "Inuit," or "Aboriginal."

References

Alarcón, R.D. 2001. Hispanic psychiatry: From margin to mainstream. *Transcultural Psychiatry* 38 (1): 5-25.

American Psychiatric Association. 2000. *Diagnostic and statistical manual of mental disorders: DSM-IV-TR.* 4th ed. Washington, DC: American Psychiatric Association.

Barrett, S.R. 1984. *The rebirth of anthropological theory.* Toronto, ON: University of Toronto Press.

–. 1996. *Anthropology: A student's guide to theory and methodology.* Toronto, ON: University of Toronto Press.

Beiser, M., and A. Gotowiec. 2000. Accounting for Native/non-Native differences in IQ scores. *Psychology in Schools* 37 (3): 237-52.

Bennion, L.J., and T. Li. 1976. Alcohol metabolism in American Indians and whites. *New England Journal of Medicine* 294 (1): 9-13.

Berry, J.W. 1970. Marginality, stress and ethnic identification in an acculturated Aboriginal community. *Journal of Cross-Cultural Psychology* 1 (3): 239-52.

–. 1975. Ecology, cultural adaptation, and psychological stress: Traditional patterning and acculturative stress. In R.W. Brislin, S. Bochner, and W.J. Lonner, eds., *Cross-cultural perspectives on learning,* 207-28. New York: John Wiley and Sons.

–. 1985. Acculturation among circumpolar peoples: Implications for health status. *Arctic Medical Research* 40: 21-27.

–. 1991. Psychology of acculturation. *Nebraska Symposium on Motivation* 39: 201-34.

–. 2003. Conceptual approaches to acculturation. In K. Chun, P. Organista, and G. Marín, eds., *Accultura-tion: Advances in theory, measurement, and applied research,* 17-37. Washington, DC: American Psychologic-al Association.

–, and R.C. Annis. 1974a. Acculturative stress: The role of ecology, culture and differentiation. *Journal of Cross-Cultural Psychology* 5 (4): 382-407.

–, and R.C. Annis. 1974b. Ecology, culture and psychological differentiation. *International Journal of Psychol-ogy* 9 (3): 173-93.

–, R.M. Wintrob, P.S. Sindell, and T.A. Mawhinney. 1982. Psychological adaptation to culture change among the James Bay Cree. *Le Naturaliste Canadien* 109 (1): 965-75.

–, J.E. Trimble, and E.L. Olmedo. 1986. Assessment of acculturation. In W.J. Lonner and J.W. Berry, eds., *Field methods in cross-cultural research,* 291-349. Thousand Oaks, CA: Sage.

–, U. Kim, T. Minde, and D. Mok. 1987. Comparative studies of acculturative stress. *International Migration Review* 21 (3): 491-511.

–, and U. Kim. 1988. Acculturation and mental health. In P. Dasen, J.W. Berry, and N. Sartorius, eds., *Health and cross-cultural psychology: Toward applications,* 207-36. Newbury Park, NJ: Sage.

Bibeau, G. 1997. Cultural psychiatry in a creolizing world: Questions for a new research agenda. *Transcultural Psychiatry* 34 (1): 9-41.

Bieder, R.E. 1986. *Science encounters the Indian, 1820-1880: The early years of American ethnology.* Norman, OK: University of Oklahoma Press.

Borofsky, R., F. Barth, R. Shweder, L. Rodseth, and N. Stolzenberg. 2001. When: A conversation about culture. *American Anthropologist* 103 (2): 432-46.

Brucker, P.S., and B.J. Perry. 1998. American Indians: Presenting concerns and considerations for family therapists. *American Journal of Family Therapy* 26 (4): 307-19.

Brumann, C. 1999. Writing for culture: Why a successful concept should not be discarded. *Current Anthropology* 40 (suppl.): S1-S27.

Chance, N.A. 1965. Acculturation, self-identification and personality adjustment. *American Anthropologist* 6 (2): 372-93.

–, and D.A. Foster. 1962. Symptom formation and patterns of psychopathology in a rapidly changing Alaskan Eskimo society. *Anthropological Papers of the University of Alaska* 11 (1): 32-43.

Chandler, M.J., and C.E. Lalonde. 1998. Cultural continuity as a hedge against suicide in Canada's First Nations. *Transcultural Psychiatry* 35 (2): 191-219.

Chapleski, E.E., J.K. Lamphere, R. Kaczynski, P.A. Lichtenberg, and J.W. Dwyer. 1997. Structure of a depression measure among American Indian Elders: Confirmatory factor analysis of the CES-D scale. *Research on Aging* 19 (4): 462-85.

Choney, S.K., E. Berryhill-Paapke, and R.R. Robbins. 1995. The acculturation of American Indians: Developing frameworks for research and practice. In J.G. Ponterotto, J.M. Casas, L.A. Suzuki, and C.M. Alexander, eds., *Handbook of multicultural counseling,* 73-92. Thousand Oaks, CA: Sage.

Christopher, J.C. 1998. Placing culture at the center of multiculturalism: Moral visions and intercultural dialogue. *Dialogues in Psychology* 1 (14 September 1998): http://www.hubcap.clemson.edu/psych/Dialogues/dialogues.html.

Cuellar, I., L.C. Harris, and R. Jasso. 1980. An acculturation scale for Mexican American normal and clinical populations. *Hispanic Journal of Behavioral Science* 3: 199-217.

Curyto, K.J., E.E. Chapleski, P.A. Lichtenberg, E. Hodges, R. Kaczynski, and J. Sobeck. 1998. Prevalence and prediction of depression in American Indian elderly. *Clinical Gerontologist* 18 (3): 19-37.

Dana, R.H. 1993. *Multicultural assessment perspectives for professional psychology.* Needham Heights, MA: Allyn and Bacon.

–, R. Hornby, and T. Hoffman. 1984. Local norms for personality assessment of Rosebud Sioux. *White Cloud Journal* 3 (2): 17-25.

Darnell, R. 2001. *Invisible genealogies: A history of Americanist anthropology.* Lincoln, NE: University of Nebraska Press.

Dawson, J.L.M. 1969. Attitude change and conflict among Australian Aborigines. *Australian Journal of Psychology* 21 (2): 101-17.

De Lacy, P.R. 1970. An index of contact for Aboriginal communities. *Australian Journal of Social Issues* 3: 219-23.

Del Pilar, J.A. 2004. Deculturation: Its lack of validity. *Cultural Diversity and Ethnic Minority Psychology* 10 (2): 169-76.

Devereux, G. 1971. Normal and abnormal: The key problem of psychiatric anthropology. In J. Casagrande and T. Goldwin, eds., *Some uses of anthropology: Theoretical and applied*, 23-48. Washington, DC: Anthropological Society of Washington.

Dillard, D.A., and S.M. Manson. 2000. Assessing and treating American Indians and Alaska Natives. In I. Cuéllar and F.A. Paniagua, eds., *Handbook of multicultural health: Assessment and treatment of diverse populations*, 225-48. San Diego, CA: Academic Press.

Dillard, J. 1983. *Multicultural counseling.* Chicago: Nelson-Hall.

Dinges, N.G., J.E. Trimble, S.M. Manson, and F.L. Pasquale. 1981. Counseling and psychotherapy with American Indians and Alaskan Natives. In A.J. Marsella and P.B. Pedersen, eds., *Cross-cultural counseling and psychotherapy*, 243-76. New York: Pergamon.

Doob, L.W. 1967. Scales for assaying psychological modernization in Africa. *Public Opinion Quarterly* 31: 415-21.

Driver, H.E. 1969. *Indians of North America.* 2nd ed. Chicago, IL: University of Chicago Press.

Fisher, G.L., and T.C. Harrison. 1997. *Substance abuse: Information for school counselors, social workers, therapists, and counselors*. Boston: Allyn and Bacon.

Fitzgerald, J.A., and W.W. Ludeman. 1926. The intelligence of Indian children. *Journal of Comparative Psychology* 6: 319-28.

Fleming, C.M. 1996. Cultural formulation of psychiatric diagnosis: An American Indian woman suffering from depression, alcoholism, and childhood trauma. *Culture, Medicine, and Psychiatry* 20 (2): 145-54.

French, L.A. 1979. Corrections and the Native American client. *Prison Journal* 59 (1): 49-60.

–. 1980. Anomie and violence among Native Americans. *International Journal of Comparative and Applied Criminal Justice* 4 (1): 75-84.

–. 1989. Native American alcoholism: A transcultural counseling perspective. *Counselling Psychology Quarterly* 2 (2): 153-66.

–. 1997. *Counseling American Indians.* Lanham, MD: University Press of America.

Fritz, W.B. 1976. Psychiatric disorders among Natives and non-Natives in Saskatchewan. *Canadian Psychiatric Association Journal* 21: 394-400.

Garbarino, M.S. 1983. *Sociocultural theory in anthropology.* Prospect Heights, IL: Waveland.

Garcia-Andrade, C., T.L. Wall, and C.L. Ehlers. 1997. The firewater myth and response to alcohol in Mission Indians. *American Journal of Psychiatry* 154 (7): 983-88.

Garrett, J.T., and M.W. Garrett. 1994. The path of good medicine: Understanding and counseling Native American Indians. *Journal of Multicultural Counseling and Development* 22 (3): 134-44.

Garth, T.R. 1921. The results of some tests on full and mixed blood Indians. *The Journal of Applied Psychology* 5: 359-372.

–. 1922. Mental fatigue of mixed and full blood Indians. *The Journal of Applied Psychology* 6: 331-41.

–. 1923. A comparison of the intelligence of mixed and full blood Indian children. *Psychological Review* 30: 388-401.

–. 1925. The intelligence of full blood Indians. *The Journal of Applied Psychology* 9: 382-98.

–. 1927. The intelligence of mixed blood Indians. *The Journal of Applied Psychology* 40: 268-75.

–, H.W. Smith, and W. Abell. 1928. A study of the intelligence and achievement of full-blood Indians. *The Journal of Applied Psychology* 12: 511-16.

Geertz, C. 1973. *The interpretation of cultures.* New York: Basic Books.

Good, B. 1997. Studying mental illness in global context: Local, global, or universal? *Ethos* 25 (2): 230-48.

Gould, S. Jay. 1996. *The mismeasure of man*. New York: W.W. Norton.

Graves, T.D. 1967a. Psychological acculturation in a tri-ethnic community. *Southwestern Journal of Anthropology* 23: 337-50.

–. 1967b. Acculturation, access, and alcohol in a tri-ethnic community. *American Anthropologist* 69: 306-21.

Green, J.W. 1999. *Cultural awareness in the human services.* 3rd ed. Boston: Allyn and Bacon.

Greenfield, P.M. 2000. What psychology can do for anthropology, or Why anthropology took postmodernism on the chin. *American Anthropologist* 102 (3): 564-76.

Heinrich, R.K., J.L. Corbine, and K.R. Thomas. 1990. Counseling Native Americans. *Journal of Counseling and Development* 69: 128-33.

Hendrie, H.C., and D. Hanson. 1972. A comparative study of the psychiatric care of Indians and Metis. *American Journal of Orthopsychiatry* 42 (3): 480-89.

Hermans, H., and H. Kempen. 1998. Moving cultures: The perilous problems of cultural dichotomies in a globalizing society. *American Psychologist* 53 (10): 1111-20.

Herring, R.D. 1989. The American Native family: Dissolution by coercion. *Journal of Multicultural Counseling and Development* 17 (1): 4-13.

–. 1990. Understanding Native-American values: Process and content concerns for counselors. *Counseling and Values* 34 (2): 134-37.

–. 1992. Seeking a new paradigm: Counseling Native Americans. *Journal of Multicultural Counseling and Development* 20: 35-43.

Ho, M.K. 1987. *Family therapy with ethnic minorities.* Thousand Oaks, CA: Sage.

–. 1992. *Minority children and adolescents in therapy.* Newbury Park, NJ: Sage.

Hoffman, T., R.H. Dana, and B. Bolton. 1985. Measured acculturation and MMPI-168 performance of Native American adults. *Journal of Cross-Cultural Psychology* 16 (2): 243-56.

Hummer, H.R. 1913. Insanity among the Indians. *American Journal of Insanity* 69: 615-23.

Inkeles, A., and D.H. Smith. 1974. *Becoming modern: Individual change in six developing countries.* Cambridge, MA: Harvard University Press.

Johnson, M.E., and K.H. Lashley. 1989. Influence of Native-Americans' cultural commitment on preferences for counselor ethnicity and expectations about counseling. *Journal of Multicultural Counseling and Development* 17: 115-22.

Keesing, R.M. 1990. Theories of culture revisited. *Canberra Anthropology* 13 (2): 46-60.

Kerckhoff, A.C., and T.C. McCormick. 1955. Marginal status and marginal personality. *Social Forces* 34 (4): 48-55.

Kirmayer, L.J., G.M. Brass, and C.L. Tait. 2000. The mental health of Aboriginal peoples: Transformations of identity and community. *Canadian Journal of Psychiatry* 45: 607-16.

–, and H. Minas. 2000. The future of cultural psychiatry: An international perspective. *Canadian Journal of Psychiatry* 45: 438-46.

Kleinman, A. 1996. How is culture important for DSM-IV. In J. Mezzich, A. Kleinman, H. Fabrega Jr., and D. Parron, eds., *Culture and psychiatric diagnosis: A DSM-IV perspective,* 15-29. Washington, DC: American Psychiatric Press.

Kluckhohn, F.R., and F.L. Strodtbeck. 1961. *Variations in value orientations.* Homewood, IL: Dorsey.

Kroeber, A.L. 1939. Cultural and natural areas of Native North America. *University of California Publications in American Archaeology and Ethnology* 38: 1-242.

LaFromboise, T.D. 1993. American Indian mental health policy. In D.R. Atkinson, G. Morten, and D. Wing Sue, eds., *Counseling American minorities: A cross-cultural perspective,* 123-43. Madison, WI: Brown and Benchmark.

–, J.E. Trimble, and G.V. Mohatt. 1990. Counseling intervention and American Indian tradition: An integrated approach. *The Counseling Psychologist.* 18 (4): 628-54.

Leland, J. 1976. *Firewater myths: North American Indian drinking and alcohol addiction.* Brunswick, NJ: Rutgers Center of Alcohol Studies.

Locke, D.C. 1992. *Increasing multicultural understanding: A comprehensive model.* Thousand Oaks, CA: Sage.

Manson, S.M. 1996. The wounded spirit: A cultural formulation of post-traumatic stress disorder. *Culture, Medicine and Psychiatry,* 20 (4): 489-98.

McMillan, A.D. 1995. *Native peoples and cultures in Canada.* 2nd ed. Vancouver, BC: Douglas and McIntyre.

McShane, D.A., and J.W. Berry. 1988. Native North Americans: Indians and Inuit abilities. In S.H. Irvine and J.W. Berry, eds., *Human abilities in cultural context,* 385-426. New York: Cambridge University Press.

Mohatt, G., and A.W. Blue. 1982. Primary prevention as it relates to traditionality and empirical measures of social deviance. In S.M. Manson, ed., *New directions in prevention among American Indian and Alaska Native communities,* 91-118. Portland, OR: Oregon Health Services University.

Morrison, R.B., and R.C. Wilson, eds. 1995. *Native peoples: The Canadian experience.* 2nd ed. Toronto, ON: McClelland and Stewart.

Norton, I.M., and S.M. Manson. 1996. Research in American Indian and Alaska Native communities: Navigating the cultural universe of values and process. *Journal of Consulting and Clinical Psychology* 64 (5): 856-60.

Nuckolls, C.W. 1998. *Culture: A problem that cannot be solved.* Madison, WI: University of Wisconsin Press.

Olmedo, E.L., J.L. Martinez Jr., and S.R. Martinez. 1978. Measure of acculturation for Chicano adolescents. *Psychological Reports* 42: 159-70.

–, and A.M. Padilla. 1978. Empirical and construct validation of a measure of acculturation for Mexican Americans. *The Journal of Social Psychology* 105: 179-87.

O'Nell, T.D. 1998. Cultural formulation of psychiatric diagnosis: Psychotic depression and alcoholism in an American Indian man. *Culture, Medicine and Psychiatry* 22: 123-36.

Phillips, M.R., and T.S. Inui. 1986. The interaction of mental illness, criminal behaviour and culture: Native Alaskan mentally ill criminal offenders. *Culture, Medicine and Psychiatry* 10 (2): 123-49.

Redfield, R., R. Linton, and M. Herskovits. 1936. Memorandum on the study of acculturation. *American Anthropologist* 38: 149-52.

Renfrey, G.S. 1992. Cognitive-behaviour therapy and the Native American client. *Behaviour Therapy* 23 (3): 321-40.

Richardson, E.H. 1981. Cultural and historical perspectives in counseling American Indians. In D. Wing Sue, ed., *Counseling the culturally different,* 216-55. New York: John Wiley and Sons.

Roy, C., A. Choudhuri, and D. Irvine. 1970. The prevalence of mental disorders among Saskatchewan Indians. *Journal of Cross-Cultural Psychology* 1 (4): 383-92.

Sack, W.H., M. Beiser, G. Clarke, and R. Redshirt. 1987. The high achieving Sioux Indian child: Some preliminary findings from the Flower of the Two Soils Project. *American Indian and Alaska Native Mental Health Research* 1 (1): 37-51.

–, M. Beiser, G. Baker-Brown, and R. Redshirt. 1994. Depressive and suicidal symptoms in Indian school children: Some findings from the Flower of Two Soils. In C.W. Duclos and S.M. Manson, eds., *Beyond the rim: Epidemiology and prevention of suicide among Indian and Native youth,* 81-94. Niwot, CO: University Press of Colorado.

Shore, B. 1996. *Culture in mind: Cognition, culture and the problem of meaning.* New York: Oxford University Press.

Shore, J.H., S.M. Manson, J.D. Bloom, G. Keepers, and G. Neligh. 1987. A pilot study of depression among American Indian patients with research diagnostic criteria. *American Indian and Alaska Native Mental Health Research* 1 (2): 1-15.

Snipp, C.M. 1997. Some observations about racial boundaries and the experiences of American Indians. *Ethnic and Racial Studies* 20 (4): 667-89.

Sue, S. 2003. Foreword. In K. Chun, P. Organista, and G. Marín, eds., *Acculturation: Advances in theory, measurement, and applied research,* xvii-xxi. Washington, DC: American Psychological Association.

Terman, L.W. 1916. *The measurement of intelligence.* Boston: Houghton-Mifflin.

Topper, M.D., and J. Curtis. 1987. Extended family therapy: A clinical approach to the treatment of synergistic dual anomic depression among Navajo agency-town adolescents. *Journal of Community Psychology* 15 (3): 334-48.

Trimble, J.E. 1975. The intrusion of Western psychological thought on Native American ethos: Divergence and conflict among the Lakota. In J.W. Berry and W.J. Lonner, eds., *Applied cross-cultural psychology: Selected papers from the Second International Conference of the International Association for Cross-Cultural Psychology*, 303-8. Amsterdam: Swets and Zeitlinger.

–. 1981. Value differentials and their importance in counseling American Indians. In P.B. Pedersen, W.J. Lonner, and J.G. Draguns, eds., *Counseling across cultures*, 1st ed., 203-26. Honolulu, HI: University Press of Hawaii.

–. 2003. Introduction: Social change and acculturation. In K. Chun, P. Organista, and G. Marín, eds., *Acculturation: Advances in theory, measurement, and applied research*, 3-13. Washington, DC: American Psychological Association.

–, and S.A. Hayes. 1984. Mental health intervention in the psychosocial contexts of American Indian communities. In W.A. O'Connor and B. Lubin, eds., *Ecological approaches to clinical and community psychology*, 293-321. New York: John Wiley and Sons.

–, and C.M. Fleming. 1989. Providing counseling services for Native American Indians: Client, counselor, and community characteristics. In P.B. Pedersen, J.G. Draguns, W.J. Lonner, and J.E. Trimble, eds., *Counseling across cultures*, 3rd ed., 177-204. Honolulu, HI: University of Hawaii Press.

–, C.M. Fleming, F. Beauvais, and P. Jumper-Thurman. 1996. Essential cultural and social strategies for counseling Native American Indians. In P.B. Pedersen, J.G. Draguns, W.J. Lonner, and J.E. Trimble, eds., *Counseling across cultures*, 4th ed., 177-209. Thousand Oaks, CA: Sage.

Uecker, A.E., L.R. Boutilier, and E.H. Richardson. 1980. "Indianism" and MMPI scores of men alcoholics. *Journal of Studies on Alcohol* 41 (3): 357-62.

Vizenor, G. 1994. *Manifest manners: Postindian warriors of survivance*. Hanover, NH: University Press of New England.

Waldram, J.B. 1997. *The way of the pipe: Aboriginal spirituality and symbolic healing in Canadian prisons*. Peterborough, ON: Broadview Press.

–. 2004. *Revenge of the Windigo: The construction of the mind and mental health of North American Aboriginal peoples*. Toronto, ON: University of Toronto Press.

–. 2006. The view from the Hogan: Cultural epidemiology and the return to ethnography. *Transcultural Psychiatry* 43 (1): 72-85.

Weaver, H.N. 2001. Indigenous identity: What is it and who *really* has it? *American Indian Quarterly* 25 (2): 240-55.

Weisner, T.S., J.C. Weibel-Orlando, and J. Long. 1984. "Serious drinking," "white man's drinking" and "teetotaling": Drinking levels and styles in an urban American Indian population. *Journal of Studies on Alcohol* 45 (3): 237-50.

Weiss, M. 1997. Explanatory model interview catalogue (EMIC): Framework for comparative study of illness. *Transcultural Psychiatry* 34 (2): 235-63.

–, S. Jadhav, R. Raguram, P. Vounatsou, and R. Littlewood. 2001. Psychiatric stigma across cultures: Local validation in Bangalore and London. *Anthropology and Medicine* 8 (1): 71-87.

Westermeyer, J.J. 1974. The drunken Indian: Myths and realities. *Psychiatric Annals* 4 (9): 29-36.

–, and J. Neider. 1985. Cultural affiliation among American Indian alcoholics: Correlations and change over a ten year period. *Journal of Operational Psychiatry* 16 (2): 17-23.

4

Social Competence and Mental Health among Aboriginal Youth: An Integrative Developmental Perspective

GRACE IAROCCI, RHODA ROOT, AND JACOB A. BURACK

Truthfully, I have created your being. Look about and see what
this world contains. It shall be your eternal duty to act as caretaker
of all that has been created upon the back of the Great Sea Turtle.

– OKWÍ:RASE, QUOTED IN L. KANE AND KANATAKTA, EDS.,
TSI NITIONKWE: NON NE KANIEN'KEHA:KA (1991), 4

The application of a developmental approach to understanding and intervening in mental health issues among Aboriginal adolescents raises the longstanding concern about the universality of psychological principles and findings (Weisz et al. 1997). On one end of the spectrum, principles of development, or of any biological or psychological realm, are considered to be applicable to all persons, regardless of culture or level of adaptability (Wyman 2003). This *universalist* framework (Kim 2000) is associated with a traditional positivistic scientific approach as researchers and practitioners apply evidence from one population to better understand other groups. At the other extreme, differences among individuals, populations, or contexts are considered so great that little can be generalized from one to another, and each needs to be studied independently (Wyman 2003). Within this *contextualist* framework (Kim 2000), general scientific conceptualizations are ignored or relegated to a minor role as the unique history, culture, and capabilities of the individual or population are emphasized. In this chapter, we attempt to chart a middle ground for the study of the development of adaptive and maladaptive behaviours among Aboriginal youth. Findings from other populations, especially those that share minority-related risk status and a background of oppression in North America, are informative within a context that is guided by the unique histories and current circumstances of the individual Aboriginal communities. The goal of this endeavour is to provide an integrated framework for understanding some of the issues that can promote wellness in children and adolescents across the many different and unique Aboriginal communities of Canada. As is the case with any type of medical or psychological intervention, success in mental health services is dependent on the identification of the relevant scientific principles as well as on the ability to tailor the information to the person for whom it is intended.

The development of social competencies that promote mental health among Aboriginal adolescents will be discussed within the perspectives of both typical development within North American culture and the uniqueness of the adolescents' own culture and heritage. This strategy is consistent with a developmental perspective (Burack 1997; Cicchetti 1984; Cicchetti and Toth 1995) in which typical and atypical development are considered to be mutually informative. It highlights the notion that Aboriginal youths not only share many characteristics and developmental issues with their peers from other cultures but also must be considered as a group or as many different groups with unique developmental concerns. We begin with a general overview of a developmental perspective in which notions of social competence and mental health are integrated with those of cultural context and examine factors relevant to developmental risk and well-being among Aboriginal youth living in Canada and elsewhere in North America. Then we assess these factors within the context of the developmental conceptualizations of resilience and risk-protective factors before concluding with a discussion of future directions for research and interventions with Aboriginal youths.

Agents of Culture and Cultural Contexts: The Dynamics of Social Competence

Within a developmental framework, social competence and mental health are considered emergent characteristics of the dynamic interplay between individuals and their environments over time (Sameroff, Seifer, and Bartko 1997; Wyman et al. 2000). The construct of social competence is typically discussed with regard to an individual's success in meeting major societal expectations at the relevant developmental stages (Luthar and Burack 2000; Luthar and Zigler 1991), whereas the related notion of mental health can be considered within the context of emotional well-being (Elias and Weissberg 2000). Individuals actively adapt to and even mould their environments as levels of both social competence and mental health change continuously within an ongoing transactional relationship that involves the biological, psychological, and behavioural aspects of the person and the physical, familial, and social aspects of the environment (Bronfenbrenner 1979; Cicchetti and Toth 1997; Sameroff 1990; Sameroff and Chandler 1975). Thus the relation between the child and the environment is collaborative, as the context does not merely influence or provide the setting for behaviour to occur but is also an essential component of the behavioural expression of competence (Cummings, Davies, and Campbell 2000). The implication is that social competence and mental health may vary dramatically as a function of the availability and compatibility of contextual supports, including community, family, and peers. Thus environments need to be considered with regard to the benefits and risks with which they are generally associated as well as with regard to the specific fit for an individual, all within a transactional process that involves constant change.

From a developmental framework, certain aspects of an environment are almost universally beneficial or detrimental, yet the impact of even these settings varies in relation to a variety of factors, including the chronicity and severity of the deleterious act, the child's age and characteristics at time of exposure, relationships with others, and additional risk or protective factors in the environment prior to, during, and after exposure. For example, poverty, in-utero exposure to certain substances or diseases, abusive or neglectful parenting, and exposure to violence and prejudice are virtually always associated with generally negative outcomes among populations of children, but a deleterious developmental outcome is rarely inevitable, as specific individuals are protected to varying extents by personality, by intellectual or emotional characteristics, and/or by environmental influences and resources (Seidman and Pederson 2003). The protective influences of certain factors prior to and during problematic periods and the ameliorative effects of specific relationships during and after exposure are evident for situations as horrific as child maltreatment (Sameroff and Chandler 1975), life in death camps during the Holocaust (Burack 1997), and exposure to brief periods of intense violence or fear (Masten, Best, and Garmezy 1990). Within this framework, the significance and impact of the detrimental influences of the risk factors and the benefits of protective factors in a specific context can vary considerably in relation to the individual and the environment (Bronfenbrenner 1979). Moreover, the impact of an event can affect an individual in different ways across the life span, as the consequences of disrupted parenting experienced during childhood may be evident only in the child's attempts as an adolescent and adult to engage in meaningful relationships and to raise his or her own children. At the most basic level, different periods in development are associated with different needs, developmental milestones, and types of relationships. Thus outcome is largely dependent on what is measured and when it is measured. The notions of resilience, risk, and protection can be evaluated only within the context of ongoing transactional relationships that include the individual and the environment, both of which are complex and multifaceted, and that change over time with regard to the occurrence, level, and type of both positive and negative outcomes.

Developmental Variation versus Deviation: Cultural Considerations

An integrative approach adheres to the notion that cultural and even developmental variations from the North American mainstream are legitimate and functional adaptations to contextual demands, being neither produced by pathology nor deviant or deficient relative to mainstream standards (Garcia Coll, Akerman, and Cicchetti 2000). For example, emotion may be a universal phenomenon, but cultural differences are evident in the specific emotions and in how and when they are elicited according to attributions and appraisal processes (Saarni 1998). In this framework, emotion is understood from the perspective of the goals of the individual and of the context within which that individual acts (Thompson 1994). This is consistent with the notion that anxiety (at the most fundamental level) in both Western and non-Western cultures is thought to be a basic survival mechanism that prepares the body for flight or fight responses to objects or situations that threaten survival (Good and Kleinman 1985; Seligman 1971). The difficulty in any cultural context, then, is to differentiate between anxiety that is adaptive and even necessary for optimal response and symptoms or syndromes of anxiety that may be debilitating and maladaptive in a specific context (Kirmayer, Young, and Hayton 1995). This tension is evident in Hallowell's (1970) observation of the cultural belief system of the Berens River Indians in Canada, which was associated with generally adaptive functioning but fostered anxieties about encounters with frogs or toads, which were commonly considered to be a bad omen. In this case, only a distortion of this belief system led to extreme fears and anxieties that disrupted the daily functioning of a community member. This is an example of the notion that emotion regulation, regardless of its culturally specific manifestation, is pathological only if it interferes with an individual's ability to meet the developmental and cultural demands for healthy adaptation.

With regard to Aboriginal emotional well-being, the type of integrated analysis that bridges the common aspects of development with those that are contextually or culturally specific is reflected in the work of Chandler and colleagues (Chandler 2000; Chandler, Lalonde, and Sokol 2000; Chandler and Lalonde, Chapter 10) on the development of identity among First Nations adolescents and the relation to cultural continuity and suicide. They view self-identity as universal at one level of explanation and culturally specific at another. For example, the notion of a continuous self over time is necessary for the development of self-identity in all cultures; however, the strategy that is used to explain self-continuity varies significantly between Euro-American and Aboriginal cultures. Generally, Euro-American cultures endorse a structural or essentialist strategy to solve the problem of self-continuity, whereas certain Aboriginal communities support a more functional and narrative-based account for personal persistence (Chandler and Lalonde 1995, 1998; Chandler et al. 2003). Although the development of a healthy conception of selfhood for both Aboriginal and mainstream adolescents relies on the ability to solve the problem of self-continuity in the face of rapid cultural change, the specific tasks that Aboriginal youth face, such as locating self-continuity within their often bleak historical narrative, renders them more vulnerable to the problem of youth suicide (Chandler et al. 2003). This reflects a type of integrative developmental paradigm that allows for the flexible and effective study of the interplay of developmental competencies and contextual demands. In this chapter, we extend this approach in discussions of a review of risk and protective factors that are relevant to the development of social competence, emotional well-being, and risk for psychopathology among Aboriginal adolescents in North America.

Risk, Resilience, and Youth: Evaluating Individual Competence in Social Contexts

The many communities of First Nations, Inuit, and Métis who collectively represent Canada's Aboriginal peoples (INAC 2002) differ in historical origins, culture, language, social organization, lifestyles, traditions, and geography but share a history of profound disruption and loss of their traditional life course through contact with Euro-American cultures. Millions of Aboriginal people and even entire communities perished due to infectious disease epidemics, were denied access to land and their livelihood, were forced to relocate and were confined to reserves, were separated from their families to be educated in institutional settings, and were forbidden to practise their native language and spirituality (Kirmayer 1994). As a result of the devastating impact on communities, families, and many individuals, the Native peoples of North America are currently a minority within the land of their ancestors (Wright 1992). These elements of history and current situation that are shared by all Aboriginal communities may be so pervasive that they elicit certain common experiences associated with specific psychological consequences, including the frequent manifestation of risk factors and mental health problems among youths. The precise expressions of the risk factors vary with regard to the unique histories and characteristics of each group and even each individual, although common themes might be identified across communities.

Preliminary evidence about Canadian Aboriginal children's mental health indicates the profound impact of cultural discontinuity that contributes to relatively high rates of depression, alcoholism, suicide, and violence in many communities (Kirmayer, Tait, and Simpson, Chapter 1). However, in the face of personal and collective hardships, certain Aboriginal communities persevered and succeeded in facing transitions on their own terms (Gotowiec and Beiser 1994). One explanation for this success is that these communities transcended the ravages of their history by actively reclaiming rights to their land, achieving autonomy to self-govern, and reviving their cultures (Chandler and Lalonde 1998). Through these efforts, they may be able to re-establish a sense of cultural continuity and ultimately protect their youth from suicide (Chandler, Lalonde, and Sokol 2000). This highlights the conceptualization of culture as an active force on development, not a passive background upon which development unfolds (Garcia Coll and Magnusson 1999). Thus Aboriginal and other minority youth may all face the same task of navigating between two cultures within a primarily Western context yet show different patterns of achieving their own cultural identity and of responding to influences from the majority culture and subcultures. In this context, personal experiences do not mirror actual events but are formed on the basis of the adolescents' perceptions of relations between their own actions and events, their previous belief systems, and the meanings that the events hold for their own well-being (Cummings, Davies, and Campbell 2000).

The Search for Identity

Perceived historical, current, and future contexts pose both constraints and opportunities in the development of problem-solving and coping strategies among adolescents. From this perspective, adaptive and maladaptive development should not be defined broadly since the meaning or adaptive value of specific behaviours is intricately intertwined with the context (Luthar and Zelazo 2003; Seidman and Pedersen 2003; Wyman 2003). This is

GRACE IAROCCI, RHODA ROOT, AND JACOB A. BURACK

evident in the struggle for the sense of belonging and connectedness that is common among all youths as they strive to integrate a sense of their individual uniqueness, a continuity of experience through connection with meaningful elements of their past, and a need for relatedness and belongingness within their peer group (Erikson 1968). Paradoxically, during this process adolescents become both more individually and socially focused as the self is differentiated from others and viewed in relation to others (Erikson 1975). Societies and more local communities facilitate the process of identity development by providing exposure to values that have stood the test of time and that are generally agreed upon by most members. Thus adolescents are free to explore the available cultural strategies set by parents and the broader community and free to settle on the more useful and satisfying ones as their own unique identities begin to form. Thus, in ideal circumstances, adolescents both shape and are shaped by their cultural context. However, during times of rapid cultural change, youths are exposed to myriad conflicting cultural values, as the values and practices of their cultural heritage may diverge considerably from those of the new culture. In these circumstances, the ability to navigate among the influences of the different cultures, often discussed within the contexts of the issues of enculturation and acculturation, is associated with a range of consequences related to social competence and mental health. The issue of adolescent development in relation to cultural conflict continues to be an essential consideration in understanding the long-term social and emotional outcomes among Aboriginal communities due to their histories and experiences with European culture and, more recently, due to the impact of global Internet communication and mass media. For example, dismissing or devaluing the significance of cultural heritage and traditions may be adaptive for increasing the probability of achieving the short-term goals of acceptance from a non-minority peer group and protecting one's self-image from the prejudices and discrimination of a mainstream society. However, within the broader context of development, this coping strategy may be maladaptive by forging negative models of self that ultimately compromise emotional well-being.

Zimmerman (1998) studied the concept of enculturation among 21 Odawa and Ojibway Native American youths with a mean age of 11.5 years. Enculturation was defined as pride in the youths' Native American cultural heritage, a strong Native American identity, and participation in Native American cultural activities. He used measures developed with members of the Odawa and Ojibway Tribes to assess whether enculturation works either to mitigate the negative effects of the risk factor of family drug problems (risk-protective mechanism) or to enhance the effects of positive self-esteem, a variable found to decrease the probability of risky behaviour (protective-protective mechanism). The significance of the conceptualization of enculturation was supported by the finding that the youths with the highest levels of both self-esteem and cultural identity reported the lowest levels of alcohol and substance use. However, the unexpected finding that youths with high levels of cultural identity but low levels of self-esteem reported the most alcohol and substance abuse reflects the complexity in the relationship between self-esteem and cultural identity and even in the assessment of each of these variables. For example, the finding that, among the three variables of enculturation, only cultural affinity predicted self-esteem and only cultural identity predicted alcohol and substance use suggests that these components may differentially affect developmental outcomes. This particular pattern of findings may be relevant only to the specific group that was studied and only to the specific period in development that was assessed. Alternatively, it reflects limitations in the measures. Thus the relations among specific components of enculturation need to be assessed more carefully by means of various methods, with groups of youth in different developmental periods, and across a wide range of communities (Zimmerman et al. 1996). This is consistent with the notion that in a culturally diverse society such as North America, youth may belong to multiple social groups on the basis of minority status, ethnicity, race, language, social class, and religion. Thus categorization according to affiliation with, for instance, one ethnic or racial group is inadequate. Alternatively, ascertaining an individual's cultural framework may be achieved through multidimensional classification systems that take into account the individual's experiences and perspectives (McLoyd 1999).

Burgeoning multiculturalism and the complexities presented by persons developing in changing contexts pose both opportunities and challenges for the study of the impact of cultural processes on the etiology and course of mental health among Aboriginal persons. The differences and similarities between minority and Aboriginal youths afford a unique opportunity to compare the course of adjustment with regard to developmental problems and competence. Comparisons in developmental profiles are valuable for providing information about risk and protective factors that are specific to a certain subculture or more generally applicable to life within mainstream North American society for those who are not raised in that community (Luthar and Burack 2000). The relations among culture, subculture, and psychopathology are highlighted as various issues are addressed. These include the prevalence of various youth problems, the specific problems for which youth are referred to mental health specialists, and the relation between referral to mental health services and adult attitudes and beliefs regarding etiology and appropriate remediation in cultures that differ markedly in beliefs and childrearing practices (Weisz et al. 1997). Accordingly, comparisons across or within the major Aboriginal cultural groups are equally valuable and may provide a better understanding of the consequences of youth problem clusters, the distribution of resources across and within communities, and differences between rural and urban settings.

School, Peer, and Family Systems and the Mental Health of Aboriginal Youth

Human development is inherently sociocultural, and thus mental health issues can best be understood within the context from which they have emerged (Bateson 1979; Wertsch and Tulviste 1992). This notion is particularly relevant in the case of children and adolescents who are inherently dependent on their parents, schools, and communities for healthy development. Moreover, the impact of sociocultural variations on development and well-being may be most pronounced during childhood and adolescence (Weisz et al. 1997), as the adolescent period is marked by fundamental developmental changes that include self-identity formation and experimentation (Zimmerman et al. 1996) and learning to understand the self in relation to peers, family, and community (Borysenko 1996). The focus on youth is practical, as early development is more malleable and thus more responsive to intervention (Nelson 2000).

Research initiatives focused on Aboriginal youth in North America are particularly timely, for recent estimates suggest that the Aboriginal population is growing at an average annual rate of about 2.3%, more than twice the rate of the rest of the Canadian population. In the Canadian census for 1996, the average age of the Aboriginal population was approximately 25.5 years, roughly 10 years younger than other Canadians. Nearly 38% of all Aboriginal people were under the age of 15 years, compared to 21% of the total Canadian population. The population of Aboriginal youth is expected to grow at a rate of about 1.4% annually through the period 1996-2011, twice that of the general population. A more rapid rate of growth (about 2.4% annually) is expected during this period in the Aboriginal labour force (aged 15 to 64 years) (National Aboriginal Youth Strategy 1999). Of greater concern, Aboriginal youths are proportionally overrepresented in any census of social-behavioural and other health problems, as they experience higher rates of school failure, encounter more risk of substance abuse, and are more likely to take their own lives than are children of the dominant, non-Native culture (Royal Commission on Aboriginal Peoples 1996).

The factors that jeopardize the well-being of Aboriginal youth are not always the same as those of the majority culture. The US National School Based Youth Risk Survey indicates that American Indian and Native Alaskan youths are more likely to carry weapons, attempt suicide, and use drugs (i.e., cigarettes, marijuana, and cocaine) more often than black or white youths (Frank and Lester 2002). In addition to differences in symptom manifestation, the developmental pattern of mental health needs may be discrepant between Aboriginal and non-Aboriginal youths. For example, Beiser and Attneave (1982) compared treatment data from the US Indian Health Service with data from hospitals and mental health clinics providing service to non-Natives in those states in which reservations are located. They found that roughly the same proportions of Aboriginal and non-Aboriginal children contacted mental health facilities before 9 years of age and that both groups showed a steady increase from then until the age of 19 years, but they also noted that the increase for Aboriginal youths was steeper than for non-Aboriginal youths. By late adolescence, the rate of contact was 4.5 times higher for Aboriginal boys than for non-Aboriginal boys and 5 times higher for Aboriginal girls than for non-Aboriginal girls. Although some of these group differences may reflect the relatively common teacher bias in reporting more mental health problems among minority youth (Beiser et al. 1998; Fisher, Bacon, and Storck 1998; Fisher, Storck, and Bacon 1999), especially among non-Aboriginal teachers (Sack et al. 1993), they highlight the difficulties that Aboriginal youth experience in their daily living abilities.

The major mental health problems of youth are usually cumulative and often recur during vulnerable periods of developmental and life transitions. With regard to Aboriginal youth, the accumulation of developmental risk factors over time may lead to particularly deleterious outcomes, for Aboriginal adolescents are 5 to 6 times more likely overall to die from suicide than is the average Canadian adolescent (Kirmayer 1994). Suicides in Aboriginal communities often occur in clusters (see Niezen, Chapter 8), and compared to suicides among non-Aboriginal persons, they are more likely to be alcohol-related, to be associated with specific stressors such as conflicts and disruptions of relationships (Duberstein, Conwell, and Caine 1993), and to involve the use of guns (Cooper et al. 1992; May 1990). Both the psychological and contextual factors related to suicide need to be delineated more precisely since the risk patterns differ between Aboriginal and non-Aboriginal groups and since incidences of suicidal behaviour can vary significantly even across Aboriginal communities (Lester 1997). Group differences with regard to psychological factors are highlighted by the finding of Sack and colleagues (1994) that First Nations elementary school students from a range of communities and regions showed fewer symptoms of depression (typically considered a risk for suicide) but higher suicidal ideation than did their non-Aboriginal peers. Although these findings may reflect either the diminished sensitivity of available assessment tools to identify more subtle signs of depression among Aboriginal youth or cultural differences in willingness to verbalize suicidal ideation, they nevertheless reflect different clinical presentations between the groups. The differential effects of community context are also evident among British Columbia's nearly 200 Native groups, in which suicide rates range from 800 times the national average in a few communities to virtually zero in others (Chandler and Lalonde 1998; Chandler and Lalonde, Chapter 10).

Resilience: Competence in the Context of Adversity

Various risk factors, such as single-parent families, poor economic conditions, and geographically isolated communities, are typically associated with the increased incidence of a wide range of negative outcomes, including teenage suicide, substance abuse, frequent incarceration, long-term unemployment, and histories of disruptive social and familial relationships among Aboriginal youths (Kirmayer 1994; Mao, Moloughney, and Seminciw 1992). Despite these risks, however, the majority of Aboriginal adolescents do not succumb to high-risk behaviours or self-destructive outcomes (Cummins et al. 1999). These outcome variations are suggestive of the potential diversity of supportive resources available within certain communities and indicate the need for a better understanding of the complex transactions among personal attributes, characteristics of the family environment, and the larger sociocultural context in determining healthy outcomes among First Nations adolescents who remain resilient in the face of adversity (Chandler and Lalonde 1998). Indeed, the widespread public perception that Aboriginal youth lead desperate and even tragic lives detracts attention from the diverse positive resources available to them within their communities. Thus the emphasis needs to be shifted from vulnerabilities, adaptational problems, and associated risk factors to potential protective factors and processes that highlight the specific strengths of Aboriginal youth and that may foster resilient development. This shift in perspective is not only theoretically and methodologically consistent with an integrative developmental approach but also relevant to individual and societal expectations regarding the health of Aboriginal youth. The task is redefined as identifying and sharing strengths rather than remediating inherently problematic youth or communities.

Within a developmental framework, resilience is the positive end of the distribution of possible outcomes and is dependent upon the individual's capacity to use internal and external resources to successfully resolve stage-salient developmental challenges despite high-risk status, chronic stress, or experiences of prolonged or severe trauma (Masten, Best, and Garmezy 1990; Rutter and Sroufe 2000; Waters and Sroufe 1983). The developmental significance is that competence in one period allows the individual to adapt to the environment and to prepare for competence in the next period (Burack 1997; Sroufe and Rutter 1984). Thus current adaptation is a product of both prevailing circumstances and developmental history (Bowlby 1980; Rutter and Sroufe 2000). However, competence in resolving issues in one developmental period does not predict later competence in a linear and deterministic way, as resilience at one time does not guarantee resilience at a later point (Coie et al. 1993). For example, inner-city youths who are considered resilient because of high IQ, academic success, or other indices of competence also show increased levels of depression and anxiety in comparison to competent adolescents from low-stress backgrounds (Luthar 1997; Luthar, Cicchetti, and Becker 2000). Children who are apparently successful in meeting the expectations of mainstream society may be shunned by their peers at a cost to their emotional well-being (Luthar and Burack 2000). This evidence that resilience in one domain may be associated with problems in another is incompatible with the notion of global resilience, for it highlights that resilience is a dynamic process that must be evaluated according to context, specific stage of development, and domain of functioning. In a study of the characteristics of resilience among 59 First Nations adolescents from a remote community in Quebec, Zygmuntowicz and colleagues (2000) found that students classified as resilient – due to their evidenced behavioural competence despite high levels of stress – reported lower levels of anxiety and similar levels of depression in comparison to behaviourally competent adolescents with low stress. Similar to non-Aboriginal inner-city youth living under high-stress conditions (Luthar 1995), behaviourally competent Aboriginal youth from a remote northern community did not experience socioemotional problems even though they reported high levels of stress. This finding highlights the importance of specifying domains of competence when defining resilience in Aboriginal youth.

The study of resilience is particularly pertinent to understanding the experience of Aboriginal adolescents who face challenges associated with the developmental transitions from infancy through adulthood within a context of physical, social, and emotional adversity yet generally manage to function adaptively (Cummins et al. 1999). The goal is to highlight the individual, family, community, and environmental factors that are associated with positive outcomes despite adversity. The individual and family factors might help to highlight the attitudes, attributes, and personality characteristics that predispose adolescents to successful adaptation and that should be the foci of intervention programs. Concordantly, the delineation of community and other environmental factors will provide information about the risk and protective factors that should be the focus of governmental and community-based programs. This range of considerations for intervention is necessary due to the multiplicity of risk factors and the complexity of the developmental process and its outcomes.

Competence in School Contexts

The numbers of Aboriginal students in the schools are increasing, but they are still considerably less likely than non-Aboriginal students to graduate from high school (Cummins et al. 1999; Tonkin et al. 1999; Hallet et al. 2004). For example, the overall dropout rate for a cohort consisting of all self-identified Aboriginal youth in the Province of British Columbia who started Grade 7 in 1995 and who lived on a reserve was 66% for those who failed to graduate within a two-year window of their final year and 41% for those who never reached Grade 12. However, rates for both these indices of school attrition for each individual band varied dramatically from 0% to 100% and were associated with a host of community-level factors (Hallet et al. 2004).

The barriers to success in the schools are typically related to a range of factors that arise from incompatibilities between the Aboriginal and majority cultures (Janosz et al. 1997). For example, the relatively small number of Aboriginals who participate in the educational system as administrators and teachers, especially in the high school years, is problematic, as it leaves the education to others and thereby diminishes the possibility of positive academic role models (Fisher et al. 1998). The increased numbers of non-Aboriginal educators results in a lack of cultural awareness by staff, which in turn leads to environments that are not particularly conducive to a positive learning experience for Aboriginal students. For example, Day (1992) found that the relationship with teachers was largely negative for many Aboriginal students, as the teachers lacked training in Aboriginal studies, knew very little about the ways that Aboriginal students differed from other students, and had low expectations and stereotypes of Aboriginal students.

Opportunities for success are also diminished by the institution of curricula that do not include the teaching of Native culture or values, the utilization of teaching methods that do not benefit from the strengths of Aboriginal students, and the creation of environments that are not consistent with Aboriginal ways of life (Yates 1987). For example, with regard to teaching methodology, education in the majority culture typically involves verbal instruction rather than imitation and also involves strategies for active participation, which are typically preferred by Aboriginal communities and consistent with greater physical activity in their societies (Brant 1990). Similarly, with regard to environment, the competition that is valued in majority-culture schools is inconsistent with Aboriginal communities' tendency toward co-operation (Beiser et al. 1998; Fisher et al. 1998).

The lack of synchrony between Aboriginal and majority cultures in the school is evident in the findings from a longitudinal study of elementary school children in which the children from the majority culture perceived themselves as increasingly competent in school, whereas the self-perceived competence of First Nations children tended to decrease over the early school years (Sack et al. 1993). The consequences of failure can often begin early for First Nations children, who often suffer from a lack of school readiness that inevitably leads to eroding self-concept (Beiser et al. 1998). During these years, the relation between children's self-perceptions and teachers' ratings tend to become stronger among non-Aboriginal children but weaker among Aboriginal youths, suggesting an asynchrony between academic setting and other areas of socialization in the Aboriginal group, for whom the importance of teacher regard and objective measures of success are diminished (Beiser et al. 1993). Beiser and colleagues (1993) suggest that First Nations youth look to areas other than academics for validation of self-perception, as school is often a place both of expected failure and of conflict with the mainstream culture. This is consistent with the notion that in the self-evaluation of competence among non-Aboriginal youths there are higher levels of integration of feelings about the home and school influences than among Aboriginal children, for whom the influence of the home environment on academic self-concept virtually disappears by the mid-elementary school grades (Beiser and Attneave 1982).

The dissociation between school and home for the students also reflects the attitudes and behaviours of their parents and other members of their communities, who are more likely to be alienated from the educational process and whose participation in decisions about and involvement in the children's education are likely to be minimized (Janosz et al. 1997; Walton 1999). Rural American Indian parents, many of whom did not enjoy successful experiences in school or did not even attend school, are less comfortable just entering the school and are less likely to interact with teachers (Fisher et al. 1999). This divide between settings is further exacerbated by the difference between the parents' and Elders' interpretations of children's behaviours and the interpretations of teachers, especially non-Aboriginal ones, who are more likely to focus on and to be critical of acting-out behaviours (Fisher et al. 1998; Fisher et al. 1999). This discrepancy is highlighted by the commentaries of Elders and members of one rural community who viewed acting out in relation to school authority not as pathological but as a valued extension of the cultural value of the "young warrior" and as an adaptive response to adverse social and living conditions (Fisher et al. 1998). Conversely, internalizing behaviours such as social withdrawal were viewed by the Elders as especially concerning and considered both potentially maladaptive and culturally incongruous (Fisher et al. 1998). This is consistent with the finding that non-Aboriginal teachers are likely to refer more Aboriginal than non-Aboriginal students for educational and psychological services (Sack et al. 1993). This confluence of school-related attitudes among children, parents, and communities that are both ambivalent and in contradiction with many of those held by the educators poses a considerable risk factor for deleterious academic and related outcomes.

The institutionalized deficiencies in the education of Aboriginal children were historically translated into repeated and widespread lack of academic success among Aboriginal Canadians throughout the twentieth century. According to Statistics Canada (2003), 59% of Inuit youth dropped out of school in 2001, compared to 66% in 1996; 42% of Métis youth dropped out, compared to 47% in 1996; and 48% of nonreserve North American Indian youth dropped out, compared to 52% in 1996. The 2001 report of Statistics Canada also revealed that 39% of Aboriginal people aged 24 to 44 residing in nonreserve areas had completed postsecondary studies. The postsecondary gap between Aboriginal people and others has narrowed slightly with time to 71 Aboriginal people for every 100 non-Aboriginal people. Even among high school graduates, fewer Aboriginal than non-Aboriginal students attended university, and, of those who attended, Aboriginal students were 2.5 times more likely than their non-Aboriginal peers to drop out (Armstrong, Kennedy, and Oberle 1990). The high failure and dropout rates suggest that school initiatives are particularly critical to Aboriginal communities (Armstrong et al. 1990; Cummins et al. 1999; LaFromboise and Low 1991; Tonkin et al. 1999). For example, in one study of American Indian students, those who dropped out were more likely to commit delinquent acts, including the use of illegal substances, as the amount of time spent in a structured and monitored setting was diminished (Beauvais 1996). In turn, an increase in delinquent behaviour further decreases adolescents' chances of returning to school and graduating, and it consequently minimizes their chances to obtain meaningful employment and ultimately places them at greater risk for incarceration (Loeber and Farrington 1998). Low self-esteem, low expectations for success, and feelings of hopelessness are common among adolescents who drop out (Jessor, Turbin, and Costa 1998). These scenarios of emotional developmental risk are evident among Aboriginal and other minority youth, for whom school dropout is implicated in lower levels of emotional health and higher rates of depression and suicide.

The necessity of fostering academic success is highlighted by the evidence that First Nations adolescents who stay in school report the same high levels of connectedness to school and families as their non-Aboriginal peers and generally do well (Tonkin et al. 1999). This effort needs to begin with basics such as school attendance, which is related to a range of variables like school achievement, school commitment, and grades (Janosz et al. 1997). In turn, perceptions of school as a community, maintenance of positive feelings toward school, and enjoyment of school protect adolescents from feelings of hopelessness and foster positive developmental outcomes (Battistich and Hom 1997; Dexheimer-Pharris, Resnick, and Blum 1997). Successful Australian Aboriginal students were found to be aware of the importance of individual effort, to accept that success at school was important to future success, and to have clear long-term goals (Day 1992). Among Aboriginal communities, variables such as a strong personal and group identity, good peer relationships and family support, participation in extracurricular activities, and involvement with traditional cultural activities are associated with reduced dropout rates (Cummins et al. 1999; Day 1992; Mahoney and Cairns 1997; McCormick 1996; Ystgaard 1997), thereby highlighting the need to provide a setting in which conventional academic curricula, nonacademic school activities, and traditional Aboriginal culture are integrated and prioritized.

Competence in Peer Contexts

Within a model of the development of social competence, peer influences are considered essential predictors of both successful adaptation and heightened risk among adolescents, as they impact the level of participation in both adaptive and maladaptive activities (Luthar 1997). In particular, the deleterious effects of the influences that foster maladaptive behaviours are magnified among youths who are initially at risk due to minority status and problematic living environments and who are thus less protected by societal safety nets (Luthar and Burack 2000). The potentially harmful aspects of peer influence include both participation in activities such as alcohol use, drug use, and unprotected sex and participation in delinquent behaviours that can lead directly to a range of problematic outcomes and to a neglect of other activities that are typically beneficial to adaptive development, such as those related to academic and extracurricular involvement.

The influence of peers on participation in potentially harmful behaviours is common across contemporary cultures, although individual differences may be evident among groups (Cushman 1990; Grob and de Rios 1992). The strongest predictor of substance abuse is one's association with a peer group whose acquisition and use of psychotropic substances are habitual (Cushman 1990).

Beauvais (1992) administered anonymous drug surveys annually from 1975 to 1990 to a US nationally representative sample of Indian youths in Grades 7 to 12 who resided on or near reservations. To obtain a sample that was representative of the range of Tribal characteristics, each year a stratified sample of 5 to 7 Tribes was drawn that varied on a number of demographic and cultural dimensions, including geographic distribution, income and education levels, and language and cultural grouping. The findings of the survey indicated that American Aboriginal youth on reservations are more likely to abuse drugs than nonreservation Aboriginals and non-Aboriginals. Youths who lived on reservations were more likely to report more friends who were heavy drug users and to be involved in risky drug-related behaviour. These types of deleterious peer influences were also evident in a study of urban-dwelling Canadian Aboriginal youth at high risk for psychosocial problems. Gfellner (1991) selected a sample of Indian youth from a database of students in Grades 5 to 12 (*N* = 3,523) who attended schools in nonurban communities in central Canada. In this population most of the students, or 88.7%, described themselves as white, 6.7% as Indian, 0.6% as black, 1.9% as Asian, and 3.1% as belonging to another group. A random sample was selected numbering 236 participants, of whom 118 Indian adolescents were matched with 118 white adolescents in terms of grade, gender, family structure, and mother's level of completed education. The mean age was 13.9 years for Indian adolescents and 14.2 years for white adolescents. Virtually all the youths who were involved in problem behaviours and delinquency maintained friendships with peers who used alcohol, drugs, or solvents and who engaged in delinquent behaviour. Within this type of milieu, the impact of peer attitudes was so strong that substance abuse seemed to be perceived as a normative behaviour among the group. The influence of these peers extended even to the effectiveness of the related intervention program, as a significant proportion, or 34%, of the participants dropped out because their friends did not attend, indicating that preventative strategies should focus on the social context of the peer group.

Grob and de Rios (1992) go beyond the issue of peer influences and argue that research on adolescent drug use is decontextualized, for it fails to consider the cultural variables of societal breakdown, meaninglessness, and social stress as well as, most important, the contextual meaning of drug use. They suggest that researchers should draw on a wealth of ethnographic data from societies ranging from foragers and hunter-gatherers to agriculturalists. They examined the adolescent ceremonial drug-use practices of the Australian Aborigine, the Shangana-Tsonga of Mozambique, and the Chumash of California. In each of these groups, a key feature of the rituals for adolescents at puberty was the cultural utilization of hallucinogenic plants. The drugs were managed by adult tutors to create states of consciousness, particularly hyper-suggestible ones, in order to enculturate the adolescents with a culturally sanctioned educational experience necessary for their survival and bonding as an adult member of the community. During the altered state of consciousness, the Elders would model culturally appropriate adolescent behaviour, religious beliefs, and secular values. The authors concluded that, based on this cross-cultural data, drug experimentation does not have to entail psychologically catastrophic implications. They emphasized the importance of the community as well as the cultural context of meaning that gives pattern and structure to the drug experience.

The role of peers extends beyond participation in substance abuse, sexual activity, and delinquent behaviours to other indices of social competence, especially school attendance and performance. For example, peer pressure is considered a primary influence on the decision by Aboriginal students to drop out of school (Narrandera High School 1986; Cavanagh 1988). Whereas the presence of friends at school initially enhances the desire to study, the incentive to stay diminishes as friends leave school (Cavanagh 1988). Thus the large dropout rates among Aboriginal students may reflect a deleterious cycle in which adolescents who leave school then influence others to also drop out and face the various consequences associated with a lack of education. Conversely, the initial findings that academic success among Aboriginal students is not associated with social rejection, as it is in inner-city minority groups, and that children can both succeed in school and maintain ties with their Native culture are indicators that peer influences are not necessarily detrimental (Burack et al. 2000). The positive relation between academic success and positive peer relationships was illustrated by the finding of Flanagan and colleagues (2002) that higher nonverbal IQs were positively associated with elevated levels of academic performance, peer preference, and positive classroom behaviour among Aboriginal adolescents attending a band school on a reserve in northern Quebec.

Competence in Family Contexts

Aboriginal families may experience many stressors, including family violence, unemployment, limited supports, injuries, and health problems throughout the life course. A sense of belonging in one's family may foster healthy self-identity development and a sense of purpose and future among Aboriginal adolescents (Carter and McGoldrick 1999). For example, parental relationships as well as family support and cohesiveness are related to school completion and plans to continue education after high school (Tonkin et al. 1999). Similarly, high levels of family involvement and connectedness are also associated with diminished risk-taking behaviours such as involvement in physical fights, alcohol abuse, and truancy (Tonkin et al. 1999). These relations point to the prioritization of programs that foster family well-being as a means to ameliorate some of the primary factors associated with developmental risk among Aboriginal youth.

The effects of single parenting is particularly relevant, as single-parent families headed by women were about twice as common among status Natives in comparison to other Canadian families during the past decade. According to Statistics Canada (2003), far fewer Aboriginal children aged 14 and under lived with two parents in 2001 than did non-Aboriginal children. Approximately 65% of Aboriginal children living on reserves lived with two parents; in contrast, almost 83% of non-Aboriginal children lived with two parents. On reserves, 32% of Aboriginal children lived with a lone parent, a rate roughly twice that of non-Aboriginal children. Approximately 5% of Aboriginal children living in large urban areas did not live with their parents, a rate 8 times that of non-Aboriginal children. The impact of single or foster parenting depends on local social and cultural factors that determine the degree of support by extended family, relatives, Elders, and other members of the community. Parenting and family variables are implicated in the adjustment of minority and non-minority adolescents (Maccoby 1992). Research on parenting styles among diverse ethnic groups in the United States provides an illustration of the ways that cultural differences can moderate the effects of protective or risk factors. Whereas high levels of authoritative parenting styles (e.g., warmth, democratically firm control, granting psychological autonomy) are associated with positive psychosocial outcomes among white and Hispanic adolescents, African American and Asian American adolescents of authoritative parents fare no better or worse than their peers of the same ethnic group who are from authoritarian homes (e.g., strict discipline, physical control, criticism) (Deater-Deckard and Dodge 1997). These findings highlight the importance of considering the "cultural meaning" of specific family-based protective factors rather than simply their surface characteristics (Chao 1994) and may be informative for understanding family resources, practices, and parenting styles among Aboriginal families. Ultimately, the goal is to identify the culture-specific family practices that contribute to school involvement and other health-promoting behaviours among Aboriginal adolescents.

Promoting Mental Health for Aboriginal Youth and Their Communities

The application of a developmental approach to the study of mental health among Aboriginal persons in Canada is based on several premises. First, certain basic principles of development are applicable across populations, and the findings from each can be informative about others. Second, development is progressive, as the individual actively evolves in a more differentiated and integrated way. Third, development is inherently systemic, given that the many different physiological and psychological components of the individual as well as the family, school, community, and physical aspects of the environment in relation to the individual's functioning affect each other and given that the individual continues to impact and be impacted by the environment. Fourth, adaptation occurs in relation both to the developmental level of the individual and to the nuances of the specific environments, including complex and continually changing patterns of risk and protective factors. Within this developmental framework, universal processes of development may be expressed in culturally specific ways and may emerge uniquely for each individual in his or her specific context. Thus the focus is on the evolving relations among the multiple factors involved in development rather than on a search either for pathology in the individual or for inherent problems in the family, community, or environment.

Protective factors at various ecological levels may contribute to adaptive outcomes among Aboriginal youth. However, the evidence is piecemeal and indirect. A more comprehensive analysis of multiple protective factors – including the community, school, peer, and family – at various ecological levels is needed to determine how protective factors serve to propel development toward more adaptive pathways. Specifically, comprehensive longitudinal studies of the development of social competence, risk, and resilience among Aboriginal youth would provide information invaluable to preventing the major mental health problems that plague some Aboriginal communities.

The primary challenge to this approach concerns the relevance of notions from other communities to specific North American Aboriginal peoples, who have historical experience that is unique in comparison to that of the persons in the majority culture or even to that of other minority groups. This is further exacerbated by the vast differences in culture, lifestyles, and histories of the hundreds of Aboriginal communities across North America, despite some shared characteristics. The challenge, then, is to highlight the ways that developmental principles can be implemented meaningfully in order to work on promoting mental health in specific communities or with particular groups. This entails collaboration with the communities through which areas of expertise are adapted and implemented, collaboration in ways that are consistent with Aboriginal values and interests and that are ultimately transmitted to members of the community.

The community is best viewed as a social influence that affects the well-being and health of individual members. Protective factors present in the community may mediate or moderate the effects of environmental stressors on development. For example, the effects of familial disruptions may be moderated by a strong sense of social support.

Social support networks, including schools, recreational centres, and places for spiritual worship, are fundamental to the functioning of any community, although the values of the dominant culture largely determine the social and economic environments of communities. Consequently, adolescents from minority cultures face greater risks, including conflicts of identity, decreased self-esteem, poor school performance, and increased depression due to marginalization, lack of access to services, and loss or devaluation of culture, language, and spirituality (Luthar and Burack 2000; Mosley-Howard 1995; Sameroff et al. 1997).

The empowerment of Aboriginal communities, including those on reserves and in cities, should enhance the availability, utilization, and effectiveness of community mental health programs. The first step is to ensure that persons who need the services are willing and able to access them, which is often not the case among Aboriginal persons (Kirmayer, Malus, and Boothroyd 1996; Kirmayer et al. 1993). These limitations extend to community facilities ranging from schools to mental health centres. The schools need to be more accessible, and the administrators and educators should reach out to parents, who often feel alienated, intimidated, or disconnected. Similarly, the relative underutilization of mental health services by Aboriginal persons suggests that the services and facilities need to be better highlighted and more positively portrayed within communities. Success in first maximizing participation and then facilitating positive outcomes in both education and mental health is largely contingent on the knowledge and incorporation of cultural, familial, and individual value systems (Sameroff and Fiese 1990; Toth and Cicchetti 1999).

The focus on life stories, both at an individual and community level, is an effective way to access cultural values and a powerful vehicle for teaching and transmitting values. Narrative approaches are grounded in the theory that humans are inherently searching for and constructing meaning from experience. Narratives serve to integrate life's events by assimilating experiences into pre-existing frames of reference and thus help to maintain a secure and enduring sense of self (White 2001). Implicit in this view is the notion that meaning is co-constructed through the process of dialogue and interpersonal exchange between active participants. Thus the focus is on the process of communication and use of language, in addition to the content imbued in the telling of the life story. Due to their consistency with Aboriginal oral traditions and practices, narrative approaches may be a particularly useful means to teach about the culture, to offer counsel about traumatic life events, or to conduct qualitative analysis in the study of Aboriginal youth (Stuhlmiller 2001; White and Epston 1994). One example is the use of narrative-based counselling for Aboriginal youth and communities who may have experienced traumatic events or witnessed an anomalous event such as a suicide. Traumatic experiences or those that are discordant with one's sense of self may disrupt the natural ability to construct a unified story that could connect the past, present, and future self across time (McAdams and Janis 2004) and that could play a protective role against suicide among Aboriginal youth (Chandler and Lalonde 1998).

The Aboriginal traditions of healing and sharing circles (McCormick 1996) and an emphasis on co-operation (Beiser et al. 1998; Fisher et al. 1998) suggest that group approaches to therapy might be particularly appropriate frameworks for intervention with Aboriginal adolescents. These approaches are especially valuable in the context of youth programs that focus on psychoeducation, counselling, and mental health problems (e.g., Brown 1993; Julian and Kilmann 1979; Scheidlinger 1985). Youths perceive group approaches as more normalizing (Aronson and Scheidlinger 2002; Scheidlinger 1985) and in these contexts report a higher degree of involvement, support, and open expression than do those who are treated in individual settings (Towberman 1993). Clinicians also report that youth who participate in group interventions are able to relate to the group leaders and peers, have more opportunity to be supportive of one another, and develop empathy toward others in the group (Towberman 1993). These benefits to children and adolescents appear concordant with the emphasis of many Aboriginal groups on community, co-operation, and narratives, and they suggest that group frameworks should be considered in the promotion of wellness.

The potential advantages of group intervention with Aboriginal youths, their peers, their families, and their communities should be considered within the contexts of current forms of intervention that might be appropriated for work with Aboriginal youths. One example is the multiple family group therapy (MFGT) approach, which involves treatment of 4 to 5 families and entails a focus on various systemic levels ranging from individual to community in a co-operative setting (Laqueur 1976). Within this framework, individual youths are viewed within their larger family and peer context, and the family is viewed within a broader community context that includes other families. Natural group-based helping processes are combined with aspects of professional helping techniques to create a therapeutic community and social network (Cassano 1989; McFarlane and Cunningham 1996). Over the course of treatment, strengths and resources within the group are highlighted and shared; thus intrafamily and interfamily interaction and helping processes increase, while professional interaction and involvement decrease (Cassano 1989). The main therapeutic elements of MFGT include an emphasis on universality in the human condition, a sense of community in confronting mental health issues (Laqueur 1972; Yalom 1995), and an opportunity for membership in a group with demonstrated capacity for autonomous functioning (Cassano 1989). The MFGT technique may be particularly useful for non-Aboriginal clinicians, who can draw on culturally specific knowledge and processes that are embedded within the therapeutic group to facilitate change within Aboriginal families. Although MFGT appears helpful when implemented with inner-city and minority youth and their families (McKay McKernan et al. 1995), its effectiveness needs to be further evaluated with Aboriginal families. In addition, the implementation of this or any other relatively intense treatment program needs to be considered with regard to community resources and participation.

The processes of highlighting strengths and communicating and sharing resources that empower youth and families to self-direct change within a therapeutic group may be

GRACE IAROCCI, RHODA ROOT, AND JACOB A. BURACK

extended to initiate positive change processes on a broader community level. Accordingly, research on the protective buffering effects of community embeddedness, family cohesion, self-identity, and self-continuity that are thought to contribute to resilience among certain Aboriginal communities may serve a similar therapeutic function by empowering communities to carry out their own therapeutic work and to promote health from within. Developmental research could extend beyond the identification of the distribution of risk and protective factors within Aboriginal communities and provide a better understanding that could be more broadly shared across Aboriginal communities. For example, each community has needs and resources and thus may both learn from and serve as a model for other communities. The unification of the many sources of "protective practices" that already operate in certain communities would provide an opportunity for other communities to learn new ways to promote mental health among their own youth. The premise of this approach is that Aboriginal communities hold the key to their own success in effectively addressing their youths' problems. Accessing the key requires information, not remediation; rather than importing solutions based on non-Aboriginal standards and values, researchers and clinicians need to uncover and harness the relevant knowledge.

An integrative developmental perspective provides a useful framework to study concurrently the myriad processes that interact and thus contribute in complex ways to fostering desirable or maladaptive mental health outcomes in Aboriginal youth. Effective policy development originates with reflective consideration of input from the community, families, and youth. This is achieved through extensive involvement of youth and community members as active participants rather than subjects of study or intervention. The ultimate goal is to provide information that will promote community-based capacities and efforts (Kirmayer, Simpson, and Cargo 2003).

The Developmental Challenges of a Budding Discipline

The integration of the two disciplines of cultural and developmental psychology involves the coalescence of contrasting worldviews and empirical frameworks, a process that, although largely beneficial and informative, is replete with difficulties in its application to empirical methodology and interpretation (Burack 1997; Weisz et al. 1997). Werner's organismic-developmental theory, originally formulated to explain increased differentiation in human development, provides a framework for conceptualizing the course of maturation of cultural and developmental psychology and its acceptance as a new discipline (Cicchetti and Cohen 1995; Werner 1957). Within Werner's framework, the initial developmental stages involve a global understanding with a preliminary focus on the apparent commonalties in development across culturally diverse groups of children and little attention to the distinctions among them. In the subsequent stage, a more precise and detailed understanding of the constituent parts of the whole is the focus, for the priority is the analysis of the finer details and differentiation among characteristics of different cultural groups. Ultimately, in the most mature stage of development, the differentiated parts are organized and integrated into the whole at a higher level of analysis as the essential unity and rich diversity of developmental phenomena are integrated into a cohesive framework. At this stage, the recognition that culture and development cannot be understood by dissecting their dynamic systems into their constituent parts emerges as the meaning and purpose of each part is embedded within the fabric of the whole. An integrative approach permits the analysis of essential aspects (i.e., interdependency and relations among the parts) that give meaning to the overall picture of development. For example, the development of persons with different cultural practices and beliefs, life histories, or living situations is uniquely informative to understanding the boundaries of typical development. And developmental guidelines provide insight about the occurrence and severity of delays and/or deviance within a specific population and context.

Within this type of integrative developmental framework, researchers identify the level at which specific cultural processes affect development and elucidate which of the many factors that distinguish cultures from one another are critical for understanding development (Bukowski and Sippola 1998). Accordingly, understanding the phenomena from within the culture entails both quantitative and qualitative methods (Sullivan 1998), such as the acquisition of multiple sources of information in multiple contexts, the use of culturally sensitive and specific measures, the comparison of specific cultural groups, dynamic assessments of interactions as they unfold over time, and multidimensional analyses and interpretations (Canino and Guarnaccia 1997; Garcia Coll and Magnusson 1999; Mohler 2001). The goal is to appropriately investigate differences and similarities in the risk and protective factors and mechanisms associated with mental health, well-being, and psychopathology at several different levels of process, including cultures and subcultures, communities, schools, families, and individuals (Cicchetti 1993; Cicchetti and Lynch 1993; Garcia Coll et al. 2000).

References

Armstrong, R., J. Kennedy, and P.R. Oberle. 1990. *University education and economic well-being: Indian achievement and prospects.* Ottawa, ON: Minister of Supply and Services Canada.

Aronson, S., and S. Scheidlinger, eds. 2002. *Group treatment of adolescents in context: Outpatient, inpatient and school.* Madison, CT: International Universities Press.

Bateson, G. 1979. *Mind and nature: A necessary unity.* New York: Dutton.

Battistich, V., and A. Hom. 1997. The relationship between students' sense of their school as community and their involvement in problem behaviors. *American Journal of Public Health* 87: 1997-2001.

Beauvais, F. 1992. Indian adolescent drug and alcohol use: Recent patterns and consequences. *American Indian and Alaska Native Mental Health Research* 5: Monograph 1.

–. 1996. Trends in drug use among American Indian students and dropouts, 1975-1994. *American Journal of Public Health* 86: 1594-98.

Beiser, M., and C. Attneave. 1982. Mental disorders among Native American children: Rates and risk periods for entering treatment. *American Journal of Psychiatry* 139: 193-98.

–, W. Lancee, A. Gotowiec, W.H. Sack, and R. Redshirt. 1993. Measuring self-perceived role competence among First Nations and non-Native children. *Canadian Journal of Psychiatry* 38: 412-19.

–, W.H. Sack, S. Manson, R. Redshirt, and R. Dion. 1998. Mental health and the academic performance of First Nations and majority culture children. *American Journal of Orthopsychiatry* 68: 455-67.

Borysenko, J. 1996. *A woman's book of life: The biology, psychology, and spirituality of the feminine life cycle.* New York: Riverhead Books.

Bowlby, J. 1980. *Attachment and loss: Loss, sadness and depression.* Vol. 3. New York: Basic Books.

Brant, C.C. 1990. Native ethics and rules of behavior. *Canadian Journal of Psychiatry* 35: 534-39.

Bronfenbrenner, U. 1979. *The ecology of human development.* Cambridge, MA: Harvard University Press.

Brown, L.N. 1993. *Group work and the environment: A systems approach.* Binghamton, UK: Haworth.

Bukowski, W.M., and L.K. Sippola. 1998. Diversity and the social mind: Goals, constructs, culture, and development. *Developmental Psychology* 34: 742-46.

Burack, J.A. 1997. The study of atypical and typical populations in developmental psychopathology: The quest for a common science. In S.S. Luthar, J.A. Burack, D. Cicchetti, and J.R. Weisz, eds., *Developmental psychopathology: Perspectives on adjustment, risk, and disorder,* 139-65. New York: Cambridge University Press.

–, C.E. Zygmuntowicz, T. Mandour, et al. July 2000. Cultural Identity as a protection against social, emotional, and behavioural problems among First Nation adolescents living in a remote community. Paper presented at the Biennial Meeting of the Jerusalem Conference in Canadian Studies, Jerusalem, Israel.

Canino, I.A., and P. Guarnaccia. 1997. Methodological challenges in the assessment of Hispanic children and adolescents. *Applied Developmental Science* 1: 124-34.

Carter, B., and M. McGoldrick, eds. 1999. *The expanded family life cycle: Individual, family and social perspectives.* 3rd ed. Boston: Allyn and Bacon.

Cassano, D.R. 1989. The multi-family therapy group: Research on patterns of interaction: II. *Social Work with Groups* 12: 15-39.

Cavanagh, P. 1988. Koories in year 12: Pressures facing Aboriginal students in senior classes in NSW high schools. *Curriculum Issues* 13: 18-26.

Chandler, M.J. 2000. Surviving time: The persistence of identity in this culture and that. *Culture and Psychology* 6: 209-31.

–, and C.E. Lalonde. 1995. The problem of self-continuity in the context of rapid personal and cultural change. In A. Oosterwegel and R.A. Wicklund, eds., *The self in European and North American culture: Development and processes,* 45-63. Boston: Kluwer.

–, and C.E. Lalonde. 1998. Cultural continuity as a hedge against suicide in Canada's First Nations. *Transcultural Psychiatry* 35: 191-219.

–, C.E. Lalonde, and B. Sokol. 2000. Continuities of selfhood in the face of radical developmental and cultural change. In L. Nucci, G. Saxe, and E. Turiel, eds., *Culture, thought, and development,* 65-84. Mahwah, NJ: Lawrence Erlbaum Associates.

–, C.E. Lalonde, B. Sokol, and D. Hallett. 2003. Personal persistence, identity development and suicide: A study of Native and non-Native North American adolescents. *Monographs of the Society for Research in Child Development* 63 (2): 1-130.

Chao, R.K. 1994. Beyond parental control and authoritarian parenting styles: Understanding Chinese parenting through the cultural notion of training. *Child Development* 65: 1111-19.

Cicchetti, D. 1984. The emergency of developmental psychopathology. *Child Development* 55: 1-7.

–. 1993. Developmental psychopathology: Reaction, reflection, projections. *Developmental Review* 13: 471-502.

–, and M. Lynch. 1993. Toward an ecological/transactional model of community violence and maltreatment: Consequences for children's development. *Psychiatry* 56: 96-118.

–, and D.J. Cohen. 1995. Perspectives on developmental psychopathology. In D. Cicchetti and D.J. Cohen, eds., *Developmental Psychopathology,* vol. 1, *Theory and method,* 3-20. New York: Wiley.

–, and S.L. Toth. 1995. Developmental psychopathology and disorders of affect. In D. Cicchetti and D.J. Cohen, eds., *Developmental psychopathology,* vol. 2, *Risk, disorder and adaptation,* 369-420. New York: Wiley.

–, and S.L. Toth. 1997. Transactional ecological systems in developmental psychopathology. In S.S. Luthar, J.A. Burack, D. Cicchetti, and J.R. Weisz, eds., *Developmental psychopathology: Perspectives on adjustment, risk and disorder,* 317-49. New York: Cambridge University Press.

Coie, J.D., N.F. Watt, S.G. West, et al. 1993. The science of prevention: A conceptual framework and some directions for a national research program. *American Psychologist* 48: 1013-22.

Cooper, M., R. Corrado, A.M. Karlberg, and L.G. Adams. 1992. Aboriginal suicide in British Columbia: An overview. *Canada's Mental Health* 40: 19-23.

Cummings, E.M., P.T. Davies, and S.B. Campbell. 2000. What is developmental psychopathology? In *Developmental psychopathology and family process: Theory, research, and clinical implications,* 17-34. New York: Guilford.

Cummins, J.R.C., M. Ireland, M.D. Resnick, and R.W. Blum. 1999. Correlates of physical and emotional health among Native American adolescents. *Journal of Adolescent Health* 24: 38-44.

Cushman, P. 1990. Why the self is empty: Toward a historically situated psychology. *American Psychologist* 45: 599-611.

Day, A. 1992. Aboriginal students succeeding in the senior high school years: A strengthening and changing Aboriginality challenges the negative stereotype. *Australasian Journal of Gifted Education* 1: 14-26.

Deater-Deckard, K., and K.A. Dodge. 1997. Externalizing behaviour problems and discipline revisited: Non-linear effects and variation by culture, context and gender. *Psychological Enquiry* 8: 161-75.

Dexheimer-Pharris, M., M.D. Resnick, and R.W. Blum. 1997. Protecting against hopelessness and suicidality in sexually abused American Indian adolescents. *Journal of Adolescent Health* 21: 400-6.

Duberstein, P.R., Y. Conwell, and E.D. Caine. 1993. Interpersonal stressors, substance abuse and suicide. *Journal of Nervous and Mental Disease* 181: 80-85.

Elias, M.J., and R.P. Weissberg. 2000. Wellness in the schools: The grandfather of primary prevention tells a story. In D. Cicchetti, J. Rappaport, I. Sandler, and R.P. Weissberg, eds., *The promotion of wellness in children and adolescents,* 243-70. Washington, DC: CWLA Press.

Erikson, E.H. 1968. *Identity, youth and crisis.* New York: Norton.

–. 1975. *Life history and the historical moment.* New York: Norton.

Fisher, P.A., J.G. Bacon, and M. Storck. 1998. Teacher, parent and youth report of problem behaviors among rural American Indian and Caucasian adolescents. *American Indian and Alaska Native Mental Health Research* 8: 1-26.

–, M. Storck, and J.G. Bacon. 1999. In the eye of the beholder: Risk and protective factors in rural American Indian and Caucasian adolescents. *American Journal of Orthopsychiatry* 69: 294-304.

Flanagan, T., C. Zygmuntowicz, J.A. Burack, B. Randolph, G. Iarocci, T. Mandour, and S. Robinson. June 2002. The pathway toward resilience in First Nations adolescents: The contribution of social perspective coordination. Paper presented at the 32nd Annual Meeting of the Jean Piaget Society, Philadelphia, Pennsylvania.

Frank, M., and D. Lester. 2002. Self destructive behaviors in American Indian and Alaska Native high school youth. *American Indian and Alaska Native Mental Health Research* 10: 24-30.

Garcia Coll, C., and K. Magnusson. 1999. Cultural influences on child development: Are we ready for a paradigm shift? In A.S. Masten, ed., *Cultural processes in child development: The Minnesota Symposia on Child Psychology,* 1-24. Mahwah, NJ: Lawrence Erlbaum Associates.

–, A. Akerman, and D. Cicchetti. 2000. Cultural influences on developmental processes and outcomes: Implications for the study of development and psychopathology. *Development and Psychopathology* 12: 333-56.

Gfellner, B.M. 1991. A profile of Aboriginal youth in a community drug program. *Canadian Journal of Native Studies* 11 (1): 25-48.

Good, B.J., and A.M. Kleinman. 1985. Culture and anxiety: Cross-cultural evidence for the patterning of anxiety disorders. In H.A. Tuma and J.D. Maser, eds., *Anxiety and the anxiety disorders*, 297-323. Hillsdale, NJ: Lawrence Erlbaum Associates.

Gotowiec, A., and M. Beiser. 1994. Aboriginal children's mental health: Unique challenges. *Canada's Mental Health* 41 (4): 7-11.

Grob, C., and M.D. de Rios. 1992. Adolescent drug use in cross-cultural perspective. *Journal of Drug Issues* 22 (1): 121-39.

Hallett, D., G. Iarocci, S. Want, L.L. Koopman, and E.C. Gehrke. June 2004. School drop-out rates and cultural continuity: Community-level protective factors in Canada's First Nations youth. Paper presented at the Thirty-Fourth Annual Meeting of the Jean Piaget Society, Toronto, Ontario.

Hallowell, A.I. 1970. Fear and anxiety as cultural and individual variables in a primitive society. In I. Al-Issa and W. Dennis, eds., *Cross-cultural studies of behaviour*, 467-75. New York: Holt, Rinehart and Winston.

Indian and Northern Affairs Canada (INAC). 2002. *First Nations in Canada*. http://www.ainc-inac.gc.ca/pr/pub/index_e.html#f.

Janosz, M., M. LeBlanc, B. Boulerice, and R.E. Tremblay. 1997. Disentangling the weight of school dropout predictors: A test on two longitudinal samples. *Journal of Youth and Adolescence* 26: 733-62.

Jessor, R., M.S. Turbin, and F.M. Costa. 1998. Risk and protection in successful outcomes among disadvantaged adolescents. *Applied Developmental Science* 2: 194-208.

Julian, A., and P.R. Kilmann. 1979. Group treatment of juvenile delinquents: A review of the outcome literature. *International Journal of Group Psychotherapy* 29: 3-37.

Kane, L., and Kanatakta, eds. 1991. *Tsi nitionkwe: Non ne Kanien'keha:ka*. Kanien'kehaka Raotitiohkwa Cultural Centre – Historic Kahnawake Series #6. Kahnawake, QC: Kanien'kehaka Raotitiohkwa Press.

Kim, U. 2000. Indigenous, cultural and cross-cultural psychology: A theoretical, conceptual and epistemological analysis. *Asian Journal of Social Psychology* 3: 265-87.

Kirmayer, L.J. 1994. Suicide among Canadian Aboriginal peoples. *Transcultural Psychiatric Research Review* 31: 3-59.

–, B.C. Hayton, M. Malus, V. Jimenez, R. Dufour, Y. Ternar, T. Yu, and N. Ferrara. 1993. *Suicide in Canadian Aboriginal populations: Emerging trends in research and intervention.* Culture and Mental Health Research Unit Report No. 1., prepared for the Royal Commission on Aboriginal Peoples.

–, A. Young, and B.C. Hayton. 1995. The cultural context of anxiety disorders. *Psychiatric Clinics of North America* 18: 503-21.

–, M. Malus, and L.J. Boothroyd. 1996. Suicide attempts among Inuit youth: A community survey of prevalence and risk factors. *Acta Psychiatrica Scandinavica* 94: 8-17.

–, C. Simpson, and M. Cargo. 2003. Healing traditions: Culture, community and mental health promotion with Canadian Aboriginal peoples. *Australasian Psychiatry* 11 (suppl.): S15-S23.

LaFromboise, T.D., and K.G. Low. 1991. American Indian and adolescents. In J.T. Gibbs and L.N. Huang, eds., *Children of color: Psychological interventions with minority youth*, 114-47. San Francisco, CA: Jossey Bass.

Laqueur, H.P. 1972. Mechanisms of change in multiple family therapy. In C.J. Sager and H.S. Kaplan, eds., *Progress in group and family therapy*, 400-15. New York: Bruner/Mazel.

–. 1976. Multiple family therapy. In P.J. Guerin, ed., *Family therapy: Theory and practice*, 405-16. New York: Gardner.

Lester, D. 1997. *Suicide in American Indians*. New York: Nova Science.

Loeber, R., and D.P. Farrington, eds. 1998. *Serious and violent juvenile offenders: Risk factors and successful interventions*. Thousand Oaks, CA: Sage.

Luthar, S.S. 1995. Social competence in the school setting: Prospective cross-domain associations among inner-city teens. *Child Development* 66: 416-29.

–. 1997. Sociodemographic disadvantage and psychosocial adjustment: Perspectives from developmental psychopathology. In S.S. Luthar, J.A. Burack, D. Cicchetti, and J.R. Weisz, eds., *Developmental psychopathology: Perspectives on adjustment, risk, and disorder*, 459-85. New York: Cambridge University Press.

–, and E. Zigler. 1991. Vulnerability and competence: A review of research on resilience in childhood. *American Journal of Orthopsychiatry* 61: 6-22.

–, and J.A. Burack. 2000. Adolescent wellness: In the eye of the beholder? In D. Cicchetti, J. Rappaport, I. Sandler, and R.P. Weissberg, eds., *The promotion of wellness in children and adolescents,* 29-58. Washington, DC: CWLA Press.

–, D. Cicchetti, and B. Becker. 2000. The construct of resilience: A critical evaluation and guidelines for future work. *Child Development* 71: 543-62.

–, and L.B. Zelazo. 2003. Research on resilience: An integrative review. In S.S. Luthar, ed., *Resilience and vulnerability: Adaptation in the context of childhood adversities,* 510-50. Cambridge: Cambridge University Press.

Maccoby, E.E. 1992. The role of parents in the socialization of children: An historical overview. *Developmental Psychology* 28: 1006-17.

Mahoney, J.L., and R.B. Cairns. 1997. Do extracurricular activities protect against early school dropout? *Developmental Psychology* 33: 241-53.

Mao, Y., B.W. Moloughney, and R.M. Seminciw. 1992. Indian reserve and registered Indian mortality in Canada. *Canadian Journal of Public Health* 83: 350-53.

Masten, A.S., K.M. Best, and N. Garmezy. 1990. Resilience and development: Contributions to the study of children who overcome adversity. *Development and Psychopathology* 2: 425-44.

May, P.A. 1990. A bibliography on suicide and suicide attempts among American Indians and Alaska Natives. *Omega* 21: 199-214.

McAdams, D.P., and L. Janis. 2004. Narrative identity and narrative therapy. In Lynne E. Angus and John McLeod, eds., *The handbook of narrative and psychotherapy: Practice, theory, and research*, 159-73. Thousand Oaks, CA: Sage.

McKay McKernan, M., J.J. Gonzales, S. Stone, D. Ryland, and K. Kohner. 1995. Multiple family therapy groups: A responsive intervention model for inner city families. *Social Work with Groups* 18: 41-56.

McCormick, R.M. 1996. Culturally appropriate means and ends of counselling as described by the Aboriginal people of British Columbia. *International Journal for the Advancement of Counselling* 18: 163-72.

–. 1997. Healing through interdependence: The role of connecting in First Nations healing practices. *Canadian Journal of Counselling* 31 (3): 172-84.

McFarlane, W.R., and K. Cunningham. 1996. Multiple-family group and psychoeducation: Creating therapeutic social networks. In J.V. Vaccaro and G.H. Clark, eds., *Practicing psychiatry in the community: A manual,* 387-406. Washington, DC: American Psychiatric Press.

McLoyd, V.C. 1999. Cultural influences in a multicultural society: Conceptual and methodological issues. In A.S. Masten, ed., *Cultural processes in child development: The Minnesota Symposia on Child Psychology,* 123-36. Mahwah, NJ: Lawrence Erlbaum Associates.

Mohler, B. 2001. Cross-cultural issues in research on child mental health. *Child and Adolescent Psychiatric Clinics of North America* 10: 763-76.

Mosley-Howard, G.S. 1995. Best practices in considering the role of culture. In A. Thomas and J. Grimes, eds., *Best practices in school psychology,* 337-45. Washington, DC: National Association of School Psychologists.

Narrandera High School. 1986. Aboriginal participation in the senior programs at Narrandera High School, 1986. Narrandera, NSW: Narrandera High School.

National Aboriginal Youth Strategy. 1999. http://publications.gc.ca/control/publicationInformation?searchAction=2&publicationId=104300.

Nelson, C. 2000. The neurobiological bases of early intervention. In J.P. Shonkoff and S.J. Meisels, eds., *Handbook of early childhood intervention,* 2nd ed., 204-27. New York: Cambridge University Press.

Royal Commission on Aboriginal Peoples. 1996. *Final report.* Ottawa: Minister of Supply and Services Canada.

Rutter, M., and L.A. Sroufe. 2000. Developmental psychopathology: Concepts and challenges. *Development and Psychopathology* 12: 265-96.

Saarni, C. 1998. Issues of cultural meaningfulness in emotional development. *Developmental Psychology* 34: 647-52.

Sack, W.H., M. Beiser, N. Phillips, and G. Baker-Brown. 1993. Co-morbid symptoms of depression and conduct disorder in First Nations children: Some findings from the Flower of Two Soils Project. *Culture, Medicine, and Psychiatry* 16: 471-86.

–, M. Beiser, G. Baker-Brown, and R. Redshirt. 1994. Depressive and suicidal symptoms in Indian school children: Findings from the Flower of Two Soils. In C.W. Duclos and S.M. Manson, eds., *Calling from the rim: Suicidal behavior among American Indian and Alaska Native adolescents,* 81-94. Niwot, CO: University Press of Colorado.

Sameroff, A.J. 1990. Neo-environmental perspectives on developmental theory. In R.M. Hodapp, J.A. Burack, and E. Zigler, eds., *Issues in the developmental approach to mental retardation,* 93-113. New York: Cambridge University Press.

–, and M.J. Chandler. 1975. Reproductive risk and the continuum of caretaking causality. In F.D. Horowitz, ed., *Review of child development research,* vol. 4, 187-244. Chicago, IL: University of Chicago Press.

–, and B.H. Fiese. 1990. Transactional regulation and early interventions. In S.J. Meisels and J.P. Shonkoff, eds., *Early intervention: A handbook of theory, practice and analysis.* New York: Cambridge University Press.

–, R. Seifer, and W.T. Bartko. 1997. Environmental perspectives on adaptation during childhood and adolescence. In S.S. Luthar, J.A. Burack, D. Cicchetti, and J.R. Weisz, eds., *Developmental psychopathology: Perspectives on adjustment, risk and disorder,* 507-26. New York: Cambridge University Press.

Scheidlinger, S. 1985. Group treatment of adolescents: An overview. *American Journal of Orthopsychiatry* 55: 102-11.

Seidman, E., and S. Pedersen. 2003. Holistic contextual perspectives on risk, protection and competence among low-income urban adolescents. In S.S. Luthar, ed., *Resilience and vulnerability: Adaptation in the context of childhood adversities,* 318-42. Cambridge: Cambridge University Press.

Seligman, M.E.P. 1971. Phobias and preparedness. *Behaviour Therapy* 2: 307-20.

Sroufe, L.A., and M. Rutter. 1984. The domain of developmental psychopathology. *Child Development* 55: 17-29.

Statistics Canada. 2003. Aboriginal peoples of Canada: A demographic profile. http://www12.statcan.ca/english/census01/products/analytic/companion/abor/pdf/96F0030XIE2001007.pdf.

Stuhlmiller, C.M. 2001. Narrative methods in qualitative research: Potential for therapeutic transformation. In K.R. Gilbert, ed., *The emotional nature of qualitative research,* 63-80. Boca Raton, FL: CRC Press LLC.

Sullivan, M.L. 1998. Integrating qualitative and quantitative methods in the study of developmental psychopathology in context. *Development and Psychopathology* 10: 377-93.

Thompson, R.A. 1994. Emotional regulation: A theme in search of definition. *Monographs of the Society for Research in Child Development* 59 (2-3): 25-52.

Towberman, D.B. 1993. Group vs. individual counseling: Treatment mode and the client's perception of the treatment environment. *Journal of Group Psychotherapy, Psychodrama and Sociometry* 45: 163-74.

Tonkin, R.S., A. Murphy, K.A. van der Woerd, G. Gosnell, A. Liebel, D. Katzenstein, B. Veitch, and S. Helin. 1999. *Raven's children.* Burnaby, BC: McCreary Centre Society.

Toth, S.L., and D. Cicchetti. 1999. Developmental psychopathology and child psychotherapy. In S. Russ and T. Ollendick, eds., *Handbook of psychotherapies with children and families,* 15-44. New York: Plenum.

Walton, P. 1999. *Toward a collective vision: An evaluation of First Nations education in North Okanagan-Shuswap S.D. 83.* http://www.bced.gov.bc.ca/abed/readings/sd83/.

Waters, E. and L.A. Sroufe. 1983. Social competence as a developmental construct. *Developmental Review* 3: 79-97.

Weisz, J.R., C.A. McCarty, K.L. Eastman, W. Chaiyasit, and S. Suwanlert. 1997. Developmental psychopathology and culture: Ten lessons from Thailand. In S.S. Luthar, J.A. Burack, D. Cicchetti, and J.R. Weisz, eds., *Developmental psychopathology: Perspectives on adjustment, risk and disorder,* 139-65. New York: Cambridge University Press.

Werner, H. 1957. The concept of development from a comparative and organismic point of view. In D. Harris, ed., *The concept of development,* 125-47. Minneapolis MN: University of Minnesota Press.

Wertsch, J.V., and P. Tulviste. 1992. L.S. Vygotsky and contemporary developmental psychology. *Developmental Psychology* 28 (4): 548-57.

White, M. 2001. Folk psychology and narrative practice. Adelaide: Dulwich Centre.

–, and D. Epston. 1994. *Narrative means to therapeutic ends.* New York: Norton.

Wright, R. 1992. *Stolen continents: The "New World" through Indian eyes.* Boston: Houghton Mifflin.

Wyman, P.A. 2003. Emerging perspectives on context specificity of children's adaptation and resilience. In S.S. Luthar, ed., *Resilience and vulnerability: Adaptation in the context of childhood adversities,* 293-317. Cambridge: Cambridge University Press.

–, I. Sandler, S. Wolchik, and K. Nelson. 2000. Resilience as cumulative competence promotion and stress protection: Theory and intervention. In D. Cicchetti, J. Rappaport, I. Sandler, and R.P. Weissberg, eds., *The promotion of wellness in children and adolescents,* 133-84. Washington, DC: CWLA Press.

Yalom I.D. 1995. *The theory and practice of group psychotherapy.* 4th ed. New York: Basic Books.

Yates, A. 1987. Current status and future directions of research on the American Indian child. *American Journal of Psychiatry* 144: 1135-42.

Ystgaard, M. 1997. Life stress, social support and psychological distress in late adolescence. *Social Psychiatry and Epidemiology* 32: 277-83.

Zimmerman, M.A. 1998. Enculturation hypothesis: Exploring direct and protective effects among Native American youth. In H.I. McCubbin, E.A. Thompson, A.I. Thompson, and J.E. Fromer, eds. *Resiliency in Native American and immigrant families,* 199-220. Thousand Oaks, CA: Sage.

–, J. Ramirez, K.M. Washienko, and M. Kathleen. 1996. The development of a measure of enculturation for Native American Youth. *American Journal of Community Psychology* 24: 295-310.

Zygmuntowicz, C.E., J.A. Burack, D.W. Evans, C. Klaiman, T. Mandour, B. Randolph, and G. Iarocci. June 2000. Cultural identity as a protective factor: A study of depression and problem behaviors in First Nations adolescents from an isolated community. Paper presented at the Thirtieth Annual Meeting of the Jean Piaget Society, Montreal, Quebec.

PART 2

Social Suffering: Origins and Representations

5

A Colonial Double-Bind: Social and Historical Contexts of Innu Mental Health

COLIN SAMSON

In his story "A short history of Indians in Canada," Thomas King (1999) describes Indians flying into the skyscrapers along Toronto's Bay Street. The Euro-Canadian protagonists who witness these nocturnal events are at first astonished but soon grow accustomed to Indians crashing to the ground along the streets and alleys of the financial district. Their shock prompts them to categorize the flying Indians according to their regalia – Cree, Ojibwa, Mohawk. After they are identified, the authorities remove the Indians from the streets in time for the day's business to begin without disturbance. Stunned Indians are tagged; the dead ones are bagged. After witnessing the spectacle, a Euro-Canadian visitor to Toronto thanks the hotel doorman for recommending a walk down Bay Street. As another Indian collides into a skyscraper, the visitor congratulates the doorman, "It's a great town ... You're doing a great job (1994 64)."

This brief "history" is a quirky but compelling commentary on the reactions of Euro-Canadians to the sudden surfeit of untimely and unnatural deaths among Aboriginal peoples, including the Innu, the people I have worked with since 1994.

Scale of the Problem

The Innu are the indigenous people of the Labrador-Quebec peninsula in Canada. Until the 1960s they were permanent nomadic hunters, living a relatively autonomous and self-reliant way of life in what is one of the most exacting physical environments on the planet. Their fortunes changed drastically when, at the promptings of the Canadian government and Roman Catholic missionaries, this interconnected people occupying vast tracts of the Labrador-Quebec peninsula were settled in the government-built villages of Sheshatshiu and Utshimassits (Davis Inlet) in Labrador and 12 other villages in Quebec. Since their sedentarization, the Innu who were settled in the Labrador villages have suffered extremely high rates of suicide, alcohol abuse, solvent abuse, and sexual abuse. Each time I return to the villages, I frequently hear that things are "worse than ever."

The scale of the largely self-destructive problems afflicting the Innu now resident in Labrador are well known and have been publicized both in Canada and internationally.

Suicide, youth gas sniffing, drug use, and alcohol-related problems are part of everyday experience. For over a decade, very high numbers of children and adolescents in Utshimassits and Sheshatshiu have been sniffing gasoline. On some occasions, there have been so many young people high on fumes that buildings, skidoos, and whatever machines are to hand have been systematically vandalized. Violent confrontations and suicide attempts have also occurred at these moments. Since the people of these villages are bound together by strong family ties across the entire Labrador-Quebec peninsula, the repercussions are widespread.

To provide a rough idea of the vast gulf between the life and death experiences of the Innu and Canadians as a whole, I went through the death registers in the two villages to find out the ages at which people were dying. From 1975 to 1995 more than half of all deaths in Innu communities were of people under 30; this was the case for only 5% of Canadians and 4% of Newfoundlanders. Conversely, while at least 80% of Canadian and Newfoundland deaths were of people over 60, only one-quarter of Innu deaths were in this age range – ages to which people are expected to live in G-8 countries (Samson 2003, 230). These figures are consistently higher than those gathered to compare Aboriginal and non-Aboriginal mortality in Canada. Comparing only status Indians and the general population of Canada and having serious limitations in the recording of information, a recent Health Canada report found that infant mortality was only 1.5 times higher among First Nations in 1999 (2003, 22). For the Innu and other Aboriginal peoples, the surfeit of untimely deaths represents a complex interplay of physical and mental health problems. The sudden eruption of diseases associated with sedentary life and junk food diets such as cancer, heart disease, obesity, and diabetes (Samson and Pretty 2006) also has a negative effect on the general well-being of the people.

Acts of self-destruction – threatened, attempted, and fatal – occur with regularity in Utshimassits and Sheshatshiu. According to an estimate of the Band Council, one-third of all adults in Utshimassits attempted suicide in 1993 (Wilson 1994). Using hospital records, Aldridge and St. John (1991, 434) calculated the rate of youth suicide (ages 10-19) for Innu and Inuit Natives of northern Labrador from 1977 to 1988 to be 180 per 100,000, compared to a non-Native rate of 11.85 per 100,000 in Labrador as a whole. In the 1980s northern Labrador as a whole, which is populated by both Inuit and Innu people, had 2 times the Canadian Native rate and almost 5 times the national rate of suicide (Wotton 1986, 141). Between 1990 and 2000 there were 8 successful suicides in Utshimassits – equivalent to a rate of 160 suicides per 100,000 people, compared to a Canadian rate of 13 per 100,000 in 1996 and a First Nations (status Indian) rate of 27.9 per 100,000 in 1999.[1] This means that the Innu of Utshimassits were almost 12 times more likely to kill themselves than the general population of Canada and almost 6 times more likely than status Indians.[2] Between 1999 and 2005 there were an additional 23 suicides in the two villages, amounting to a rate of 182.6 per 100,000 in a population of 2,300 for both villages.

Although these numbers alert us to the scale of suffering, there are undoubtedly methodological and other problems related to establishing comparable suicide rates among

Aboriginal peoples in Canada, between them, and between them and non-Aboriginal Canadians (Kirmayer 1994, 6-7). Much of the problem lies in the lack of research into this sensitive topic in individual communities and the poor quality of most of the health and mortality records in small Aboriginal villages. The anguish that results is further exacerbated by what many Innu see as the indifference of the Canadian authorities.

Many of the suicide-related activities in Aboriginal communities, of course, never make it into any public record. I know from my own time in the village of Sheshatshiu and from the reports of my friends there that, over the past decade, there has been at least one major suicide attempt per month. During certain periods when heavy drinking occurs en masse, there can be several in any given week. Nearly all successful suicides and suicide attempts are those of teenagers and young adults, both male and female. A further complicating factor is that significant numbers of Innu also die in what are called accidents, even though the dividing line between accident and wilful harm or death to oneself and others is a very fine one. Many deaths occur when individuals who have been drinking heavily fall through ice, are run over on the road, or simply pass out and freeze to death. There are also well-known cases of parents whose descents into alcohol abuse and other forms of self-destruction have been precipitated by the suicide of a child.

Forms of Misunderstanding: The Local Health Professional

The impression I reached from interviewing numerous health professionals working with the Innu in the 1990s, including those at the highest levels, is that they either cannot or will not acknowledge the larger contexts of the misery occurring all around them (Samson 2003, 231-55). Many of them are perplexed as to why the Innu do not live according to the same values as they do, why they socialize their children differently, and why Innu standards of hygiene are not the same as theirs. Many also share a common Newfoundland-settler view of Native people: that they have been dealt with humanely and even generously by the state and that this goodwill has been squandered by irresponsibly unhealthy and self-destructive behaviour.

The narratives of health professionals tend to circle around a concept of blame. Innu suffering is deemed to be in large part a function of negligence on the part of the Innu themselves – a failure to live up to even the minimal standards attained by the normal health-conscious citizen. Aboriginal peoples are seen to have benefited from free and improved health care facilities as well as from technological and pharmaceutical means to deal with their health overall. From these observations, it is a short step to the calculation of individual and collective fault for the numerous casualties of drinking, smoking, suicide, gas sniffing, and drug abuse.

Some professionals undoubtedly have perceptive and sincere views that convey a deep empathy and concern for the Innu, and the tireless work of some of them demonstrates that they have been willing to make many personal sacrifices to help Innu patients. But even among conscientious professionals, much of the larger context of Innu suffering is simply ignored. To illustrate this, I will use the example of Dr. Jane McGillivray, who was the general practitioner in Sheshatshiu for most of the 1990s until her resignation in 2000.

Dr. McGillivray's resignation was a very public affair involving a published letter to the Innu Nation on the reasons for her decision, newspaper reports, and a CBC radio interview. In her various statements to the press and the Innu Nation (Lindgren 2000; CBC 2000), it was clear that Dr. McGillivray found her work emotionally draining, thankless, and frustrating. She found herself in the position of attending to huge amounts of self-inflicted suffering, noting in the press report cases such as a gas-sniffing 9-year-old with a perforated bowel and a child whom she had delivered being burned alive in a house fire while the parents were drinking. The blame for much of this, Dr. McGillivray argued, should be placed upon the Innu adults, "who are presently engaging so willfully in drunkenness, debauchery, and denial." Dr. McGillivray urged the Innu "to take charge of their lives, to care for their children" (Lindgren 2000). In the radio interview, the problem was framed in the libertarian language of individual freewill and choice – "every single person is responsible for taking care of their own life." The implication of these remarks was that these troubled Innu could extricate themselves from their afflictions through taking positive actions, exercising restraint, and facing up to their personal problems.

In McGillivray's account, the Canadian government was also indicted as contributing to the catastrophe of the Innu. The government had responded to the situation by pouring money into the community to establish what she considered "bogus" counselling services, thus fostering a "culture of addiction" and further removing health from personal responsibility. Here, the doctor was referring to the work of pan-Native healing organizations such as the Nechi Institute, based in Edmonton. Nechi was funded through Health Canada to instigate "treatment" for the Innu, beginning with a crisis that emerged in 1992-93, when the scale of the alcohol and gas-sniffing problems became widely publicized. On the whole, such organizations have employed popular psychology, New Age thinking, and Alcoholics Anonymous "addiction" models to the problems of the Innu. Although there have been some successes with addiction-oriented therapies among the Innu (Degnen 2001), there has also been a tendency to ignore that the culturally alien treatment methods have had the effect of pushing aside more genuinely indigenous healing techniques. Such interventions have been made at great expense and with few concrete results for non-urbanized Aboriginal peoples such as the Innu.

While adapting the addiction ideology of popular therapies, Nechi and other organizations convey their healing techniques to troubled Innu through Plains Indian cultural practices involving herbal smudging and sweat lodges. Although there is some resonance between these ideas and practices and those of the Innu, most of the methods are at variance with Innu customs. However therapeutic the sweat lodge might be for particular individuals, the way that it is now used in the villages varies from the way that the Innu used the sweat lodge while hunting. Several Tshenut (older Innu people) I have spoken to object to sweat lodges on the basis that those who partake of them are not "sick," that it is misplaced to erect them in the village (instead of in the country), and that the participants are "playing with" the powerful spiritual forces that sweat lodges can harness. To a large extent, then, the foreign culture of addiction has been promoted with state funding as a means to assist in healing the damage inflicted by the rampant self-destructive activities that followed sedentarization. Promoting these kinds of interventions is ideologically useful for the state since it neatly removes the issues from the arena of collective human rights and reduces them to a matter of individual failing. This was not, however, the point of Dr. McGillivray's observations about the culture of addiction. Limiting herself to commenting on the lack of efficacy and self-indulgent qualities of these techniques, she stopped well short of any wider political and cultural analysis of the effects of pan-Native healing.

However, the Innu leaders did come under McGillivray's microscope. She charged them with contributing to the suffering of the people by buying votes with alcohol and creating a general alcoholic frenzy around election times. The corruption of some Aboriginal political bodies is a topic that is rarely discussed publicly. However, when the local settler population – and here I include Dr. McGillivray – level criticism against Aboriginal leadership, the source of the problem tends to be depicted as a flaw in the character of the leaders themselves. Typically, little consideration is given to how these individuals may have found themselves in a position to exploit and become dependent on non-Aboriginal forms of power in the first place (Alfred 1999, 41-46).

If these leadership positions and institutions were derived from the customary Aboriginal political structure, it would be another matter. The fact is that the current Aboriginal political system was imposed. It relies on alien conceptions of power and authority, and all this has been deeply divisive and socially disruptive for the Innu and other indigenous peoples (Samson 2003, 33-39). As Mohawk scholar Taiaiake Alfred points out, "the people who dominate in most Native communities and organizations today model themselves on the most vulgar European power-wielders" (1999, xvi). That this is the case, however, is a direct consequence of colonial policies designed to extract the consent of Aboriginal peoples for Euro-Canadian occupation and "development" of land. In part, this was accomplished through creating institutions of permanent authority such as band councils, elevating certain individuals above others as "chiefs," and legitimizing such authority through divisive ballots. After the *Calder* Supreme Court case in 1970, there also arose a need on the part of the state to deal with the "land claims" of Aboriginal peoples such as the Innu who had not signed treaties.[3] Aboriginal political bodies based on the statist Euro-Canadian model – a model deeply antithetical to the consensus orientation and personal autonomy characteristic of traditional Innu decision making – were thus funded so that Canada would have a party on the other side of the table with which to negotiate (Samson 2001). Even the money used to procure alcohol for election campaigning comes either from the state through its funding of these political bodies, resource extraction industries, or local non-Native entrepreneurs hoping for certain kinds of Innu economic co-operation.

Beginning with the historical context, I now turn to some of the broader issues that Dr. McGillivray and other settlers frequently downplay.

The Historical Context: The Impacts of Relocation and Sedentarization

The first observation one should make in any assessment of the mental health of the Innu is that they are a transplanted people. Within relatively recent times, the Innu have had to rapidly adjust to their transition from being permanent nomadic hunters, enmeshed in a vibrant, largely healthy, and meaningful way of life, to being village dwellers, partially cut off from the land, largely unemployed, and subject to the imposition of alien authority structures. Although as hunters the Innu had to endure extreme climatic and environmental conditions and highly variable supplies of animals, it is undeniable that as a people they were much healthier prior to settlement. It is not through some romantic nostalgia that Tshenut point out the superiority of the mobile Innu way of life over the villages. Apart from the obvious benefits of a healthy diet of wild foods, physical exercise, and the necessary co-operative ethos of camp life, it was self-reliance that gave the Innu much of their vitality. As Shushep Mark of Sheshatshiu remarked in a conversation in 2003: "We were very happy in the past in the country. Then, there was no government or wildlife officers. The government did not support the Innu. We supported ourselves on the land. There were no child benefits or welfare then ... In this community, I have seen a lot of changes, such as suicide, violence, and drinking. We never saw any of that before."

The accounts of older Innu such as Shushep Mark and others (Innu Nation and Mushuau Innu Band Council 1995, 25-33) accord with those of nineteenth- and twentieth-century explorers and anthropologists, who found the Innu to be a largely vigorous and independent people. The situation gradually changed as the numbers of European missionaries and traders along the coasts increased and as forays into the interior of the Labrador-Quebec peninsula were made from the mid-nineteenth century onward. Closer contact with Europeans brought infectious diseases such as tuberculosis, influenza, and red measles to which the Innu had no immunity (Samson 2003, 265-69).

However, as Shushep Mark confirms, it was not until sedentarization that more social and psychological afflictions related to alcohol, gas sniffing, and suicide appeared. In Sheshatshiu the turning point came in the late 1950s, when the missionaries, trading officers, and some Newfoundland officials convinced the Innu who came to the North West River trading post and camped at Sheshatshiu and neighbouring environs that they should stay in one place. Soon a school was created for the tent-dwelling Innu. In the 1960s houses were built, and the Innu became progressively ensnared in welfare dependency and a "psychology of fear" created by the missionaries (Samson 2003, 32-33, 172-78). The origins of the current problems in Sheshatshiu are often traced to this first act of sedentarization, especially with the influence of the missionary-inspired school, the most important instrument of assimilation. As Dominic Pokue, a Tshenu, told me in 2003: "The changes came about first in 1959 when the school was built. This changed our way of life. With education came the loss of interest in the country, materialism, foreign values, alcohol, and suicide among teenagers. All these things were never known in the country."

Before they were situated at Davis Inlet on Iluikoyak Island, the Mushuau Innu had suffered a previous relocation. In the first relocation, Innu camping at the trading post at Davis Inlet were transported to Nutak on the coast of northern Labrador in the cargo hold of a ship. While at Nutak, the men were engaged in servile labour, cutting firewood for the small Inuit community there. Although the details are sketchy, so apparently severe were the conditions and so high the mortality (allegedly only 7 births and 70 deaths) among the Innu in this treeless coastal area that all the survivors walked back to the Davis Inlet trading post on foot (Canadian Human Rights Commission 1993, 34-38; Royal Commission on Aboriginal Peoples 1996, vol. 1, 448-54). Neither the Innu nor the Inuit of coastal Labrador were mentioned in the terms of agreement by which Newfoundland entered Confederation in 1949. They were not registered under the Indian Act and, as a result, became the responsibility of bureaucrats in the distant capital of St. John's.

The second relocation in 1967 was really an act of sedentarization since it put a final stop to permanent nomadic hunting and brought the Innu fully under the control of the state. Once at the new settlement of Davis Inlet, the authorities never ensured that running water and sanitation were provided to the shacks built for the Innu. The Canadian Human Rights Commission concluded that the 1967 relocation took place without any meaningful consultation. Furthermore, it was motivated by a desire to redirect the Innu away from their traditional way of life. Since 1967, the report continued, the authorities have failed to remedy the unsanitary living conditions of the people in the community (Canadian Human Rights Commission 1993, 46). Basic services that would be required of any village or town were also not provided. One of the most important reasons for the extensive loss of life in Davis Inlet from house fires, for example, was the failure to provide even a rudimentary fire-protection service.

Although it was not planned with any degree of precision, the effects of the sedentarization of the Innu share characteristics with other actions to relocate or resettle peoples deemed to be in the way of industrial development. Virtually all such enterprises, including that involving the Innu, were justified under the banner of progress. Indigenous and tribal peoples across North America and in many other parts of the world were thought to be deficient in the social, economic, and psychological qualities deemed necessary to achieve greater material prosperity. One of the individuals responsible for the sedentarization of the Innu, Walter Rockwood, the director of the Division of Northern Labrador Affairs, provided a stirring rendition of this view when he remarked of the Inuit ("Eskimo") and Innu ("Indian") Natives of the territory: "But one fact seems clear, Civilization is on the northward march, and for the Eskimo and the Indian there is no escape. The last bridges of isolation were destroyed with the coming of the airplane and the radio. The only course now open, for there can be no turning back, is to fit him as soon as may be to take his full place as a citizen in our society. There is no time to lose. No effort must be spared in the fields of Health, Education, Welfare and Economics" (1957, 6).

Despite numerous indications from prior experiences with indigenous peoples that "fitting them into our society" might be a disastrous course of action, Rockwood, along with priests and some members of the philanthropic society the International Grenfell Association, were fairly single-minded in taking this decision.[4] In doing so, there seemed to have been almost no acknowledgment of adverse social consequences. To the contrary, records indicate that the authorities were full of certainties concerning the perceived evolutionary leap of "the Indian" through schooling and industrial employment (Samson 2003, 143-48).

In the late 1960s, at the time that the Innu were being settled in villages, the Norwegian anthropologist Georg Henriksen (1973, 73-117) depicted the Mushuau Innu as living in "two worlds": the coastal trading post at what is now called "old" Davis Inlet, across the bay from Iluikoyak Island, and the tundra and forest territories inland. He found that, whereas a communitarian spirit existed in the hunting camps, coastal life was marked by individualism, the pursuit of cash, and interpersonal conflict. In the country, much of the activity was governed by observances to the Animal Gods, which entailed *mukushan* feasts and respect accorded to animals in hunting, such as using their meat and skins while disposing of their bones according to prescribed practice. The hunters whom Henriksen travelled with lived in flexible family groupings. Individual hunting expeditions were under the temporary leadership of *utshimaut* (literally "first men"). Both camp life and relations between the numerous groups of Innu in the country were highly convivial and sociable, often "celebratory." Relatively stable gender relations prevailed without patriarchal power. This social order was broken up on the coast by the imposed authority of the missionary, storekeeper, and government agents. Whereas alcohol was largely absent from the hunting camps, it became the centre of social life at Davis Inlet and, predictably, precipitated conflicts and quarrelling (Henriksen 1973, 74).

Like so many other hunting peoples, there are remarkable bonds connecting the Innu people to the animals and the physical environment. These bonds, which are based on thousands of years of experience in this landscape and which form the basis of Innu religion, have been fundamental to their social and psychological stability. Villages have provided no substitutes for the sense of well-being and social solidarity experienced by the Innu on the land. In fact, village social organization, imposed authority, and physical conditions have actually worked to undermine collective well-being. In part, this has occurred through schooling and employment, both predicated on an imposed competitive ethos. Furthermore, the fractious institutions of self-government, which function on the basis of individuals competing with each other at alcohol-fuelled elections and vying for monies from the state, have only deepened the splits within the Innu community. However, the major obstacle to any amelioration of the trauma of the Innu lies in the failure of the authorities to recognize the larger historical dimensions of the problem. As argued by the

Royal Commission on Aboriginal Peoples (1995, 2) in a special report on suicide, the root cause of these cultural dislocations lies in the history of colonial relations between Aboriginal peoples and the authorities and settlers who went on to establish "Canada" and in the distortion of Aboriginal lives that resulted from that history.

Similarly, other studies of "social pathologies" in Northern communities have stressed how Native peoples see these problems as intimately associated with the intrusion of Europeans. In regard to the Whapmagoostui Cree, a people closely related to Innu families in both Utshimassits and Sheshatshiu, Adelson has argued that many Cree "view the larger societal pathologies present in the community as either a direct or indirect result of interferences of 'whiteman.' Immediate social problems such as interpersonal violence or substance abuse are thus viewed as agonizing symptoms of a much larger disorder and people regularly express the conviction that one cannot 'be alive well' as a result of the past and continuing encroachments upon Cree lives" (1998, 15).

Part of the reason for this is that the important links between indigenous peoples and land are so vital to the notion of the self. Speaking of the fact that the Navajo were required to move as a consequence of the US government's resolution of the Navajo-Hopi land dispute, Schwarz argues that "forced relocation constitutes a breach of personhood – a severing of the vital connection between the individual and place" (2001, 46). In another study of this relocation, Lassiter found "loss of memory, disorientation, an inability to concentrate, cases of partial paralysis ... severe depression and physical deterioration" to be common among Navajo relocatees and potential relocatees (1987, 225-26). With this sort of evidence, much of the extreme self-destructive behaviour of the Innu becomes intelligible. A person who has lost vital connections with the sources of his or her personhood is easily prey to all these manifestations of psychic destabilization. In this regard, Northern hunting peoples such as the Innu are particularly vulnerable because of the wholesale changes brought upon by sedenterization.

Looking through the examples cited above, it is evident that the experience of the Innu is one instance of a repeating pattern of circumstances, events, and reactions that occur when indigenous peoples are relocated and sedentarized. Despite differences among specific groups, common outcomes include an exacerbation of factionalism, a breakdown of communication and identity, loss of land, a shift in gender roles,[5] an undermining of customary leadership functions, and an increase in both aberrant behaviour and mortality. Typically, resettlements were carried out to make way for industrialization and to induct indigenous peoples into what state authorities claimed was a superior civilization. In countless cases, the people who were relocated were given false promises as to the circumstances in the new settlement (Tester and Kulchyski 1994; Royal Commission on Aboriginal Peoples 1996, vol. 1, ch. 11; Bussidor and Bilgen-Reinart 1997). Because those overseeing the changes often had strong ethnocentric beliefs in the validity of social engineering, especially in the light of views declaiming hunting as an evolutionary precursor to industrial society, little time was devoted to understanding the worldview or history of those affected by relocation.

The Political Context: Industrial Development and the Loss of Personhood

Clearly, the mental health problems of the Innu are inseparable from their relations with the state. The state itself engineered their settlement and supported the extensive transformation of their lives. Initially, sedentarization weakened the bonds between families who had previously travelled the entire Labrador-Quebec peninsula, as people were settled in various villages on the north shore of the St. Lawrence, in the interior of northern Quebec, and along the Labrador coast. However, the role of Canada did not end when these settlements were established. After settlement, the lands that the Innu occupied on a permanent basis were continually appropriated for industrial development.

Labrador has long been seen as having great potential for resource extraction. Explorers and geographers throughout the nineteenth and early twentieth centuries commented on the bounties available to adventurous pioneers (Hind 1863, v; Gosling 1910, 427; Tanner 1947, 826). However, it was not until the Innu territories came under the authority of the Canadian state that organized efforts were made to industrialize Innu lands. To date, Innu lands have been sequestered for dozens of hydroelectric projects, the largest of which is the Churchill Falls generating station, a $2.9 billion nickel-mining development, as well as for thousands of other mineral claims and for roads that will make settlement and industrial development more attractive. In addition to this, low-altitude military flight training and target practice have sullied the Innu's experience of hunting life in their territories in the interior. More minor but no less offensive intrusions include the building of settler cabins and commercial fish camps, many of which appear at locations that have been favoured by Innu families for generations. These are often places with significant historical, cultural, and personal associations – burial sites, former campsites, and archeological sites. To add further to the sense of humiliation, the provincial government has renamed Innu lands, lakes, rivers, and mountains with names derived from the recent experience of Labrador settlers and transient Newfoundlanders.

To slow down the pace at which Innu land is confiscated, the Innu Nation has been in the process of negotiating a Comprehensive Land Claims Agreement for over a decade. Numerous industrial developments are within the area of the Innu Nation claim, and the land upon which these industrial developments have been authorized is by law unextinguished Aboriginal title land. The territories have not been ceded by any agreement, and the state can produce no document in support of either its sovereignty or its authority to approve the sale of the land within them. Despite this, the government has operated since 1949 as though the Innu have no pre-existing Aboriginal rights whatsoever and has actively encouraged the development of Innu lands.[6]

The Innu have interpreted these actions not merely, at their most transparent level, as theft but also as a loss of their personhood since their identity as hunters and as human beings is inseparable from the land. There is a very wide consensus among the Innu that industrial activities damage health not only by their potentially toxic by-products (mercury in rivers from dams, air and noise pollution from military jets, tailings from mines) but also by disrupting the existing ecological balance and causing adverse changes to the animal population. At a social and psychological level, industrial development brings with it influxes of settlers and workers whose influences are widely seen as disruptive of Innu family and community ties, while also encouraging alcohol consumption and sexual permissiveness. Innu predictions of the corrosive effects of the expansion of the Goose Bay air base for low-altitude flight training (Armitage 1989, xxvii) have already been borne out, as Goose Bay is now a magnet for Innu drinking and gambling that contributes to family destabilization.

In the mid-1990s, Innu in Davis Inlet believed that the imminent Voisey's Bay mine would simply exacerbate problems of alcohol abuse and ill-health. During the early exploration phase of the mine, reports were coming back that the Innu workers who were hired – significantly, at the very lowest occupational levels – were often bypassing their families on payday for the bars of Goose Bay. Predictions from the Tshenut and health workers in the two communities were of rapid erosion of the Innu way of life, not simply from the influence of Newfoundlanders, who constituted most of the workers, but also from Innu avoiding this prime hunting, fishing, and gathering area.

In 1996 the Innu Nation set up a taskforce on mining activities, which was published in a pamphlet called *Ntesinan nteshiniman nteniunan: Between a rock and a hard place*. Although there were diverse opinions represented among the Innu canvassed, a remarkable number of people drew a direct link between mining and an increase in social and psychological problems. The crucial connection was almost always articulated as a loss of the Innu way of life that would be occasioned by the taking of Innu land and the influence of the development itself, with all its industrial and capitalistic values (Innu Nation 1996, 51, 56, 57):

> We might get a big sum of money from mining companies, but that will only increase our problems. The land and the animals are the most important. If we protect them from being destroyed, we can continue to use the land. But once it is destroyed, we will no longer be able to go to nutshimit (the country). We will be a lost people. (Hank Penashue, Sheshatshiu)

> The problem will be that land will be destroyed if the mining goes ahead and there will be a lot of white people, and a lot of Innu people will be drinking especially for those who stopped drinking in the last couple of years, and have worked on their healing journey. (Judith Rich, Utshimassits)

> On the Hobbema Reserve, the oil field on their land has made them very rich, but there are a lot of negative results from it – gangs, drugs, social problems, population explosion of non-Natives, guns, shootings, watchdogs, jealousies ... There may be many jobs and lots of money from a mine but it does not necessarily mean good things." (Sheshatshiu workshop)[7]

In addition, many people have observed that the social cohesion of the Innu as a people has been damaged as a consequence of the courting of Innu leaders for "joint ventures" with the extractive industries. As a result of various financial overtures, very large sums of money have been paid out to Innu "shareholders," binding them into the process of resource extraction and creating ever greater chasms of material wealth between these individuals and the vast bulk of Innu who survive on welfare.

Although the influx of money from these joint ventures as well as from the Voisey's Bay Impact Benefit Agreements and the anticipated land claims agreement is in many respects welcome, it is a very mixed blessing for the Innu. Indeed, as the example of Hobbema above indicates, other indigenous communities that have been subject to newfound wealth have not necessarily fared well. The problem with material affluence, at least as it is conveyed in the present capitalistic context, is that it is largely distributed unevenly and becomes a further basis for emphasizing individual rather than collective well-being. As more emphasis is placed on entrepreneurship, joint ventures, and shareholding as the way forward for the Innu (Dyson 2003), the communal attachments Innu have by virtue of their being Innu will diminish. This is not because the Innu cannot "adapt" to a more nakedly commercial social order but because this new social order rewards personal qualities such as materialism and the quest for personal gain, which the Innu have hitherto found maladaptive to the cohesion of their society. Those few Innu who are able to benefit from this wealth may not be as susceptible as others to the problems of suicide, heavy drinking, and solvent abuse, at least while the bonanzas hold up, but others will not be so lucky. Even in the unlikely event that this new wealth "trickles down," money will not be able to replace the manifold communal attachments that have bound Innu together by virtue of their relationships to the land. When looked at historically, what is represented by these changes is a move from a high degree of communal economic self-reliance, prior to sedentarization, to dependency on resource extraction for a modicum of unequally distributed monetary security.

Moreover, not only is money coldly silent to suffering, but it can be seen to strike a bargain, which, at least in the eyes of those distributing it, redeems the crimes of the past. In what many Tshenut see as a sleight of hand, money is offered as a replacement for confiscated land and for the human tragedies that followed from the loss of land. But the exchange is unequal; it is a trade of something ultimately transient and ephemeral for something that sustained Innu permanently. In the Innu Nation's inquiry into the opinions of members of the villages on land claims, the overwhelming majority of Tshenut were hostile to the idea of striking any such bargain. As the late Tshenish Pasteen of Utshimassits remarked, "money will not last, but land will always be there. I don't want government money. I want to protect my land. The government doesn't like losing money. I certainly don't like losing my land" (Innu Nation 1998, 25).

Although now over a century old, Émile Durkheim's sociological theories can be used to illuminate some of the human consequences of this type of rapid social change. For

Durkheim, society is a set of ideas and sentiments, something that resides within us as a source of morality and arbiter of action. As Durkheim pointed out, societal institutions are symbols of the bonds between the individual and the group (1951, 212). When these institutions are broken down, as they obviously are in Innu society, "the bond attaching man to life relaxes because that attaching him to society is itself slack" (214). The configuration of circumstances Durkheim identifies as surrounding "anomic" suicide is almost identical to those affecting the Innu. These include a disturbance in the collective order, a breakdown of traditional authority, an attenuation of religion, and a rise in individualism. Eventually, "the more the family and community become foreign to the individual, so much the more does he become a mystery to himself, unable to escape the exasperating and agonizing question: to what purpose?" (212).

Suicides are experienced as communal tragedies. Most people recognize the frequency of youth suicide as a commentary on the health of the community itself. And here it is not simply the proximate problems of drinking and parental neglect that are singled out as factors but also the whole predicament of a people who have been removed from one way of life in which they had independent, meaningful, and purposeful activity to another that, after just two generations, holds little for most of them as an alternative. For many of the younger people, the community life is dull and devoid of purposeful activity. There are television, video games, and visiting friends but very little that provides them with any sense of self-esteem either as Innu (since they are becoming increasingly severed from the land) or as Canadians (since employment is extremely scarce and educational opportunities necessitate leaving their communities and immersing themselves in an alien and often hostile environment). Few find ways to latch hold of anything that will make them feel good about themselves. There is often no exit from the purposelessness, and unfortunately, for some, the gun or the noose provides release. As Jean-Charles Pietacho, of the Innu community of Ekuantshit (Mingan) in Quebec, remarked in a submission to the Royal Commission report on Aboriginal suicide, "suicide is the ultimate denunciation of the absence of choice for an individual or a community" (Royal Commission on Aboriginal Peoples 1995, 39). This "absence of choice" is not an impersonal force of history but a result of conscious social engineering.

Forms of Misunderstanding: Recent Interventions of the State

Another form of misunderstanding the Innu predicament is manifest in state strategies to cope with the suffering in the villages. This is done primarily by providing what are considered material benefits to the people. In this section, I will discuss two examples of this: the move of the Mushuau Innu to Natuashish and the medicalization of gas sniffing.

It is undeniable that the further relocation in the winter of 2002-3 of the Mushuau Innu to Natuashish on the mainland has gone some way to addressing the housing problems the Innu faced by virtue of not having access to running water and sanitation at Utshimassits. The Innu are no longer cut off from hunting areas on the mainland for significant lengths of time, and the country life can now be enjoyed year round. However, pessimism in Davis Inlet about the curative effects of the move to Natuashish was fairly high throughout the 1990s. Few in Davis Inlet believed that the move alone would be able to heal the psychological scars caused by living for some 35 years on Iluikoyak Island. Indeed, even the auditor general of Canada, Denis Desautels, was equally pessimistic. In a report to Parliament on 17 October 2000, Desautels observed that the federal government had failed to identify what remedies were needed to address the "social pathologies" of the Innu: "There is a significant risk that the causes of these conditions will not be adequately addressed through the relocation" (Office of the Auditor General of Canada 2000).

A few months after the move, there were reports of an upsurge in drinking, vandalism, and other kinds of dysfunction. Echoing many of the motifs of dispossession mentioned above, a little over 6 months after the move, George Rich of Natuashish made the following statement:

> There are new headlines for the Innu in our community right now such as *Innu Vandalize Their New Homes, $130 Million Wasted In The New Community, and Heavy, And Increased Alcoholism In The New Community.* Do you think a piece of plywood or piece of lumber and new road would automatically cure all of our problems, such as alcoholism and drug problems. Are all white people cured when they build new homes, with water and sewage? First they took our land at the Voisey's Bay, then they corrupted our leaders with money, buying them new skidoos, and then they locked us into the new Indian Act policy. We will be jailed for life, we will never live like white people, even if they build million dollar houses. They should have concentrated on getting people to live their way of life. We are Innu. (2003, original emphasis)

Although the new houses at Natuashish are preferable to the shacks the Innu endured at Davis Inlet, they do not deliver meaning and purpose. The houses do not replace the sense of pride and accomplishment in living the Innu way of life, and they certainly do not compensate for the loss of the land at Voisey's Bay and elsewhere. Nor do the new houses do anything to alleviate the chronic boredom of the younger generation in the new village. Many, if not most, Innu youth are in the unenviable position of only sporadically participating in the Innu hunting life, while simultaneously not having the requisite education or opportunities to participate in the non-Innu society. In some ways, the new houses, replete with basements, garages, and other accoutrements of suburban living, can be viewed as symbolic of the containment and domestication of the Innu. Perhaps it was this idea of being "jailed for life" that provoked vandalism damages totalling around $500,000 soon after the move (Blackmore 2003).

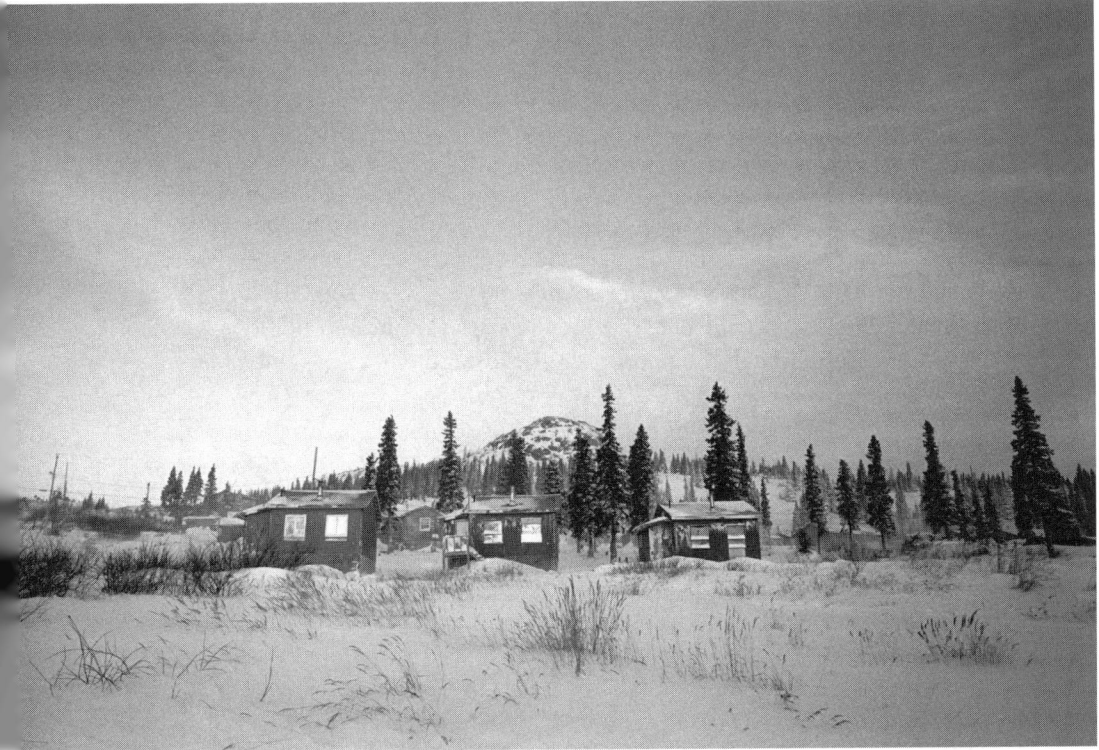

FIGURE 5.1   Early evening in Davis Inlet, 2002. (Photo: D. Tyler)

The overarching reaction of the state to publicized crises in Aboriginal communities throughout Canada has been to spend more money on the community infrastructure. However, even progress here is shockingly slow. As the recent report *Statistical Profile on the Health of First Nations in Canada* (Health Canada 2003) confirmed, quality-of-life indicators for First Nations peoples – such as infant mortality, rates of infectious diseases, rates of long-term chronic diseases, access to basic sanitation, environmental conditions, and rates of suicide and alcoholism – lag a long way behind those for the rest of Canada. For example, almost half of First Nations homes were considered inadequate in 1999-2000, and overcrowding affected almost 1 in 5 First Nations families (65). Although the move to Natuashish was designed to address some of these problems, even here, a cursory inspection of the houses themselves would reveal that the non-union construction crew cut many corners in the building of the houses. After only a few months, cracks were appearing in walls, screws and bolts were exposed, and the sheetrock walls provided little defence against the subarctic winds. The much-heralded provision of potable water also turned out to be a mirage, as many Innu initially found the heavily salted water undrinkable, and some were hauling water from brooks once again.

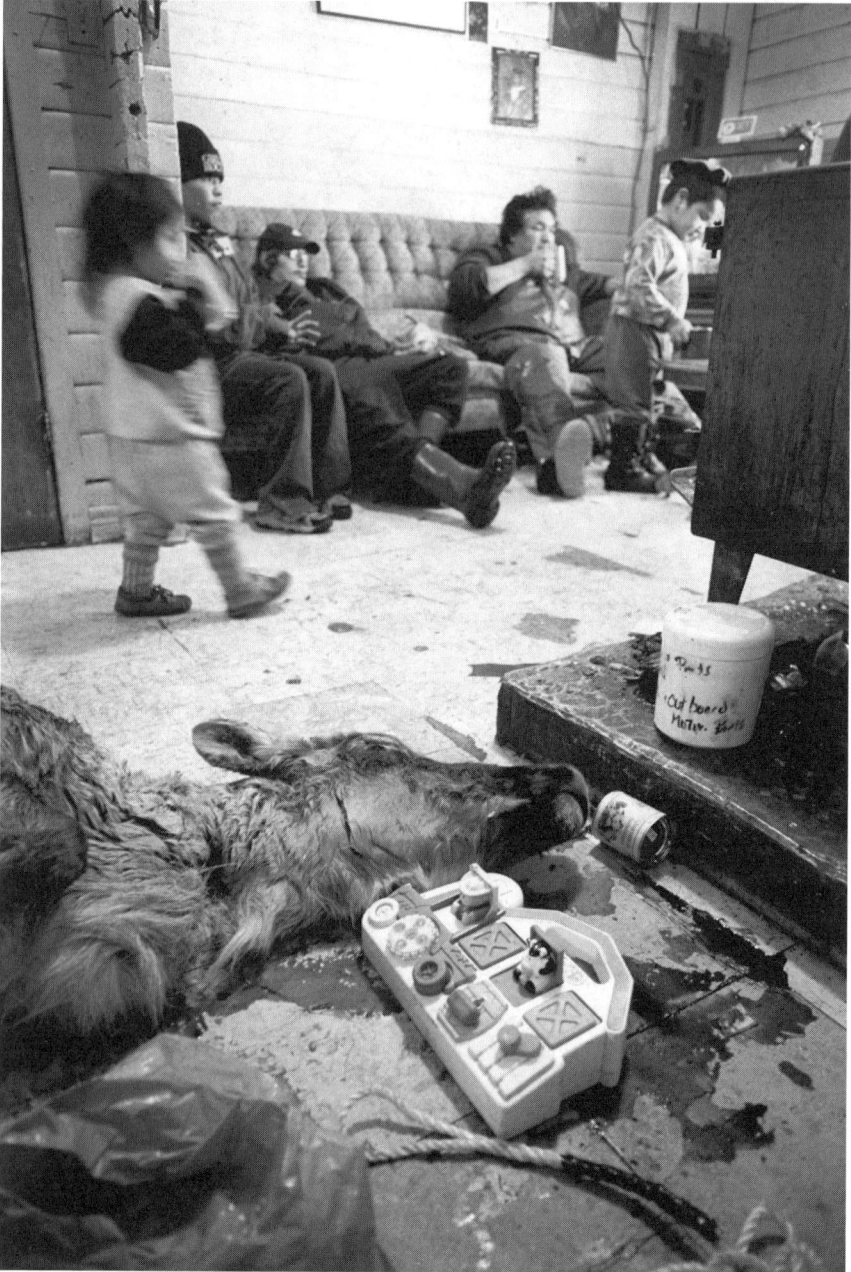

FIGURE 5.2   A caribou carcass thaws on the floor of a house in Davis Inlet while the returned hunters drink tea. The takings of a hunt are traditionally shared among the community, with the choicest cuts going to the Elders and the leg bones of caribou reserved to make a *mokushan* feast, 2002. (Photo: D. Tyler)

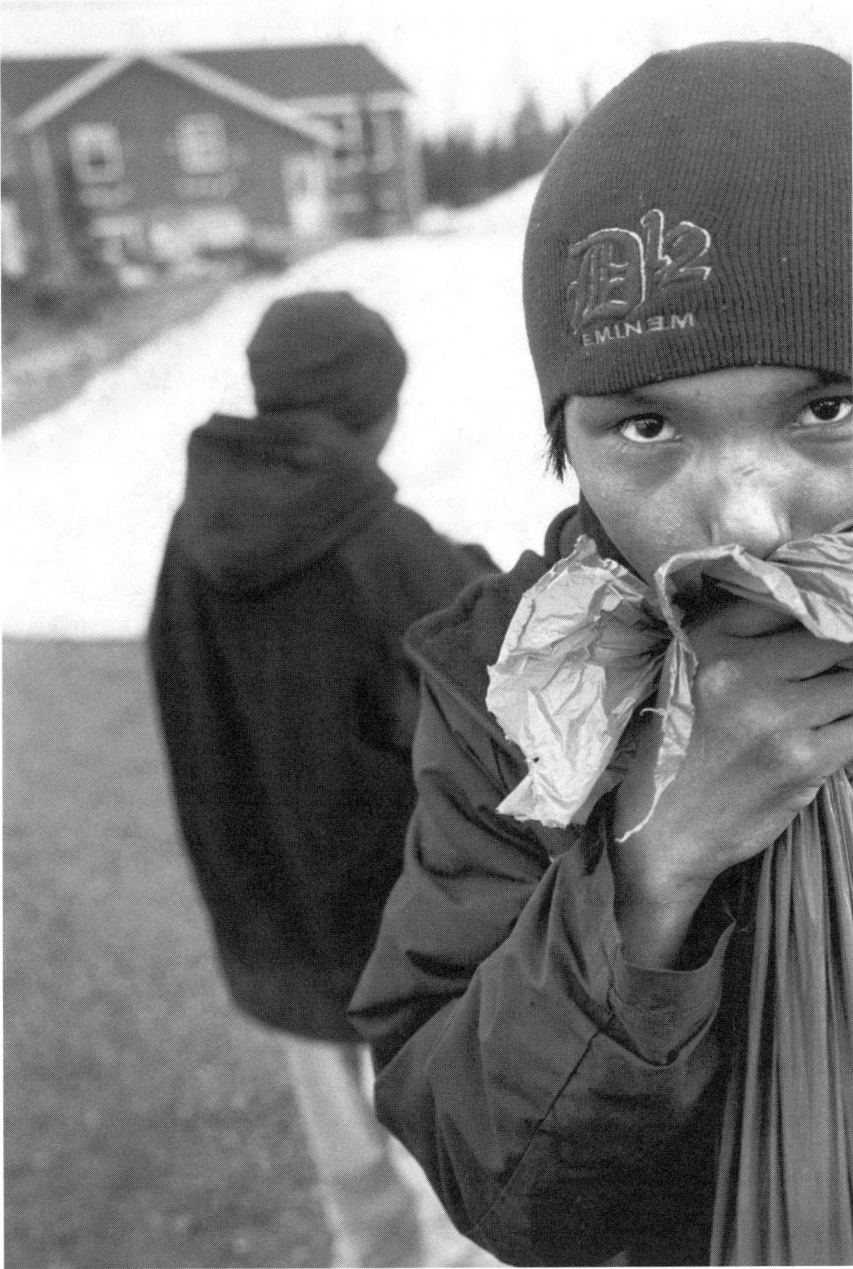

FIGURE 5.3   Innu boys sniffing gasoline on the street in Natuashish, 2005.
(Photo: D. Tyler)

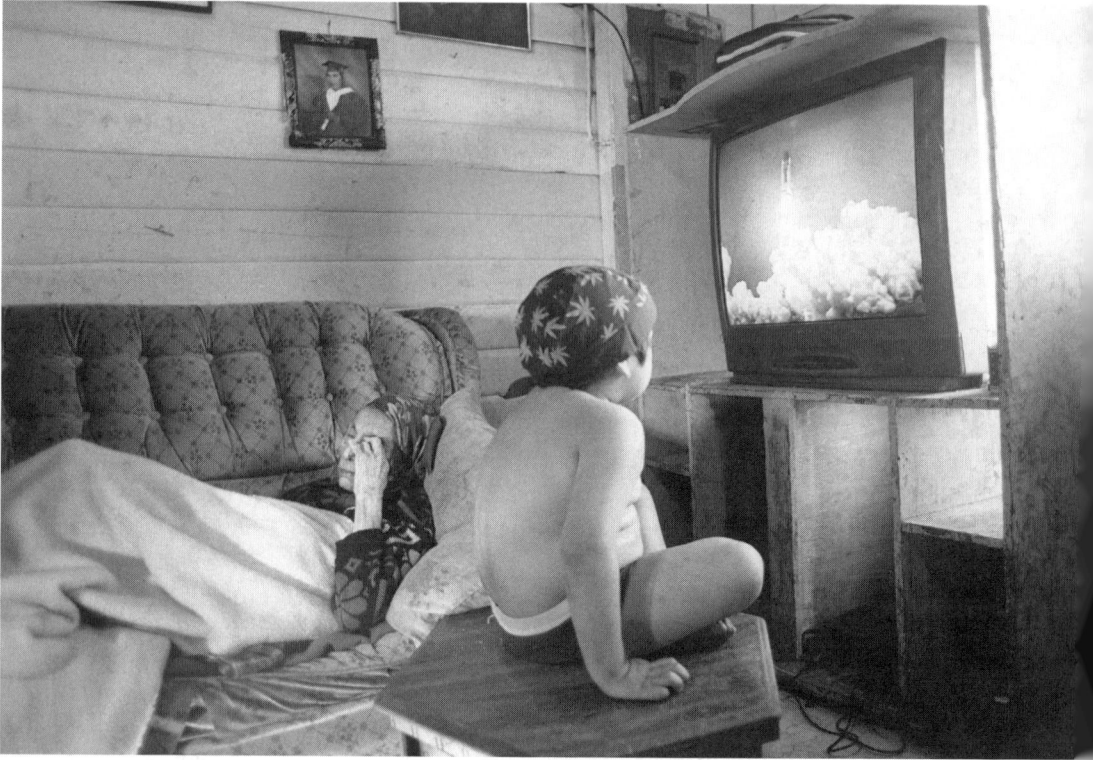

FIGURE 5.4   Elizabeth Napeo rests on the sofa while her great-nephew Kirby watches a space
shuttle launch on TV. When Elizabeth was Kirby's age, she and her family were still nomadic,
travelling across Labrador along traditional routes that mirrored the availability of seasonal foods
and animal migrations, 2002. (Photo: D. Tyler)

Undoubtedly, material poverty – in the terms in which this is understood in the dominant society – is a source of unhappiness to the Innu, as it is to other peoples who have
not had easy access to potable water, sanitation, employment, health care facilities, and
dignified housing. But to limit policies to these side effects of their relationship to Canada
is to stop far short of any alleviation of the suffering. Durkheim argued that material poverty itself, at least within a socially stable society, can have protective effects against suicide, while sudden injections of monetary wealth can be associated with quite dramatic
increases in the suicide rates (1951, 244-46). This is because the social order is thrown out
of balance. It is also the case, as Sahlins (1974) argued, that hunter-gatherers' notions of
wealth are necessarily not the same as those whose criteria are based on the teachings of
Adam Smith. Since wealth among the Innu, in the form of meat and fish, as well as other
necessities, was almost always shared, it was intrinsically related to respect for a good
hunter rather than to any accumulation of possessions, which would hinder mobility and

COLIN SAMSON

imperil survival. By contrast, the focus on material wealth and poverty on the part of the state functions to reinforce the materialistic values that the governmental and church authorities have been trying to instill for so long. When this becomes the primary means by which the state deals with collective trauma, it has the effect of further eroding the communitarian values that helped the Innu to create solidarity and well-being among themselves.

At the same time, the focus on cash to deal with poverty and pathology sidelines the profound denial of nationhood that is apparent in Canada's past and present policies of extinguishment (Alfred 1999, xv; Epstein 2002; Saganash, Orkin, and Orkin 2003). This is one of the reasons why the efforts of the state to engineer material and monetary prosperity have so often coincided with a further deterioration in the mental health of indigenous peoples. As Napoleon remarks of his own Yup'ik people of Alaska: "As their physical lives have improved, the quality of their lives has deteriorated ... Since the 1960s there has been a dramatic rise in alcohol abuse, alcoholism, and associated violent behaviors, which have resulted in physical and psychological injury, death, and imprisonment ... One thing we do know – the primary cause of the epidemic is not physical deprivation" (1999, 325).

A similar situation exists in other indigenous communities where a sudden infusion of money has been precipitated by compensation packages from resource-extraction industries. As York remarks of the Plains Cree of Hobbema, Alberta, where substantial oil revenues were handed out to each family, "when the money came pouring into Hobbema, alcohol and drug abuse grew steadily worse. In the 1980s, most of the suicides and other health problems at Hobbema were linked directly or indirectly to alcohol, solvent abuse, cocaine, and other drugs" (1990, 95).

A second, and linked, strategy of the state has been to tacitly assume that the physical and mental health problems of the Innu are primarily medical issues. This is done by financing medical facilities or treatment programs for gas sniffing and alcohol abuse. From the Nechi training sessions to the building of ever more medically oriented institutions in the villages, this trend continues to gather momentum. A crisis point was reached in the winter of 2000-1, when large numbers of Innu children and adolescents in both villages were filmed in the woods and on the ice sniffing gas. Some children were reportedly 6 or 7 years of age. Images of Innu youth speaking to reporters while holding plastic bags of gasoline in one hand and lit cigarettes in the other were beamed across Canada and, to the embarrassment of the state, around the world.

At the height of this crisis in December 2000, I accompanied members of the Mushuau Innu Band Council to meet with the federal Departments of Health and Indian Affairs in Ottawa. Simeon Tshakapesh, the chief, began one meeting by showing a short amateur video made by two young Innu. In this film, the life of young gas sniffers was portrayed realistically, yet empathically, through testimonies of Innu youth. It conveyed the sense of hopelessness and futurelessness for the young people of Sheshatshiu and Davis Inlet. After the viewing, the minister of health, Allan Rock, was the first to respond: "Thanks for showing the film. It was very moving ... The film is appropriate. It puts a sharp light on the *children*. The most important thing is to get the social workers and trained personnel into the community to get them the *attention* they need. We should agree tonight that that is going to happen. Do we share that objective?" (original emphasis intoned).

The chief's response was a muted and unenthusiastic "sure." Although the Innu recognized that there was a place for the medical assessment of the large numbers of gas-sniffing children in the village, they were also looking for some understanding. Instead, they received a rather brusque response urging that treatment begin immediately and that this be bureaucratically facilitated through various legal channels such as the Newfoundland Child Welfare Protection Act, which would ensure that the non-Innu social workers could make assessments of the children. While the government negotiators continually uttered their "respect" for "Aboriginal traditions," it was clear the provincial statutes were non-negotiable. This was salient because at previous meetings numerous Innu had reminded the government of the unhappy experience of having children removed by social workers in the past. Until the 1970s many Innu children were forcibly dispatched to Newfoundland and other areas of Canada, where they were raised by non-Native foster parents. In these meetings, the Mushuau Innu leadership had pointed out that they had jurisdiction over their own children and that, in the co-operation they desired with Newfoundland's Social Services Department, Innu parents would be the final arbiters of whether a child ought to be removed from his or her family.

The end results – the placement of a number of Mushuau Innu children in a treatment program in St. John's, the funding of a variety of treatment programs (the most important of which has still to materialize almost 8 years later), and the entrenchment of the notion that the Innu do not have primary jurisdiction over their own children – were expedients that fundamentally misunderstood the problems of the Innu. Whereas the children in crisis were taken off into new environments, tested with the latest biomedical technologies, housed, fed, and given treats unimaginable in Davis Inlet, such as trips to shopping malls, hockey games, and restaurants, the wider contexts of the problem were left unattended. The tests may well have been essential to establish whether the children had suffered any organic damage, but the state's response functioned to suffocate the deeper *political* dimensions of the crisis. It did this by insisting on a medical remedy for what was perceived as solely a medical problem and by insisting on the primacy of its own laws over Innu children. By doing so, it quashed any Innu aspirations to limited political autonomy in the matter.

It is also the case that diverting the suffering of the Innu children into state-approved medical channels was a means to obscure a perception of gas sniffing as an effect of a long chain of events – sedentarization, imposition of alien institutions and values, sexual abuse by priests and teachers (Samson 2000/1; Samson 2003, 178-80), theft of Innu land, and chronic unemployment – which were ultimately authored by Canada.[8] In dealing with this and similar situations, government officials did not recognize the interconnectedness of the problems experienced by Innu. If this were a case of a simple misunderstanding,

COLIN SAMSON

we might leave the matter there. However, to a certain extent, this lack of recognition is staged and strategic since the interconnectedness of the problems is constantly exposed to these officials by Innu leaders and their attorneys, human rights groups, a vast quantity of literature, and the voices of the Innu sufferers themselves on television and film.

By resorting to medical and pan-Native healing techniques, the Innu villages are starting to gear up for what is in relative terms a massive institutionalization of the problems of gas sniffing, alcoholism, suicide, domestic violence, and sexual abuse. Whereas the specifically Innu therapeutic experience of *nutshimit* (the country) has gradually attenuated – the Outpost Program, which transports families to the country, has virtually ground to a halt, with fewer families going to the country each year and funds for an "alternative school" to teach Innu youth in the country (Innu Tshiskutamashun) having been terminated – specialized medical or pan-Native programs have proliferated in Sheshatshiu in the past decade. At the same time, the closely entwined structures of Innu medicine and spirituality, which had previously helped the people in times of crisis, have been systematically discredited by generations of missionaries and rendered secondary to biomedicine in the villages.[9] When the state has funded specifically Innu-oriented programs – such as a recent Health Canada initiative called Strengthening Communities, in which Innu Elders were funded to spend time with children in the country – the funds have often been only short-term. In the case of Strengthening Communities, the project was discontinued after only one year, allowing no time to gauge how successful such a nonmedical alternative might be.

The Psychological Context: Authenticity and the Double-Bind

What has been said up to now should not be taken to mean that Innu or any Aboriginal people are static. Peoples obviously change, make pragmatic adaptations to new circumstances, and abandon customs. However, it is important to distinguish between forced and voluntary changes. On the whole, immigrants to North America made voluntary adjustments as a result of their settlement across the continent. Aboriginal peoples, by comparison, have been required to make changes as a result of having had to deal with colonizers who first usurped their lands and then embarked upon an aggressive program of assimilation. As is so often observed, Aboriginal peoples such as the Innu now find themselves precariously wedged between two very different societies. "How do we begin to balance the two?" asked the participants at a workshop in Sheshatshiu. "We are experiencing an identity crisis and confusion" (Innu Nation and Mushuau Innu Band Council 1995, 54).

These "two worlds" of the Innu, which Henriksen (1973) drew attention to in the 1960s, can still be discerned almost a half-century later. However, they are nowhere near as discrete as they were in the days that Henriksen was travelling by dogsled with the Mushuau Innu. If there were only two self-contained "worlds" – nutshimit, which is Innu; and the community, which is Akaneshau (non-Aboriginal) – and only two selves that were adapted to each, the Innu predicament would be less complicated. It is not simply that many Innu have to be able to move between the two relatively incompatible spheres of hunting and sedentary village life. Although this is surely a tough test of the fortitude of any individual, it is not all they face. Subject to the pervasive intrusion of industrial developments, and given the constant pressures on the Innu to return to the community for money and other reasons, the country is gradually becoming almost an appendage to the settlements. Simultaneously, with the building of ever more medical or quasi-medical institutions – clinics, treatment centres, shelters – as well as the increasing demands of the state and justice system, the Innu are becoming entrenched in an externally imposed disciplinary order.

The consolidation of the settlements, however, has not eradicated Innu norms and values – sharing, hunting skills, respect for the animals, storytelling, and command of the Innu-aimun language. Although these customs are valued by most Innu, to a large extent they are diminished, contradicted, and/or rendered irrelevant by the standards for education, employability, justice, and the like that must be met to enable any degree of survival beyond welfare. Hence, for the masses of Innu mired in welfare dependency, encouragement to relinquish Innu identity lurks at every turn. Local Akaneshaut (plural of Akaneshau) are keen observers of this predicament. Instead of dwelling on the exertion of power that brought this into being in the first place, their tendency is to play down the differences between Innu and non-Innu. This occurs in part through a kind of folding of Innu historical experience into a larger universalism guided by linear time and constrained by laws of cultural evolution. In the two Labrador villages, this manifests itself in a kind of cheerful championing of skilful "adaptation" to life in the community. The tragedies that continually beset the Innu are spoken of only in terms of momentary lapses, correctable by shrewd political tactics of leadership and with the intervention of outside services.

That there is not very much *significantly* different about the Innu is presupposed by the widespread evolutionary metaphors that were used to justify the sedentarization of the Innu (Samson 2003, 142-50). Differences pertained only to the details of the trajectory of progress since the transition from hunting to industrial society was seen as universal and inevitable. For example, the notion that while in the country the Innu now employ knowledge and technologies derived from elsewhere is often used by Akaneshaut to signify such a leap. The assumption is that by using snowmobiles, driving trucks, or using radios, they are made less Innu. This places the Innu in an impossible situation. Even though they have, like other indigenous peoples, used some ideas and practices to their own benefit very effectively, Innu may be made to feel that this is, in the most charitable interpretation, a borrowing from another people. In turn, the borrowings and adaptations are often perceived to make them less authentically indigenous. The Akaneshaut whom I have met in Goose Bay and elsewhere in Labrador seldom tire of pointing out what they see as the contradictions in a seemingly proud people increasingly adapting the ideas, practices, and languages of Euro-Canada.

A drunken young Innu man, after beckoning me up to his mother's house, once told me several interconnected stories. He was sitting at the kitchen table, looking around blankly at the detritus strewn around the living room. Several cans of beer sat on the table next to what looked like the remains of a plate of fried eggs smeared with tomato ketchup. While continually checking my eyes, he spoke slowly, some physical pain occasionally coursing across his face. He told me of his separation from his wife. Having recently returned from nutshimit, he was reflecting on the contrast in the ways of life. Already, he was embarking on what would be a long spell of drinking. But, now upon his return, he reflected on his separation. How sad it was to see his brother taking his children in his canoe, while his kids were hundreds of miles away in Uashat. He went on to tell me how unhappy he was to be back in Sheshatshiu. Waving his arms toward the window, he said that all the people we saw walking the beach road were *Indians*, those who live in houses, have jobs with the Band Council, and fly to nutshimit. The Innu really lived only before 1950. To be an Innu was to be nomadic, to be a hunter, before sedentarization.

This melancholy reflection folded itself into a story about his first encounter with an Akaneshau after returning to the village. As he was fixing leaks on a canoe with silicone along the beach at Sheshatshiu, the man approached him. Tapping the outboard motor, the white man told him that this machinery was not Innu and that he would be dead without it. The young man said that the Akaneshau's words paralyzed him. He suddenly felt that he couldn't get up from the ground, as if he should sink into the sand.

Most Innu know from their own experience that there is wisdom, pleasure, and meaning in the Innu way of life. Yet they live under every possible mode of persuasion and coercion to operate in the manner of Akaneshaut – this was the original function of imposed institutions such as the school – and when they do so, they are vulnerable to the charge that they are no longer Innu. If they attempt to live what they see as the closest thing to an Innu way of life, like the young man at the kitchen table, this is labelled inauthentic by whites when non-Innu technologies are employed. If they stay in the community, they are said to have simply adopted the Euro-Canadian sedentary lifestyle and to be on the road to becoming whites in all but outward appearance. The more they do this, the more they are perceived as a success in Euro-Canadian terms. This is no longer depicted as a victory of civilization over savagery but euphemistically as a troubled Aboriginal people sharing in what my friend the hunter Napes Ashini calls "the good life." In the eyes of settlers or colonists, the turning point always comes when the Native group begins to employ some technology, attend school and church, or go along with some or all of the demands of Europeans. As Frantz Fanon wrote, "if ... the colonized society expresses its agreement on any point with the colonizing society, there will at once begin to be talk about successful integration" (1965, 126). Only then can settlers gleefully point out, as one did to the young hunter repairing his boat, that the Natives would be dead without the whites, are now living a lie, and would be better off admitting that they and whites are the same.

What we have, then, is a rather complicated double-bind. In the classic formulation of the concept by Bateson and colleagues (1972, 178-79), a double-bind involves the creation of a "no-win" situation for a person who is the subject of repeated and contradictory demands that he or she cannot escape or comment on. Bateson and colleagues argued that, "when a person is caught in a double bind situation, they will respond defensively in a manner similar to a schizophrenic" (180).

Although the double-bind theory has long been contested as an explanation of schizophrenia, it provides a striking metaphor for the contradictions faced by contemporary Innu. Their repeated experiences with the state and its agents are characterized by the insistence that they adapt to foreign institutions and the Euro-Canadian sedentary society. Through the imposition of law, justice, health care, social services, the church, and other institutions, the Innu receive a strong message that in order to survive they will have to start thinking and operating in ways that are often in deep contradiction with Innu morals, values, and practices. If they do not, a host of punishments and reprimands flow – including jail sentences if they do not comply with the law, withdrawal of funds if they do not follow the regulations of Social Services, further sequestration of their land if they do not comply with the various land claims processes, and even the instilling of guilt by the clergy and judges for various acts of noncompliance. This is contradicted by the wishes of most Innu to remain, at least in some degree, Innu. To do so, however, is often very difficult, given the need to conform to the contradictory assumptions both of the law and of the regulations imposed by the institutions that the authorities have established in the villages. Psychologically, the Innu are in a collective no-win situation.

Keeping in mind Bateson's double-bind, we can see that Innu are prevented from exiting this no-win situation, for it is now impossible to break off their relationships with the state and Euro-Canadians. When the Innu attempted to exercise autonomy by evicting an insensitive and racist judge from Davis Inlet in 1993, land claims negotiations were abruptly suspended by the government. In effect, disobedience to the state was countered by the removal of the right to the fundamental element of Innu personhood – their relationship to the land. They were eventually dragged back into line and conceded to bring themselves under the authority of a justice system that they believed violated their cultural integrity and human rights.

Bateson and colleagues claimed that "almost any part of a double bind sequence may ... be sufficient to precipitate panic or rage" (1972, 179). Under the pressure of confusing communications and meta-communications to which no response would be adequate, the researchers argued, the boundaries of the self could dissolve. Individually, the young Innu in the settlements are also in such a no-win position. As many older Innu observe, the young have already begun to internalize Euro-Canadian values and to diminish the import of what is Innu. As Elizabeth Penashue of Sheshatshiu said, "some kids don't want to go to the country. They think they are not Innu. They feel ashamed to say they are Innu" (E. Penashue, pers. comm.) But this rejection of Innu identity is neither comfort nor resolution, as the numbers of young Innu gas sniffers, drinkers, and suicide victims have mushroomed since settlement. Nevertheless, it is not simply a rejection of what is Innu that really affects many of these children. It is a rejection of everything in the society that they have grown into. Many children, like those who are kept in the group home in Sheshatshiu, "don't like school, the community, or *nutshimit*," as the Innu assistant there once told me. In many ways, this points to an important reason why self-destructive activities are rife. Many young people are not integrated into the Innu way of life and do not fully understand or accept the worldview upon which it is based. At the same time, they are not offered an acceptable Euro-Canadian lifestyle and likewise find the premises of much of the dominant worldview – competition, capitalism, urban life, even "multiculturalism" – either remote or objectionable.[10]

The Importance of Cultural Continuity

Both the state and the medical personnel who have been drafted to help deal with all the new mental health problems that have arisen in the Labrador Innu villages have failed to grasp how loss of culture has played a role in the ubiquitous suffering of the people. Yet we know that one of the most important determinants of psychological resilience is cultural continuity.

In the mid-1990s Nutshimiu Atusseun, a forerunner of the "alternative school," Tshiskutamashun, was established as an Innu "school" in the country for Innu youth desperately caught up in cycles of depression and dysfunction within the village. With the help of many hunting families, the program taught young Innu the history of their people, the geography of their lands, and the practical skills needed to live in the country. This assisted in both the transmission of Innu skills and the strengthening of Innu identity among the youth. As a result, those who set up the projects argued that the young people who participated in the program became some of the healthiest and strongest individuals in the communities. According to the organizers, several spontaneous initiatives of the Innu to expose gas-sniffing youth to country life also resulted in vastly enhanced self-esteem and confidence. In all their meetings and conversations on this matter, no one mentioned an instance in which a gas-sniffing child from the community continued to abuse the substance when he or she was placed in the very different environment of the country.[11]

Apart from the obvious benefits of social cohesiveness from which these young people have benefited, they have also been learning in an active rather than a passive way. The development of the senses in the country further helps to reverse the atrophying of many of these same senses through passive and television-mediated education (Nabhan and St. Antoine 1993, 242). Furthermore, it is likely that language fluency and oratory are also stimulated. Taken together, these factors can only assist in enhancing mental well-being. There is also evidence from Tribal educational institutions in the United States that learning about Native American histories, as well as such issues as colonization, political oppression, and violence, can help Native Americans to make sense of the trauma they see around them (Ambler 2003). This is significant because it is precisely these issues that are ignored by the current Labrador School Board's educational system.

There is a growing body of research in social psychology and epidemiology relating to other Aboriginal communities in Canada that backs up the observations of those who have worked with Innu youth on these projects. Some of these studies indicate that a command of traditional knowledge is associated with less self-destructive tendencies. Looking at youth solvent abuse and treatment approaches in two Native centres, Dell and colleagues (2002) argue that young people who have connections with Aboriginal spirituality and have good community support are less likely to be solvent abusers. Chandler and Lalonde (1998; Chapter 10) show that those Aboriginal peoples in British Columbia with higher levels of "cultural continuity" have lower suicide rates than those who have, for various reasons, lost control over their lands and communities. Waldram (Chapter 3) further argues that efforts to reassert autonomy from external institutions is critical to well-being. In observing the close association between suicide and rapid social and cultural change, Kral recommends that "activities directed towards continuity of valued practices ... continue to be developed" (2003, 38). All this makes perfect sense in the contexts in which I have tried to locate the mental health problems of the Innu. It is not simply contact with Europeans that has precipitated the crisis but also the continually invasive and destructive type of contact. Because of the undermining of Innu society and the spiritual dispossession that it occasions, the Innu have lost confidence in their own ways of dealing with conflict, suffering, and affliction. Hence, as Niezen points out, "the decline of local healing resources ... is an obstacle to recovery when crisis does occur." This means that "a vacuum is created by the absence of locally meaningful strategies for dealing with relatively new pathologies of reservation and urban life" (2000, 122). To combat this, Kirmayer, Simpson, and Cargo recommend a "recovery of tradition" as a means to heal the manifold mental health problems in Aboriginal communities (2003, S16). This means that the communal vitality of Innu society will need to be strengthened along the lines of such projects as the alternative school as a defence against the continuing assimilationist pressures, which have the effect of weakening it.

Conclusion

Much of the evidence from ethnographic studies and from the testimonies of Aboriginal peoples themselves suggests that we can address Native self-destructive activities only by taking in a wider span of considerations. Concentrating on pathologies alone and isolating them as medical conditions, although sometimes expedient, ignores that these signs of affliction are part of a larger whole that must first be understood.

The Innu, like several other Northern peoples, stand at a crossroads. From kindergarten classes at the local schools to the latest offer of ameliorative action by the federal government, they are increasingly being handed every possible encouragement to abandon not only the land-based Innu way of life but also the values that have made them unique as a people. It is obvious that assimilation is not a simple matter of "fitting him into our society," as Walter Rockwood (1957) contended, but involves destroying the self that was intimately identified with the indigenous way of life. Thus the older generation of Innu who were socialized as hunters have found it virtually impossible to find any fulfillment in the life of the village. Although they have had the fortitude to eke out livings on welfare, they have not been immune to problem drinking, and many respected Tshenut have died alcohol-related deaths in indignity. The younger generations, however, have had much looser moorings in nutshimit and more intense exposure to the institutions of assimilation. These individuals have often been in the position of being successful in neither the Innu world nor the Akaneshau world, where the local schools have proved woefully inadequate at educating them for the various opportunities in the wider Canadian society.[12] Consequently, the young, feeling they are failures in both worlds, often live out their existences in the villages in a sort of torpor punctuated by drinking, gas sniffing, random and depersonalized sex, and violence. The most recent report to the Canadian Human Rights Commission faults the government both for failing to provide full and continuous support for Innu-directed educational activities and for supporting a Newfoundland educational system that "clearly does not work" (Backhouse and McCrae 2002, 62, 53).

Any understanding of why the Innu and other similarly situated people suffer so much from gas sniffing, suicide, and alcohol-related mortality must start by confronting what it means to deliberately destroy a well-functioning society. To begin with a search for individual medical or psychological pathologies is to start at the end of a historical process, not at the beginning. This lack of attention to the social context hinders the Innu in overcoming their various losses and traumas because they are aware that the reasons why there is so much *communal* dysfunction are related to wider historical, political, and socially generated psychological processes. Similarly, a focus on cash investments in the absence of considerations for cultural continuity may be only a kind of "bagging and tagging" in the imagery of Thomas King's short story described at the start of this chapter. If this continues, the Innu could become, like Thomas King's Indians, curiosities that simply self-destruct.

Acknowledgments
This chapter reflects work done with the Innu from 1994 to 2006. I would like to thank especially George Rich, Napes Ashini, Shushep Mark, Dominic Pokue, Anthony Jenkinson, Simon Claridge, Jules Pretty, and Laurence Kirmayer for assistance with this chapter.

Notes
1 See Table 1.4.19.2 Suicide (ICD-9 E950 E-959), rate per 100,000 population and confidence interval by sex, Canada, provinces, territories, and health regions, on the Statistics Canada website: http://www.stat.ca/english/freepub/82-221-XIE/01201/tables/html/P14192.htm (accessed 2001).
2 It should be noted that the Davis Inlet figure is derived from an average baseline population of 500, and potentially large fluctuations in rates can occur in small samples. The First Nations rate was calculated by Health Canada (2003, 34).
3 The *Calder* case involving the Nisga'a of British Columbia led to the instigation of the Comprehensive Land Claims Policy, which has dealt with the land claims of those Aboriginal groups such as the Innu that have not signed treaties. The ruling established that in these cases Aboriginal title *may* exist and consequently that, once proven, such title needs to be extinguished to establish "certainty" over the disposal and ownership of the lands in question (Asch 1984, 47-51; Berger 1991, 140-53).

4   For example, as early as the 1930s, when sedentarization was beginning to be contemplated, the trader and settler Richard White (1931), who interacted regularly with the Mushuau Innu, predicted that halting the movements of the Innu would have catastrophic consequences.

5   In the Innu case, this gender-role shift involved moving away from the more egalitarian model, common among Northern hunters, and toward a more patriarchal model: the Innu became inducted into the fur trade, missionaries appointed men as "chiefs," and the Canadian welfare system favoured male authority. Eleanor Burke Leacock (1981, 1982) has pointed out that this shift represents a considerable change from the past. Seventeenth-century records show that women were highly autonomous within a largely egalitarian Innu society.

6   This was the case with Premier Smallwood's promotion of the Churchill Falls hydroelectric project in the 1950s and 1960s, Premier Brian Tobin's campaign for a massive extension to this project in 1996, the provincial government's policy of "map-staking" mineral claims, and the federal government's lease of the Goose Bay airbase to NATO (Samson 2003, 96-111).

7   Indeed, the observations of these Innu accord with the prior experiences of indigenous peoples who have been evicted from their lands for mining around the world. In Guyana, for example, among the Amerindian peoples whose lands have been sequestered for mining, the "old values of sharing and cooperation have been replaced by cash values and monetary exchange ... Sophisticated arts and crafts have fallen into disuse, thereby increasing dependency on mining as a mainstay of the economy" (Colchester 1997, 69).

8   As Nancy Scheper-Hughes reports of an analogous situation in the northeast of Brazil, "medicine is, among other things, a technical practice for 'rationalizing' human misery and for containing it to safe quarters, keeping it 'in its place,' and so cutting off its potential for active critique" (1992, 199).

9   This "medical evangelism," combining the forces of Christianity with biomedicine, occurred across Canada as an instrument of dispossession and assimilation (Kelm 1998, 104-6; Niezen 2000, ch. 4).

10 A number of researchers have suggested that this kind of "deculturation" is a particularly important risk factor in Aboriginal suicide and other self-destructive tendencies (Kirmayer 1994, 30; Young 1994, 215).

11 The families associated with the alternative school went on to establish the Tshikapisk Foundation, which has started to organize similar land-based activities for Innu youth. See http://www.tshikapisk.ca/home (accessed 17 June 2008).

12 A study of the two schools in Sheshatshiu and Natuashish found attendance at the schools is typically under 50%, that all 15-year-olds tested were at least 5 years behind equivalent pupils in Canada, that only 17 students had graduated over a 10-year period from both communities, and that 35% of Innu youth display learning difficulties associated with fetal alcohol syndrome (Philpott et al. 2004).

References

Adelson, N. 1998. Health beliefs and the politics of Cree well-being. *Health* 2 (1): 5-22.

Aldridge, D., and K. St. John. 1991. Adolescent and preadolescent suicide in Newfoundland and Labrador. *Canadian Journal of Psychiatry* 36 (6): 432-36.

Alfred, T. 1999. *Peace, power, righteousness: An indigenous manifesto*. Don Mills, ON: Oxford University Press.

Ambler, M. 2003. Cultural resiliency. *Tribal College Journal* 14 (4): 8-9.

Armitage, P. 1989. *Homeland or wasteland? Contemporary land use and occupancy among the Innu of Utshimassit and Sheshatshit and the impact of military expansion*. Sheshatshiu: Innu Nation.

Asch, M. 1984, *Home and native land: Aboriginal rights and the Canadian Constitution*. Toronto: Methuen.

Backhouse, C., and D. McCrae. 2002. *Report to the Canadian Human Rights Commission on the treatment of the Innu of Labrador by the Government of Canada*. Ottawa, ON: University of Ottawa, Faculty of Law.

Bateson, G., D. Jackson, J. Haley, and J. Weakland. 1972. Towards a theory of schizophrenia. In G. Bateson, ed., *Steps to an ecology of mind*, 173-98. London: Paladin.

Berger, T. 1991, *A long and terrible shadow: White values, Native rights in the Americas*. Vancouver: Douglas and McIntyre.

Blackmore, K. 9 June 2003. A cry for help: The new community of Natuashish is experiencing severe growing pains. Editorial. *Labradorian*. http://labradorian.optipresspublishing.com/June09-03/articles/labedit.htm.

Bussidor, I., and U. Bilgen-Reinart. 1997. *Night spirits: The story of the relocation of the Sayisi Dene*. Winnipeg: University of Manitoba Press.

Canadian Broadcasting Corporation (CBC). 7 December 2000. Radio interview with Dr. Jane McGillivray. *This Morning with Shelagh Rogers*.

Canadian Human Rights Commission. 1993. *Violations of law and human rights by the Governments of Canada and Newfoundland in regard to the Mushuau Innu: A documentation of injustice in Utshimassits (Davis Inlet)*. Ottawa, ON: Canadian Human Rights Commission.

Chandler, M., and C. Lalonde. 1998. Cultural continuity as a hedge against suicide in Canada's First Nations. *Transcultural Psychiatry* 35 (2): 191-219.

Colchester, M. 1997. *Guyana: Fragile frontier*. London: Latin America Bureau.

Degnen, C. 2001. Country space as a healing place: Community healing at Sheshatshiu. In C. Scott, ed., *Aboriginal autonomy and development in northern Quebec and Labrador,* 357-78. Vancouver, BC: UBC Press.

Dell, D., et. al. 2002. Resiliency and holistic inhalant abuse treatment. http://www.naho.ca/english/documents/JournalVol2No1ENG3abusetreatment.pdf.

Durkheim, É. 1951. *Suicide: A study in sociology*. Trans. J. Spaulding and G. Simpson. Glencoe, IL: Free Press.

Dyson, J. 30 June 2003. A boost for Innu business: Development center gets $499,035 from ACOA. *Labradorian*, A3.

Epstein, R. 2002. The role of extinguishment in the cosmology of dispossession. In G. Alfredsson and M. Stavropolou, eds., *Justice pending: Indigenous peoples and other good causes,* 45-56. Amsterdam: Kluwer.

Fanon, F. 1965. *A dying colonialism*. New York: Grove Press.

Gosling, W.G. 1910. *Labrador: Its discovery, exploration, and development*. London: Alston Rivers.

Health Canada. 2003. *Statistical profile on the health of First Nations in Canada*. Ottawa, ON: Health Canada.

Henriksen, G. 1973. *Hunters in the barrens: The Naskapi on the edge of the white man's world*. St. John's, NL: ISER Books.

Hind, H.Y. 1863. *Explorations in the interior of the Labrador Peninsula: The country of the Montagnais and Nasquapee Indians*. London: Longman, Green, Longman, Roberts, and Green.

Innu Nation. 1996. *Ntesinan nteshiniman nteniunan: Between a rock and a hard place*. Sheshatshiu: Innu Nation.

–. 1998. *Money doesn't last: The land is forever.* Final report, Innu Nation Community Consultation on Land Rights Negotiations. Sheshatshiu: Innu Nation.

–, and Mushuau Innu Band Council. 1995. *Gathering voices: Finding strength to help our children*. Vancouver, BC: Douglas and McIntyre.

Kelm, M.-E. 1998. *Colonizing bodies: Aboriginal health and healing in British Columbia, 1900-1950*. Vancouver, BC: UBC Press.

King, T. 1999. A short history of Indians in Canada. *Canadian Literature* 161/162 (Summer/Autumn): 62-64.

Kirmayer, L.J. 1994. Suicide among Canadian Aboriginal peoples. *Transcultural Psychiatric Research Review* 31 (1): 3-58.

–, C. Simpson, and M. Cargo. 2003. Healing traditions: Culture, community and mental health promotion with Canadian Aboriginal peoples. *Australasian Psychiatry* 11 (suppl.): S15-S23.

Kral, M. 2003. *Unikkaartuit: Meanings of well-being, sadness, suicide, and change in two Inuit communities*. Final report to the National Health Research and Development Programs, Health Canada. Ottawa, ON: Health Canada.

Lassiter, C. 1987. Relocation and illness: The plight of the Navajo. In D. Levin, ed., *Pathologies of the modern self,* 221-30. New York: New York University Press.

Leacock, E.B. 1981. *Myths of male dominance: Collected articles on women cross-culturally.* New York: Monthly Review Press.

–. 1982. Relations of production in band society. In E.B. Leacock and R. Lee, eds., *Politics and history in band societies,* 159-70. Cambridge: Cambridge University Press.

Lindgren, A. 4 December 2000. Doctor says parents must change. *St. John's Telegram.*

Nabhan, G., and S. St. Antoine. 1993. The loss of floral and faunal story: The extinction of experience. In S. Kellert and E.O. Wilson, eds., *The biophilia hypothesis,* 229-50. Covelo, CA: Island Press.

Napoleon, H. 1999. Yuuyaraq: The way of the human being. In C. Samson, ed., *Health studies: A critical multidisciplinary reader,* 311-37. Oxford, UK: Blackwell.

Niezen, R. 2000. *Spirit wars: Native North American religions in the age of nation building.* Berkeley, CA: University of California Press.

Office of the Auditor General of Canada. 17 October 2000. Other audit observations. Press release.

Philpott, D., W. Nesbit, M. Cahill, and G. Jeffery. 2004. *An educational profile of the learning needs of Innu youth.* St. John's: Memorial University of Newfoundland.

Rich, G. 23-25 June 2003. Statement to the regional meeting of experts on Indigenous rights in Canada and the Commonwealth Caribbean Region. Georgetown, Guyana.

Rockwood, W. 1957. *General policy in respect of the Indians and Eskimos of northern Labrador.* St. John's, NL: Provincial Archives of Newfoundland and Labrador.

Royal Commission on Aboriginal Peoples. 1995. *Choosing life: Special report on suicide among Aboriginal people.* Ottawa, ON: Minister of Supply and Services Canada.

–. 1996. *Looking forward, looking backward.* Vol. 1. Ottawa, ON: Minister of Supply and Services Canada.

Saganash, R., A. Orkin, and J. Orkin. 25 June 2003. *A study in contrasts: A new vision of Aboriginal inclusion in Quebec and the continuing federal government imposition of extinguishment of Aboriginal rights across Canada.* Submission of the Grand Council of the Crees (Eeyou Istchee) to the Indigenous Rights in the Americas Project meeting. Georgetown, Guyana.

Sahlins, M. 1974. *Stone age economics.* London: Tavistock.

Samson, C. 2000/1. Teaching lies: The Innu experience of schooling. *London Journal of Canadian Studies* 16 (special issue Continuities and changing realities: Meanings and identities among Canada's Aboriginal Peoples): 83-102.

–. 2001. Sameness as a requirement for the recognition of the rights of the Innu of Canada: The colonial context. In J. Cowan, M.-B. Dembour, and R. Wilson, eds., *Culture and rights: Anthropological perspectives,* 226-48. Cambridge: Cambridge University Press.

–. 2003. *A way of life that does not exist: Canada and the extinguishment of the Innu.* St. John's, NL: ISER Books.

–, and J. Pretty. 2006. Environmental and health benefits of hunting lifestyles and diets for the Innu of Labrador. *Food Policy* 31 (6): 528-53.

Scheper-Hughes, N. 1992. *Death without weeping: The violence of everyday life in Brazil.* Berkeley, CA: University of California Press.

Schwarz, M.T. 2001. *Navajo lifeways: Contemporary issues, ancient knowledge.* Norman, OK: University of Oklahoma Press.

Tanner, V. 1947. *Outlines of the geography, life, and customs of Newfoundland-Labrador: The eastern part of the Labrador Peninsula.* 2 vols. Cambridge: Cambridge University Press.

Tester, F.J., and P. Kulchyski. 1994. *Tammarniit (Mistakes): Inuit relocation in the eastern Arctic, 1939-1963.* Vancouver, BC: UBC Press.

White, R. 1931. The Naskapi Indians: Notes compiled for Dr. Frank G. Speck. St. John's, NL: Centre for Newfoundland Studies.

Wilson, J. (writer), and K. Kirby (producer). 7 August 1994. *The two worlds of the Innu.* BBC2 documentary film.

Wotton, K. 1986. Mortality of Labrador Innu and Inuit, 1971-82. In R. Fortuine, ed., *Circumpolar health '84: Proceedings of the Sixth International Symposium on Circumpolar Health,* 139-42. Seattle, WA: University of Washington Press.

York, G. 1990. *The dispossessed: Life and death in Native Canada.* London, UK: Vintage.

Young, T.K. 1994. *The health of Native Americans.* New York: Oxford University Press.

6

Placing Violence against First Nations Children: The Use of Space and Place to Construct the (In)credible Violated Subject

JO-ANNE FISKE

Residential schools for First Nations children, operated for more than a century by religious institutions on behalf of the Canadian government, confined young children and adolescents within physical and symbolic boundaries. Sequestered from families and communities, First Nations children lived a regimented life that reflected European penal and seminary practices: strict gender separation, rigid routines, hard physical labour, humiliating surveillance and corporeal punishments, and cultural and social deprivation. Native languages were forbidden, cultural practices condemned, and family organization deemed primitive and immoral (Deiter 1999; Jaine 1993; Milloy 1999). Religious instruction and domestic training – girls for household work and boys for agricultural and industrial trades – took precedence over classroom learning. The consequences of this bounded life have been revealed in recent decades with disclosures of sexual, physical, mental, and spiritual abuses (Jaine 1993; Knockwood 1992; Milloy 1999). Public revelations, protests, and litigation in the 1980s led the churches involved to apologize not only for cases of criminal abuse but also for the core practices of residential schooling. By the close of the last century, as the media reported on court cases and negotiations for redress and as First Nations authors wrote of their personal and collective schooling experiences, there emerged a new understanding of the schools as a dehumanizing legacy that disrupted families and communities through successive generations (Deiter 1999; Milloy 1999). In this new discourse, First Nations people were constituted as violated subjects (Chrisjohn and Young 1997).

In this chapter, I want to show how the violated subject of the residential school was created by the social production of place – that is, quite literally, how the violated subject is *located*. Stated otherwise, the violated subject comes into focus through a complex set of spatial practices – positioning, naming, locating, and mapping – that are simultaneously ideological, theological, political, cultural, and structural. Stated otherwise, our understanding of subjectivity is mediated through place. To show this, I will compare the location of domestic violence to that of colonial violence situated within a residential space – the "Indian residential school." Drawing on anthropological and postcolonial theories of spatiality interwoven with feminist praxis, I develop my argument in five steps. First, I discuss the spatial production of the subject – that is, the ways that different forms of subjectivity are created by configurations of spatial boundaries and locations. Boundaries simultaneously divide and connect concepts of space and place as they function to oppose the habitable to inhabitable, domestic to wild, secular to sacred. Second, I consider the spatial production of the *violated* subject in the domestic realm and follow this with an examination of the spatial production of the violated subject in the colonial institution. Here, I draw on the notion of the religious community as an extension of the "domestic" realm to explore the role of this domesticity in displacing the "wild" as a marked feature of "civilization." Fourth, I take up the production of privacy and denial, of "not seeing" the interior of domestic space, which makes it an "invisible landscape" and leads to a refusal to accept social-collective responsibility. I argue that what unites the domestic and the colonial institutions are commonsense perceptions of the home and the residential school as moral places bounded by privacy and a naturalized, gendered hierarchy. Finally, I make the claim that in these perceptions each site/location is understood to be separated from the public site (and hence from the public gaze) of common responsibility by a naturalized boundary between chaos and order. My interest lies in linking popularized gendered images and cultural templates to a particular neo-conservative politics that disavows justice claims arising from bodily and mental harm suffered in intimate spaces and that reverses the claims of injustice so that the churches – not the Aboriginal children, families, or communities – are positioned as victims.

Representing Place and Space

> *Man is a wanderer. Woman holds him back. A land without woman, fit only for passing through, a country uninhabited because it lacked a place to plant the stake the restless animal is tethered to.*
>
> – JACQUES FERRON, *CHRONICLE OF ANSE SAINT-ROCH* (1997), 172

Theoretical concepts of place are currently a "contested terrain." As theorists have sought to locate the construction of social relations, they have moved our understanding of place and space beyond that of a conventional geographical mapping of concrete materiality to what Walter has called the *expressive place*: "a specific milieu laded with emotional and symbolic features of experience; a place that contains feelings and meanings, which may be expressed through objects, structure, forms, surfaces, images, stories myths, memories, and dreams" (1988, 215). In focusing on place as a location and mode of expression, we move from understanding place as a container or location of social relations and lived reality to perceiving spatial practices as constructing and being constructed by social relations. Walter distinguishes place as "a location of experience; the container of shapes, powers, feelings, and meanings," from space, which lies outside of experience (1988, 215). I build on Walter's application of the ancient Greek notion of *theoria* as the holistic grasping of the whole experience of place, linking sight with insight as a way to grasp experience that involves all the senses and feelings (4). Lying beyond senses and feelings, space connotes wilderness, a vast emptiness, a location of the unsettled, and hence a site of chaos. To invoke space is to locate the imagination beyond experience, to invoke darkness within a moral topography.

In exploring more broadly the relationships between place and subjectivity, I wish to work through the dichotomy of space/place as constituted in colonial subjugation and settlement, in which the notion of home represents an absolute sense of belonging to place (Rose 1993). Colonial discourses were grounded in "scientific claims constituted by, and then made to bear the weight of, moralistic judgments about both people and place" (Livingstone 1994, 136). The association of wilderness with amorality by colonial powers gave rise to a "moral geography" that persisted from the mid-nineteenth century through the late Victorian era and into the twentieth century (Livingstone 1994; Smith 1996). Juxtaposing the amoral space of wilderness to the "moral place" of domesticity and civilization allowed the frontier to be concretized by the cartographic representation of settled, domestic place. From this viewpoint, residential schools marked the moral obligation of the British Empire – as expressed in 1842 by W.R. Hamilton, a fellow of the Royal Society – "for enlarging her powers of civilizing the yet benighted portions of the globe, and for bearing her part in forwarding and directing the destinies of manhood" (quoted in Livingstone 1994, 135). Residential schools for the Aboriginal children marked the transformation of unsettled wildness to settled experience. To the social evolutionists, space and its inhabitants represented concretely "the blind powers of nature" over which civilization triumphed (Buckle 1882), and to this end residential schools were designed to transform children from "the natural condition to that of civilization" through displacement of Aboriginal culture and reorientation in a place imbued by European meaning – that is, in a "circle of civilization that would operate as a 'home' to the children" (Milloy 1999, 25, 33).

Place is not inert; place and being are, as Heidegger (1962) postulated, intimately connected. In Jager's words, "dwelling ... becomes itself the fundamental human activity, in light of which both place and space find their first clarification" (1983, 154). Drawing on Heidegger, Jager argues that architecture is the embodiment of place, as it "comes to accentuate a certain sense of bodily possibilities." "A building," he asserts, "shapes our movements and leads us to a certain outlook or assures us a certain grasp ... [it] is a codified dance, an insistent invitation to live our bodily being in a certain manner ... Place therefore, the 'place' of the 'subject,' throws light upon subjectivity itself" (155). Following Augé, we can conceive of the residential school as an "anthropological place" characterized by "identity, relations, and history." Anthropological places embody social identity and spatial representations of the past – that is, they constitute the history of a people and their place, geographically and socially (Augé 1995, 52). Located on the frontier, residential schools constitute simultaneously the subjectivity of the colonizer and the colonized. They index multiple meanings within a moral geography: the colonizers' topography of benevolent civilization and the colonized topography of violation and loss.

JO-ANNE FISKE

As postcolonial theorists have pointed out in the past decades, place emerges not only through actions and inhabitation but also through language and naming. "Place is thus the concomitant of difference, the continual reminder of separation, and yet of the hybrid interpenetration of the coloniser and the colonised ... The theory of place ... indicates that in some sense place *is* language, something in constant flux, a discourse in process" (Ashcroft, Gareth, and Tiffin 1995, 391, original emphasis). Understanding place as discourse leads us to recognize the discontinuous and imagined nature of place. This resonates with Walter's concept of expressive place, for "it is precisely within the parameters of place and its separateness that the process of subjectivity can be conducted" (1988, 392).

Domestic Place

> *This is the true nature of home – it is the place of Peace; the shelter, not only from all injury, but from all terror, doubt and division. In so far as it is not this it is not home; so far as the anxieties of the outer life penetrate into it, and the inconsistently minded, unknown, unloved, or hostile society of the outer world is allowed by either the husband or the wife to cross the threshold, it ceases to be home; it is then only a part of that outer world which you have roofed over, and lighted fire in. But so far as it is a sacred place, a vestal temple, a temple of the hearth watched over by Household Gods ... so far as it is this, and roof and fire are types only of a nobler shade and light, shade as of the rock in a weary land, and light as of the Pharos in the stormy sea; – so far it vindicates the name, and fulfils the praise, of Home.*
>
> – JOHN RUSKIN, *SESAME AND LILIES* (1865), PARA. 68

In its original meaning, *domestic* refers literally to the attachment of animals to the house. Husbandry of tame animals is set in civilization narratives as the opposition of the human to the wild. In European thought, the female domestic subject emerges from dichotomous spatial practices of private/public realms whose meanings are encoded in ideological discourses of civilization and the rise of the state. The state constitutes the private sphere but concedes its authority to father/husband and thereby defines the domestic interior as a place of male liberty beyond public law. Within this duality, the domestic dwelling emerges as an expressive place that marks gender status relations through the enclosure of woman and the confinement of sexuality to the private realm. Burdened by the legacy of coverture, in which marriage traditionally marks the "civil death" of wife through loss of identity and full adulthood, the woman is positioned in relation to husband. Her legal position is relative, not based on individual rights as citizen, as is her husband's, but on her status as a subservient and subordinate subject.[1]

The private dwelling signifies the sphere of acceptable sensuality and control of sexuality. Because privacy contains desires, containment within the private dwelling marks female submission to moral rules (see Douglas 1991). The logic of the female body is incorporated through the occupation of the private; through enclosure in the private realm women learn enclosure/privacy of the body. Their morality is incorporated in the moral architecture of home lived spatially through degrees of privacy and exclusion. The privacy of the bedroom encodes the privacy of the female body. From the male perspective, ownership of place signifies ownership of the female body contained within it (Grosz 1995).

As a site of incorporated experience, the private dwelling is the choreographer of routine feminized labour, which, when trivialized, constitutes female subjectivity as inferior and lacking autonomy and, when valorized, constitutes female nurture as the boundary between the civilized and the barbarian. Thus female subjectivity is forever contradictory. At once inferior and superior, the female subject emerges as an *incredible* violated and violating subject. Her claims of abuse are discounted as she is represented either as misrepresenting harms done to her or as constituting a threat to social well-being.[2] It is within the home, the private domain, where a woman comes to know herself as a victim of *domestic violence,* not a victim of violence *per se.* Discourses of the domestic place her as a victim violated by the intimacy that is engendered to protect her. The place of idealized safety is now embodied as the site of double jeopardy: physical endangerment as hidden by the veil of privacy does not abate with public visibility. Instead, emerging into public gaze, the "domestic" violated subject is located as an incredible subject. She is trapped within contradictory discourses of superficial wounding and intimate commitment and their extreme opposite, which frames violated women as having a stoic forbearance of danger that defies rationality (Grosz 1995; Koshan 1997; Mahoney 1991; Schneider 1994).

Located as a victim of domestic violence, the violated subject cannot help but be simultaneously located as a violator: victims become victimizers. As the site of male domination, the home signifies a "safe haven" for men; emerging discourses of male victimology seek to reclaim this safe haven of naturalized power, even as they view the public sphere as a newly appropriated site of unbridled female power. If the home is no longer the protected domain of women, it is no longer the safe haven of men whose power remains undisputed. The verbally assaulted ("male bashed") man replaces the physically violated woman as an object of concern. In discourses linking displacement of men in the public sphere to violence against women in the private sphere, roles are semantically reversed and encoded in exaggeration and distortion. Public space displaces the home as the safe haven of men seeking refuge from women's words as men are represented as victims of women's powers. A plethora of websites trumpeting "father's rights" and "men's rights" claim to represent true manhood, which they say is threatened by changing sexual morals and the emergence of women in public places. In semantic reversal of the powerful and dominated, men are located as victims in domestic and public realms.

> The epidemic rate of malicious false sexual harassment and other charges
> clearly demonstrate that men need the right to "safe havens." Nowhere is safe
> for a man at present, especially with record levels of sexual harassment charges

at work. Some men may experience constant day long verbal abuse in the home from their partners and with record male unemployment the traditional safe havens such as bars and working men's clubs may be unavailable to them. (UK Men and Father's Rights 1996)

Aggressive rhetoric, which is meant to alarm, is commonplace on websites protesting men's loss of power and rights. From the United States, Gerald Rowles, who holds a doctorate, ruptures illusions that belligerent rhetoric is linked to poor education or is merely wild rant that can be easily dismissed. As with the advocates of men's rights in Britain, Rowles associates power of men with civilization and asserts that without the uncontested supremacy of the former, the latter will be destroyed:

> It's time to attack the forces that are trying to destroy the American culture.
> It's time for men to aggressively retake manhood and fatherhood from the usurpers. It's time to take your children back from the socialists, the sexual hedonists and the sodomy lobby. It's time to tell the Feminihilists to just shut up, and stop calling men vicious names. It's time to raise some legal hell that makes your voice heard. (2002)

Fear of women-occupied public space has been expressed in less strident but no less hostile terms when public figures were brought to account for past violence against women, particularly when the women were marginalized by race and class. In 1999 in Canada, textual reversals and coded stereotypes explicitly racialized women's sexuality in media coverage and political comment following the rape trial of member of Parliament Jack Ramsay, then justice critic of the Reform Party. Found guilty of attempted rape of an Aboriginal teenaged girl while serving in the RCMP in her First Nations community, Ramsay (who after an appeal pleaded guilty on a lesser charge) was depicted in the national media as the "saint," his victim as the "sinner" (Sampert 2002). His political supporters decried the plaintiff's actions against the "family man" with a life lived well and deployed rhetorical strategies of exaggeration: they warned Canadians that all men are now threatened by the ease with which women of their pasts could accuse them of sexual predation and racialization, and they drew lurid images of domestic life in First Nations communities. The president of Ramsay's riding association averred: "Every male in Canada should check the skeletons in their closet because what this means is any lady can accuse you of rape, and even when you haven't done it, it's your word against theirs" (Henry and Tator 2002, 213).[3]

Like the ancient Greek playwrights Sophocles, Euripedes, and Aeschylus, who construed Athenian women as barbarians by likening them to the Persian invaders, and Aristotle, who argued that women's rights led to the downfall of Sparta, those who now disavow the credibility of the violated domestic subject constitute the uncontrolled woman as the "barbarian within" when she asserts her rights to citizenship and public space. Citing

Newt Gingrich as an example, Patterson demonstrates the link as lying in the neo-conservative view that "practices that aid women or members of minority groups should either be placed in the control of men, restricted, or criminalized" (1997, 124).

The violent language found on websites may be absent from academic texts but not the fear that recognition of the credibility of violated subjects will threaten civilization as the sphere of masculinity. John Fekete, a Canadian cultural theorist, targets loss of male power within domestic space as an index of emasculation. He condemns feminist understandings of gender as a "biopolitics," which he considers an "anti-politics; a regression *from* politics to a new primitivism which promotes self-identification through groups defined by categories like race or sex" (1994, 22, original emphasis). Through denigration of women as primitive, Fekete conflates racial and gender identities to mock claims for equitable citizenship. Thus he displaces attention from experienced injustices and violence onto abstract political goals. His framing of women as a primitive danger within and to civilization deflects attention from the very real consequences of abuse of women in all it forms.

As a minority within a minority, Aboriginal women are triply victimized in this regard. First, they are subjected to extraordinary levels of physical and sexual violence within and outside the domestic realm.[4] Second, when they disclose their suffering and seek justice, they are positioned as a threat to civilization in a politics of nationalism that raises spectres of primitivism and atavistic violence. Third, in the process, Aboriginal strategies to regain control over community processes through revitalizing traditional legal orders and healing practices are implicitly denigrated.

Colonial Space

> Remember that ... England is ... the nation which above all others has conquered nature by obeying her; that it pleased God ... that we, Lord Bacon's countrymen, should improve that precious heirloom of science, inventing, producing, exporting, importing, till it seems as if the whole human race, and every land from the equator to the pole must hence forth bear the indelible impress and sign of English science ... the glorious work which God seems to have laid on the English to replenish the world and subdue it.
>
> – CHARLES KINGSLEY, *SCIENTIFIC LECTURES AND ESSAYS* (1880), 308

Just as the violated domestic subject emerges from dichotomous spatial practices of public/private realms, so the violated colonial subject emerges from spatial dichotomies of unsettled space/settled place. As suggested above, within colonial worldviews the notion of space evoked a sense of an empty wilderness that lay outside of civilization (Livingstone 1994; Smith 1996). "Wilderness" was marked as vast, empty space, dark and hostile. It was imagined to be beyond the location of experience and fantasized to be the unknown and as yet unconquered.[5] In contradistinction, colonialists understood place as the site of settled experience. Place connoted the very representation of lived reality; wilderness marked a mysterious space haunted by wild beasts – Anglo Saxon *wylder ness* has been glossed as the nest or lair of the wild beast and the Old English *wilddeoren* as the place where beasts ran wild (Sluyler 2002, 185). Once it was understood as the location of the "other," wilderness came to mark nomadic territory, and colonial texts are replete with references to the inhabitants of the "wilderness" as wild and untamed. The colonial dichotomy of wilderness/civilization is foregrounded today in historical, geographical, and ecological narratives that draw their titles and themes directly from colonial texts, signalling the enduring appeal that notions of exile and emptiness retain (Cole 1979, 2001; Livingstone 1994; McNab 1999). In the colonial mind, place-naming and space-bounding symbolically transformed *space* into *place;* the expressive places of colonial history marked the (im)moral boundary of imperial penetration (Burghardt 1996; Sluyler 2002; Smith 1996).[6]

The colonial awe of wilderness was founded on the Christian representation of wilderness as a site of temptation and darkness, a place of exile. As a site of civilization on the colonial frontier, the missionary residential school took on multiple, often contrary meanings. It stood at the intersection of the real and the imagined, of sacred dreams and sacrilegious memories. Imagined in the colonial consciousness as the antithesis to wilderness, as sociosacred place – containing chapels, consecrated cemeteries, and secular common areas of study and work – the residential school marked, and continues to mark, the site of struggle between nature and nation, between colonized and colonizer symbolized in the juncture of male authority and female nurture (Fiske 1981; Rutherdale 2002, 103-5, 120). The building and lands of the residential school shaped domestic relations of work and social interaction in a "codified dance" that enscripted power/knowledge relations. At the level of concrete lived experience, the spatial arrangements of the school marked a series of dichotomous domesticated social relations through inclusion/exclusion: priest versus nuns, teaching staff versus farm help, workers versus students, and male versus female. The principal as patriarch separated himself from the subjugated and inferior staff and students through his occupation of spaces of power: office and private rooms, which included dining and sitting areas. Sisters/matrons lived also within a space dichotomized not only from the principal but also among themselves: the mother superior/matron had her position of authority distinct from the living and social spaces of her subordinates, the sisters who taught and nursed the children. Physical boundaries marked repressed emotional expression as children filed to meals in silence, confined themselves to gender specific areas, and governed the speed of their movements to conform to the coercive and often brutal discipline (Fiske 2005).

Children's domestic roles, encoded in gender servitude, played out in the distinct tasks of boys and girls. Outdoor spaces were masculine; boys worked in fields, "just like bulldozers" (Fiske 1981, 25), and carried out routine tasks in barns and other outbuildings. Indoors was a female space; in the infirmary, kitchen, and sewing rooms, girls learned

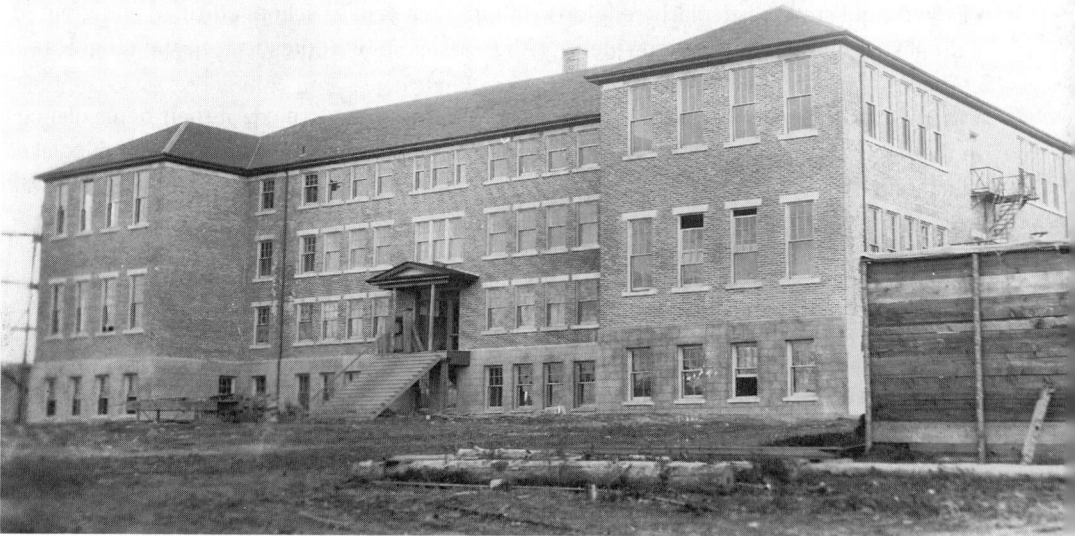

FIGURE 6.1   Lejac residential school at Fraser Lake, BC. *Courtesy of The Exploration Place at the Fraser-Fort George Regional Museum, Fraser-Fort George Museum Society, P982.33.91*

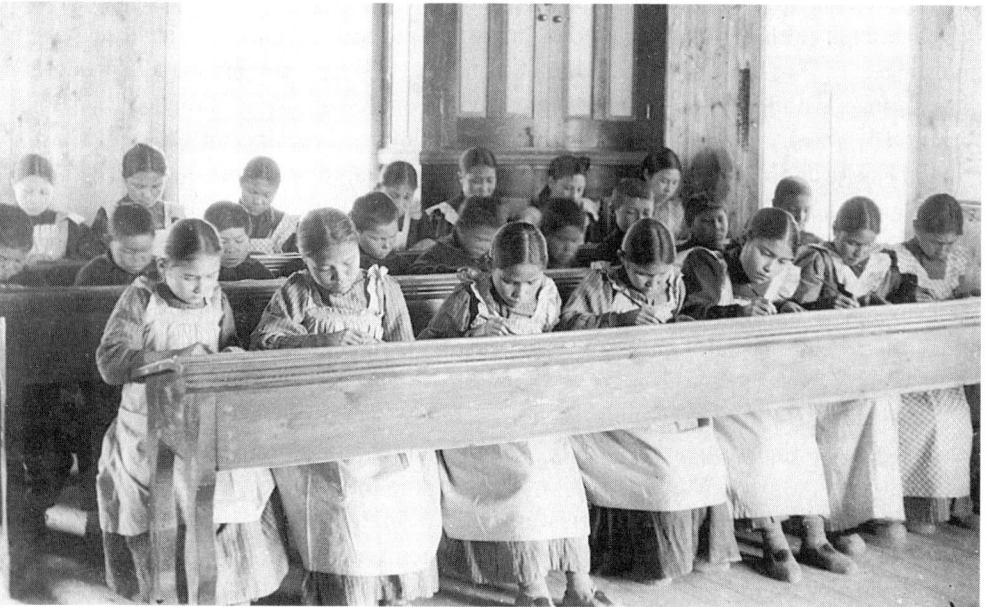

FIGURE 6.2   Study time, Indian residential school, Fort Resolution, NWT. *Courtesy of Library and Archives Canada, Department of Mines and Technical Surveys, PA-042133*

their gender roles through the embodiment of domestic tasks (Fiske 1981). Thus the school's architecture was imaged as domestic, with spatial arrangements woven through notions of fictive and sacred kinship and the social processes of family. In the lived reality of the school staff, particularly religious staff, the residential school affirmed and granted a domestic, moral, and religious identity, the extension of domesticity to the religious community (Rutherdale 2002, 100ff).

For staff, the school was the site of their suffering and sacrifice, of their benevolence in their personal and collective crusade against the wilderness and its wandering, unplaced inhabitants. Personal sacrifice was indexed within the very architecture of the school: staff lived in small, sparse quarters, confined themselves to gender-specific areas, and endured poorly heated and ventilated rooms. What the children suffered as abuse and privation could be conceived by the staff as being no different from their self-abnegation: lack of privacy, austerity, physical discomfort, isolation from family and community, meager diet, and the like. In this manner, children's deprivations, mental and emotional stress, and even prevailing hunger were read, and continue to be read, within the narratives of altruistic femininity as the deprivations and the mental and emotional stress of the subjugated house-wife – that is, as a spatial relation of socioreligiously mandated subordination (Fiske 2005).

Domesticity was incorporated not only by those who dwelt within but also by the mission societies that sponsored the staff. Neighbours passing by in their daily routines took for granted the expressive symbols of domestic life. The fences, fields, gardens, and barns bore the conventional arrangement of rural places and replicated the farmers' lived patterns of daily life. The neatness of fields and buildings, richness of gardens, and even flapping of full clotheslines all marked meaning and purpose sought by agricultural settlers and suggested that life within the school was normal and predictable. The neat cemetery with its small wooden crosses spoke to the rhythm of life embodied in the nearby farms. As noted by a woman rancher, after her half-century of passing along the highway adjacent to the Lejac residential school in central British Columbia, the cemetery was particularly reassuring to her that life within the institution played out in predictable routines. Shocked by former residents' allegations of deprivation, hunger, loneliness, and abuse, she wondered how a place that so clearly cared for the dead souls could be accused of violating the living. "There were no signs," she said, "that anything was wrong. Just a lovely farm site with its beautiful fields and lakeshore. I never imagined that they could have wanted more."[7]

This inability to imagine life inside the school reveals the power of "buildings themselves [to] make their appearance as a certain embodied grasp on the world, as possible human stances, as particular manners of taking up the body and the world, as specific orientations disclosing certain aspects of a worldly horizon" (Jager 1983, 154). Through their everyday interactions with one another as a community that dwelt beyond the boundaries of the "other," the neighbouring farmers reproduced the social structure that subordinated First Nations children in an ideology of civilized domesticity. The spatio-social continuum of domesticity in an agricultural household was read into the lives of

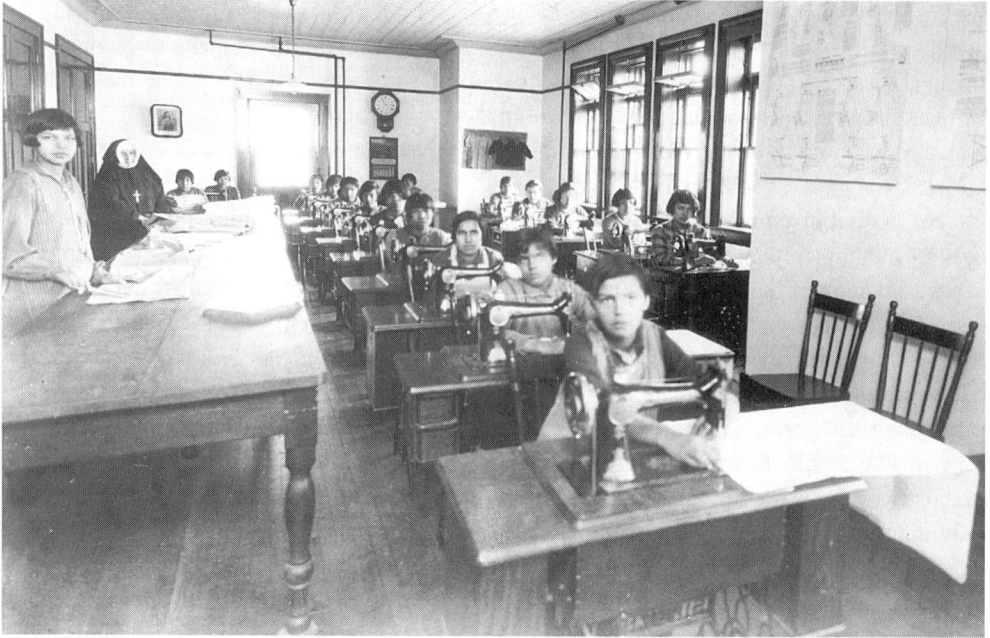

FIGURE 6.3
Sewing class, Indian residential school. *Courtesy of the Aboriginal Healing Foundation*

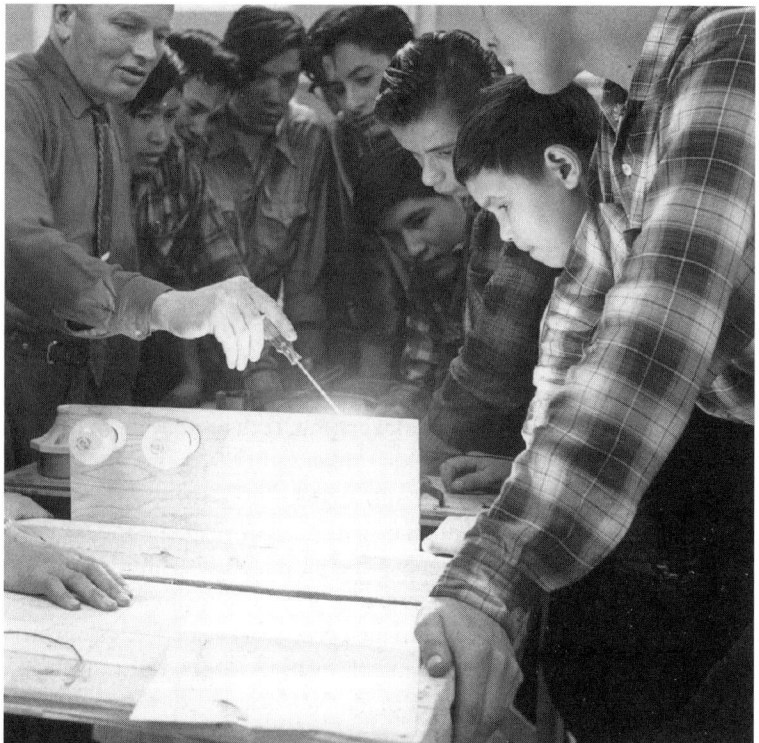

FIGURE 6.4
Shop class, Indian residential school. *Courtesy of the Aboriginal Healing Foundation*

the residents of the school so that neighbours could not "see" a life other than one mirrored in their own as they read conventional spatial arrangements as proof of normal
social relations. In this context of domestication, tales of suffering and abuse are received
with the same skepticism as recovered memories of sexual abuses in the private home
and are thus prey to repudiation as confabulations, exaggerations, or conscious deceit
for personal gain or political posturing.[8]

The spatial discourse of domesticity radiated beyond the mundane routine of daily
lives to ideological and theological spheres. Residential schools marked the presumptive
frontier of settler society. Fields and barn, united with church, stood against the wilderness and stood for settlement. The cross above the chapel and in the graveyard, the sight
of religious sisters in their black habits, and the routine pastimes of Sunday worship and
country walks all served to justify to the passersby their own claims to the vast lands,
which were to be transformed from wilderness to field. Residential schools also served
to remind settlers of their own historical origins in the "old countries" and the enduring
authority of the Christian faith. The domesticity of the residential school therefore not
only shaped settlers' complacency that all was well with the children but also reinforced
the colonial ideological supposition that the children *needed* domestic confinement. Placed
beyond the public gaze, children were rendered invisible by the imagined moral frontier.

The very existence of the school and its placement beyond the boundaries of community on the margin reflected back to the children their subjectification as uncivilized,
barbarous, and wild. Fences not only delineated the boundaries of wilderness and domesticity but also imprisoned the students, while the cemetery and its fences – a deathscape
– communicated loss and suffering to the little inmates.

In the paradoxical deployment of colonial subjugation, spatial containment of children
represented their presumed imposed subjectivity as the transformers of the very wildness
they were accused of embodying; sociospatial transformation lay in their own processes
of subjectivity. Set beyond the boundaries of settlement, the residential school was a liminal space, a site of transcendence through domestication of wild children and cultivation
of the soil. Just as the domesticated woman is held in a paradoxical subjectivity as both
socially inferior and morally superior, so the children of residential schools were viewed
simultaneously as needing containment in order to regulate their desires and as the potential agent of a civilizing transformation of their people. In the words of Milloy, "they
would be the leaven of civilization, moving their communities along to a fully civilized
and self-sufficient state" (1999, 17).

If we accept Aristotle's maxim that to know oneself, one must know one's place, two
principles must follow. To know oneself as a violated subject, one must experience the
violation of place; to envision a new subject position, one must envision a new sense of
place. If in memories of the former residences, the school takes on meaning as a sick or
bad place – in Walter's terms a *cacotope* (1988, 215) – the transition of the residential
school site to a good or healing place (as has been the case when First Nations reclaim
the buildings as education or healing centres under their own control) takes on meaning

as a spatial politics of resistance.[9] Spatial discourses give differential substance to memories of abuse as they shift membership from domestic to public relationships. Continuous renaming of the "place" – from mission or residential school to prison (Milloy 1999); from concentration camp (Crow Dog and Erdoes 1990) or genocidal battlefield (Chrisjohn and Young 1997; Churchill 1998) to holy site of pilgrimage (Fiske 1996) – reinvents colonial place and its inhabitants as something other than violated subjects. Renaming shifts subjectivity from wild child to student, from student to victim and inmate, from victim to survivor, from survivor to warrior and even to saint.[10] References to the deadly consequences of residential schools (school records provide evidence of death rates ranging from 11% to 47% due to epidemics and other causes)[11] as a holocaust redefines the schools as "concentration camps," no longer places of colonial altruism and Christian sacrifice but places of misbegotten benevolence, whose intent had a dark side (Furniss 1995). The subject position as survivor marks a personal strength and endurance that inscribes a moral affinity with other kinds of survivors recognized at the global level and reconstitutes the individual memories of abuse and subjugation of victimhood as a collective memory of national scale. Narratives of school memories – arising as testimonials in conferences, law courts, and healing circles and published in a plethora of Aboriginal news magazines and biographies, particularly as an avowed resistance to the assimilationist intent of the school regime – constitute a historic landscape that creates empathy for past generations by honouring the heroics of cultural warriors (e.g., Deiter 1999; Knockwood 1992). The location of the problems of contemporary life, fraught with dysfunction and personal suffering, at the site of collective abuse reconfigures marginalized experiences as an honourable collective history and in doing so dishonours the official history of the colonial regime. This discursive shift aims to move the experience of abuse out of the domesticated realm of childhood and into a political sphere of ethnopolitics and national identity, thus opening the way for a new meaning of experience within the consciousness of an oppressed people: history of place emerges as history of power (Chrisjohn and Young 1997).

The residential school, unveiled of its mystique of domestic altruism, becomes the most poignant symbol of colonial violence. It is revealed as a torturous landscape of common suffering. The shift from the private place of childhood abuse to the social place of political oppression offers validation of personal suffering and grants credibility to tales of abuse and valorization through public disclosure, as Kirmayer has noted in comparing the incredibility of childhood victims' memories of sexual abuse with the legitimacy eventually accorded Holocaust survivors' narratives of suffering. A public space of trauma provides a consensual reality and collective memory through which the fragments of personal memory can be assembled, reconstructed, and displayed with a tacit assumption of validity. A private space of trauma places the victim in a predicament since the validation of suffering depends on recovering enough memory to make it real for others, but this memory can be retrieved only by reliving or re-presenting the place of victimization (Kirmayer 1996, 190).

JO-ANNE FISKE

Kirmayer goes on to assert that "the fundamental difference [between accounts of childhood abuse and Holocaust testimonies] lies in the social context of retelling. In the case of Holocaust testimony, the enormity of the event always precedes the individual story, so that every detail becomes portentous. In the case of the victim of childhood abuse, the retelling involves an idiosyncratic personal history whose moral implications attack our complacent image of family life" (1996, 190).

To this, I would add that difference arises from location. Unlike a colonial regime of education and purported advancement and assimilation, the public evil of the massacre of millions of Jews, gypsies, and other peoples cannot be disavowed by reference to domesticity. Renaming and reconstitution of subjectivity are no easier for the violated subjects of colonial power than they are for victims/survivors of domestic abuse. In the current struggle over the meanings and consequences of residential schooling, faith in altruistic sacrifice of a colonial regime threatens to override First Nations' quest for citizenship, human rights, and universal justice.

Narratives of abuse are once again located within a domestic realm, and victims of violence are made out to be threats to the established moral and political order. Disavowal of the legitimacy of survivors' claims phrased in a discourse of space versus place arises in defence of "civilization." In sanctioned ignorance or approved denial, survivors' calls for justice are repudiated with calls to honour self-abnegation. In a letter to the *Globe and Mail,* Larry Bennett responded defensively to a column by former residents of the schools: "I was absolutely stunned at the ingratitude of Aboriginals toward people, most of them decent, hard-working souls, who gave their lives to the cause of native peoples. It couldn't have been easy spending your life in isolated communities, trying to guide a stone-age people into the atomic age. Most nuns and priests treated the children as though they were the ones they never had; now they are treated like this" (2001, A12).

In a similar vein, *The Report Newsmagazine* opined that "the group that many express concern for is those who gave their entire lives to the church and are now feeling devalued, tarred by the same brush as the pedophiles" (McLean 2000, 23). Neo-colonial[12] recuperations such as this not only echo the gestures of benevolent colonizing of the late nineteenth century but also echo the very evolutionary premises of space and place that led the residential school regime of more than a century ago to congratulate itself on its program of civilizing children:

> The circumstances of Indian existence prevents him following that course
> of evolution which has produced from the barbarian of the past the civilized
> man of today. It is not possible for him to be allowed slowly to pass through
> successive stages, from pastoral to an agricultural life and from an agricultural
> one, to one of manufacturing, commerce or trade as we have done. He has
> been called upon suddenly and without warning to enter upon a new existence.
> Without the assistance of the Government, he must have failed and perished

miserably and he would have died hard entailing expense and disgrace upon the Country. (J.A. Macrae 1886, quoted in Milloy 1999, 27)

Efforts to relocate the site of abuses from the private to the public realm are read not necessarily as the discourse of an honourable collective history but as the dishonouring of colonial moral history. This neo-colonial reading relocates First Nations as the enemy within – returning them to the position of wildness as their lives and homelands are depicted as "primitive" sites where missionaries with skills and sentiments reserved for the "most cultured circles" of London "live on, love on, labour on in this vast expanse, little trodden but by the Indians for whom they live and will die" (McLean 2000, 24). A writer to the *Globe and Mail* captures this position: "Do you even see the hypocrisy your life is? You say you have been in the military, and yet you advocate native land claims? Doesn't that go against your military training? You were supposed to protect the integrity of Canada from its enemies, without and within. This includes groups that would take land that belongs to Canada, yes this means natives" (Colonel 2000, A24).

Far from granting the vindication and empathy sought by rendering abuses public in discourses of genocide and trauma, neo-colonial discourse confronts First Nations people in a vitriolic backlash; like women who are positioned as threats to male safe havens, both the litigants against residential schools and the church leaders who apologize for the residential school regime are placed as robbers of Christian largesse by journalists and academics seeking to restore past colonial paternalism. Not the First Nations victim of abuse but the churches themselves are now the ones who would be the survivors, as abuse settlements push Christian dioceses toward sale of church buildings, liquidation of assets, and loss of congregations. Professor emeritus of law Ian Hunter, himself an Anglican, in responding to the Anglican primate, Michael Peers, denounces the apologies and gestures of reconciliation offered by the church hierarchy in his protest of the consequent likelihood of widespread loss of church assets. In a letter to the editor of the *National Post,* Hunter writes: "The real church of Christ need not fear a bushel of lawsuits that, if tried, might be held to consist largely of historical revisionism and false memory syndrome" (Hunter 2000, A18).

Just as women seeking rights in fifth-century Greece were mocked as the barbarous threat within, so the former residents of residential schools are reviled as a den of thieves with genocidal power:

> "Cultural genocide" is a very simple matter. A large number of natives have decided to blame the white man for their lives – for their problems with booze, drugs, women, the law ... "Follow me," said Christ, "and I will make you fishers of men." But that's a tad strong, isn't it? Much easier to concede that yes, doing the Lord's work for over a century is, indeed, cultural genocide, and the only question is whether our victims will accept a post-dated cheque ... I'm not a litigious type, but if I were touting a class-action genocide

JO-ANNE FISKE

suit that would materially change Aboriginal lives, I'd suggest one against the federal government for the ruinous policies it's inflicted on natives since it abandoned the evils of "Eurocentrism." (Steyn 2001, A12)

Conclusion

A rabble is created only when there is joined to poverty a disposition of mind, an inner indignation against the rich, against society, against the government, etc.

> – HEGEL, *LECTURES ON THE PHILOSOPHY OF RIGHT* (1942), PARA. 244

As Jager as argued, "any thought concerning the body affects our understanding of the home, the office, the hospital, the laboratioure and the city itself. All of these places of inhabitation come to share in the mystery which is the mystery of the body. An understanding of inhabiting becomes inseparable from an understanding of incorporation" (1983 153). In this chapter, I have carried this understanding of space and body further to argue that how we incorporate the violated subject is inherent to the social production of space/place. Social production of residential space, whether it be the space of the "private" family or the religious community as the extended family, hides individuals from view and renders them as less than fully participating citizens for whom and with whom we share a common collective responsibility of care. Once hidden from view behind a facade of "moral" protection, women and children are neither accorded respect nor positioned as credible subjects in their own right.

The spatial production of the violated subject within the private nuclear family and within the extended family of residential institutions is marked by parallels in sociospatial continua. This has been demonstrated by illustrating an understanding of expressive spatiality as experienced and imagined. Expressive space of domesticity is extended to colonial institutions by marking the latter as sites of altruistic nurture. Just as the colonial sensibility drew on a binary positioning of public and private in its conceptualization of the domestic subject, so did it draw on a binary positioning of wild space and domestic place in its conceptualization of civilizing progress.

The politics of resistance to domesticated violence are a politics of spatiality; they seek to redefine the ideological sense of dwelling place and are contested by counter-narratives of morality and Christendom. Counter-narratives of subjectivity challenge narratives of national identity by disrupting conventional shared memories of space/place. First Nations' desires for an honourable history are thwarted when they re-emerge in a neo-colonial text of social evolution as an aggrieved rabble, a den of thieves in the "piety-scape" that once again links church and state in a crusade for civilization.

The very idea of civilization, and the social hierarchy on which it rests, is encoded in separation of space and place, wilderness and settlement. As Jager expresses it, "body and soul, earth and people, cave and inhabitants make their appearance only as unities of mutual implication, as poles of an indissoluble unity of reciprocal reference" (1983, 156). Home thus inscribes a specific way to take up outlooks and sensibilities. In European traditions, home encodes civilization, as taken by its proponents to mean "the highest cultural grouping of a people and the broadest level of cultural identity people have short of that which distinguishes humans from other species. It is defined both by objective elements, such as language, history, religion, customs, institutions, and by the subjective self-identification of people ... The civilization to which he belongs is the broadest level of identification with which he intensely identifies" (Huntington 1993, 24).

To question the sanctity of domesticated place is to threaten civilization itself: neither woman nor child can unequivocally move beyond private shame to public suffering without disrupting the spatial symbolics of the narrative of civilization. Thus the private shame of domestic abuse is placed on the body of the First Nations child of the residential school in an effort to reclaim the colonial signification of the im/moral frontier.

Notes

1 The eighteenth- and nineteenth-century literature on domestication and subjugation of women is extensive, including works by Herbert Spencer (1861), Edmund Burke (1955), Frederick Engels (1985), and John Stuart Mill (1869). For postcolonial and postmodern, gendered critiques of the underlying political philosophy and its impact on colonial thinking and ruling relations, see Ann Stoler (1995) and Robert Young (1995); for gendered analysis of the political contract, see Carole Pateman (1990); and for an erudite reading of the philosophical underpinnings of contemporary embodiment, see Grosz (1995).

2 Representations of women making fraudulent claims of being violently abused and as constituting a threat to civilization are common on websites and in other media that take an antifeminist stance. For Canadian expressions of these views, see BC Fathers (http://www.bcfathers.bc.ca), Fathers are Capable Too (FACT) (http://www.fact.on.ca), and *Everyman Online: A Men's Journal* (http://www.everyman.org). These sites, among others representing British, Australian, and American men's groups, cite studies arguing that domestic violence is as frequently perpetrated by women as by men (although they have no statistics to demonstrate that the effects on men are as great as on women), that women are more likely to abuse children than are men, and that purported rising rates in criminality and mental illness are a direct consequence of lone-mother families. The most extreme expression of vehemence against women who step outside of patriarchal subjugation is the discursive framing of women as "family terrorists" and white men as the new "nigger" (http://www.fathers.bc.ca). Statistics on family violence can be found in *Family violence in Canada: A statistical profile* (Statistics Canada 2005).

3 For similar accounts of the case, see *The Report Newsmagazine,* 3 July 2000, 12; Bunner (2000, 11); Byfield (2000, 60); and *North Shore News,* 6 December 1999, 1.

4 Rates of reported domestic violence in Aboriginal households vary across Canada; in 1989, in a frequently cited report, the Ontario Native Women's Association estimated that more than 80% of First Nations women suffered domestic violence. Koshan (1997, 101 n. 3) cites a number of studies with estimates ranging from 33% to 80%, with one study reporting that 60.6% of violent acts against Aboriginal women are committed by family members.

5 The use of the past tense here is not meant to mislead. Colonial notions of wilderness as vast and empty persist, as is clear from the legal judgment in *Delgamuukw v. British Columbia*. In his reasons for judgment, the BC Supreme Court justice in the case, Allan McEachern, described the Aboriginal territory in its present state in just these terms: a vast, empty wilderness.

6 The practice of juxtaposing indigenous peoples and settlers through tropes of wildness flourished in the mid-twentieth century in an outpouring of nostalgic frontier and pioneer history written for a popular audience, a particular gendered view of settler women's moral domesticity. Andrew Sluyler's (2002) critical reading of colonial landscape practices reveals their Biblical routes.

7 This statement was made in an interview I conducted in 2000 as part of a larger project on the contested meanings of residential schools and their twentieth-century legacy. For this project, "The im/moral frontier: Contested histories of the 'Indian Residential School,'" I interviewed former students, staff, and neighbours of schools in British Columbia as well as members of churches, lawyers, and public servants engaged in processes of reconciliation and litigation.

8 It is difficult to assess the degree to which Canadians hold these positions. I collected more than 300 articles, letters to editors, and editorials from the major Canadian newspapers over a five-year period, 1995-2000. It is striking that when news of abuses at the residential schools was headlined in these papers, in each case readers' responses included one or more of the following: denunciations of claims of abuse, defences of the residential school as necessary for civilized progress, and depictions of school staff as self-sacrificing heroes. Of all the print media, *The Report Newsmagazine* and its affiliated newsmagazines, *BC Report, Alberta Report,* and *Western Report,* were the most persistent in denouncing claims of social, cultural, linguistic, and spiritual abuses and strongest in their defence of the purpose and practices of residential schooling.

9 For example, in British Columbia, Saint Mary residential school at Mission now houses centres for early-childhood education; a former school in the south-eastern part of the province is a tourist site; and Coqualeetza has housed an adult learning centre and research archives.

10 An annual pilgrimage is held at the site of the now razed Lejac residential school in Fraser Lake, British Columbia, where a former student, Rose Prince, is buried. Currently, efforts are underway to move to her sainthood. See Fiske (1996).

11 It is difficult to estimate an average rate of mortality; data are not always available or transparent. Often schools discharged very ill children, realizing their deaths were imminent. John Milloy (1999) and James R. Miller (1996) provide data on individual schools and cite official estimates of deaths across the system.

12 Neo-colonialism has a range of meanings. In this chapter, I employ the concept of neo-colonialism to refer to current strategies that seek to entrench liberal values of individualism, constrain state policies of collective obligations and public services, and advance the cause of corporate capitalism. Neo-colonialism draws its power to disrupt Aboriginal claims for autonomy from the capacity of discourse to shape identity. It frames itself within neo-liberal discourses that deny politics of identity based on difference, collective membership, social justice, collective Aboriginal rights, and gendered politics advancing women's well-being. In the particular case of Aboriginal/non-Aboriginal relations, it reaffirms the colonial goals of the past while justifying corporate powers on a global basis.

References

Ashcroft, B., G. Gareth, and H. Tiffin, eds. 1995. *The post-colonial studies reader*. London: Rutledge.

Augé, M. 1995. *Non-places: Introduction to anthropology of supermodernity*. London: Verso.

Bennett, L. 2 March 2001. Letter to the editor. *Globe and Mail,* A12.

Buckle, H.T. 1882. *History of civilization in England*. London: New Edition.

Bunner, P. 3 July 2000. Ramsay's trial moves to Crowfoot. *The Report Newsmagazine* 27 (5): 10-11.

Burghardt, A.F. 1996. Boundaries: Setting limits to political areas. In C. Earle, K. Mathewson, and M.S. Kenzer, eds., *Concepts in human geography*, 213-30. London: Rowman and Littlefield.

Burke, E. 1955 [1791]. *Reflections on the revolution in France*. Ed. T.H.D. Mahoney. Indianapolis, IN: Bobbs-Merril.

Byfield, Ted. 3 July 2000. The whole phenomenon of the new Canada may be about to go on trial in Crowfoot. *The Report Newsmagazine* 27 (5): 60.

Chrisjohn, R., and S. Young. 1997. *The circle game: Shadows and substance in the residential school experience in Canada*. Penticton, BC: Theytus.

Churchill, W. 1998. *A little matter of genocide: Holocaust and denial in the Americas, 1492 to the present*. Winnipeg, MB: Arbeiter Ring.

Cole, J.M. 1979. *Exile in the wilderness: The Biography of Chief Factor Archibald McDonald, 1790-1853*. Seattle, WA: University of Washington Press.

—. 2001. *This blessed wilderness: Archibald McDonald's letters from the Columbia, 1822-1844*. Vancouver, BC: UBC Press.

Colonel. 3 August 2000. National Issues Forum. *Globe and Mail*, A24.

Crow Dog, M., and R. Erodes. 1990. *Lakota woman*. New York: Harper Perennial.

Deiter, C. 1999. *From our mother's arms: The intergenerational impact of residential schools in Saskatchewan*. Toronto, ON: United Church Publishing House.

Douglas, M. 1991. The idea of a home: A kind of space. *Social Research* 46: 287-303.

Editorial. 6 December 1999. *North Shore News*, 1.

Engels, F. 1985 [1884]. *The origin of the family, private property, and the state*. Harmondsworth, UK: Penguin.

Everyman Online: A Men's Journal. N.d. http://www.everyman.org.

Fekete, J. 1994. *Moral panic: Biopolitics rising*. Montreal, QC: Robert Davies.

Ferron, J. 1997. The chronicle of Anse Saint-Roch. In D. Lampe, ed., *Myths and voices: Contemporary Canadian fictions*, 162-75. Buffalo, NY: White Pine.

Fiske, J. 1981. "And then we prayed again": Carrier women, colonization and mission schools. MA thesis, University of British Columbia.

—. 1996. Pocahontas's granddaughters: Spiritual tradition and transition of Carrier women of British Columbia. *Ethnohistory* 43 (4): 663-82.

—. 2005. Spirited subjects and wounded souls: Political representations of an im/moral frontier. In K. Pickles and M. Rutherford, eds., *Contact Zones: Aboriginal and settler women in Canada's colonial past*, 90-105. Vancouver, BC: UBC Press.

Furniss, E. 1995. *Victims of benevolence: The dark legacy of the Williams Lake residential school*. Vancouver, BC: Arsenal Pulp Press.

Grosz, E. 1995. *Space, time and perversion*. London: Routledge.

Hegel, G.W.F. 1942. *Lectures on the philosophy of right*. Trans. T.M. Knox. Oxford, UK: Oxford University Press.

Heidegger, M. 1962. *Being and time*. Trans. John Macquarrie and Edward Robinson. New York: Harper and Row.

Henry, F., and C. Tator. 2002. *Discourses of domination: Racial bias in the Canadian English-language press*. Toronto, ON: University of Toronto Press.

Hunter, I. 15 June 2000. Letter to the editor. *National Post*, A18.

Huntington, S.P. 1993. The clash of civilizations? *Foreign Affairs* 72 (3): 22-49.

Jager, B. 1983. Theorizing and the elaboration of place: Inquiry into Galileo and Freud in Duquesne studies. In A. Giorgi, A. Barton, and C. Maes, eds., *Duquesne studies I: Phenomenological psychology*, 153-80. Pittsburgh, PA: Duquesne University Press.

Jaine, L. 1993. *Residential schools: The stolen years*. Saskatoon, SK: University of Saskatchewan Extension Press.

Kingsley, C. 1880. *The works of Charles Kingsley: Scientific lectures and essays*. London, UK: McMillan.

Kirmayer, L. 1996. Landscapes of memory: Trauma, narrative, and dissociation. In P. Antze and M. Lambek, eds., *Tense past: Cultural essays in trauma and memory*, 173-98. New York: Routledge.

Knockwood, I. 1992. *Out of the depths: The experiences of Mi'kmaw at the Indian residential school at Schubenacadie*. Lockeport, NS: Roseway.

Koshan, J. 1997. Sounds of silence: The public/private dichotomy, violence, and Aboriginal women. In S. Boyd, ed., *Challenging the public/private divide: Feminism, law and public policy*, 87-112. Toronto, ON: University of Toronto Press.

Livingstone, D. 1994. Climate's moral economy: Science, race and place in post-Darwinian British and American geography. In A. Godlewska and N. Smith, eds., *Geography and empire,* 132-54. Oxford, UK: Blackwell.

Mahoney, M. 1991. Legal images of battered women: Redefining the issue of separation. *Michigan Law Review* 90 (1): 1-94.

McLean, C. 3 July 2000. Circling like wolves: Lawyers and Indians team up to take down the Anglican church ... and the church cheers them on. *The Report Newsmagazine* 27 (5): 18-24.

McNab, D. 1999. *Circles of time: Aboriginal land rights and resistance in Ontario.* Waterloo, ON: Wilfred Laurier University Press.

Mill, J.S. 1869. *The subjection of women.* London: Parker. http://etext.library.adelaide.edu.au.

Miller, J.R. 1996. *Shingwauk's vision: A history of Native residential schools.* Toronto, ON: University of Toronto Press.

Milloy, J. 1999. *A national crime: The Canadian government and the residential school system, 1879 to 1986.* Winnipeg, MB: University of Manitoba Press.

Pateman, C. 1990. *The disorder of women: Democracy, feminism and political theory.* Cambridge, UK: Polity Press.

Patterson, T.C. 1997. *Inventing Western civilization.* New York: Monthly Review Press.

Rose, G. 1993. *Feminism and geography: The limits of geographical knowledge.* Cambridge, UK: Polity Press.

Rowles, G. 2002. Whither manhood and fatherhood: It's time to yell "Fire" in this theater. http://www.fathers.bc.ca/whither_manhood.htm.

Ruskin. J. 1865. *Sesame and lilies.* http://ruskin.classicauthors.net/SesameAndLilies.

Rutherdale, M. 2002. *Women and the white man's God: Gender and race in the Canadian mission field.* Vancouver, BC: UBC Press.

Sampert, S. 2002. Saints, sinners and squaws: The media framing of the Jack Ramsay trial. Unpublished ms.

Schneider, E. 1994. The violence of privacy. In M. Fineman and R. Mykitiuk, eds., *The public nature of private violence,* 36-53. New York: Routledge.

Sluyler, A. 2002. *Colonialism and landscape: Postcolonial theory and applications.* Boulder, CO: Rowman and Littlefield.

Smith, J.M. 1996. Ramification of region and senses of place. In C. Earle, K. Mathewson, and M.S. Kenzer, eds., *Concepts in human geography,* 189-212. London: Rowman and Littlefield.

Spencer, H. 1861. *Education: Intellectual, moral and physical.* London: Williams and Norgate.

Statistics Canada. 2005. *Family violence in Canada: A statistical profile.* Ottawa, ON: Minister of Industry.

Steyn, M. 9 April 2001. I'll give you cultural genocide. *National Post,* A12.

Stoler, A.L. 1995. *Race and the education of desire: Foucault's* History of Sexuality *and the colonial order of things.* Durham, NC: Duke University Press.

UK Men and Father's Rights. 1996. A male manifesto. http://www.coeffic.demon.co.uk/manifest.htm.

Walter, E.V. 1988. *Placeways: A theory of the human environment.* Chapel Hill, NC: University of North Carolina Press.

Young, R.J.C. 1995. *Colonial desire: Hybridity in theory, culture and race.* London: Routledge.

7

Narratives of Hope and Despair in Downtown Eastside Vancouver

DARA CULHANE

A Peopled Place: Downtown Eastside Vancouver

The intersection of Main and Hastings streets marks the heart of Vancouver's now in-famous inner-city neighbourhood: the Downtown Eastside. Approximately 16,000 people live in Downtown Eastside Vancouver, and around 3,000 of the 5,000 Aboriginal residents are women (Vancouver/Richmond Health Board 1999). Often labelled "Canada's poorest postal code," the average income in the neighbourhood is $12,000 per year (City of Vancouver 2000).

In 1997 epidemiologists working with the Centre for Excellence for HIV+/AIDS reported that rates of HIV+ infection among neighbourhood residents exceeded those any-where else in the "developed" world. In response, the City of Vancouver Health Department declared the inner city a public health emergency zone. Downtown Eastside Vancouver has since become a focal point in emerging local, national, and international debates about the causes of, and solutions to, widespread practices of intravenous-drug injection and the spread of HIV+/AIDS. A somewhat less publicized aspect of Vancouver's IV-drug and HIV+/AIDS crisis is that rates of HIV infection are significantly higher among women than among men and about 2 times higher among both male and female Aboriginal intravenous-drug users than among non-Aboriginals (Spittal et al. 2002). Although neither HIV+/AIDS nor IV-drug use are restricted to impoverished and marginalized communities, it is the case that the burden of these epidemics is disproportionately borne by those with the least economic and political power across the globe (Kane and Mason 2001; Lawless, Kippas, and Crawford 1996; Parker 2001; Ship and Norton 2000; Singer 2001; Zierler and Krieger 1997).

That so many people living in poverty in Downtown Eastside Vancouver are Aboriginal women and that a disproportionate number of these women are intravenous-drug users afflicted by HIV+/AIDS are neither accidents nor coincidences (Benoit, Carroll, and Chaudhry 2003). The social origins of distress among inner-city Aboriginal women can be traced through colonial policies and practices that are implicated in the lives of most Aboriginal people in Canada in diverse ways. The present-day "City of Vancouver" is con-structed on land that has been owned and occupied by indigenous peoples of Coast

Salish Nations for many thousands of years. Some contemporary residents of the inner city are descendants of ancestors who have lived in this particular space for thousands of years. Others come from all over Canada: dislocated and relocated, they and their ancestors have moved and been moved through space and over time.

Two caveats are in order when seeking to understand Aboriginal emplacement in the inner city. First, not all Aboriginal people in the City of Vancouver live in the Downtown Eastside. Reliable demographic data are hard to establish, but estimates can provide an overview. In 1998-99, hoping to obtain a more accurate assessment of the Aboriginal population of the City of Vancouver, the Vancouver/Richmond Health Board commissioned a "capture/recapture study" based on Census Canada 1996 figures (Vancouver/Richmond Health Board 1999). This study, entitled *Healing ways,* estimated a total population of 28,000 Aboriginal people living in the City of Vancouver. Of these, approximately 5,000 (17%) reside in the Downtown Eastside; 14,000 (50%) live in the adjacent neighbourhoods of Northeast, East, and Southeast Vancouver; and the remaining 9,000 (33%) are scattered throughout other neighbourhoods. Over 50% of urban Aboriginal households in Vancouver are headed by women, and these are concentrated in the low-income sectors of East Vancouver.

Second, statistics – particularly those that describe Aboriginal women who already bear heavy burdens created by long histories of negative stereotyping – must be read and interpreted carefully. We should ask about relationships between diagnostic labels, racialized categories, and epidemiological statistics: who do they represent, what do they connote, and what knowledge and information do they fail to convey? For example, in Vancouver, as elsewhere, young women with few options for making a living other than working in the sex industry are classified as a group at high risk for contracting the HIV virus. A recent study in the Downtown Eastside reported that 70% of the 350 street sex workers identified as working on the "lowest track" of this global industry were Aboriginal women under the age of 26, most of whom were mothers (Currie 2000). Such quantitative estimates are important for drawing attention to the racialized nature of the sex trade and to the disproportionate number of young Aboriginal women working in the most violent and dangerous echelons of it. However, the majority of Aboriginal women living in Downtown Eastside Vancouver are not current sex-trade workers (a deeply stigmatized employment category) or consumers of illicit drugs (a description of an equally stigmatized and illegal practice), nor are they infected with HIV/AIDS (an illness diagnostic category). The minority for whom one or more of these labels is applicable, however, are also grandmothers, mothers, daughters, sisters, aunts, nieces, wives, friends, lovers. Many neighbourhood residents – Aboriginal and non-Aboriginal – are poor and/or elderly and cannot afford to live anywhere else in Canada's highest-rent city. Neighbourhood Aboriginal women are often members of local and far-flung extended kinship networks and/or of shared communities. Neither human life and dignity nor social relationships and identities are quantifiable values. The challenge is to take meaningful account, simultaneously, of the significance of all these figures and of the relationships between them.

Beginning in 1999, I became involved in longitudinal ethnographic research focused on a series of in-depth interviews with Aboriginal and non-Aboriginal women living in Downtown Eastside Vancouver. In this chapter, I present stories about two Aboriginal women: Jeanette and Marlene.[1] Both Jeanette and Marlene are labelled – and identify themselves as – "drug addicts," and both have engaged in commercial sex work at various times in their lives; Marlene has been diagnosed with HIV/AIDS, but Jeanette has not. Like many of the women we spoke with, Jeanette and Marlene had fallen – or been pushed – through every crack in mainstream Canadian and Aboriginal social structures. Rarely had any person or community, or social safety net, or indigenous practice been there to break their falls. At the same time, these women's stories demonstrate persistent practices of mutual aid, care, compassion, and community building in the face of tremendous obstacles.[2]

I compiled and edited the accounts set out here from several formal interviews and informal conversations that Jeanette and Marlene courageously shared with Health and Home Project researchers.[3] I have two primary goals in retelling these women's stories. First, I propose that by attending to autobiographies we can better understand how the health effects of colonialism and economic and social exclusion are not only produced and embodied but also resisted. Second, I hope to demonstrate that embedded in the stories that Jeanette and Marlene recount about their everyday/everynight lives are thoughtful analyses and pragmatic recommendations that can offer directions to advocates, care providers, policymakers, and politicians. By locating these specific women's stories within the social context of their telling, my writing, and your reading, I hope to facilitate the construction of more effective roadblocks on the pathways between social inequalities and health disparities.

I will return to Jeanette's and Marlene's stories in the second half of this paper. Before doing so, I offer brief discussions about pertinent issues in Aboriginal health scholarship in Canada, discussions about linkages between poverty and health, and debates about research and representation with marginalized populations.

Aboriginal Health

Over the past 20 years or so, a field of research and practice has emerged in Canada and elsewhere that can be descriptively identified as "Aboriginal (or Indigenous) Health Studies."[4] While diverse in its interests and directions, and a site of frequent and often vigorous debate, a foundational premise of Aboriginal health work is that health and illness are irreducibly interrelated with, and interconnected to, the social, cultural, economic, and political contexts in which Aboriginal people(s) live. These contexts include natural, supernatural, and built environments; material and social living conditions; and political relations among and between Aboriginal and non-Aboriginal peoples. This "holistic" concept of health and health care is counter-posed to more narrow biomedical definitions that view health as contained within individual minds and bodies and evidenced by an absence of disease. At the policy and service-delivery level, Aboriginal representatives argue against fragmented bureaucratic models and for integrated and innovative approaches that reflect a holistic foundation. The common listing of social determinants of health found in Health Canada's population-health grid now reflects Aboriginal health's focus on the iatrogenic effects of past and present Canadian "Indian" policy, whose disastrous consequences are outlined in the introduction to this volume. And access to health care services and pathways to healing are now complemented by Aboriginal health's concern with spirituality and struggles for social justice.

Many of the Aboriginal women who shared their stories with the Health and Home Project recounted longstanding practices in their own lives and in those of their families and communities of seeking escape, comfort, companionship, and community through the use of intoxicants and narcotics. These patterns, reproduced in generation after generation, also distinguish, in a general way, most but not all Aboriginal from non-Aboriginal participants in the Health and Home Project. A more common pattern among non-Aboriginal female injection-drug users, for example, is for their drug use to render them relatively unique among – and often isolated from, rather than closer to – their mothers, daughters, grandmothers, aunts, nieces, and sisters.

Aboriginal women participants in the Health and Home Project also talked about their aspirations for change and renewal. They spoke of utilizing detoxification services, residential and out-patient treatment programs, and other Aboriginal and non-Aboriginal health services, including 12-step and other self-help groups and healing circles, but they also told stories about "informal" care provided for them by recovering users and Elders: "street Moms" and healers. What Aboriginal and non-Aboriginal women in the Downtown Eastside do share is contemporary material poverty.

Poverty and Health

In their review of literature on linkages between poverty and disease, anthropologists Vinh-Kim Nguyen and Karine Peschard (2003) discuss the importance of distinguishing between *absolute poverty* (inadequate access to basic subsistence, shelter, and sanitation) and *relative poverty* (inequalities in distribution of material resources within and between populations). Some sectors of the Canadian public, and some politicians, argue that absolute poverty has been eradicated in Canada through income-assistance programs and social services. However, increasing numbers of homeless and hungry citizens visible on the streets of both rural villages and metropolitan centres challenge these assumptions and call attention to health implications of the growing gap between *haves* and *have-nots* that constitutes "relative poverty."

The Aboriginal and non-Aboriginal population of the Downtown Eastside is characterized by low levels of formal educational attainment, little training or employment experience, and high levels of residential mobility and stress. Social assistance and/or low-wage service-sector employment are their legitimate options for obtaining subsistence. Rates of reliance on income assistance and/or disability allowances vary considerably from one recipient to the next, and allocations vary over time. Individual social workers and financial assistance workers have some discretion, for example, in whether to approve applications for crisis grants and nutritional supplements. Doctors may successfully support patients in obtaining support for special transportation needs, clothing, or household goods. These variations make it difficult to assess precise dollar amounts that accurately represent income-support rates. In 2000 and 2001, when the Health and Home Project interviews were conducted, the basic income-assistance rate for a single, unemployed person designated "employable" was $325 per month as a shelter allowance from the provincial income-assistance program. Rent for a small basement apartment in the working-class and low-income neighbourhood of East Vancouver begins at around $600 per month. Hotels with single-room occupancy and rooming houses – often in poor repair and lacking locked doors and private bathrooms – in the Downtown Eastside are available at welfare-shelter rates. Another option is to find one of the few available spaces in social housing. Employment at British Columbia's minimum wage of $8 per hour is the other legitimate option available to people with little education or training. Most of these positions are part-time and temporary, and they include no benefits or possibilities for skill development or career advancement. These figures offer heuristic insights into relationships between average cost of living and government income support.

Federal, provincial, and municipal social-policy decisions determine income-assistance rates, minimum wage levels, and accessibility of affordable housing, factors that shape the living conditions for many Aboriginal people, particularly those living off-reserve and in urban areas. The well-documented relationship between absolute and relative poverty and poor health make these government policies important determinants of Aboriginal and non-Aboriginal health in Canada (Coburn 2000).

Nguyen and Peschard go on to stress the importance of balancing class-based analyses with those of gender, ethnicity, and colonialism when analyzing health and social inequality. They argue that "the concept of social class, although a conceptually robust first approximation of social inequality, is too blunt an instrument to capture the fine-grained differences that occur within groups that share the same material conditions of reproduction" (2003, 449).

Geographer Evelyn Peters (1998) notes that dominant discourses in academia, government, and the public have tended to take a polarized either/or approach to the relationship between Aboriginal health and poverty. Aboriginal people have been characterized and acted upon as though they are "only poor" and not simultaneously culturally distinct and subject to racism and colonial domination. Alternatively, some attempts to rectify deterministic class-based theories result in analyses that focus on cultural distinctiveness, considering poverty a backdrop to – or worse, an outcome of – cultural difference (Richards 1995, 2000). One-dimensional causal theories lead to inadequate proposals for decreasing health disparities: assimilation and upward mobility of individuals within the dominant Canadian society *or* symbolic recognition of cultural difference in the absence of effective redistribution of wealth and resources (McCovey 1998). In the case of marginalized inner-city Aboriginal women, the analytic and practical effectiveness of abstract and fragmented categories debated by academics and politicians are challenged by the realities of everyday life in which Aboriginality, female gender, racism, sexism, and poverty are lived and experienced simultaneously, not sequentially.

The Health and Home Project documented some shared experiences in the biographies of many Aboriginal and non-Aboriginal women in the Downtown Eastside – the most common being histories of poverty, child abuse, domestic violence, and sexual assault. However, culturally and historically specific patterns in the life stories of the Aboriginal women who participated in this research are evident: influences of diverse and complex ways of being rooted in precolonial life-ways; experiences of radical and repeated dislocation from home communities and disconnection from families through residential schools and/or foster-care systems; legacies of Indian Act-related policies that have resulted in further alienation and exclusion; and frequent experiences of racial discrimination in public institutions and in everyday life (see Benoit et al. 2003; Currie 2000; McDonald 2002; Native Women's Association of Canada 1997; Razack 2000; Ship and Norton 2000; Tait and Prairie Women's Health Collective 2000). Simply put, health and illness among Aboriginal women in Downtown Eastside Vancouver cannot be adequately addressed by reference only to the material deprivation they share with non-Aboriginal women living in the same neighbourhood.

Although it is important to recognize the significant differences between impoverished Aboriginal people and impoverished non-Aboriginals, other factors that complicate analyses, policies, and interventions in the field of Aboriginal health are differences within and among Aboriginal populations. These include a multiplicity of nations of origin; diverse experiences of colonialism across time and space; implications of gender relations and sexuality; divergent community, family, and individual histories; and varied positions in socioeconomic hierarchies within Aboriginal communities that are articulated in complex ways through global and national class relations (Hull 2001; Slowey 2001).

Most relevant to the subject of this chapter are descriptions and analyses of diversity within inner-city Aboriginal populations in Canada. Carol LaPrairie, in her study *Aboriginal over-representation in the criminal justice system: A tale of nine cities,* writes that "even within the inner cores of the ... cities, class differences existed" (2001, 3). Although inner-city Aboriginal residents as a whole are more disadvantaged than their non-Aboriginal neighbours, the most impoverished group – both absolutely and relatively – in relation to both Aboriginal and non-Aboriginal social and economic hierarchies are Aboriginal women. Intravenous-drug use, dangerous sex work, and HIV/AIDS infection enact and embody a matrix of exploitation, pain, and marginalization described by anthropologists Arthur Kleinman, Veena Das, and Margaret Lock (1997) as "social suffering."

Researching and Representing Social Suffering

The clustering of substance abuse, street violence, domestic violence, suicide, depression, post traumatic stress disorder, sexually transmitted disorders, AIDS and tuberculosis among people living in disintegrating communities ... points to the often close linkage of personal problems with societal problems ... This is not merely a statistical correlation, but a causal web in the global political economy.

– A. KLEINMAN, V. DAS, AND M. LOCK, EDS., *SOCIAL SUFFERING* (1997), IX

Socioeconomic, epidemiological, and media profiles of Downtown Eastside Vancouver represent the neighbourhood as a space of social suffering, similar in many ways to the clusters described above by Kleinman, Das, and Lock. These authors, and others, also discuss the complex ethical and political questions that arise when working with people experiencing high levels of distress. Researchers' challenges revolve around questions of voice, representation, and audiences.[5] Who should we tell about the social suffering we witness? How should we tell these stories, if at all? Most important, will telling change anything?

On the one hand, based on the simple premise that people can act only on what they know, and with the enduring hope that when confronted by suffering most human beings will feel compassion and be moved to ameliorative action, it seems imperative to describe the ways that structured inequality limits opportunities for women, Aboriginal people, and poor people. This responsibility seems increasingly urgent in the face of contemporary neo-liberal social and policy environments where individuals are increasingly blamed and stigmatized for being poor – as though living in poverty is a "lifestyle choice" they made from a full range of other opportunities available to them.

On the other hand, there is always a danger that such descriptions and representations may result in confirming the very stereotypes they seek to subvert. In conditions of ongoing relations of radical inequality, focusing on the destructive impacts of historically and socially produced experiences and conditions runs the risk of paying insufficient attention to the complexities, the wisdom, and the capacity of people to survive disadvantage. Researchers and advocates working in the field of Aboriginal health point out that endless repetition of statistics about illness, disease, violence, and dysfunctional communities and of "horror stories" about painful personal experiences of trauma misrepresents the diversity and complexity of Aboriginal experience by excluding those who survive through extraordinary strength and resilience. Kimberly Scott notes: "Even in those scenarios, which seem despairing, many robust, balanced individuals survive and are usually at the forefront of community development. In fact, an increasing number of individuals in such contexts are finding the resolve to change their lives through personal empowerment. In the process, they are having an impact on their families and friends, or in some cases are leading community health endeavours" (2001, 5).

DARA CULHANE

Jeanette and Marlene are women who, at the time they were interviewed, were still struggling – with varying degrees of success – to become "robust and balanced individuals." Their stories chronicle their efforts and their errors.

Reading behind the Labels

Sally Zierler and Nancy Krieger, discussing their work with female injection-drug users in American inner cities, write that the challenge for researchers is

> to keep in the forefront a vision of women capable of passion and playfulness, of hard work and creativity, of loving parenting and strong kinship, people who desire full participation in society, to be generative and to make a difference in the world, these are the women about whom we are writing. Pushing against such vital possibility are the challenges of economic and political forces and structures that threaten and often take these lives and the lives of their loved ones. Women's struggles with and resistance to social and economic subordination include strategies for survival that bear the burden of drug use, violence, hunger, social disintegration, and sexual risk. (1997, 404)

How can we create spaces where the most marginalized may speak their truths to power? Experiences of poverty, exclusion, drug use, violence, or mental illness may significantly compromise peoples' capacity to act productively in their own or others' interests, to feel they are people of worth with anything of value to offer themselves or others, and to tell their stories in language that can be heard and understood by those who do not share these experiences.

In the Health and Home Project we attempted to create relatively open spaces for women like Jeanette and Marlene to tell their stories, recognizing at the same time that our work is still shot through with unequal power relations: that Jeanette's and Marlene's voices are still constructed and constrained in myriad and complex ways, still translated and represented by researchers.

More often than not, women who participated in the Health and Home Project judged themselves and their behaviour harshly and did not seek to justify or excuse the harm they may have done to others, particularly their children. Motivated by the hope that in telling their stories they would help others in similar situations to make healthier choices, they engaged in purposeful truth telling that was often a painful process. As witnesses, we researchers were frequently overwhelmed by the relentless brutality and injustice chronicled in the women's stories, by their sorrow, their strength, their hope and despair. As re-presenters and translators of these stories, we struggled with ethical concerns about the potential consequences of publication, of exposing these women's lives to the gaze and inevitable judgment of diverse readers. However, the women who participated in the

Health and Home Project are likely the most intrusively observed population in Canada. Their lives are monitored by apparatuses of law enforcement and criminal justice, their access to subsistence and their private lives are monitored by social-service agencies, their minds and bodies are examined by medical institutions, and their appearances in public space are sensationalized by media.

Many women held little hope for their own individual fate, but all were deeply concerned about the increasing numbers of young people who are becoming involved in drug use, sex work, and street life. These young people constituted the most important audience for Jeanette and Marlene, who hoped their stories would warn youth and inspire them to take different paths through life.

Jeanette

Jeanette was 44 years old at the time of our conversations. She came from a large family in northern Canada and spent most of her childhood and adolescence being moved between residential and boarding schools:

> When I was six years old I was sent into boarding school. There were seventeen of us kids, and my parents had gotten into that alcohol that just came to our town then, all of a sudden like. I was pushed around from one town to the next town to the next town, going in residential schools, and it was very hard for me to pick up my education. I remember I was in boarding schools or residential schools in five different places up north, that I remember. I have no idea why they moved me around so much. The residential schools were too full, and then there was another opening in another town so ... well, I think they shipped us around here and there, and it was just by chance that it was me.

On her sixteenth birthday, authorities determined it was time for her to leave school, so there she was: alone and penniless in a small northern town. She found her way to a sister in a prairie city. With neither experience, nor skills, nor confidence, Jeanette survived as well as she could. She met a man, fell in love, and had three children. Jeanette left her children's father after he attacked her, and her children were apprehended while she was hospitalized for a week as a result of the beating. Her children were 2, 4, and 5 when Jeanette fled with them to Vancouver.

Jeannette's stories of the years 1985-95 describe many hardships. But they also describe a ferociously independent woman struggling to survive and determined above all to raise her own children. In her accounts of those years, Jeanette repeats over and over in various ways three goals that drove her: not to lose her kids, to shelter them, to feed them. The apprehension of her children that had precipitated her flight to Vancouver had been traumatic for her (see also McDonald 2002). Her main goal in relation to social and health services was to achieve maximum invisibility. Jeanette went to great lengths to stay out of the gaze of authorities. Her family was one of few Aboriginal households in the racially mixed, working-class neighbourhood in which Jeanette chose to live. She stayed in one house for six years despite repeated conflicts with an abusive landlord so that the kids could stay both at one school *and* in one house. Like many unemployed parents, Jeannette spent a lot of her time working to supplement her income: combing thrift stores for clothes and toys, going to food banks for subsistence, doing babysitting and house cleaning for others, signing her children up for subsidized activities.

Jeanette drank a lot during these years and had several unhappy relationships with men who often brought alcohol, drugs, crime, and violence into her home. Cycles consisting of periods of heavy drinking and bad relationships that ended in violence, followed by efforts to focus on her home and children and to abstain from alcohol, repeat over and over again in Jeanette's life story. Despite her hard work, as her children entered adolescence, Jeanette's fragile independence and the home she struggled to maintain began to unravel.

Her eldest son was arrested a number of times for robbery and sent to a juvenile detention centre. Her daughters entered government care voluntarily. Jeanette was heartbroken. She felt she had lost everything and had been defeated in the battle that had sustained her. For Jeanette, the daily struggle to provide basic shelter and nutrition had been a hard one. As the children became teenagers, they began to desire and demand more and more expensive consumer goods, like brand-name clothing, and to rage against their mother who could not provide them. This is a story most parents of teenagers could tell. For many poor parents in this situation, that foster parents are paid 3 to 4 times as much as a single parent's welfare allowance adds insult to injury.

The girls were rebellious, Jeanette told me, and they said she was too strict. Like many mothers living in low-income drug- and crime-saturated neighbourhoods, Jeanette often felt she was living under siege as she desperately tried to keep her children away from the street and the fast money offered by the drug and petty-crime economy. Jeanette's attempts to protect her children were often experienced by them as overly restrictive and confining. And the girls were angry, Jeanette acknowledged, about experiences they had suffered during the times when she had lost control of her drinking.

With the children gone, the shelter (or rent) portion of Jeanette's income-assistance cheque was reduced to $325 per month: single rate. She had to move out of her house and into the only place she could now afford: a hotel with single-room occupancy (SRO) in the Downtown Eastside. This is another common pattern that creates a vicious circle: children are apprehended, a mother has to move to accommodations that are deemed inappropriate for children or teenagers, and she can't hope to regain custody unless she has appropriate housing. Jeannette added drugs – cocaine specifically – to her drinking binges and spiralled downhill.

At the time she participated in the Health and Home Project, Jeanette had been living in and around the Downtown Eastside for about 10 years. She had stayed in close touch with her children and had seen them often, but she hadn't lived with them again. Mostly, Jeanette's time in SRO hotels has been punctuated by periods of homelessness when she has stayed with friends and relatives. Although she has applied for various forms of social housing, her strong sense of independence and her wariness of institutions of all sorts make Jeanette chafe against the rules, regulations, curfews, and surveillance that characterize most housing projects.

Food was a significant theme in all Jeanette's stories about her past and her present. She had an encyclopaedic knowledge of where and how to acquire food, and she spent the better part of many of her days doing so (see also Sinclaire 1997). Not only did Jeanette know the hours and locations of food banks, soup kitchens, and service agencies that provided meals or snacks and which stores marked items down at 6:00 p.m. in the Downtown Eastside, but she could also recite most of the Skytrain[6] route and deliver a detailed inventory of when certain stores, restaurants, or community centres within walking distance of each station offered free or bargain food. Being a reliable and knowledgeable food provider became one of Jeanette's means of economic survival and provided her a respected role in the community, one she took very seriously. Jeanette taught others her food-gathering skills and knowledge, she shared food with people who were hungry, she bartered it, she sold some of it sometimes, and she traded it for drugs when she was on a binge.

When her daughters were moved out of their group homes and into "independent living," Jeanette trained them rigorously, dragging them with her on her rounds, shopping bags in hand. Always worrying that her daughters and nieces and nephews eat too much junk food, Jeannette frequently drops off food for them at their apartments or rooms.

Jeanette was proud of the fact that she never went anywhere empty-handed. When she was in between secure housing and relying on friends and relatives for couch or floor space, she paid her way with food. When she had her own housing, she was a generous host.

Independence, self-sufficiency, and generosity are important to Jeanette's sense of self. She works hard. In the two years she was involved in the Health and Home Project, Jeanette earned a small monthly stipend working in a community-service agency, was a volunteer in a women's housing project, and enrolled in an adult basic-education course for residential school survivors. She also took various short-term jobs, including dishwashing, cleaning, and house demolition. Of these, she enjoyed the last most. She earned good wages and enjoyed the physical work. Jeanette participated in numerous healing circles and ceremonies, went to a range of workshops offered by diverse agencies to learn crafts like beading and making dream catchers and drums, and took classes in meditation, yoga, video making, and journal writing.

Jeanette struggles mightily with her addictions. She can stay away from crack cocaine for weeks at a time and is very motivated to free herself of this habit. When she has work and activities, and when her relationships with her children and her partner are going well, she can stay clean. But holding on to a sense of well-being is difficult. "It's just all the things that have happened to me, and I feel so sad and so alone sometimes," she says. "I'm learning to know when I start feeling that way, and I know that's when I want that drug to just shine a little light in my darkness."

Marlene

Marlene was a self-described and medically labelled crack cocaine addict when we met in 2001. She was born in a western Canadian city in the early 1960s, the youngest of 15 children. Her parents were heavy drinkers, and periods of Marlene's childhood were spent with grandparents on a northern reserve where she learned to speak her Aboriginal language. Her parents died when she was a child, and she was placed in foster care. Her older siblings tried to look after her, but "they couldn't handle me," she says with some pride. "I always ran away." She was not sure when she started using alcohol, but she remembers a time when she was nine and was kicked out of school for showing up high on cough syrup. She was injecting heroin before she left the city of her birth at the age of 13 and drifted to Vancouver, where she met a Native American man. She travelled around the United States with him for about 10 years. She used drugs all this time. But, she says, "it wasn't like now. The drugs wasn't all I had going for me then." Marlene eventually returned to Canada, to Vancouver, with 5 children. There were two reasons for returning, she said: her partner was sentenced to 15 years in prison, and Marlene missed her family.

After she returned to Vancouver in 1985 and during the years she tried to raise her five children, Marlene's heroin use was heavy (see also Hardesty and Black 1999). She served several stints in jail on drug-related charges. Marlene's children moved in and out of foster care and back and forth between their parents' relatives during these years. In an attempt to keep her oldest son off the street and away from drugs, she sent him to live with her family in northern Canada, where he died, high on gas, in a snowmobile accident. A few years later, one daughter died in a house fire and another of a drug overdose. This pattern of recurring and devastating loss was a common one among the women who participated in the Health and Home Project (see also Roberts 1999).

Marlene thought about quitting drugs often. She admits that she *thought* about it more often than she actually tried to *do* it. She said that thinking about giving up drugs filled her with terror. She imagined being consumed by emotional and physical pain and really did not think she would live through the experience. "My drugs are my best friends," she said. "They never let me down."

The times that Marlene did reach out for help were discouraging. There is a "window of opportunity" between coming down from a high and becoming "dope sick" and desperate for another fix when regular users are open to accessing help and treatment. It usually lasts a few hours, until more drugs can be accessed. Waiting lists to get into detox facilities are weeks and sometimes months long. Abstinence-based residential and outpatient treatment programs require an individual to be clean and sober for a period of time before being admitted. This lack of fit between the reality of addicts' experiences and treatment services has led to a persistent demand by advocates for "treatment on demand": facilities that will welcome an addict *the moment* they reach out.

In 1995 Marlene was diagnosed with HIV. Since then, she hadn't seriously considered giving up drug use. In an effort to be responsible and not infect others, however, she gave up injecting heroin and switched to snorting powder cocaine and, increasingly, to smoking crack. She also went on methadone. Methadone helps to soften the crash experienced coming down from cocaine highs. It helps to dull cravings and thus reduces the amount of illicit drugs many addicts need. A smaller habit, in turn, particularly for women, means less sex work is required to support it. "That's a good thing about methadone, especially as you get older," Marlene explained. "Yeah, I hated that. You never know what a guy is going to do." But methadone never "fills up that big hole inside me. It just doesn't ... I don't know ... doesn't give you that feeling, you know, that you're OK, everything's OK" (see also Bourgois 2000).

When she received the HIV+ diagnosis, Marlene surrendered custody of her two remaining children to their father's family. "They'll be stronger if they're raised there," she said. "Not with me. I'm too, you know, just too fucked up. And, now, well, I won't be around long, hey? It's better this way. It won't be so hard on them when ... when ... I go. I see them though. They come here. I go there. They know I love them. They know that."

Although her everyday life during the time we worked together was overdetermined by her use of crack, and increasingly by frequent periods of hospitalization for bouts of endocarditis and pneumonia, Marlene would rally herself for two events. First, visits from or to her children were reasons to clean up and stay straight for as long as she could. Second, she held "Marlene's Give-Aways" – gatherings that she organized herself and held in the small but self-contained subsidized apartment she had been allocated after she was diagnosed HIV+. During the time I worked with her, she organized one such give-away, but she described others previously held.

Planning for a give-away began with Marlene identifying a few people whom she considered were in worse shape than her. She would make the rounds of thrift stores and free-clothing outlets, assembling complete sets of clothes for each person. She took great care shopping, finding a cowboy shirt for one, a slinky skirt for another, warm jackets, and funky hats. Between her own runs (binges) and the care she took in finding things she thought would really suit the particular individuals she had in mind, the preparation she told me about took a few months. Once these packages of clothes were accumulated and she had washed everything in the free laundromat in her housing project, she began to plan the give-away event itself. This involved collecting and hoarding enough food from the soup kitchens and food banks to be able to feed everyone at one time, a project that took considerable time and effort in Marlene's situation. With everything ready, she rounded up her guests and brought them to her apartment. They each showered and changed into their new duds. They smudged, prayed, and "ate until we were ready to burst," she said.

Hospitality, sharing food, and distributing gifts are characteristic activities of many diverse indigenous celebrations, including Potlatches, feasts, and Pow-Wows. The process of preparing for and hosting one of her give-aways was a lifeline and a social practice through which Marlene claimed dignity and moral worth as a contributing member of a community. During our interviews, she repeatedly turned the conversation away from her past and present sorrows, away from her illness or her drug use, and to detailed descriptions of her "finds" and of her plans for the give-away. This linked her with Aboriginal cultural practices and reaffirmed her identity as an Aboriginal woman engaged in care giving and community building.

Like most of the women interviewed in the Health and Home Project, Marlene was deeply concerned about the increasing numbers of young people, particularly young Aboriginal women, engaged in street life in the Downtown Eastside. "I make a point of trying to connect with them when I first see them down here. I tell them '*Go home; get out of here.*' I show them all the pills I gotta take. I show them my tracks all over my body, my scars. I tell them 'Look at me. I'm just skin and bones. You're looking at a woman who is going to die soon. Is this what you want?' They don't listen. They think it's all just a big party."

When I asked Marlene what she thought would "work" to keep young people away from drugs or to help people who were already addicted, she said: "Love ... just lots and lots of love ... to know you're OK ... you're not alone. Sounds stupid hey? Corny, like. L-O-V-E – *LOVE. (Laughs.)* But, hey, it's all I have to say. And for our Indian people, we got to get ourselves back, our ways ... And food! *(Laughs.)* Lots of food."

Marlene died in 2002 of AIDS-related pneumonia. At her funeral people remembered her kindness, her humour, and her love for her children. She made a difference in the lives she touched.

Conclusion

We need to tell the stories from the side of policy that is never asked to speak out, to interrupt the hegemony of elite voices dictating what is good for this segment of the population."

– M. FINE AND L. WEISS, "WRITING THE 'WRONGS' OF
FIELDWORK" (1996), 269

Even the most well-intentioned health and social policies and programs consistently fail to meet their objectives because they do not take seriously the experiences and the self-defined and self-recommended strategies of target populations. Although rates of HIV/AIDS infection among Aboriginal women who are injection-drug users are higher than for any other identified group in Downtown Eastside Vancouver, these women's voices, experiences, and analyses and those of their families tend to be excluded from serious discussions both about the routes people take to injection-drug use and about possible solutions to the problems resulting from such a practice.

Jeanette's and Marlene's stories propose a wide range of comprehensive directions and concrete programs that may inform policymakers. At the broadest level, they support longstanding proposals advocated by Aboriginal health researchers, practitioners, and political representatives concerning the necessary linkages between historical, cultural, and political relations and health. The failure of fragmented approaches that, for example, treat education, employment, housing, and health as separate issues is evidenced by these women's daily life experiences. A consistent theme in their stories and those of other women who participated in the Health and Home Project is that "addiction" is not a disease with a simple etiology or cure and that "recovery" is a multifaceted process. Formal treatment programs and centres are crucial aspects of this proces, but without broad supports, their effectiveness is limited. A common experience among the women we interviewed was that of emerging from a treatment program hopeful and determined to change their lives, only to be undermined by problems in obtaining housing, in surviving on income assistance, or of being relied upon too heavily by others. Women stressed the importance of building strong support networks, of access to safe housing, of protection from interpersonal violence, and of opportunities for education. Both active and recovering drug users emphasized the importance for healing of reconnecting with children, homes, families, and communities, of claiming pride in Aboriginal identity, and of obtaining economic relief and security.

I hope that by enabling women to tell their stories and by linking their stories to contexts of social injustice and hopes for transformation in my representation of them, I will have honoured Jeanette's and Marlene's stated desire to contribute to changes that will ensure future generations of Aboriginal women have different life stories to tell.

Notes

1   These are pseudonyms. The Health and Home Project endeavoured to develop an ethical practice of considering informed consent a process rather than an event. The women about whom I am writing initially gave signed, informed consent for their real names to be used, and each reviewed the transcript of her interview. They live in a criminalized community where, particularly in the past six years, use of illicit drugs and other illegal practices are carried on in full view of the public and the police. Hence the women interviewed saw no need to protect themselves in this regard. However, I have opted to change their names and other identifying information in what some may interpret as a "maternalistic" gesture. It is not possible to consult with their children or their families, and I felt that I could not evaluate or anticipate the myriad consequences that publishing these stories might have for them. And although illicit drug use does not attract criminal punishment, new provincial regulations have come into effect since these interviews were conducted that criminalize earning money and/or acquiring goods in kind to supplement income assistance.

2   Health and Home Project researchers also interviewed Aboriginal and non-Aboriginal health care providers; conducted participant observation at diverse community events and at numerous forums, conferences, and discussions; and reviewed countless studies, media reports, program proposals, and policy documents. We endeavour to link our work with the emergent fields of Aboriginal/indigenous health studies, international comparative research on "inner-city health" that examines global forces that shape significant commonalities and meaningful differences between and among inner-city populations around the world, and critical feminist analyses of linkages between gender, race, and class relations and health (see, for example, Blankenship 1998; Bourgois 2000, 2002, 2003; Coburn 2000; Farmer 2000; Hardesty and Black

1999; Jacobs and Gill 2002; Kane and Mason 2001; Parker 2001; Roberts 1999; Singer 2001; Whiteis 1998; Zierler and Krieger 1997).

3 In an effort to develop mutually respectful relationships and to put into practice the idea that "gaining informed consent" should be considered an evolving process rather than an event, beginning with the second interview (and at each subsequent meeting), women were given typed transcripts of previous interviews and invited to review these either in privacy or with researchers. Most women chose to edit their stories to ensure that no one else would be identified or hurt by their publication.

4 The literature in this field is developing rapidly. Central works most pertinent to this chapter include Adelson (2003); Dieter and Otway (2001); Dion-Stout, Kipling, and Stout (2001); Elias et al., and O'Neil (2000); Scott (2001); Tait and Prairie Women's Health Collective (2000).

5 See Fine et al. (2000) for a provocative discussion of these issues.

6 "The Skytrain" is the local name for Vancouver's elevated rapid-transit system.

References

Adelson, N. 21-23 September 2003. Aboriginal Canada. Draft synthesis paper presented at the International Think Tank on Reducing Health Disparities and Promoting Equity in Vulnerable Populations, Canadian Institutes of Health Research, Ottawa, ON.

Benoit, C., D. Carroll, and M. Chaudhry. 2003. In search of a healing place: Aboriginal women in Vancouver's Downtown Eastside. *Social Science and Medicine* 56 (6): 821-83.

Blankenship, K.M. 1998. A race, class, and gender analysis of thriving. *Journal of Social Issues* 54 (2): 393-404.

Bourgois, P. 2000. Disciplining addiction: The bio-politics of methadone and heroin in the United States. *Culture, Medicine and Psychiatry* 24 (2): 165-95.

–. 2002. Understanding inner-city poverty: Resistance and self-destruction under U.S. apartheid. In J. MacClancy, ed., *Exotic no more: Anthropology on the front lines*, 15-32. Chicago, IL: University of Chicago Press.

–. 2003. Crack and the political economy of social suffering. *Addiction Research and Theory* 11 (1): 31-37.

City of Vancouver. 2001. *Downtown Eastside monitoriing report*. Vancouver, BC: Social Planning Department, City of Vancouver.

Coburn, D. 2000. Income inequality, social cohesion and the health status of populations: The role of neo-liberalism. *Social Science and Medicine* 51 (1): 135-49.

Currie, S. 2000. *Assessing the violence against street involved women in the Downtown Eastside/Strathcona community*. Report for the Ministry of Women's Equality. Vancouver, BC: Province of British Columbia.

Dieter, C., and L. Otway. 2001. *Sharing our stories on promoting health and community healing: An Aboriginal women's health project*. Winnipeg, MB: Prairie Women's Health Centre of Excellence.

Dion-Stout, M., G.D. Kipling, and R. Stout. 2001. *Aboriginal Women's Health Research Synthesis Project*. Ottawa, ON: Centres of Excellence for Women's Health.

Elias, B., A. Leader, D. Sanderson, and J. O'Neil. 2000. *Living in balance: Gender, structural inequalities, and health promoting behaviours in Manitoba First Nations communities*. Winnipeg, MB: Prairie Women's Health Centre of Excellence.

Farmer, P. 2000. The consumption of the poor: Tuberculosis in the 21st century. *Ethnography* 1 (2): 183-216.

Fine, M., and L. Weiss. 1996. Writing the "wrongs" of fieldwork: Confronting our own research/writing dilemmas in urban ethnographies. *Qualitative Inquiry* 2 (3): 251-74.

Fine, M., L. Weis, S. Weseen, and L. Wong. 2000. For whom? Qualitative research, representations, and social responsibilities. In N.K. Denzin and Y.S. Lincoln, eds., *Handbook of qualitative research,* 107-31. Thousand Oaks, CA: Sage.

Hardesty, M., and T. Black. 1999. Mothering through addiction: A survival strategy among Puerto Rican addicts. *Qualitative Health Research* 9 (5): 602-19.

Hull, J. 2001. *Aboriginal people and social classes in Manitoba*. Ottawa, ON: Canadian Centre for Policy Alternatives.

Jacobs, K., and K. Gill. 2002. Substance abuse in an urban Aboriginal population: Social, legal, and psychological consequences. *Journal of Ethnicity in Substance Abuse* 1 (1): 7-25.

Kane, S., and T. Mason. 2001. AIDS and criminal justice. *Annual Review of Anthropology* 30: 457-79.

Kleinman, A., V. Das, and M. Lock. 1997. Introduction. In A. Kleinman, V. Das, and M. Lock, eds., *Social suffering*, ix-xxvii. Berkeley, CA: University of California Press.

LaPrairie, C. 2001. *Aboriginal over-representation in the criminal justice system: A tale of nine cities*. Ottawa, ON: Department of Justice.

Lawless, S., S. Kippas, and J. Crawford. 1996. Dirty, diseased and undeserving: The positioning of HIV+ women. *Social Science and Medicine* 43 (9): 1371-77.

McCovey, S. 1998. Ascending poverty and inequality in Native America: An alternative perspective. In E.A. Segal, K. Kilty, and M. Kilty, eds., *Pressing issues of inequality and American Indian communities,* 85-88. New York: Haworth Press.

McDonald, K.A. 2002. *Missing voices: Aboriginal mothers who have been at risk of or who have had their children removed from their care*. Phase 2 report. Vancouver, BC: Legal Services Society of British Columbia and Law Foundation of British Columbia.

Native Women's Association of Canada. 1997. *Hear their stories: 40 Aboriginal women speak*. Ottawa, ON: Native Women's Association of Canada.

Nguyen, V.-K., and K. Peschard. 2003. Anthropology, inequality and disease. *Annual Review of Anthropology* 32: 447-74.

Parker, R. 2001. Sexuality, culture, and power in HIV/AIDS research. *Annual Review of Anthropology* 30: 163-79.

Peters, E.J. 1998. Subversive spaces: First Nations women and the city in Canada. *Society and Space* 16 (6): 665-85.

Razack, S. 2000. Gendered racial violence and spatialized justice: The murder of Pamela George. *Canadian Journal of Law and Society* 15 (2): 91-130.

Richards, J. 1995. Comment. In H. Drost, B.L. Crowley, and R. Schwindt, eds., *Market solutions for Native poverty,* 8-13. Toronto, ON: C.D. Howe Institute.

–. 2000. Reserves are only good for some people. *Journal of Canadian Studies* 35 (1): 190-204.

Roberts, C.A. 1999. Drug use among inner city African-American women: The process of managing loss. *Qualitative Health Research* 9 (5): 620-38.

Scott, K.A. 2001. Balance as a method to promote healthy indigenous communities. Canada Health Action: Building on the Legacy Papers. Commissioned by the NFH Determinants of Health. *Settings and Issues* 3: 147-79.

Ship, S., and L. Norton. 2000. It's hard to be a woman: First Nations women living with HIV/AIDS. *Native Social Work Journal* 3 (1): 69-85.

Sinclaire, M. 1997. Barriers to food procurement: The experiences of urban Aboriginal women in Winnipeg (Manitoba). MS thesis, University of Manitoba.

Singer, M. 2001. Toward a bio-cultural and political economic integration of alcohol, tobacco and drug studies in the coming century. *Social Science and Medicine* 53: 199-213.

Slowey, G. 2001. Globalization and self-government: Impacts and implications for First Nations in Canada. *American Review of Canadian Studies* 31 (1-2): 265-81.

Spittal, P.M., K.J.P. Craib, E. Wood, N. Laliberté, K. Li, M.W. Tyndall, M.V. O'Shaughnessy, and M.T. Schechter. 2002. Risk factors for elevated HIV incidence rates among female injection drug users in Vancouver. *Canadian Medical Association Journal* 166 (7): 894-99.

Tait, C., and Prairie Women's Health Collective. 2000. *A study of the service needs of pregnant addicted women in Manitoba*. Winnipeg, MB: Prairie Women's Health Centre of Excellence.

DARA CULHANE

Vancouver/Richmond Health Board. 1999. *Healing ways: Aboriginal health and service review*. Vancouver, BC: Vancouver/Richmond Health Board.

Whiteis, D.G. 1998. Third World medicine in First World cities: Capital accumulation, uneven development and public health. *Social Science and Medicine* 47 (6): 795-808.

Zierler, S., and N. Krieger. 1997. Reframing women's risk: Social inequalities and HIV infection. *Annual Review of Public Health* 18: 401-36.

8
Suicide as a Way of Belonging: Causes and Consequences of Cluster Suicides in Aboriginal Communities

RONALD NIEZEN

Whatever insight I might have into Aboriginal suicide I acquired unintentionally during two years that I lived as an ethnographic researcher in Cross Lake, Manitoba, a northern Aboriginal reserve community. I had initially intended to do a long-term study of the community's campaign, then in its early stages, to redress grievances following from the construction of a large-scale hydroelectric project in the early 1970s and from the failure of a compensation treaty, the Northern Flood Agreement, signed in 1977. The strategy of implementing the Northern Flood Agreement, mainly through petty claims of compensation for broken boat propellers caused by floating debris or snowmobiles lost or damaged in weakened ice conditions, was clearly not meeting anyone's aspirations for the treaty's promises of employment and community development. A commitment to public transparency in a new political process was the principal reason for the community's review of my curriculum vitae in a public meeting and their subsequent request that my family and I live with them for two years to witness and report on the conditions of their lives and on their campaign to change these conditions through defining new relationships with the federal and provincial governments and with the Crown corporation Manitoba Hydro. It was in this context that I began my work as an ethnographic researcher, concentrating most of my attention on the complex, shifting political dynamics brought about by a new strategy of legal pressure and public lobbying.

But when, in 1999, three suicide-related deaths and a spate of suicide attempts occurred in close succession, my attention and involvement in events went in quite another direction. It was clear that locally staffed institutions – the Pimicikamak Cree Nation Health Services and the Awasis Child and Family Agency – were already overwhelmed by the extent of their responsibilities, having inherited a clientele that had a high frequency of addictions, mental illness, and family crises. Consequently, they were wholly unprepared for the occurrence of several suicides and numerous suicide attempts in close succession. A hastily prepared application by the Health Authority to the federal government for funding of an intervention program was categorically rejected, without any offer of assistance to clarify the application format and procedures. It took several months for the Health Authority to submit a new application, for the proposal to be negotiated with federal officials, and for an intervention program – reduced in scope to a telephone crisis line – to be implemented. Meanwhile, the nursing station, on the front line of response to the crisis, faced even greater constraints, with staff shortages so severe that during several weeks in 1999 it became necessary to close the building and accept only emergency cases, with a hand-lettered sign on the inside window of the locked main entrance calling for patients to self-triage in accordance with very basic criteria: "Life or death situations, e.g., heart attack; uncontrolled bleeding; choking."[1] Community leaders, faced with what they regarded as an unresponsive government, were forced to accept a situation in which to garner the resources they needed they would have to reveal the extent of the crisis to a wider public in an appeal to justice, opening their situation of suffering and incapacity to distant sympathizers and, through that sympathy, exerting pressure on public officials to act responsibly. It was under these circumstances that my attention turned more urgently to Aboriginal youth suicide.[2]

I begin my effort to understand cluster suicide among Aboriginal youth with the premise that suicide can be both an individual act – perhaps the ultimate expression of individual will and struggle with conscience – and a social phenomenon, influenced by common conditions and experiences and by shared values, beliefs, symbols, and practices. The social influences on suicidal behaviour, although not as immediate as the individual act of self-destruction, are attested to by the phenomenon sometimes referred to as the *contagion effect* – evident, for example, in high rates of suicide among those who witness media reports on completed suicides. And it is especially evident in *suicide clusters,* a pattern of concentrated self-destruction that occurs in particular communities, such as campuses, barracks, and in the instances I will explore here, Aboriginal villages.

The term "suicide cluster" has much the same meaning as the popular concept of an "outbreak": a high number of self-inflicted deaths occurring in temporal *and* geographical proximity (Gould, Wallenstein, and Davidson 1989, 17) – bringing with it the discomforting idea that suicide can somehow be contracted from others through an "epidemic" in a way analogous to disease. The most obvious explanation for such intense episodes of self-destruction does in fact centre on a "contagion" effect, with one self-inflicted death appearing to be connected by emotional disturbance and imitation to other suicidal acts, apparently resulting in (and from) dramatic increases in depression and anxiety disorders among surviving community members. But it is not at all clear how suicidal acts can produce such a contagion effect. It could be that some who are shocked, disturbed, and aggrieved by the suicide or attempted suicide of a friend or family member become more distressed, but not suicidal, after the event. Others who are already depressed, anxious, hopeless, or angry may be strongly influenced by an idea or action derived from the suicidal behaviour of others, while the degree of their distress remains essentially unchanged.[3] Cluster suicides seem to involve a central paradox that follows from the fact that those who commit or attempt suicide are often driven by profound loneliness, neglect, or a sense of being unimportant and invisible, while, at the same time, this condition of loneliness becomes directly or indirectly shared with others. There appears to be a kind of perverse sociability at work in which self-destruction itself becomes a basis for linkage between individuals, a source of group behaviour beyond more widely accepted social norms (Coleman 1987, 3).

Public knowledge of such events in some of Canada's Aboriginal communities has in recent years greatly increased at the same time that it has become contracted and over-simplified. When an unusually high number of self-inflicted deaths occur in a small reserve village in a short space of time, the media occasionally respond with coverage communi-cated to a wide public, breaking down the barriers of community isolation with stark im-ages of poverty and grief, bringing immediate attention to the occurrence of the deaths and the social circumstances in which they took place. Today, virtually anyone in the world who has regularly read a daily newspaper or visited Internet news sites is in some way aware of the exceptionally high rates of suicide in some Aboriginal communities in Canada. For those who do not look beyond what is of necessity selected and superficial informa-tion, Aboriginal people come to be seen as typically impoverished, depressed, and suicidal.

But comparison of national statistics with those of Aboriginal communities in crisis dispels the idea that cluster suicides are the norm for the Aboriginal population as a whole. The generally high suicide rate for so-called status Indians nationwide – approxi-mately 29:100,000 compared to 13:100,000 for Canada as a whole – is actually a conse-quence of very high frequencies in particular Aboriginal communities or regions, whereas other areas report no suicides at all. Ward and Fox (1977), for example, investigated a "chain of deaths" in which 8 suicides took place over a 12-month period from 1974 to 1975 in a large reserve community in northern Ontario, resulting in a rate of 267:100,000 for that year. Other communities in northern Ontario have more recently faced comparable crises. Preliminary data from the Sioux Lookout First Nations Health Authority, respon-sible for 15 reserve communities that have experienced suicide "epidemics" or "clusters" within the past 10 years, reveal the occurrence of some 270 self-inflicted deaths within a population of 15,000, comprising a suicide rate of approximately 180:100,000.[4] Very high rates of suicide, concentrated in space and time, were also reported from northern Mani-toba, before the 1999 crisis in Cross Lake. Norway House, a reserve community approxi-mately 100 kilometres by road from Cross Lake, experienced 8 youth suicides from 1981 to 1984, resulting in an overall rate of 77:100,000 (Ross and Davis 1986); and Cross Lake itself, as I discuss below, experienced a similar crisis from 1986 to 1987. A central issue raised by such suicide clusters becomes apparent only when they are viewed in the con-text of national statistics. Clearly, if crises of this kind were the norm for Native commun-ities nationwide, the suicide statistic for Canada's Aboriginal population would be much higher than it is. Suicide rates are not evenly shared by all Aboriginal communities but tend to be sharply elevated in some and substantially lower than that of the general population in others.[5]

One of the potential reasons for this variability is that self-destruction can in some circumstances become central to group belonging. Suicidal behaviour occurs with great-est intensity where the idea of purposefully ending one's life has become an aspect of a shared outlook on life, particularly within youth groups that are isolated from usual pathways to socialization with older generations. To fully understand the phenomenon of suicide clusters, we must therefore abandon the (often implicit) idea of community as necessarily associated with the values of comfort, consolation, and security. In some circumstances, particularly among some groups of young men, self-destruction can itself become a central value of social life. In the absence of life-affirming examples of security and hope, young people will occasionally construct their own forms of solidarity, premised on rejecting security, abandoning expectations of a better future, and, ultimately, negating their personal attachments to life itself.

Part of what I intend to do here is to reduce the social distance between analyst and actor in the study of collective suicide. Having lived in an Aboriginal community as a social-science researcher during a time when a suicide crisis occurred, I can now act on an opportunity to present a perspective that is informed over the long term by an understanding of the social background, events, and people in which a heavy concentration of suicide attempts and completed suicides took place. Such a crisis cannot, of course, be anticipated from the point of view of planned research, and in the thick of events it did not occur to me to apply formal methods that might reveal, with professionally recognized standards of precision, such things as the extent of depression or suicide ideation in the community. But there is still much that can be gained from a more interpretive ethnographic approach, one that begins with the accidental circumstances of being in a time and place in which a suicide cluster could be, as much as possible, witnessed and experienced. I intend to draw on this experience in an effort to better understand the occurrence – in *some* Aboriginal communities – of a socially concentrated will to die.

Cross Lake's Crises

During the two years that I lived in Cross Lake, Manitoba, from 1998 to 2000, there were altogether 9 deaths from suicide, most of them occurring in a 6-month period, this in a community of a little more than 4,500 residents.[6] The suicide crisis swept through the village with the force of a natural disaster, only without the minimal consolation of an explanation for the ruin and suffering left in its wake. There was no tornado, no earthquake, to account for loved ones lost and no recognizable possibility of rebuilding and restoration, only unanswered and unanswerable questions. Besides the strong emotions that followed from the premature end of life, the acts of suicide left friends and families with little understanding of their cause, inviting regret, guilt, and above all widespread anxiety about the apparent willingness to die among some of those in the victim's circle of friends and siblings.

Added to the emotional injury of completed suicides were the anxiety, sorrow, guilt, and impotent anger that followed from a simultaneous spate of suicide attempts and threats of suicide. During the Cross Lake crisis, "survivals" from attempted suicide were far more common than deaths by suicide. The Royal Canadian Mounted Police reported to the press that in Cross Lake in 1999 there were 144 requests for assistance involving threatened or attempted suicide, and the local nursing station acted on many other cases of self-harm in which the police were not called in.[7] These ranged from such incidents as "calls for help" involving mild overdoses of over-the-counter medication to more serious events, such as miraculous, timely survivals from hanging. Each of these events added itself to the community's networks of news, sorrow, and anxiety.

The results of an intervention program further revealed the manner and extent to which the idea of suicide had taken hold. The Cross Lake Band Office reports on its website that a 24-hour suicide crisis line established in September 1999 logged 18,688 calls in its first three years, a rate of approximately one call every 84 minutes.[8] If the events of suicide completions and attempts were not enough to create an impression of a widespread potential for self-destruction, this remarkable figure seems retrospectively to confirm the fact of its existence.

This impression of deep-seated suicidality was further reinforced by considering the records and recollections of suicide in Cross Lake. Some 10 years earlier, in 1986 and 1987, the same thing had happened, the same pattern of deaths, attempts, rescues, and frantic efforts to intervene by volunteer counsellors who, before long, had worked themselves to the point of "burnout." In a 6-month period between 1986 and 1987, there were approximately 60 police and nursing-station interventions in suicide attempts and 7 completed suicides.[9] One of the members of this group of suicidal youth, who himself attempted suicide three times, recalled that at this time suicidal behaviour "was becoming like a norm, where you hear about it and you go 'ha!' and people would laugh and joke about it. Kind of like a normal thing" (Cross Lake, 31 March 1999).

Nevertheless, in a courageous effort to counteract the influence of this "norm" in Cross Lake, a handful of volunteer counsellors formed an impromptu Crisis Committee and worked themselves to exhaustion, with little political support and too great a burden of young clients who saw no place for themselves in the future, seemingly nurturing the will to end their lives.[10] Since most suicide attempts occurred within 3 or 4 hours after midnight (possibly because this is a time of diminished social activity), volunteers would often be up at night dealing with threats of suicide, then return home in the morning to get their children ready for school and get themselves to the jobs that they continued to hold in addition to their volunteer counselling. One of these counsellors recalled the effects of emotional pressure and overwork that went along with close involvement with a core group of suicidal youth: "It got to the point for me that every time I heard a loud noise, like a door slamming or something, I thought it was another shot gun going off" (Cross Lake, 13 November 1998).

Former counsellors from this earlier crisis were those who first recognized in 1999 that the pattern of self-destruction was repeating itself. The only essential difference was that the second crisis tended to involve people in their late twenties or early thirties, whereas the crisis a decade earlier most commonly involved those in their late teens and early twenties. In other words, in Cross Lake a pattern is evident, with a particular group more often dangerously or lethally committing acts of self-destruction.

Once we recognize that an unusually high number of suicides have occurred within a relatively short period of time and in a clearly defined community, the task of explanation can no longer be accomplished by focusing exclusively on the "proximal" factors, the life events and circumstances of individuals. With so many threatened, attempted, and completed acts of suicide happening in such proximity, we are forced to recognize the occurrence of a crisis that goes beyond the usual manifestation of mental illness, that is larger than individual life histories, and that can be explained only by considering the social context in which suicide somehow gained wide currency.

Suicide is a notoriously difficult phenomenon to understand, above all in those cases that seem to follow from the effects of social contagion. But our knowledge can be advanced when we highlight this complexity by pointing to the difficulties and multiple possibilities, both in the realm of mental health crisis and in the realm of ideas, inherent in trying to understand cluster suicides in Canada's Aboriginal communities.

Interpreting Cluster Suicides

The wide differences in rates of suicide between Aboriginal populations as a whole and those places in which suicide clusters have occurred is one of the strongest indications we have of a social origin to suicide, encouraging an approach that is more encompassing than the focus on the suicide victim and his or her immediate family or social entourage. Where self-destruction is most concentrated, the possibility is greatest that it is being influenced by shared ideas and values.

The idea of a collective dimension to suicide among the peoples of Australia and New Zealand was considered in 1926 in a comparative study by Marcel Mauss, "Effet physique chez l'Individu de l'idée de mort suggérée par la collectivité" (The physical effect in individuals of the idea of death suggested by the collectivity). According to Mauss, suicide can sometimes result from the elaboration of collective ideas, above all moral and religious ideas, that compel individuals toward self-destruction "by suggestion." This influence on individual behaviour of shared ideas about acceptable or inevitable death resulting from spiritual forces is, he proposed, a clear indication of the influence of social life on the motives and behaviour of individuals. Group pressure and education can create a foundation of belief that, under the least provocation, can unleash "ravages or overexcitement of forces" (2004, 315). Although contemporary suicide research has largely dispensed with the colonial cultural stereotypes built into the material invoked by Mauss, his general observation of a collective dimension to self-destructive behaviour, traceable largely to the influence of shared ideas, remains a significant, yet largely overlooked, point of analytical departure.

This influence is evident from accounts of Cross Lake's suicides in 1986 and 1987. This crisis appears to have first occurred principally among members of a close-knit group of friends who had grown up in abusive homes, who were then separated when some of them were sent to distant foster homes, and who were reunited in Cross Lake in their mid- to late teens. As often occurs in such groups, security and comfort were provided by one among them – let us call him George. As one of this group of friends remembered, their parents' drinking parties were dangerous events in families with histories of violence and sexual abuse: "We'd have to sneak out the window and go sleep in the bush in the middle of the night ... come out in the morning when everyone was passed out." It was in these circumstances that George gave hope to his younger siblings. "He was telling my brothers and my sisters not to worry, that he was going to take care of them" (Cross Lake, 31 March 1999).

George, who had become the focus of a youth group's security, was the first to die by suicide in 1986, suffering a traumatic and public death in the local nursing station from a self-inflicted gunshot wound. Soon, another of the same group survived a self-inflicted gunshot wound from a 303 British rifle. The self-inflicted deaths and attempts at suicide from this point seemed to gain momentum: "After that there just seemed to be lots and lots of suicides. It wasn't too long after that [that] my ... she hung herself. [And another of our friends] shot himself a couple of months after that too. They tried to stop him. The only thing he said was, 'Hey, I'll say hi to all those guys for you,' and pulled the trigger" (Cross Lake, 31 March 1999).

One of the striking things to emerge from this narrative is the very public nature of self-inflicted death in this suicide crisis. In a remote community surrounded by wilderness, those who took their lives did not do so distantly and quietly but died in ways that were sure to be witnessed by others. Suicides that occurred in crowded reservation housing, especially in the context of house parties, gave the widest possible exposure to the fait accompli of self-destruction. The most direct way to communicate the *idea* of suicide was through one's choice in the *act* of suicide. Nor was the nursing station a setting that offered privacy during a situation of crisis; rather, it offered self-destruction to public view in crowded facilities, in which a significant number of spectators of the violent consequences of suicidal acts were almost certain to be friends or relatives of the victim.

The point seems to emerge from this case material that there can be a group dynamic involved in the development of a suicide cluster and that the idea of suicide can be directly or indirectly promoted through group dynamics. This is an aspect of the study of suicide that is not adequately understood. The social or cultural processes or "routes of exposure" by which susceptible individuals come to seriously accept the idea of suicide are tremendously significant but remain unclear (Gould, Wallenstein, and Davidson 1989). In some instances at least, there can be much more happening behind the events of cluster suicides than an unusually intense and unresolved form of collective grief or individual identification. How does the idea of suicide become so entrenched, so widely accepted as an escape from unbearable distress, that it can be acted on by many or most members of a community? It would appear from Cross Lake's experience that the thought of suicide can in some circumstances become normalized and, I would argue, even become part of a group's self-image.

This observation takes us in a direction that has not been adequately explored in the study of suicide. Michael Kral has convincingly pointed out that a strong emphasis in suicide research has been on some notion of individual "perturbation," on the state of intolerable psychological distress in all its myriad forms that creates a motivation for suicide, but that "we know next to nothing about lethality: how the idea of suicide becomes internalized and later selected as a course of action by some people" (1998, 223). Distress, no matter how severe, is not always acted upon in lethal acts of self-destruction, so why is it that conditions of unbearable suffering will lead some to take their own lives while others do not? Kral suggests that "the only direct 'cause' of suicide is the *idea* of suicide and ways to do it, and that in order to better understand suicide we need to know more about how ideas are spread throughout society and become part of an individual's repertoire" (1994, 253). The social study of suicide, then, involves the complex task of accounting for historical and social conditions that might contribute to "perturbation" *and* the often less tangible influence of culture on the currency and form of the idea of suicide. Understanding how the idea of suicide becomes internalized is particularly relevant for suicide clusters because the very nature of the phenomenon suggests the influence of collective ideas, even the possible influence of collective self-image or identity, on the frequency of suicide.

Historical Etiology

Virtually everyone who tries to understand the social origins of suicide in indigenous communities now pays particular attention to their distinctive historical background, marked very often by the impacts of political domination, displacement, and economic marginalization, which can be seen as having widely ramifying effects on nearly every aspect of life and society. Such histories are often invoked as sources of explanation for high frequencies of mental illness, addictions, family violence, and self-destruction. But the nature of the connection between past trauma and present crisis is not well understood, and most of those who link history with self-destruction seem to simply assume an effect of collective psychological disturbance that follows naturally and predictably from a colonial legacy or from more immediate disruptions to community autonomy and viability. If, as the findings of psychology have long revealed, the events and memories that shape individual personality are ambiguous and complex, how much more equivocal and subject to variability and reinvention must be the collective interpretations of a community's history.

There are two questions to consider when we look at this historical background. First, if the pattern of colonial occupation and displacement by nation-states is essentially similar for all indigenous people and if this legacy is in fact part of how they define themselves, does this create a different "background noise," aside from human nature or possible genetic predispositions toward psychiatric illness, that would explain overall high frequencies of suicide in indigenous populations? And second, over and above this general background to Aboriginal suicide, are there significant variations in the historical experience of different regions, communities, or extended families, particular traumas of collective displacement, that can be seen to correlate consistently with the occurrence of suicide clusters? It is certainly possible to show that some communities have been historically subject to particularly acute collective traumas such as forced relocation, loss of subsistence in conjunction with large-scale resource extraction, or the lasting effects of a particularly abusive residential school. If such distinct traumas can be shown to create a social experience that combines what Joiner refers to as "noxious stimuli" (1999, 92) with decreased social support, we would have the plausible beginnings of an explanation for the origin and distribution of cluster suicides.

One does not have to agree on the particulars of the historical record or on the extent to which events or policies might have contributed to lasting collective trauma to see that the experiences shared by many Aboriginal people in Canada – shared, for that matter, by indigenous people in many parts of the world – have brought about extraordinary challenges to the viability of families and communities. On a nearly global scale, there is an apparent correlation between the common historical experiences that define indigenous peoples – which boil down to forced removal from territory and removal from intergenerational transmission of knowledge – and the contemporary experiences of mental health crises.

The Elders whom I came to know in Cross Lake and other places in Canada's North remember their youth as a time when most families lived for 6 to 10 months of the year in isolated bush camps, coming into small settlements only in the summer months. As children, they learned such things as how to set snares, how to string fish nets under a layer of ice, and how to navigate by the stars. In their lifetimes they have seen the rapid centralization and growth of villages, the arrival of modern medicine, increased participation in formal education, including the now widely recognized traumas of residential schools, profound social and environmental changes brought about by large-scale extractive industries, and a historically sudden increase in the complexity and sophistication of local political structures and processes.

Turning to the particular historical experience of Cross Lake, we can clearly see these patterns of removal and abrupt cultural discontinuity. The imposition of residential school education with the establishment of the St. Joseph Christian School in 1919 until the phasing out of residential education in the early 1970s stands out as one plausible source of collective trauma with a possible connection to later manifestations of suicide. A theme that ran through my many interviews with social-service workers in Cross Lake and several other northern reservation villages centred on the problems Aboriginal people encounter today in bringing up children. The skills of parenting were lost through the separation of children from their families. Children were not given a sense of pride in themselves and their social origins but were taught the iniquity of their families and forebears. Their education was grounded in inherently contradictory efforts to impart autonomy and self-sufficiency through the imposition of alien values. The notorious cruelty inflicted on incarcerated children in some residential schools became in later years a background to failed families in which parents were unable to express affection, having only the abusive model of their own childhood as a basis for interacting with their children. The churches, in large measure through their failed efforts at cultural engineering, are widely seen as responsible for the decline of traditional values, the loss of effective curing ceremonies, and a legacy of confusion and sorrow resulting from the institutional abuses of residential schools. And this legacy, directly or indirectly, would appear to be a significant part of the background to and explanation for the self-destructive behaviour of youth in some communities.

The imposition of large-scale resource extraction is another theme that commonly runs through historical explanations of mental illness and suicide in indigenous societies. In Cross Lake the injustices and discontinuities caused by a large-scale hydroelectric project constructed in the 1970s seem to be tangibly represented by the Jenpeg generating station some nine miles upstream from the village. Here too they have something in common with many other Aboriginal peoples. Most mental health experts who work in Canada's North agree, at least according to anecdotal observation, that where communities have been displaced to make room for large-scale projects, there is likely to be a marked increase in so-called pathological behaviour: drug and alcohol addictions, family violence, child neglect, juvenile crime, and, of course, suicide. The social displacements caused by large-scale resource extraction, resulting in forced resettlement, loss of territory, and loss of subsistence, are commonly invoked sources of collective trauma in the historical backgrounds of many people from many parts of the world who today refer to themselves as "indigenous." This history seems in particular to be directly relevant to the etiology of Aboriginal suicide.

The first difficulty we encounter when we try to connect the specific historical traumas of indigenous people with later manifestations of social crisis, however, is not that the impact of imposed change is indeterminate or negligible but that it is multiple. Very often in colonial history, it is not just one event that can be seen as stretching the elastic limits of people and communities beyond their capacity to adapt but several significant dislocations that seem to plausibly account for widespread depression. As in the case of Cross Lake, there are often successions of losses and social disconnections that cumulatively seem to lie behind a community's inability to transmit knowledge, values, and well-being to new generations.[11] With the long unfolding of colonial relationships, state-sponsored programs of removal and assimilation, and the newer obstacles posed by marginalization and dependency, virtually every Aboriginal community can invoke a troubled historical legacy as an explanation for present afflictions.

Why doesn't every historical ordeal of domination and disjuncture leave a similar legacy of social crisis? If the suicide crises of particular communities seem to be explained by the cumulative impact of grief following, at least in part, from the events of historical trauma, why does the same pattern not happen uniformly in every village with a similar legacy of disrupted social networks or with a similar history of political marginalization and economic dependency? Why, for example, among the Nishnawbe communities of the Sioux Lookout zone in northern Ontario, which share essential features of culture and history with Cross Lake, are some communities afflicted with pervasive and seemingly intractable cycles of grief and self-harm, while others are not?

So we return to our original question: Why do some Aboriginal communities or families seem especially susceptible to collective manifestations of self-harm? If the severity of historical trauma is not sufficient on its own to explain why suicide is high in some places and virtually nonexistent in others, what remains to be considered? And if, as seems to be the case, the way historical memory is constructed is open to more creativity, variability, contest, and cultural boundary-crossing (or trespass) than is commonly supposed, how might this realization be applied to better understanding the cultural conditions of suicide?

Heritage and Healing

An alternative approach to Aboriginal suicide might better explain the wide variability in frequencies of social pathologies within communities that have basically similar historical backgrounds, forms of social organization, and spiritual practices. It is premised on the idea that people, as individuals or collectivities, destroy themselves not merely because they are in a state of social instability and isolation but above all because they are unable to find their way out of uncertainty, unable to *create* a new collective awareness of pride, permanence, and security. Consistent with this observation, heritage has become a focal point of studies that attempt either to predict, and possibly alleviate, conditions in which Aboriginal communities spiral out of control or to uncover conditions in which communities have corrected self-destructive tendencies in youth by creating new foundations of social solidarity based on distinct identity. This approach stresses that it is not so much the historical background to social dislocation that correlates with suicidal behaviour as whether, and in what way, communities are able to overcome a traumatic historical inheritance. Conditions of social reform and renewal of identity are every bit as important in determining the frequencies of social pathologies as are the foundational conditions of social displacement, marginalization, and exclusion.

This perspective is evident, for example, in the work of Michael Chandler and Chris Lalonde (1998; Chapter 10), which highlights the importance of "cultural continuity" as a protective factor for Aboriginal youth. The central markers of cultural continuity – the pursuit of land claims, regimes of self-government that include local control of education, police, and health services, the development of Aboriginal cultural facilities, and the active participation of women in the position of chief or band councillor – are shown by Chandler and Lalonde to protect the personal identities of youth and therefore to cumulatively act as a hedge against suicide and self-destructive behaviour.[12] The literature on Aboriginal youth suicide broadly confirms that there are specific local strategies and resources available to those Aboriginal communities that set out to develop their own suicide-prevention programs.[13]

If indeed such programs are broadly effective in reducing suicide frequency, it might be possible at the same time to arrive at a more complete understanding of the factors contributing to high rates of suicide in some Aboriginal communities. The specific social conditions and intervention measures that are effective in reducing frequencies of suicide can at the same time reveal the most likely causes of suicide. If connecting with family and community is an important part of the healing process, a condition of disconnection from family and community is evidently a significant part of the background to high suicidality. If being close to nature and spirituality has therapeutic value, remoteness from nature and detachment from spiritual traditions must factor into the way we understand self-destruction. The literature on youth suicide in Canada's Aboriginal population seems to approach a single, central conclusion from several directions: the affirmation of life is enhanced by an unambiguous understanding of one's place in a social world. Self-destruction does not often reach a point of crisis in societies that have anchorages to history or tradition and in which the political realm creates a secure environment. A community or society that is clearly able to answer the question "who are we?" for its members and for the outside world is better able to give its individual members an answer to "who am I?" – or perhaps more important, "*why* am I?" – and to enhance their ability to overcome obstacles to personal growth and find purpose in living.

Self-Destruction and Collective Identity

As it now appears, suicide crises do not always come to a definitive end when they taper off into a semblance of normality. As the example of the progression from youth to young-adult suicide in Cross Lake illustrates, if one age group was once particularly afflicted by a suicide crisis, those same people seem to carry with them a self-destructive fragility throughout their lives, which can emerge again in times of particular stress, set off, perhaps, by only one incident of self-harm among their peers.

To better understand the occurrence of suicide clusters, we should therefore consider those features of cultural life that contribute to the durability of the idea of suicide. If one of our principal concerns is to understand how the idea of suicide can become deeply embedded in the repertoire of ideas (Kral 1998, 225), one prominent feature of Aboriginal cultural life that we should consider is the collective expression of grief. Colin Samson, reflecting on an apparently socially connected series of suicides among the Innu of Davis Inlet, remarks that "suicide is a communal tragedy. Almost every Innu in Sheshatshiu and Utshimassits attends the long and emotional funerals. Because members of the community are closely related to each other by blood and marriage, funerals are reminders of the collective trauma of the Innu as a people" (2003, 228; see also Chapter 5). In any Aboriginal community, in which the social network of every individual ramifies broadly, there is a far-reaching effect of public mourning that follows from a self-inflicted death, and if one adds to this the many, sometimes highly traumatic, suicide attempts, an entire community can arrive at what seems to be a self-reinforcing cycle of emotional injury and self-harm.

But collective suffering does not provide a complete explanation of socially intense suicide. Simply correlating shared misery with a high frequency of suicide does not give sufficient place to the kind of creativity we find in almost every common human venture, especially those ventures undertaken in the face of oppression. Once we establish that suicide has a collective dimension, it is quite simply inconceivable that it would be exclusively the result of unadorned grief rather than influenced by shared ideas, cultural dynamics, and a process of reshaping collective self-definition and self-presentation.

This is my sense of what has occurred in places stricken by intensely concentrated self-destruction. Youth groups often first form around binge drinking or solvent abuse, moving progressively to greater severity of self-harm, sometimes to the point at which death itself becomes a focus of belonging. The influence of shared ideas on suicide occasionally seems so pervasive that we might appropriately refer to suicide clusters as a graduated form of mass suicide – collective manifestations of self-destruction that are an apparent response to inescapable oppression provoked by repressive forces outside a closed community. Understood in these terms, suicide clusters are "typical of defeated and colonized populations that are forced to escape from a reality in which human dignity is not acknowledged" (Mancinelli et al. 2002, 91-92). These deaths do not always occur under the direction of a charismatic leader, nor do they appear to be inspired by a single powerful idea that validates an ultimate collective end to immediate, inescapable oppression. Rather, the frequent occurrence of suicides among members of a youth group seems to be inspired by more nebulous, purposeless acceptance of self-imposed risk, self-injury, and self-inflicted death as part of the way one lives.

Suicide is often narrowly seen as occurring most often where there is an absence of anchorages to tradition, where collective and individual identities are fragile, inconsistent, or subject to doubt and crisis. But in some communities, above all those with marked indicators of a self-destructive youth, the disengagement of young people from older generations and the absence of almost any channel for productive activity can contribute to a distinct form of identity that begins with the normalization of suffering and goes on to give positive value to self-harm and self-destruction. In the context of cultural confusion, there can develop a collective normalization of self-destruction among youth who are cut off from the example and social persuasion of older generations, accompanied by a readiness to turn instead to the negation of life, to a rejection of healing and nurturing. Where all other avenues to a secure sense of self are blocked or rejected, where there are few recognized outlets for establishing oneself as a memorable person, it is still possible to express oneself through self-negation. It is not adequately recognized by those seeking to understand Aboriginal suicide that in some circumstances and in some social circles, identities can be constructed around the negation of life, the absence of a future, and acceptance of the idea, if not the positive appeal, of self-harm and premature death.

The idea of suicide gains widest currency when intergenerational transmission of knowledge and values has been interrupted and when institutions of socialization outside the family – most commonly schools and churches – have failed to provide a broadly legitimate sense of collective selfhood. It is not just that the violence and abuse of the worst residential schools left legacies of grief and self-destruction but also that, largely through this abuse, the schools made it impossible for children to see themselves in the future as noteworthy individuals or as people of honour. Whether or not we see concentrated self-destruction as a form of resistance to conditions of oppression, it occurs in circumstances in which accepted forms of self-expression are disconnected from opportunity. Taking one's own life is the ultimate rejection of all that has been offered – and of all that has been taken away – as a prospect in life. In the absence of other viable possibilities, it becomes a way to achieve recognition, to make one's mark, to belong to a sympathetic and accepting community of peers.[14]

The literature on Aboriginal heritage as a source of community healing supports the idea that suicide has cultural determinants from another direction. Cluster suicides occur not where there are relatively stable patterns of conformity and pathways for each individual's life but where there are historical backgrounds of social disintegration and confusion of personal and collective identity.

Self-destruction becomes socially intense not just where anchorages to tradition are weak or nonexistent but above all where they are misdirected, where death becomes one of the only avenues toward sympathy, notoriety, and love. Prominent, emotional burials constitute displays of affection after death that were largely absent in life. Community-based healing programs can proclaim in public forums that suicide is a call to action, a "wake-up call," and can thereby transmit the secondary idea that premature death brings to life a collective sense of purpose that was previously lacking. And media attention brings home the similar idea that one has greater value through death than one could ever hope to achieve through a lifetime of struggle for other forms of recognition.

Suicide is therefore deeply implicated in ideas about collective selfhood. Erik Erikson's formative insights into personal growth and identity in the 1950s have spilled over into a more recent concern with collective ideas of self in the political-science literature, in which identity attachments are almost always seen as a necessary outcome of individual and collective human growth, perhaps resolving themselves into groups that are, if anything, *too* cohesive and strident in their struggle for the exclusion or domination of others. But when we look more closely at the cultural context of youth suicide in some Aboriginal communities, we are confronted with the possibility that identity attachments can also form around suffering and self-negation. My sense is that collective suicide occurs not always in the absence of healing efforts but sometimes as a group-sanctioned alternative or resistance to healing. It occurs not because of personal obstacles or losses that create a sense of the impossibility of overcoming grief but because of a collective rejection of the possibility that grief might end. Where all other avenues for human cultural expression and belonging have been blocked or rejected, a group's identity can form around the will to die. This occurs among those who see that they are not like their Elders and cannot be like those in the dominant society. Where there is little or no connection between youth and their parents or grandparents, no relevant model for growth and aspirations, no immediate answer to the question "who are we?" – except perhaps a recognition of the pervasiveness of grief and despair – the thoughts and emotions associated with suicide can themselves provide a model for belonging and a semblance of an answer to the problems of identity.

Notes

1 The nursing shortage, as reported in the *Winnipeg Free Press* (Nurse shortage 1999), was precipitated by the simultaneous departure of four nurses on "stress leave." At the time, staffing levels in some 20 northern nursing stations were inadequate because of job insecurity, social isolation, and high workloads.

2 I undertook the investigation of suicide in Cross Lake with the support of the Pimicikamak Cree Nation Health Authority and the Cross Lake First Nation Band Office. To both these institutions I am grateful. I am aware of an ethical dilemma that arises in community-based studies of suicide. Depictions of mental health crises can have a stigmatizing effect and can even contribute to the currency of ideas that are implicated in high frequencies of suicide. This is particularly true of depictions in popular media. At the same time, without a more complete understanding of the causes and consequences of Aboriginal youth suicide, communities like Cross Lake will be at a disadvantage when it comes to developing effective intervention strategies. Cross Lake's leadership in the crisis of 1999-2000 opted to communicate the community's plight to the public by inviting the news media to report on it (which resulted in articles in a variety of Canadian newspapers, a report by Global Television, and a mini-documentary on CBC's national news program *24 Hours*). They also requested, and were refused, a coroner's inquest into one of the suicides. I have contributed to this volume in the hope that this chapter can in some small way, consistent with the spirit of seeking a formal inquest, contribute to a deeper understanding of Aboriginal youth suicide and eventually to more effective ways to prevent it.

3 I am grateful to Laurence Kirmayer for this latter observation (personal communication, 3 January 2007).

4 I am grateful to Arnold Devlin of the Dilco Ojibway Child and Family Services for this estimate of the rate of suicide in the Sioux Lookout zone of northern Ontario.

5 Chandler and Lalonde (Chapter 10) report findings from two studies that reveal a pattern in British Columbia in which high rates of suicide occur in a few Aboriginal communities, whereas most others actually have low rates of suicide. From 1993 to 2000, "roughly 90% of the suicides occurred in only 12% of the bands, and more than half of all Native communities suffered no youth suicides during this 8-year reporting period."

RONALD NIEZEN

6 Population statistics for those living on Aboriginal reserves are difficult to determine with precision because of a fluctuating population of registered band members living "off-reserve." The figure of 4,500 is
therefore a rough estimate.

7 One of the more informative of these press articles, "Cross Lake needs reasons to hope," was published
in December 1999 when there were 120 reported attempts.

8 http://www.crosslake.fn.ca/health.html (17 December 2005).

9 This included one notation of a suicide that was thinly disguised in the death record as originating from a
"self-inflicted disease." There is a further irregularity in the death record: it shows the 7 suicides occurring
over a 17-month period. This figure is inconsistent with the memories of those who were active in a volunteer association formed to deal with the crisis. They consistently assert that the crisis took place over
a 6-month period. The disparity is possibly the result of delays in formally reporting the causes of self-
inflicted deaths and entering them in the death record. (These records were made available to me by the
Cross Lake First Nation Band Office.)

10 Representatives of Haid Smith Counselling, a Winnipeg-based organization that provides training for
mental health workers in Aboriginal communities, recalled in a letter to the Cross Lake Education Authority that since the 1980s Cross Lake had not responded to suicide-intervention training with the same
level of commitment as in neighbouring communities: "When we have been invited by other communities
to do similar development we have found excellent response, sustained enthusiasm and attendance at
our trainings and workshops. In Cross Lake very few persons attended unless mandated to do so –
enthusiasm was lacking with little follow through ... This is our evidence that this community is in 'crisis'
and the rate of suicides and attempted suicides confirms this fact" (Haid and Smith 2000).

11 This was made particularly clear by the investigative efforts of the Royal Commission on Aboriginal
Peoples, in which an almost bewildering array of injustices and sorrows were laid at the feet of those who
came to the villages to listen sympathetically with the intention of assembling a public document based
on what they heard.

12 This finding is seconded by Rod McCormick's (1997b; Chapter 15) examination of Aboriginal community-
based healing initiatives, which suggests that culturally sanctioned healing practices that focus on natural
methods are more effective for Aboriginal people than are orthodox forms of clinical counselling. Among
McCormick's sample of First Nations people from British Columbia, "connecting with family, community,
culture, nature, and spirituality seems important in successful healing" (McCormick 1997a, 183). Laurence
Kirmayer and his team of researchers find another point of specificity in this general finding by pointing
to the forest economy and way of life as a source of collective healing: "Increased time in the bush may
confer mental health benefits by increasing family solidarity and social support, reinforcing cultural identity, improving physical health with nutritious bush foods and exercise, or providing respite from the
pressures of settlement life" (2000, 50).

13 It is at the same time necessary to recognize and investigate a number of potential obstacles to incorporating cultural and spiritual restoration in healing processes that might more effectively address suicide
among Aboriginal youth. First, "tradition" does not refer to a single source of inspiration that can be incorporated in healing strategies that are applied uniformly to all Aboriginal communities, at least not
without oversimplification, promotion of stereotypes, encouragement of cultural misunderstanding, and
confusion of healing processes. Rather, Aboriginal ways of life – including the ways that suffering is expressed and healing effectively carried out – are highly diverse and, at the same time, capable of change
through borrowing and innovation. The diversity and malleability of culture means that, to be effective,
healing strategies based on cultural and spiritual restoration cannot be approached in a way that is too
widely generalized and inflexible. It is not an easy matter, and probably not possible at all, to find specific
community-based healing strategies with proven effectiveness for all Aboriginal communities. The challenge of finding forms of prevention and intervention that contribute to resolving suicide crises must

therefore take into account the diversity and flexibility of Aboriginal cultures while isolating conditions in which community-based strategies are elaborated and implemented that might be more broadly conducive to effective healing.

Another complication in the study of community-based responses to youth suicide lies in the potential for cultural dissent within the Aboriginal communities themselves. Berlin finds that among south-western Pueblos, healing strategies are not as likely to get off the ground "where pressures to acculturate are great and there is extensive tribal conflict about maintaining traditional religion, governmental structure, clans, societies, and extended families" (1987, 224). Under these circumstances, more mental health problems occur, and not coincidentally, the suicide rate in the adolescent and young-adult population is high. This observation might equally apply to those communities in northern Canada in which rapid social change has brought about an erosion of knowledge of healing methods, of language, and of the environment; in which reciprocal sharing of resources has been replaced by competition for limited opportunities in the formal economy; and in which reliance on recognized Elders for healing and mediation of conflict has been replaced by the services of formal administrations. The development of local responses to suicide prevention sometimes occurs in village settings in which helping traditions are not securely defined or communicated between generations (Niezen 1993, 6).

14 J.E. Levy and S. Kunitz (1971), in a study of suicide among Hopi youth, similarly arrive at the observation that suicide is associated with pressure to conform.

References

Berlin, I. 1987. Suicide among American Indian adolescents: An overview. *Suicide and Life Threatening Behavior* 17 (3): 218-32.

Chandler, M., and C. Lalonde. 1998. Cultural continuity as a hedge against suicide in Canada's First Nations. *Transcultural Psychiatry* 35 (2): 193-211.

Coleman, L. 1987. *Suicide clusters.* London: Faber and Faber.

Cross Lake needs reasons to hope. 12 December 1999. *Winnipeg Free Press,* B4.

Gould, M., S. Wallenstein, and L. Davidson. 1989. Suicide clusters: A critical review. *Suicide and Life-Threatening Behavior* 19 (1): 17-29.

Haid, J., and M. Smith. 11 January 2000. Letter to Cross Lake Education Authority. Unpublished.

Joiner, T. 1999. The clustering and contagion of suicide. *Current Directions in Psychological Science* 8 (3): 89-92.

Kirmayer, L.J., L. Boothroyd, A. Tanner, N. Adelson, and R. Robinson. 2000. Psychological distress among the Cree of James Bay. *Transcultural Psychiatry* 37 (1): 35-56.

Kral, M. 1994. Suicide as social logic. *Suicide and Life-Threatening Behavior* 24 (3): 245-55.

–. 1998. Suicide and the internalization of culture: Three questions. *Transcultural Psychiatry* 35 (2): 221-33.

Levy, J.E., and S. Kunitz. 1971. Indian reservations, anomie, and social pathologies. *Southwestern Journal of Anthropology* 27 (2): 97-128.

Mancinelli, I., A. Comparelli, P. Girardi, and R. Tatarelli. 2002. Mass suicide: Historical and psychological considerations. *Suicide and Life-Threatening Behavior* 32 (2): 91-100.

Mauss, M. 2004 [1950]. Effet physique chez l'Individu de l'idée de mort suggérée par la collectivité [1926]. In *Sociologie et anthropologie,* 313-22. Paris: Presses Universitaires de France.

McCormick, R.M. 1997a. First Nations counsellor training in British Columbia: Strengthening the circle. *Canadian Journal of Community Mental Health* 16 (2) (special issue Mental health and Aboriginal communities): 91-99.

–. 1997b. Healing through interdependence: The role of connecting in First Nations healing practices. *Canadian Journal of Counselling* 31 (3): 172-84.

Niezen, R. 1993. *Traditional helping systems and social services among the James Bay Cree.* James Bay: Cree Board of Health and Social Services of James Bay.

Nurse shortage shuts northern health centre. 17 September 1999. *Winnipeg Free Press,* A9.

Ross, C., and B. Davis. 1986. Suicide and parasuicide in a northern Canadian Native community. *Canadian Journal of Psychiatry* 31 (4): 331-34.

Samson, C. 2003. *A way of life that does not exist: Canada and the extinguishment of the Innu.* St. John's, NL: ISER Books.

Ward, J.A., and J. Fox. 1977. A suicide epidemic on an Indian reserve. *Canadian Psychiatric Association Journal* 22 (8): 423-26.

9

Disruptions in Nature, Disruptions in Society: Aboriginal Peoples of Canada and the "Making" of Fetal Alcohol Syndrome

CAROLINE L. TAIT

You've seen lots of kids with FAS [fetal alchohol syndrome] and FAE [fetal alcohol effects]. They are the giggling, howling, glue-sniffing ghost children from Sheshatshiu who so shocked the nation that the Governor-General herself paid a visit to their ruined community ... They [FAS and FAE] are the leading known cause of mental retardation. And they are the common denominator for many of the plagues of native communities. Alcohol-damaged kids have poor impulse control, significant learning disabilities, and impaired judgment ... Even if they never drink themselves, their difficulties are life long. As they get older, their sexual behaviour is also impulsive. Among native communities, rates of child sexual abuse and teenage pregnancy are very high. Heavy drinking (and its effects) are responsible ... But the facts about our most vulnerable citizens ought to break your heart. There are around 300,000 Aboriginal kids in Canada under the age of 15 (and high birth rates mean the numbers are soaring). The guesses about the prevalence of FAS and FAE in native communities go as high as 40 per cent.

– MARGARET WENTE, "FINALLY, WE'RE TALKING ABOUT FAS,"
GLOBE AND MAIL, 1 FEBRUARY 2001

In recent decades, the diagnostic label fetal alcohol syndrome has emerged in Canada as a common framework for defining mental and social distress experienced by Aboriginal peoples. Central to this framework is the belief that Canadian Aboriginal women are at significantly higher risk than any other group of women to give birth to an alcohol-affected child. By the mid-1980s, this assumption resulted in claims that an epidemic of FAS was affecting upwards of 10% to 50% of the population in some Aboriginal communities and that, as a result, whole communities were paralyzed and dysfunctional.

In this chapter I explore how, despite a lack of sound scientific evidence, the dominant Canadian society came to conceive the issue of pregnancy and substance use as predominantly a health and social problem of Aboriginal populations. The politicized discourse of Aboriginal drinking and its association with FAS in the 1980s and 1990s reconfigured the long history of inequality and racism in the lives of Aboriginal communities. Particularly, the construction of FAS as a public health issue unduly stigmatized and blamed impoverished Aboriginal women for elevated rates of mental and social distress unfolding in their communities while simultaneously ignoring historical, social, and environmental factors that could account for the same outcomes. However, while the dangers associated with prenatal alcohol exposure encouraged increased health and social-service surveillance of Aboriginal women, only limited changes were made to improve either front-line support services or addiction-referral, treatment, and aftercare programs for women struggling with substance-abuse problems. Although such an investment would have significantly reduced fetal and maternal risk among the highest risk group of women, government programming was largely directed toward public health education campaigns targeting all pregnant women.

With increased attention in the 1980s to the danger of alcohol and pregnancy came the belief that large numbers of pregnant Aboriginal women across the country were exposing their fetuses to dangerous levels of alcohol and other toxic drugs and that, across generations, prenatal alcohol birth effects were not only common but also represented a major mental health crisis in many Aboriginal communities. Emerging out of this discourse was not only a new image of the "Indian" as someone who could not "recover" or be "healed" but also a medicalized explanation that linked prenatal alcohol exposure with social distress and malaise found in reserve and urban Aboriginal communities.

In the following pages, I explore from several vantage points the links made in popular and scientific discourse between FAS and Aboriginal peoples. However, despite my critique of FAS-related research, interventions, and public health policy, my argument in no way is meant to diminish or dismiss the seriousness of FAS or to deflect attention from its impact on individuals and families. Rather, my aim is to provide a cautionary tale on the potential dangers of claims to certainty where very little certainty exists. History teaches Aboriginal peoples that the naming of our distress by others can have far-reaching and unexpected effects; diagnostic labels and explanations that single out particular causes for complex problems may help to organize an effective response, but they can also be used to justify our individual and collective marginalization and disenfranchisement.

Disruptions in Nature, Disruptions in Society

Treaty Indians receive billions of dollars a year in aid; their food, housing, university, college and medicine is free; they pay no taxes; they can hunt and fish whenever they want to: and they are accorded special treatment by the courts, the schools and employers. Despite all of this largesse – okay, probably because of it – their society is a shambles. Rates of addiction to alcohol, cocaine, gambling, glue are eight to 10 times the norm. Birthrates, encouraged by child welfare benefits, are three times the

non-Indian level and the progeny are typically fathered by several men, usually absent.
A disproportionate number of native children are born with fetal alcohol syndrome, a
condition that predisposes them to not working or to the drug-oriented criminal
world.

– RIC DOPHIN, "NO SIMPLE SOLUTIONS TO NATIVE PROBLEMS,"
CALGARY HERALD, 11 JUNE 2002

Anthropologist Margaret Lock (1997) argues that disruptions of what are assumed to be the "natural" human relations basic to moral order in any given society will undoubtedly create national concern. This concern is certainly evident in situations involving pregnant Aboriginal women who consume alcohol because their use of alcohol is seen to not only "disrupt" the natural responses that a pregnant woman is expected to feel toward her unborn child but also to inscribe on and within the fetal body a lifelong trajectory of physical and social suffering. Persons with FAS are conceptualized as being "made" during pregnancy because the natural life course of the person who will come into being has been irreparably altered (Streissguth 1997; Robinson 1988; Dophin 2002).

Prenatal drinking has come to signify not only a breakdown in the natural relationship between the mother and child but, by extension, also a societal breakdown of significant proportion, whereby children with FAS are described as "society's children" (Buxton 2000). From this point of view, persons with FAS and the mothers who give birth to them are not considered contributing members of the population but are seen to be a significant and preventable financial and social drain on the larger society (Streissguth 1997; Szabo 2000; Wente 2001). Ann Streissguth, a leading North American FAS researcher, writes: "Our children, our families, our schools, and our communities are suffering because of FAS/FAE ... Misunderstood children are dropping out of school and often having babies for whom they can't care. Their parents are unable to cope with their problems, which go beyond the demands of normal parenting ... Communities are uncertain how to respond ... it is essential and urgent that we as a society spend resources to attack this problem" (1997, xxiii).

Similar to children with FAS, Aboriginal peoples have been conceived of as "society's children" within the context of longstanding relationships with European colonizers and the Canadian state. The governing Euro-Canadian view has always held that Aboriginal peoples' "future" is best served under the control and regulation of the dominant society. The relationship between colonialist and neo-colonialist governments and Aboriginal peoples has been characterized by imperialist control and two overlapping constructions of Aboriginal peoples.

The first construction of Aboriginal peoples is as a problem *for* government, manifested in unrest and resistance to colonialist expansion and government policies – specifically, resistance to loss of control over land and resources and loss of collective autonomy through legislation known as the Indian Act. Protest by First Nations, Inuit, and Métis

CAROLINE L. TAIT

groups has generally been viewed as a barrier to assimilation, progress, and modernization within Aboriginal communities. Resistance to government strategies of assimilation, along with calls from Aboriginal groups for justice, apology, and compensation for past assimilation strategies such as the residential school system remain contentious and controversial issues that significantly influence Aboriginal and non-Aboriginal relations. Calls by Aboriginal leaders for negotiations of self-government and settling of land claims generate strong, often emotional, responses from many Canadians who picture reserve and urban Aboriginal communities as "nests of hopelessness" (Dophin 2002) in which social problems such as alcohol abuse, chronic poverty, violence, crime, and FAS are endemic. Within this context, Aboriginal self-determination appears misguided to most Canadians.

The second construction of the "Indian problem" is played out through arguments about appropriate resolutions for various health and social issues that are perceived to be endemic in First Nations, Inuit, and Métis communities. From this perspective, Aboriginal peoples are seen to *have* problems, and it is the moral responsibility or, worse, the moral burden of the dominant society to come up with solutions to address these problems.

From the latter half of the twentieth century, overt discourse about the "civilizing" of the minds and bodies of Aboriginal peoples has increasingly been replaced with the "neutral" language of science and medicine, with a focus on "inferior" health (epitomized by lower life expectancy and higher infectious-disease rates) and social problems, including high rates of teen pregnancies, alcohol abuse, school dropout, and criminal behaviour. Fetal alcohol syndrome is but one example of this transformation in the master narrative of the "Indian problem" from a civilizing discourse to one of identification, prevention, and treatment/intervention.

While health and social problems have drawn the greatest attention in recent decades, economic problems also loom large in this context. However, the dominant society generally views economic problems as *outcomes* of health and social problems rather than regarding them as the source. For example, the chronic poverty experienced by many Aboriginal people is often attributed to social/cultural problems such as defects in the character of individuals and/or Aboriginal belief systems and the inability of Aboriginal peoples to deal with the stressors of civilization and modernization (see Samson, Chapter 5).

Anthropologist John O'Neil points out that, for Aboriginal peoples, there is a contradiction inherent in the increased medicalization of the physical and social embodiment of poverty and inequality – one that has serious implications even in light of ongoing resistance by Aboriginal peoples to dominant representations and understandings of Aboriginal health and social circumstances (O'Neil 1993; O'Neil, Reading, and Leader 1998). He argues that "public health surveillance systems perform disciplinary and regulatory functions in society independent of their overt purpose of tracking health conditions." Therefore, they can construct knowledge about "sectors of society that reinforce unequal power relationships; in other words, an image of sick, disorganized communities can be used to justify paternalism and dependency." O'Neil adds that "external agencies and academics that analyze data also have the power to interpret the data and to construct an image of

Aboriginal communities as desperate, disorganized, and depressed environments. This image is created ostensibly to support lobbying efforts to secure a larger share of national resources for community development. However, this image is reflected through the Canadian media and general public and is to some extent internalized by Aboriginal communities, reinforcing dependency relationships" (1993, 34).

O'Neil and colleagues argue that a discourse on difference in health and social conditions in Aboriginal communities inevitably finds its way into the experience of community members. In some ways, this is quite overt (O'Neil, Reading, and Leader 1998, 231), but in other ways interference in the lives of individuals and communities is subtle. They write, "less obvious perhaps is the way that this discourse has been, and continues to be, used to suppress the legitimate claims of Aboriginal people for full participation in Canadian society. The portrait of a sick, disorganized community implicit in this epidemiological discourse is increasingly dangerous in a tough world of negotiation for self-government and economic development. As justification for continued marginalization and paternalism, the repressive implications of the discourse are apparent" (231).

Indigenizing FAS in the Social Imagination: The "G" Case

> *Drinking in Canada is most common in the northern territories and western provinces and children with alcohol-related birth defects are more frequently seen in these regions. One mother has had seven children with FAS. Tragically, the pattern is more common among the Aboriginal peoples, a lingering reminder of the economic and cultural injustices of the colonial past. We anticipated criticism from some native people to the effect that this conference placed unfair emphasis on native drinking and that the stereotype of Indian drinking patterns was perpetuated ... The fact is, however, that FAS is largely a problem of the native children in British Columbia and there is nothing to be gained by pretending otherwise. Rather we must continue to do everything we can to stop this ecological tragedy.*

> – DR. GEOFFREY C. ROBINSON, "OPENING REMARKS" (1988)

In 1996 the association between Aboriginal women and FAS took on greater significance when Winnipeg Child and Family Services filed two petitions to detain a young First Nations woman who was 5 months pregnant and reportedly regularly sniffing paint thinner, glue, and other substances. Even though the petitions were filed against "Ms. G"[1] because of her solvent abuse, alcohol use by pregnant women and the FAS diagnosis became the central focus of media attention.

The legal debate generated by the case of Ms. G eventually ended up in the Supreme Court of Canada in 1997, where it was widely reported on by media across the country. The implication that substance abuse would critically damage the unborn child challenged existing legal and moral debates over abortion and fetal rights, particularly how the legal system should or should not be used to regulate the actions of pregnant women. Images of Ms. G's "devastatingly thin" pregnant body entered the public imagination, along with knowledge of her "addiction" to glue sniffing and her "overall poor health."[2] But this image bore little resemblance to the everyday woman whose rights to autonomy and bodily integrity were being challenged by the petitions. National media further reported that the 22-year-old had previously given birth to three children, all of whom were in the care of social services and two of whom had been permanently "injured by her glue-sniffing addiction" (Chisholm 1996; Coyne 1997). This information made the argument that her rights should supercede those of her unborn child even less plausible.

Representations of Ms. G, however, did have a certain familiarity for Canadians. Her image signified a notable contrast to the symbolic image of women whose rights are in need of protection. Her abuse of glue, descriptions of her poor health, and the revelations that her three other children were in the care of social services collectively reinforced racial and gendered stereotypes that the behaviour of Aboriginal women was placing a significant burden on government resources. For the dominant society, images of Ms. G validated growing concerns about increasing numbers of young Aboriginal people living in urban ghettos characterized by high fertility rates, high unemployment, widespread substance abuse, and violence. No longer hidden away on reserves or in residential schools, the "Indian problem," as exemplified by Ms. G, was an increasing threat to the dominant society. It was also a threat that served to undermine the arguments of Aboriginal leaders that the federal and provincial governments should cease withholding Aboriginal people's rights to self-determination.

In this contemporary context, the case of Ms. G came to exemplify Aboriginal fetal development as both risky and precarious when left unchecked by medical and legal surveillance. The case also came to represent internal disruptions of "natural" human relations within Aboriginal families and communities. This challenged the moral fabric of Canadian society and called for more state surveillance and control over Aboriginal women. There was growing national attention to the problem of alcohol and pregnancy as well as repeated claims by prominent government officials (Szabo 2000) and members of the medical community that Aboriginal populations were most at risk. Along with this media coverage came widespread acceptance by Aboriginal groups (particularly those living in the northern and western regions of Canada) that alcohol had come to harm their people in yet another way (Fournier and Crey 1997; Royal Commission on Aboriginal Peoples 1996).

Information from Health Canada's First Nations and Inuit Health Branch (FNIHB) was reinforced by the scientific-medical community. This professional consensus encouraged Aboriginal groups to respond quickly to funding opportunities from the federal and provincial/territorial governments, which targeted the "FAS problem" in their communities. While funding for FAS prevention and interventions flowed into Aboriginal communities, almost none of the funding sought to directly improve or expand referral, treatment, or aftercare services for women struggling with alcohol abuse. Rather, governments steered funding toward public health education in the form of posters, pamphlets, and presentation strategies targeting the general population and toward primary prevention aimed at all pregnant women. Further, within local communities, limited knowledge existed about the true extent of the problem: in most circumstances, not a single individual had been diagnosed with FAS. Although neither local nor regional information about the levels and patterns of alcohol use by pregnant women existed, this uncertainty did not bring into question the assumption that the problem was widespread and growing. The FNIHB and the scientific-medical community promoted the idea of a nationwide epidemic in the Aboriginal population despite only a limited body of research characterized by methodological problems, unfounded speculations about Aboriginal drinking, and quasi-scientific conjectures about the effects of prenatal alcohol use (Tait 2003b).

Fetal Alcohol Syndrome

> Experience with the FAS diagnosis remains somewhat circular at this time which is a typical problem in clinical syndromology and hardly unique to FAS. Clinical experts assert that certain patients have fetal alcohol syndrome and the abnormalities found in those patients are then used to refine the diagnosis. A truer case definition will be established only when a reliable biologic marker for alcohol teratogenesis is found or when a diagnostic tool is developed that can demonstrate high sensitivity and specificity in identifying dysmorphic individuals who are exposed in utero to potentially teratogenic doses of alcohol.

> – COMMITTEE TO STUDY FETAL ALCOHOL SYNDROME, THE AMERICAN
> INSTITUTE OF MEDICINE, QUOTED IN K. STRATTON, C. HOWE, AND
> F. BATTAGLIA, EDS., *FETAL ALCOHOL SYNDROME* (1996), 71-72

The introduction of a new diagnostic category brings with it the power to reshape our understandings of individuals and populations. On the surface, medical diagnosis appears to occur in a value-free domain situated apart from the influence of larger historical and sociocultural processes. Moreover, as with any new diagnosis, medical researchers and clinicians are encouraged to set their sights on determining where risk is located and how best to reduce the conditions that create it. The immediate and long-term risks that an illness is believed to pose to individuals and the broader society generally determine the level, type, and urgency of resources directed toward prevention. Strategies developed attempt to reduce the conditions that produce risk and to manage the needs of patient populations. In some cases, new illnesses take on an added moral dimension, most notably those that are believed to be preventable or better managed through changes in individual behaviour and lifestyle, such as the case of alcohol use by pregnant women (Armstrong 2003).

American researchers Kenneth L. Jones and David W. Smith (1973) first described fetal alcohol syndrome in the scientific literature in 1973.[3] The hallmark features of FAS are a characteristic set of facial features, evidence of growth deficiency, evidence of structural or organic brain dysfunction, and confirmed maternal alcohol exposure. Of these anomalies, the "facial gestalt" is thought to be clinically unique, and damage to the central nervous system (CNS) is considered the most significant abnormality (Stratton, Howe, and Battaglia 1996, 71). Because none of the diagnostic characteristics are unique to FAS, clinicians have found it difficult to apply diagnostic criteria to patients, resulting in diagnostic inconsistencies across clinical contexts (Abel 1998).

A number of fundamental questions framed early FAS-related research; however, more than 30 years after the introduction of the diagnosis, researchers still lack evidence that would enable them conclusively to answer key questions related to alcohol and pregnancy. For example, although it is well acknowledged that alcohol is teratogenic, the threshold at which maternal alcohol consumption becomes dangerous to the developing fetus and the specific mechanisms through which this occurs are unknown. Controversy remains over the relationship between dose, timing, and patterns of exposure in producing prenatal effects, as well as over whether alcohol is both necessary *and* sufficient to cause the syndrome (Abel 1998).

A central problem in FAS research is that it is difficult to confirm causal links between prenatal alcohol exposure and certain anomalies, particularly cognitive and behavioural problems found in alcohol-exposed offspring. However, despite this uncertainty, the research literature strongly associates FAS with chronic maternal alcohol abuse, higher maternal age and lower education levels, prenatal exposure to cocaine and tobacco, custody changes, lower socioeconomic status, paternal drinking and drug use at the time of pregnancy, reduced access to prenatal and postnatal care and services, inadequate nutrition, and a poor developmental environment (i.e., one characterized by stress, abuse, and neglect) (Chudley et al. 2005; Abel 1998; Abel and Hannigan 1995; Armstrong 2003; Astley et al. 2000). That alcohol alone is not sufficient to cause FAS is further suggested by the observation that anywhere from 4.7% to 21% of the babies born to women who drink heavily during pregnancy have FAS (Armstrong 2003, 4; Grant et al. 2005).

Fetal alcohol syndrome research faces a number of barriers that prevent accurate diagnostic assessment, particularly in patients who do not exhibit the full-blown syndrome.[4] These include the difficulties of differential diagnosis, the lack of standardized measurements and tools that can be readily applied in clinical assessments, an insufficient number of physicians trained in FAS diagnostic assessment, and financial and logistical constraints in assembling the multidisciplinary teams necessary to make accurate diagnoses (Abel 1998; Tait 2003a, 2003b). Ernest Abel, a leading American FAS researcher, directly associates diagnostic challenges with a mistaken impression that minimal amounts of in-utero alcohol exposure can cause individual birth anomalies. He writes: "The simple fact is that the term fetal alcohol syndrome has created such a false impression that large numbers of clinicians now believe even minimal amounts of alcohol consumption during pregnancy can produce the syndrome. Because no cases of this syndrome have ever been found outside of the context of alcohol abuse, renaming it fetal alcohol abuse syndrome should, at the very least, preclude glib diagnosis ... More importantly, it should also keep many children from being misdiagnosed and receiving treatment, if any, for a condition they do not have" (1998, 8).

As a result of the uncertainties, controversy, and logistical challenges that characterize fetal alcohol spectrum disorder (FASD) diagnosis, very few individuals in Canada are systematically assessed. Instead, most individuals who are identified as being alcohol-affected lack a clinical diagnosis but have been labelled through other means (e.g., by nonmedical professionals such as teachers, social workers, front-line addiction workers, and judges or through screening associated with front-line programming or incarceration)[5] (Tait 2003b).

Despite the uncertainty that surrounds the diagnostic spectrum, FASD has not resulted in cautious statements about the unknown magnitude of the problem in Aboriginal populations, as might be expected to arise around such a sensitive issue. This is a rather unique situation, one in which diagnostic and research challenges to documenting the incidence and prevalence rates of alcohol-related birth effects are thought to be masking the true extent of the problem. In turn, labelling impoverished Aboriginal individuals in crisis – children, adolescents, and adults – with FAS or FAE has become common practice. In western and northern regions in particular, nonmedical professionals have increasingly adopted the category of FASD to describe, label, and manage the misfortune of impoverished Aboriginal people.

Labelling non-Aboriginal people with FAS or FAE does not happen to any significant degree, with the exception of children born to impoverished women who are alcohol abusers. Despite government figures showing that fewer Aboriginal women (60.6%)[6] than non-Aboriginal women (67%)[7] choose to drink alcohol, the drinking behaviours of Aboriginal women, as well as the behavioural problems exhibited by Aboriginal youth and adults, have come under significantly greater scrutiny by the human-service sector – education, health, social welfare, justice – in relation to FASD.

Perceptions of Prenatal Alcohol Exposure and Aboriginal Drinking

> *FAS is implicated in most adoptions that go bad. Virtually every native child adopted over the past 20 years has some degree of alcohol damage. It is that, and not the pain of alienation from white society, that accounts for their frequent estrangement from their adoptive families and their terrible problems in life. The failure of cross-cultural adoptions is one of the most tragically misunderstood stories of recent years. It has wreaked havoc in some of Canada's most prominent families ... And yet adoptive families everywhere are still being told their children were ruined by a cultural identity crisis.*
>
> – MARGARET WENTE, "OUR POOR RUINED BABIES: THE HIDDEN
> EPIDEMIC," *GLOBE AND MAIL,* 7 OCTOBER 2000

CAROLINE L. TAIT

The significant attention given to FAS in both Canada and the United States has been provoked by public health messages warning pregnant women to abstain from all alcohol use. Because researchers have not determined the threshold at which maternal alcohol becomes dangerous to the fetus, this public health message counsels pregnant women to err on the side of caution. In effect, this message marks a shift away from broader understandings of FAS as a problem of alcohol abuse and toward a more pervasive concern with preventing the potential risk to every pregnant woman who drinks alcohol. This reconfiguration of risk to include any amount of alcohol implies that the prevalence of alcohol-related birth defects is much higher than recognized and supports the growing assumption that current rates of FASD reflect only the tip of the iceberg of a much larger problem (Tait 2003b).

From the initial stages of FAS research, evidence strongly suggested that alcohol use alone was insufficient cause for the observed birth anomalies (Abel 1998; Armstrong 2003; Armstrong and Abel 2000); however, American researchers in the 1970s and 1980s singled out alcohol as both necessary and sufficient to cause the spectrum of birth effects associated with the condition (Clarren 1981; Clarren, Astley, and Bowden 1988; Clarren and Smith 1978; Streissguth 1977). And this perspective has continued to dominate research (Astley and Clarren 1999; Boland, Duwyn, and Serin 2000; Streissguth 1997) and reports on the topic (BC FAS Resource Society 1998; Boland et al. 1998; McCuen 1994; Szabo 2000). Sociologist Elizabeth Armstrong points out that, "even today, despite the emphasis on evidence-based medicine, dubious medical findings [in FAS research] may be speedily and widely accepted within the medical community." It is difficult, she adds, "to extirpate such medical 'knowledge' once it has taken hold. In addition, the bias toward positive results in the scientific literature is exacerbated when there is an overt moral dimension to the research question at hand, as in the case of substance use in pregnancy" (2003, 82-83).

Growing awareness in the early 1970s about female alcoholism coincided in Canada and the United States with the introduction of FAS diagnosis. Canadian researchers and providers of health care service generally took a less alarmist position on both issues than did their American counterparts (Tait 2003b), but the more benign view of alcohol use did not extend to their understandings of alcohol use by Aboriginal women.

Anthropologist James Waldram observes that, in the area of Aboriginal mental health, no other topic has "dominated the research and discourse as much as alcohol, and none has generated such a combination of perverse curiosity, genuine concern, and outright absurdity, not to mention racism" (2004, 134). Waldram points out that, from the early contact period onward in North America, Aboriginal drinking patterns were constructed as homogeneous in nature while simultaneously being portrayed as "wildly different" from non-Aboriginal norms (136). This portrait led to several theories that posited a biological susceptibility of North American Aboriginal peoples to alcohol abuse. Waldram writes: "It has been suggested that the belief that Aboriginal peoples metabolize alcohol differently, and that this explains how they drink, why they drink, and the problems that drinking causes, has led to the 'myth of the drunken Indian' ... or 'firewater myths' ... The pervasiveness of the biological explanation is impressive; not only do many non-Aboriginal North Americans believe in it, but it has been argued that many Aboriginal peoples have bought into the explanation as well" (2004, 135).

Waldram adds that researchers concentrating on single Aboriginal communities have been attracted to the exoticism of the "drinking party," thus reinforcing the "myth of the drunken Indian" engaging in "raucous bouts of binge drinking lasting days." This myth, Waldram concludes, reinforces the perception that Aboriginal people not only drink differently but somehow also react to alcohol in a manner biologically different from their non-Aboriginal counterparts, thus supporting arguments that Aboriginal persons have different outcomes in response to alcohol use (2004, 136).

Waldram's argument helps us to understand contemporary perceptions of FAS and Aboriginal women. Two intersecting factors – the single-minded focus on alcohol as the sole cause of observed effects (Armstrong 2003) and mainstream perceptions of Aboriginal drinking patterns – led Canadian FAS researchers, government health ministries, and the human-service sector to focus their attention on the drinking behaviours of Aboriginal women. By the mid-1990s, FAS-prevention activities were dominated by an assumption that alcohol abuse by pregnant women was common across Aboriginal communities. Fuelling this perception were studies of FAS that not only portrayed the alcohol-drinking patterns of First Nations, Inuit, and Métis women as relatively homogeneous across community and regional divides but also portrayed binge drinking, a pattern of drinking found to be especially dangerous to the fetus, as typical Aboriginal drinking behaviour. For example, K.O. Asante, a physician working in northern British Columbia, argued in 1981 that First Nations and Métis women in northern British Columbia and Yukon engaged in binge drinking more frequently than non-Aboriginal women, behaviour that he claimed was "a common part of the northern lifestyle" (1981, 335). The same year, American researcher Jon Aase (1981) argued that "cultural attitudes towards drinking" meant that American Indian women living on reservations in the south-western United States were more likely to engage in binge drinking patterns of alcohol use than any other group of American women. In both instances, the authors provided limited or no research data to confirm that binge drinking was a common practice among Aboriginal women. Nor did they specify whether the communities under study exhibited a higher incidence of binge drinking compared to the general population or indicate to what *degree* the communities participated in binge drinking, if indeed they did.

In contrast, the Aboriginal Peoples Survey (Statistics Canada 1993), which questioned Aboriginal people about their consumption of alcohol, found that a lower proportion of Aboriginal than non-Aboriginal Canadians drink daily (2% Aboriginal versus 3% other Canadians) or weekly (35% Aboriginal versus 46% other Canadians). Abstinence was also reported to be twice as common among Aboriginal people (15% Aboriginal versus 8% other Canadians). Similar results, in which abstinence was more common among Aboriginal people, were found in self-report surveys in the Yukon (Yukon Government 1991) and in Cree communities in northern Quebec (Santé Québec 1994). However, the latter two studies found that of people who reported alcohol use, heavy drinking was more common than moderate consumption. This suggests the value of targeting this subgroup of women to determine their patterns of alcohol use when pregnant and, at a minimum, the creation of services to support women in accessing and completing substance-abuse treatment and aftercare programs.

In the arena of public health and pregnancy outreach, Aboriginal women were not only singled out as a high-risk group but were also simultaneously portrayed as representing the main locus of risk in Canada for FAS. Some researchers suggested that Aboriginal belief systems reinforced high-risk drinking patterns (e.g., Asante 1981; Robinson, Conry, and Conry 1987). True to broader arguments about Aboriginal drinking, researchers also described risks for FAS in North American Aboriginal populations as fundamentally different from the risk for other populations. A statement made by Jon Aase illustrates this point of view: "The American Indian population possesses several unusual cultural, social and possibly environmental and biological traits which may work together to increase the risk for FAS in this group. If studies now underway substantiate the increased incidence suggested by anecdotal reports, we will be presented with a situation resembling the Hopi Kachina doll which has two faces: on the one side, a public health problem of massive proportion to be dealt with, on the other, new insights about the causation and possible prevention of this devastating congenital disorder" (1981, 155).

As concern over the risk of alcohol use during pregnancy grew in the 1990s, two further assumptions arose: first, that a unidirectional link could be made between the colonization of Aboriginal peoples and present-day rates of FAS; and second, that many of the Aboriginal women believed to be at risk for giving birth to a child with FAS were themselves alcohol-affected (e.g., Children's Commission of BC 2001, 24).

In the broader context of Aboriginal health care, the 1990s was a period when Aboriginal peoples and the human-service sector invoked the Indian residential school system as a primary source of contemporary mental health problems and social suffering found in Aboriginal populations. This attention to the impact of residential schools was quickly incorporated into discussions of alcohol, pregnancy, and FAS. For example, in an interview with journalist David Square, Jack Armstrong, former president of the Canadian Medical Association, stated: "The white population cannot point smugly at Aboriginals and claim fetal alcohol syndrome is just a native problem. For one thing, we [Europeans] helped to create the problem by refusing to acknowledge Aboriginal culture and by sending Indian children to residential schools. People with low self-esteem often turn to alcohol for consolation" (quoted in Square 1997, 60).

This type of argument helped to forge a unidirectional link between the experience of residential school students and the "problem" of FAS through the use of phrases such as "low self-esteem" and "self-medication." Armstrong's statement suggested that the task of physicians, as well as that of government and other health and social-service providers, was to treat the consequences of past oppression as located within the individual and collective bodies and minds of Aboriginal peoples.

In "postcolonial" Canada, federal, provincial, and territorial governments assume the role of altruistic caregivers who, being more "enlightened," set themselves apart from their colonizing predecessors. Oppression of Aboriginal peoples is located in the past, and the intergenerational effects of colonization are relabelled as "treatable conditions," like FAS, low self-esteem, and alcohol abuse – conditions that mainstream health and social services are poised to address in their efforts to improve the lives of Aboriginal peoples. Various sources of mental distress – endemic poverty; racism; food, water, and housing insecurities; social and economic marginalization – are put aside for explanations of individual pathology and calls for individualized interventions.

By 2000 prenatal alcohol exposure was increasingly identified as a widespread threat to the health of unborn Aboriginal children, and claims were also being made that elevated rates of FASD were having a negative societal impact by creating and sustaining social problems in Aboriginal communities. Media images of urban and reserve Aboriginal communities plagued by alcoholic-affected adolescents and adults with "little or no ability to comprehend the difference between right and wrong" became commonplace (e.g., Dophin 2002; Wente 2001). Many sources speculated that alcohol-related birth effects (ARBE) were causally linked to elevated rates of school dropout, unemployment, poverty, substance abuse, mental health problems, suicide, teen pregnancy, homelessness, incarceration, and recidivism in Aboriginal populations (e.g., Barnett 1997; Boland et al. 1998; Boland et al. 2000; Roberts 1998, A3; Szabo 2000).

More important, while FAS was evolving into a catchall category for Aboriginal distress, the same association did not occur in relation to other populations, despite knowledge that actual cases of prenatal alcohol exposure were higher among non-Aboriginal women.[8] Unlike in the United States, where a "moral panic" ensued around all pregnant women and any amount of alcohol use (Armstrong 2003), in Canada attention fixated on Aboriginal women, fuelling an invented epidemic that was believed to span geographical and generational divides (Tait 2003b).

Creating an Epidemic of Fetal Alcohol Syndrome

> *A recent study on a First Nations Reserve in Manitoba indicates that 1 in 10 children is the victim of alcohol teratogenesis. And that, says a researcher involved in a seminal investigation of fetal alcohol syndrome (FAS) and possible fetal alcohol effects (FAE) in Canada's Aboriginal population, is just the tip of the iceberg.*[9]
>
> – DAVID SQUARE, "FETAL ALCOHOL SYNDROME EPIDEMIC ON
> MANITOBA RESERVE" (1997), 59-60

Following the introduction of FAS as a diagnostic category in 1973, Canadian researchers specifically targeted Aboriginal communities to examine rates of FAS prevalence. The characteristics of certain reserve communities made them perfect sites for this type of research (e.g., alcohol abuse was known to be high, suggesting that rates of detection would be elevated; a defined population based on a band membership who share similar genetics and socioeconomic and cultural characteristics; potential for control groups to determine local standards for comparative use in diagnostic assessment; and access to patient medical charts and records). This narrowing of focus quickly led to an overrepresentation of Aboriginal people in cohort- and population-based studies completed in Canada and helped to solidify the perception that the problem of alcohol and pregnancy and FAS was widespread among Aboriginal women and their children.

However, in dealing with the information obtained from studies with Aboriginal peoples, American and Canadian researchers and governments took very different directions. In the United States, researchers looked beyond Native American communities in attempts to "democratize" the risks associated with alcohol and pregnancy. Armstrong and Abel point out that American researchers argued that, regardless of ethnic, "racial," and socioeconomic group, pregnant women who drank alcohol were equally at risk for giving birth to children with FAS (Armstrong 2003; Armstrong and Abel 2000). Although Native American women remained overrepresented in FAS-related research, so too were African American and Hispanic women, supporting claims that ethnicity or "race" was not a determining factor in producing the illness (Abel 1998).

Even though early Canadian studies were limited in scope and methodology (Tait 2003a, 2003b), these limitations did not prevent researchers from taking an alarmist position and interpreting their data as representative of *all* Aboriginal communities. This perception has had far-reaching consequences, most specifically to redefine and narrow the cause of behavioural problems found in Aboriginal children, adolescents, and those who come into contact with the criminal justice system. It has also shifted focus away from other known risks to fetal development. For instance, despite sound evidence linking environmental toxins and contaminants to uranium and other forms of mining, despite further evidence linking birth defects to mercury and lead exposure, and despite Aboriginal groups living in some of the most exposed and polluted environments in Canada, these causal links are rarely ever mentioned in relation to Aboriginal pregnant women and fetal development.

By contrast, the dangers associated with alcohol and pregnancy appear to have raised only limited concern within broader Canadian society. For example, virtually no attention has been given by researchers to determining national and regional prevalence and incidence rates of prenatal alcohol exposure or FAS.[10] Arguments, such as those found for Aboriginal groups, suggesting that FAS could contribute to increased social problems like crime are absent from research, policy, and media arenas. In a manner similar to other public health messages targeting pregnant women, warnings about the dangers of alcohol use during pregnancy have been incorporated into general prenatal care and broad-based public health campaigns, whereas, as stated previously, only limited improvements have been made to referral, treatment, and aftercare services for pregnant women struggling with alcohol abuse.

By the late 1980s, North American Aboriginal peoples, specifically those living in north-western Canada, were clearly identified in the FAS literature as "high-risk" populations. In 1989 Bray and Anderson conducted an appraisal of the epidemiological research on FAS involving Canadian Aboriginal populations, raising several questions about detection bias and the overrepresentation of Aboriginal peoples in the research literature. They began by asking two questions: "Is it merely coincidental that Indians are [over]represented in various case studies or is there reason to believe that Native children suffer an increased prevalence of FAS? *Is there epidemiological evidence that suggests FAS occurs more frequently in Native populations?*" (Bray and Anderson 1989, 42, original emphasis). Bray and Anderson also expressed concern about the difficulties that researchers face when applying a standard diagnostic criterion for FAS to Aboriginal groups: "Since anthropomorphic features of Indian children generally differ from Caucasian children, the use of facial characteristics as a diagnostic criteria is questionable. Educational assessment across cultures, especially the use of IQ tests in the evaluation of CNS dysfunction as a criterion, requires special attention" (44).

In their appraisal, Bray and Anderson pointed to the lack of published research in Canada on the prevalence of FAS in non-Aboriginal populations. They argued that the absence of this research made it difficult, if not impossible, to make valid comparisons of prevalence rates for Aboriginal and non-Aboriginal populations or to draw inferences regarding high prevalence rates (1989, 44). This shortcoming in the research literature has persisted, in part because Canadian researchers continue to focus on either Aboriginal communities or geographical areas with large concentrations of Aboriginal people (e.g., Godel et al. 1992; Williams and Gloster 1999).

At the time of Bray and Anderson's publication, only two studies estimating overall prevalence rates of FAS in Canada existed. Both studies involved subpopulations of Aboriginal people living in the West Coast region of Canada and were therefore representative of neither the general Canadian population nor Aboriginal Canadian populations (Bray and Anderson 1989, 44). Despite this limited sample, the high prevalence rates of FAS/FAE estimated for the studies' target populations – 25:1,000 (northwest British Columbia) and 46:1,000 (Yukon) in the study by Asante and Nelms-Matzke (1985), and 190:1,000 (northern British Columbia) in the study by Robinson and colleagues (1987) – continue to be interpreted as representative of prevalence rates for the *general* Aboriginal population. In discussing the studies' findings, Bray and Anderson cautioned: "The investigations themselves may lack methodological sophistication and therefore warrant scientific conservatism in accepting the prevalence rates prima facie ... Native peoples should not be stigmatized by a condition such as FAS which is difficult to prove as factual and which may have a negative impact within the Native community. Caution is warranted before we conclude that FAS is more prevalent in any Native peoples" (1989, 44).

Although governments claimed to base their funding and program-development strategies on arguments made in early FAS studies, they ignored Bray and Anderson's notable critique of the studies' research methods and conclusions. Even the increasing government emphasis on "evidence-based medicine" to inform policies and programming, which in this case should have directed policymakers to focus more narrowly on alcoholic women and their children, had no impact on the direction of government policy and funding. Instead, the methodological shortcomings, inconclusiveness, and lack of evidence found in general within the FAS literature was overlooked and replaced with the argument that an epidemic of FAS was unfolding in Aboriginal populations across the country. However, despite the alarmist position taken by various levels of government, funding allocated for FAS-related prevention and intervention programming was minimal compared to the presumed scope of the problem.

"Secondary Disabilities" and Aboriginal Peoples

> *Mr. Linden issued a warning about the growing number of crimes in which the accused suffers from fetal alcohol syndrome – a physical brain disorder caused by mother's ingestion of alcohol during pregnancy. He predicted an entire generation of FAS youths are about to enter the criminal justice system – youngsters with little or no ability to comprehend the difference between right and wrong. These youngsters have little hope of rehabilitation, experts have said. About 79 per cent of inmates in Manitoba's prison system are native, as are 45 per cent of federal prisoners in Manitoba. Prison officials suggest at least half of these native inmates suffer from FAS or less severe fetal alcohol effects.*
>
> – D. ROBERTS, "NATIVE MURDER RATE IN MANITOBA ALARMING,
STUDY SHOWS," GLOBE AND MAIL, 2 NOVEMBER 1998

In the late 1990s signs of prenatal alcohol-related pathology, specifically dysfunctional behaviour, were closely associated with "secondary disabilities" in Aboriginal adolescents and adults (Conry and Fast 2000; Fast, Conry, and Loock 1999). Secondary disabilities are believed to arise from the interaction between primary disabilities, especially neuro-developmental anomalies, and negative environmental influences. Characteristics include mental health problems, disrupted school experience (e.g., suspension, expulsion, early departure), trouble with the law, confinement (e.g., incarceration, in-patient treatment for mental health and addiction problems), inappropriate sexual behaviour, and alcohol/drug problems (Streissguth et al. 1997, 34). Risk factors that magnify the severity of primary disabilities in alcohol-affected persons include living in an unstable home environment, multiple foster placements, child abuse/neglect, late diagnosis (after 6 years of age), and absence of special health, social, and educational services (Streissguth et al. 1997).

Critiques that point to the limitations of the small body of research examining the occurrence of secondary disabilities in patients have generally been ignored. Instead, the argument that FAS is a root cause of a range of interrelated social problems in Aboriginal communities has emerged as both compelling and convincing in the arenas of research and the human-service sector (Tait 2003a, 2003b). Furthermore, the occurrence of secondary disabilities is portrayed as especially elevated in persons who have not been medically assessed – the majority of people assumed to have FAS – and who are therefore unable to access support services (Streissguth et al. 1997). When a direct causal link between prenatal alcohol exposure and secondary disabilities is taken at face value and when this link is coupled with assumed prevalence rates of FASD ranging from 1% in the general population to 10% in some Aboriginal populations, alcohol-related birth effects are perceived to reach far beyond the lives of affected individuals and to be responsible for certain manifestations of social disruption and disharmony.

In this context a tautological argument suggests that the presence of considerable social distress in urban Aboriginal and reserve communities is evidence of high prevalence rates of FASD. In turn, claims that FASD is common among Aboriginal adolescent and adult populations are used to account for the same set of social problems. However, the myriad social and environmental factors that influence both individual and collective experience and behaviour are, for the most part, ignored or increasingly rescripted as secondary disabilities.

The collapsing of the concepts of "culture," "poverty," and "pathology" into a single collective identity that is inscribed upon Aboriginal peoples weaves its way through this argument and is illustrated in a statement made by Ann Streissguth in her book *Fetal alcohol syndrome: A guide for families and communities*. She states: "On some Indian reservations, where alcohol abuse is common among women, FAS has been reported in 1 in 100 children ... In one small Native American [Canadian] community, the incidence of FAS was 1 in 8 ... At that frequency, FAS is a community catastrophe that threatens to wipe out any culture in just a few generations. However, FAS is not a Native problem or a problem of poverty per se. It is an *alcohol* problem, and it is *our* problem" (1997, 8-9, original emphasis). In Streissguth's vision, whole communities are at risk of being transformed into a postcultural state characterized by widespread pathology and marked especially by a loss of what distinguishes human beings, namely culture. Replacing moral values, social structures, and institutions that are inherent to any group's culture is a "community catastrophe" that manifests itself as individual brain dysfunction and collective malaise, as an inability to self-govern, and as an internal perpetuation of both abject poverty and the social problems that accompany this level of despair.

Arguments such as this embody a tone of certainty, urgency, and a dangerous logic that effectively masks underlying prejudices about Aboriginal peoples. For example, according to Streissguth's argument, when the prevalence rate of FASD reaches a certain threshold, the group is no longer able to sustain its belief system and cultural identity. As a result, the social body enters a perpetual state of pathology with "catastrophic" consequences for the group. Furthermore, this transformation to a postcultural state is conceived as placing a significant social and economic burden on the broader society as a "FAS community" becomes incapable of contributing positively to its own or the collective good.

CAROLINE L. TAIT

This incapacity, the argument runs, morally justifies increased intervention and surveillance from the outside world.

By linking FASD with social disharmony and arguing that "FAS is not a Native problem or a problem of poverty per se" but an "alcohol problem" that burdens the larger society, Streissguth and others (e.g., Asante 1981; Dophin 2002; Robinson 1988; Square 1997; Wente 2001) seek to accomplish four things: (1) to reconfigure the source of problems experienced by Aboriginal populations as grounded in biology and caused by a single etiology – alcohol consumption by pregnant women; (2) effectively to marginalize the importance of historical processes of colonization, especially family and community disruption, in the form of residential schooling, foster care, land appropriation, and disease epidemics; (3) to marginalize the role of present-day challenges faced by many Aboriginal families and communities, such as daily acts of racism directed toward Aboriginal peoples, the difficulties of living in abject poverty, and, in many cases, daily environmental toxin and contamination exposure; and (4) to reconfigure FAS from a health issue that affects a segment of the population to a societal issue that involves all members of the community and provides a morally justifiable entry point into the collective life of Aboriginal communities that supercedes consideration of Aboriginal autonomy and identity.

Conclusion

> *Jason isn't sure how prevalent FAS/E is in the community, since no detailed formal studies have been done, but it's safe to say it's significant. A lot of the kids he works with have not been diagnosed, and many don't seek out diagnosis, although CHIP does make referrals for FAS diagnostic assessments. However, CHIP staff can see the patterns with clients in the community. Sometimes the birth mother shares that she consumed alcohol during her pregnancy. Because CHIP is community-based, the workers may also know or hear through the grapevine that a mother drank during pregnancy. They also know that if a child was adopted there's also a good chance that alcohol was involved.*

> – D. ANDERSON AND J. WEMIGWANS, "HEALING WITH A DEEP HEART" (2002), 8

In a sociopolitical climate in which Aboriginal groups regularly invoke health as a political issue, it is surprising that the wholesale promotion of the FAS diagnosis has gone largely unchallenged. The portrayal of Aboriginal people in Canada as suffering disproportionately from a chronic disabling brain dysfunction has failed to generate concern that they may be unduly targeted or stigmatized. In fact, because of its place within medical nomenclature and the history of Aboriginal peoples and alcohol, FAS largely exists as an uncontested label (e.g., Anderson and Wemigwans 2002; Fournier and Crey 1997). For example, the Assembly of First Nations, a political umbrella organization, identifies FAS as a health priority among their constituents, the *Report of the Royal Commission on Aboriginal Peoples* describes FAS as a "serious problem" (Royal Commission on Aboriginal Peoples 1996),[11] and FAS was one of three priorities in a recent call from the Institute of Aboriginal Peoples' Health for research proposals.[12]

As a theory that focuses on a single causal factor for complex mental health problems yet simultaneously furnishes an explanation for profound disparities in the health and social status of Aboriginal populations, FAS may be compelling and convincing for many both because it has the authority of medical science and because it deflects attention from other historical and social structural problems in the relationship of Aboriginal peoples to the dominant society. For similar reasons, this explanation may also appeal to many Aboriginal people who struggle to understand and cope with the realities that they see and experience in their communities. For Aboriginal people, it is not surprising that alcohol has once again negatively impacted their communities, so FAS has been added to a litany of alcohol-related problems that they associate more broadly with colonization, marginalization, and oppression (e.g., Royal Commission on Aboriginal Peoples 1995; Tait 2003a). As the spectrum of alcohol-related birth effects is assumed to account for broad-based individual and collective distress and to be preventable simply by having pregnant women abstain from alcohol use, it offers hope for a better future within a single generation and suggests at least a partial solution to the enormous problems faced by many Aboriginal communities.

The solution, however, may not be so straightforward. In her arguments for effective interventions, Streissguth (1997) suggests a shift in the focus of prevention and treatment services for FAS and prenatal and family support from the "person with FAS" to the "FAS community." While a community-based approach is laudable when the situation calls for it, labelling a whole community "FAS" may confer an enduring stigma and undermine ongoing efforts to achieve greater autonomy and collective well-being. Broader goals of community development and control, including calls for self-determination, risk falling prey to the assumption that the individual, social, and political bodies that make up the community are collectively and chronically damaged.

Alarmist arguments that characterize Aboriginal communities as dysfunctional and pathologic ignore the historical resilience and resistance of Aboriginal peoples in the face of adversity brought on by European colonization, including the many individuals and communities that have rejected alcohol use altogether. An unfortunate and tragic side effect is that a growing number of Aboriginal people and communities have internalized the FAS explanation as a way to make sense of their misfortune and suffering (Anderson and Wemigwans 2002). Furthermore, because all prenatal alcohol exposure is viewed as potentially causing brain damage, the needs and circumstances of those Aboriginal and non-Aboriginal women in Canada most at risk for giving birth to a child with prenatal alcohol-related birth defects – those who are alcoholic – get lost in a racially focused discourse of epidemics and widespread risk and pathology. Increased awareness of the social and political implications of FAS discourse on Canada's ideology of Aboriginal women, pregnancy, and alcohol use is absolutely necessary to the creation of meaningful and effective support and treatment services that respond to FAS as a complex interaction of physiological and environmental factors with prenatal alcohol abuse, not as a predetermined characteristic of Canadian Aboriginal cultures and communities.

Notes

This chapter is based on research conducted in the 1990s as part of my doctoral project. At the time I was also involved in government working groups, research meetings, and conferences focused on the issue of FAS, and I was doing research on FAS for the Aboriginal Healing Foundation and Manitoba Health.

1 The woman's name was not used during the court case in efforts to protect the identity of her children.

2 Inhalants or solvents as substances of choice are very difficult for most Canadians to imagine using, even those with addiction problems. The positioning by the Winnipeg Child Welfare Agency of Ms. G as so distinctly "other" made it easier for the general public to feel outrage about her behaviour and to consider punitive sanctions against her than if she had been a pregnant, middle-class Caucasian woman who was abusing alcohol.

3 Lemoine and colleagues (1968) were first to publish on birth defects and developmental disabilities in offspring born to alcoholic parents.

4 New classifications, such as fetal alcohol effects (FAE) and alcohol-related birth defects (ARBDs), were adopted in the 1970s and 1980s to describe the presence of alcohol effects in the absence of the full-blown syndrome. These categories generated significant controversy because of their lack of specificity, making it even more difficult to apply them consistently across clinical settings than to apply a diagnosis of FAS. Although FAE is a commonly used label, it is not officially recognized as a medical diagnosis. Different diagnostic nomenclatures have been developed (Chudley et al. 2005), but consensus does not exist as to a "gold standard." In recent years "fetal alcohol spectrum disorder" (FASD), which is not a medical diagnosis but a term used to describe the full spectrum of alcohol-related birth defects, has become a widely used term.

5 Screening tools for alcohol-related birth effects are being developed in various clinical and research settings, but standardization of these tools has not yet occurred (Chudley et al. 2005). In many cases, particularly in prison populations or front-line service delivery, a person will screen positive but because of the inaccessibly of medical diagnosis, further assessment does not occur. High rates of false positive are likely with these tools, which can result in perceptions that the prevalence rates in certain populations are extremely high.

6 Statistics Canada (1993).

7 Poole (1997, 5); see also Addiction Research Foundation of Ontario (1996).

8 Comparative figures of prenatal alcohol exposure between Aboriginal and non-Aboriginal women do not exist. The Canadian Centre on Substance Abuse reports that 14.4% of pregnant Canadian women drank at some point during their pregnancy.

9 The study was never published in a scientific peer-reviewed journal or elsewhere. However, Square's reference to prevalence rates that were reported to him as a journalist are quoted in other peer-reviewed publications as though the study were peer-reviewed and published (see for example, Chudley et al. 2005).

10 Canadian incidence and prevalence rates for the general population are still drawn from American studies. Only a handful of Canadian studies completed in the 1980s and 1990s, all involving small populations, exist. In these studies all, or the large majority, of the population is Aboriginal (Chudley et al. 2005, S1).

11 See http://www.ainc-inac.gc.ca/ch/rcap/sg/si13_e.html#1.2%20Physical%20Health.

12 The Institute of Aboriginal Peoples' Health is 1 of 13 Canadian Institutes for Health Research. It draws on the expertise of Aboriginal researchers and health experts to set annual research priorities.

References

Aase, J.M. 1981. The fetal alcohol syndrome in American Indians: A high risk group. *Neurobehavioral Toxicology and Teratology* 3 (2): 153-56.

Abel, E.L. 1998. *Fetal alcohol abuse syndrome*. New York: Plenum.

–, and J.H. Hannigan. 1995. Maternal risk factors in fetal alcohol syndrome: Provocative and permissive influences. *Neurotoxicology and Teratology* 17 (4): 445-62.

Addiction Research Foundation of Ontario. 1996. *The hidden majority: A guidebook on alcohol and other drug issues for counselors who work with women*. Toronto: Addiction Research Foundation of Ontario.

Anderson, D., and J. Wemigwans. 2002. Healing with a deep heart: A community-based approach to living with FAS/E. *Aboriginal approaches to fetal alcohol syndrome/effects*. Toronto, ON: Ontario Federation of Friendship Centres.

Armstrong, E.M. 2003. *Conceiving risk, bearing responsibility: Fetal alcohol syndrome and the diagnosis of moral disorder*. Baltimore, MD: Johns Hopkins University Press.

–, and E.L. Abel. 2000. Fetal alcohol syndrome: The origins of a moral panic. *Alcohol and Alcoholism* 35 (3): 276-82.

Asante, K.O. 1981. FAS in northwest BC and the Yukon. *British Columbia Medical Journal* 23 (7): 331-35.

–, and J. Nelms-Matzke. 1985. *Survey of children with chronic handicaps and fetal alcohol syndrome in Yukon and British Columbia*. Ottawa, ON: National Native Advisory Council on Alcohol and Drug Abuse, Health and Welfare Canada.

Astley, S.J., and S.K. Clarren. 1999. *Diagnostic guide for fetal alcohol syndrome (FAS) and related conditions: The 4-digit diagnostic code*. 2nd ed. Seattle, WA: University of Washington Press.

–, D. Bailey, C. Talbot, and S.K. Clarren. 2000. Fetal alcohol syndrome (FAS) primary prevention through FAS diagnosis, part 2, A comprehensive profile of 80 birth mothers of children with FAS. *Alcohol and Alcoholism* 35 (5): 509-19.

Barnett, C.C. 1997. A judicial perspective on FAS: Memories of the making of *Nanook of the North*. In A.P. Streissguth and J. Kanter, eds., *The challenge of fetal alcohol syndrome: Overcoming secondary disabilities*, 134-45. Seattle, WA: University of Washington Press.

BC FAS Resource Society. 1998. *Community action guide: Working together for the prevention of fetal alcohol syndrome*. Victoria, BC: British Columbia Ministry for Children and Families.

Boland, F.J., R. Burrill, M. Duwyn, and J. Karp. 1998. *Fetal alcohol syndrome: Implications for correctional service*. Ottawa, ON: Correctional Service Canada.

–, M. Duwyn, and R. Serin. 2000. Fetal alcohol syndrome: Understanding its impact. *Forum on Correctional Research* 12 (1): 16-18.

Bray, D.L., and P.D. Anderson. 1989. Appraisal of the epidemiology of fetal alcohol syndrome among Canadian Native peoples. *Canadian Journal of Public Health* 80 (1): 42-45.

Buxton, B. March 2000. Society's child. *Elm Street,* 114-20.

Children's Commission of BC. 2001. *Fetal alcohol syndrome: A call for action in B.C.* Victoria, BC: British Columbia Ministry for Children and Families.

Chisholm, P. 19 August 1996. Does a fetus have rights? *Maclean's,* 16-19.

Chudley, A.E., J. Conry, J.L. Cook, C. Loock, T. Rosales, and N. LeBlanc. 2005. Fetal alcohol spectrum disorder: Canadian guidelines for diagnosis. *Canadian Medical Association Journal* 172 (suppl. 5): S1-S21.

Clarren, S.K. 1981. Recognition of fetal alcohol syndrome. *Journal of the American Medical Association* 245 (23): 2436-39.

–, and D.W. Smith. 1978. The fetal alcohol syndrome. *New England Journal of Medicine* 298 (19): 1063-67.

–, S.J. Astley, and D.M. Bowden. 1988. Physical anomalies and developmental delays in nonhuman primate infants exposed to weekly doses of ethanol during gestation. *Teratology* 37 (6): 561-69.

Conry, J., and D.K. Fast. 2000. *Fetal alcohol syndrome and the criminal justice system*. Vancouver, BC: Fetal Alcohol Syndrome Resource Society, Law Foundation of British Columbia.

Coyne, A. 4 November 1997. Court's conundrum. *Montreal Gazette,* B3.

Dophin, R. 11 June 2002. No simple solutions to Native problems. *Calgary Herald,* A5.

Fast, D.K., J. Conry, and C.A. Loock. 1999. Identifying fetal alcohol syndrome among youth in the criminal justice system. *Developmental and Behavioral Pediatrics* 20 (5): 370-72.

Fournier, S., and E. Crey. 1997. *Stolen from our embrace: The abduction of First Nations children and the restoration of Aboriginal communities*. Vancouver, BC: Douglas and McIntyre.

Godel, J.C., H.F. Pabst, P.E. Hodges, K.E. Johnson, G.J. Froese, and M.R. Joffres. 1992. Smoking and caffeine and alcohol intake during pregnancy in a northern population: Effect on fetal growth. *Canadian Medical Association Journal* 147 (2): 181-88.

Grant, T.M., C.C. Ernst, A.P. Streissguth, and K. Stark. 2005. Preventing alcohol and drug exposed births in Washington state: Intervention findings from three parent-child assistance program sites. *American Journal of Drugs and Alcohol Abuse* 31 (3): 471-90.

Jones, K.L., and D.W. Smith. 1973. Recognition of the fetal alcohol syndrome in early infancy. *Lancet* 2: 999-1001.

Lemoine, P., H. Harousseau, J.P. Borteryu, and J.C. Menuet. 1968. Les enfants de parents alcooliques: Anomalies observées a propos de 127 cas [The children of alcoholic parents: Anomalies observed in 127 cases]. *Quest Médicale* 2: 476-82.

Lock, M. 1997. Decentering the natural body: Making difference matter. *Configurations* 5 (2): 267-92.

McCuen, G.E. 1994. *Born hooked: Poisoned in the womb*. Hudson, WI: Gary E. McCuen.

O'Neil, J.D. 1993. Aboriginal health policy for the next century. In *The path of healing: Report of the National Roundtable on Aboriginal Health and Social Issues,* 27-48. Ottawa, ON: Minister of Supply and Services Canada.

–, J. Reading, and A. Leader. 1998. Changing the relations of surveillance: The development of a discourse of resistance in Aboriginal epidemiology. *Human Organisation* 57 (2): 230-37.

Poole, N. 1997. *Alcohol and other drug problems and BC women: A report to the minister of health from the minister's Advisory Council on Women's Health*. Victoria, BC: British Columbia Ministry of Health and Ministry Responsible for Seniors.

Roberts, D. 2 November 1998. Native murder rate in Manitoba alarming, study shows. *Globe and Mail,* A3.

Robinson, G.C. 28-29 October 1988. Opening remarks. Paper presented at the conference Alcohol and Child/Family Health, Vancouver, British Columbia.

–, J.L. Conry, and R.F. Conry. 1987. Clinical profile and prevalence of fetal alcohol syndrome in an isolated community in British Columbia. *Canadian Medical Association Journal* 137 (3): 203-7.

Royal Commission on Aboriginal Peoples. 1995. *Choosing life: Special report on suicide among Aboriginal peoples*. Ottawa, ON: Minister of Supply and Services Canada.

–. 1996. Health and healing. In *Gathering strength: Report of the Royal Commission on Aboriginal Peoples*. Ottawa, ON: Minister of Supply and Services Canada.

Santé Québec. 1994. *A Health profile of the Cree: Report of the Santé Québec Health Survey of the James Bay Cree 1991*. Ed. C. Daveluy, C. Lavallée, M. Clarkson, and E. Robinson. Montreal, QC: Ministère de la Santé et des Services sociaux, Government du Québec.

Square, D. 1997. Fetal alcohol syndrome epidemic on Manitoba reserve. *Canadian Medical Association Journal* 157 (1): 59-60.

Statistics Canada. 1993. Language, tradition, health, lifestyle and social issues. In *1991, Aboriginal Peoples Survey,* 1-8. Ottawa, ON: Statistics Canada.

Stratton, K., C. Howe, and F. Battaglia, eds. 1996. *Fetal alcohol syndrome: Diagnosis, epidemiology, prevention, and treatment*. Washington, DC: National Academy Press.

Streissguth, A.P. 1977. Maternal drinking and the outcome of pregnancy: Implications of child mental health. *American Journal of Orthopsychiatry* 47 (3): 422-31.

–. 1997. *Fetal alcohol syndrome: A guide for families and communities*. Toronto, ON: Paul H. Brooks.

–, H.M. Barr, J. Kogan, and F.L. Bookstein. 1997. Primary and secondary disabilities in fetal alcohol syndrome. In A.P. Streissguth and J. Kanter, eds., *The challenge of fetal alcohol syndrome: Overcoming secondary disabilities,* 25-39. Seattle, WA: University of Washington Press.

Szabo, P. 2000. Fetal alcohol syndrome. Unpublished manuscript. http://www.paulszabo.com/images/pdf_books/BKFAS.pdf.

Tait, C.L. 2003a. *Fetal alcohol syndrome among Canadian Aboriginal peoples: Review and analysis of the intergenerational links to residential schools*. Ottawa, ON: Aboriginal Healing Foundation.

–. 2003b. The tip of the iceberg: The "making" of fetal alcohol syndrome in Canada. PhD diss., McGill University.

Yukon Government. 1991. *Yukon Alcohol and Drug Survey,* vol. 1, *Technical report*. Whitehorse: Yukon Government Executive Council Office, Bureau of Statistics.

Waldram, J.B. 2004. *Revenge of the Windigo: The construction of the mind and mental health of North American Aboriginal peoples*. Toronto, ON: University of Toronto Press.

Wente, M. 7 October 2000. Our poor ruined babies: The hidden epidemic. *Globe and Mail,* A17.

–. 1 February 2001. Finally, we're talking about FAS. *Globe and Mail*. http://archives.theglobeandmail.com.

Williams, R.J., and S.P. Gloster. 1999. Knowledge of fetal alcohol syndrome (FAS) among Natives in northern Manitoba. *Journal of Studies on Alcohol* 60 (6): 833-36.

PART 3

Resilience: Transformations of Identity and Community

10

Cultural Continuity as a Moderator of Suicide Risk among Canada's First Nations

MICHAEL J. CHANDLER AND CHRISTOPHER E. LALONDE

Ten years ago the journal *Transcultural Psychiatry* published the results of an epidemiological study (Chandler and Lalonde 1998) in which the highly variable rates of youth suicide among British Columbia's First Nations were related to six markers of "cultural continuity" – community-level variables meant to document the extent to which each of the province's almost 200 Aboriginal "bands" had taken steps to preserve their cultural past and to secure future control of their civic lives. Two key findings emerged from these earlier efforts.

The first was that, although the province-wide rate of Aboriginal youth suicide was sharply elevated (more than 5 times the national average), this commonly reported summary statistic was labelled an "actuarial fiction" that failed to capture the local reality of even one of the province's First Nations communities. Counting up all of the deaths by suicide and then simply dividing through by the total number of available Aboriginal youth obscures what is really interesting – the dramatic differences in the incidence of youth suicide that actually distinguish one band or tribal council from the next. In fact, more than half of the province's bands reported no youth suicides during the 6-year period (1987-92) covered by this study, while more than 90% of the suicides occurred in less than 10% of the bands. Clearly, our data demonstrated, youth suicide is not an "Aboriginal" problem per se but a problem confined to only some Aboriginal communities.

Second, all six of the "cultural continuity" factors originally identified – measures intended to mark the degree to which individual Aboriginal communities had successfully taken steps to secure their cultural past in light of an imagined future – proved to be strongly related to the presence or absence of youth suicide. Every community characterized by all six of these protective factors experienced no youth suicides during the 6-year reporting period, whereas those bands in which none of these factors were present suffered suicide rates more than 10 times the national average. Because these findings were seen by us, and have come to be seen by others,[1] not only as clarifying the link between cultural continuity and reduced suicide risk but also as having important policy implications, we have undertaken to replicate and broaden our earlier research efforts. We have done this in three ways. First, we have extended our earlier examination of the community-by-community incidence of Aboriginal youth suicides to include also the additional 8-year period from 1993 to 2000. Second, we collected comparable information on adult as well as youth suicides. Finally, we worked to expand the list of cultural continuity factors from the original six included in our 1998 study to a current total of nine. The full details of these new efforts are currently being compiled for separate publication. The present chapter will paint, in broad strokes, the general outline of these new findings, set them in relation to the results of our earlier 1998 publication, and bring out some of the practical implications flowing from these two studies.

Because the rationale and conceptual underpinnings that inform this ongoing program of research are already elaborated elsewhere (e.g., Chandler 2001; Chandler and Lalonde 1998; Chandler et al. 2003), we begin, in the first of the three sections to follow, with just enough about the theoretical foundations that undergird these efforts to make it clear why our search for insights concerning the roots of Aboriginal suicide is as focused as it is. The second section summarizes key empirical findings from our studies of the relation between cultural continuity and community-level rates of Aboriginal suicide – data that now cover the 14-year period from 1987 to 2000. Finally, in the third section, we emphasize what we take to be some of the action or policy implications of this work.

Working Out Which Stones Are Worth Turning Over

The program of research to be summarized here had its beginnings nearly 20 years ago with work aimed at better understanding the linchpin role that convictions about personal persistence play in the general identity-formation process (Chandler et al. 1987). Persuaded by these early results that disruptions in the maintenance of self-continuity were associated with a failure on the part of young persons to maintain a serious stake in their own future, we subsequently turned attention to the study of actively suicidal adolescents who behave in deadly serious ways as though there were no tomorrow (Ball and Chandler 1989; Chandler and Ball 1990). More recently (e.g., Chandler 1994, 2000, 2001; Chandler and Lalonde 1995, 1998; Chandler et al. 2003; Lalonde and Chandler 2004), we have aimed to extend this line of inquiry by focusing attention not on individual suicidal behaviours but on the differential rates of actual suicide found to characterize whole communities. In all these research contexts, we have been guided by the working theoretical assumption that the risk of suicide (whether at the individual or the community level) rises as a consequence of disruptions to those key identity-preserving practices that are required to sustain responsible ownership of a past and a hopeful commitment to the future.

On this evolving theoretical account, the successful development and maintenance of an "identity" (any "identity" – including the self-identities of individual persons and the shared cultural identities of whole communities) necessarily requires that there always be in place some workable personal or collective continuity-preserving mechanism capable of vouchsafing necessary claims of persistence in the face of inevitable change. Life (whether personal life or cultural life) is of course temporally vectored and thus always awash in a stream of exceptionless change. Identities are stobs in this changing stream and stand as the test of, and the limit for, change (Bynum 2001). Identities do this by insisting that something (some entity, some process) remains in common, connecting one moment of inevitable transformation to the next. The battles we as individuals and as cultural groups wage against the currents of change – battles that when won allow both persistent persons and persistent peoples to be identified and re-identified as one and the same across time – are however never decisive but form parts of an ongoing project aimed at sustaining a measure of temporal coherence or biographical continuity. This is true, we have argued, not only because so many (classic and contemporary) touchstone figures before us have insisted that it is so (e.g., Harré 1979; James 1891; Locke 1956; MacIntyre 1977; Parfit 1971; Strawson 1999; Taylor 1988; Wiggins 1980) but also because, in a world otherwise on the move, notions of personal persistence and cultural continuity are deeply constitutive of what it could possibly mean to be a person or to have a culture. That is, any claims made on behalf of enduring personhood or cultural continuity would prove fundamentally nonsensical unless some such identity-preserving project was successfully in place (Cassirer 1923). This follows for the reason that every conceivable form of moral order requires an accounting system that allows individuals and communities to be held responsible for their own past actions (Locke 1956), just as every planful action commits both individuals and collectives to the prospect of a future in which they are the legitimate inheritors of their own just desserts (Unger 1975).

Although all that has just been said is meant to help build the case that a secure sense of personal and cultural continuity are necessary conditions for personal or cultural identity, more still needs to be said about the high costs associated with failing to meet these identity-securing requirements and about the reasons that such failures might sometimes occur. If, owing to some train of personal or collective mishaps, single individuals or whole communities lose track of themselves in time and thus suffer some disconnect with their past or future, life becomes cheap. On this account, what ordinarily keeps us all from impulsively shuffling off our respective mortal coils whenever (as so regularly happens) life seems hardly worth living are all those responsibilities owed to a past that we carry with us and all the still optimistic expectations we hold out for the persons we are en route to becoming. As seen from this perspective, individual persons and whole communities that successfully maintain a sense of personal persistence or cultural continuity are shielded from at least some of the slings and arrows that outrageous fortune regularly holds in store and thus ordinarily choose life over death. By contrast, when circumstances (whether developmental or sociocultural) turn in such a way as to undermine self- or cultural continuity, a sense of ownership of the past is easily lost, and the future (because it no longer seems one's own) loses much of its consequentiality. To the extent, then, that the temporal course of one's individual or cultural identity is somehow fractured or disabled, those persons and those whole communities that have suffered such broken ties to their past and future are put at special risk to suicide, just as achievements that serve to preserve or rebuild such ties work as protective factors that shield them from the threat of self-harm.

Any really adequate test of these theoretical expectations will require an extended program of research that examines the train of causal relations connecting measures of personal and cultural persistence with negative outcomes such as youth suicide. A necessary early step in detailing this causal chain is to show that suicide and other health-related problems do in fact co-occur with failures in the maintenance of personal persistence and cultural continuity. The program of research to be detailed below begins this search process.

From Theory to Practice

Two broad sets of implications flow from the theoretical account just outlined: one of these is diagnostic, whereas the other concerns "prevention," intervention, or otherwise minimizing the risks of suicide, especially in First Nations communities.

The first of these prospects having to do with risk assessment arises from the fact that, because suicides remain rare even when "epidemic," individual suicidal acts effectively defy prediction. Things that happen 10 or even a 100 times per 100,000 cases are simply too rare to ever get any predictive purchase upon. Still, it continues to make sense to try to ferret out which subgroups from the general population run markedly elevated risks of killing themselves. The likely utility of such information is strongly dependent upon: (1) the extent to which such efforts actually work to pick out persons or groups that are sufficiently at risk to warrant intervening in their lives and (2) the degree to which such profiling efforts actually recommend, or realistically afford, any sort of remedial action.

As it turns out, not everything known to be statistically associated with suicide actually fits the criteria just outlined. For example, boys are, on the average, about 4 times more likely to die by suicide than are girls (BC Vital Statistics Agency 2001), and Aboriginal persons, adolescents, and people living in poverty are at somewhat greater risk to suicide than are their richer or younger or older or culturally mainstream counterparts (Cooper et al. 1992). Although not without interest, such broad demographic markers are, in most cases, of only marginal utility. The obvious problem is that any serious suggestion that someone might be actively suicidal obliges us to intervene. Such preventative steps are of course the sort of things one undertakes not lightly but soberly and discreetly. Clearly, before limiting individuals' personal freedoms (as is commonly the case when suicide is seriously suspected), stronger evidence is required than, for example, simply noticing that an individual's risk to suicide quadruples (from something like 10:100,000 to 40:100,000) simply because he is young or male. Similarly, wholesale economic reform, although almost guaranteed to work, is unlikely to be judged as a politically expedient suicide-prevention strategy. What seems required instead, given the futility of going on naming things that can't or won't be changed, is not another blind troll through yet another sea of low-yield actuarial details but a theory-guided search for individual and cultural practices that are subject to possible reform and that stand in some interpretable relation to actual decisions about life and death.

Adolescent Development and Self-Continuity

Our initial work on suicidal behaviours, carried out in the late 1980s and early 1990s (Ball and Chandler 1989; Chandler and Ball 1990), built on still earlier research (e.g., Chandler et al. 1987) aimed at tracking routine developmental changes in the course of identity development – in particular, changes in the way that young people lay claim to, and attempt to warrant, the common conviction that they somehow remain one and the same person despite often dramatic changes. Relying on procedures that required young respondents to justify their claims to personal persistence, both in their own lives and in the changing lives of various characters drawn from classic works of fiction, we generated an age-graded typology of the increasingly complex ways that ordinary, culturally mainstream adolescents justify their own claims of personal persistence in time.

Although everyone we tested was quick to claim some measure of personal persistence, most got better at defending such claims as they grew older. The preteens we interviewed commonly imagined, for example, that they and various story protagonists retained their identity across large-scale changes in appearance, behaviour, and belief simply because their names or fingerprints or some other concrete part of their make-up somehow stood apart from time and served as tangible proof of their continuing identity. By contrast, their older teenage counterparts tended to subscribe to altogether different and more sophisticated claims for sameness in the face of change by insisting, for example, that the real personal transformations that they and others routinely suffered represented only surface changes that were easily trumped by the presence of some other deep-lying core (e.g., their personality, or character, or soul) that was thought to go on being self-same through thick and thin.

Our earliest research made two things especially clear. One of these was that, essentially without exception, all of the more than 200 ordinary young people that we individually interviewed were strongly committed to the view that, despite what was commonly recognized to be wholesale change, they and others were personally persistent (i.e., numerically identical with themselves) and thus deserved to be counted only once. Second, although the particular strategies that our young participants adopted in backing their claims for self-continuity varied in systematic ways, with older respondents typically employing more adequate and cognitively complex arguments, all were able to make some clear case for why the changes in their lives deserved to be discounted in favour of an identity that remained recognizably the same.

From Self-Continuity to Suicide

One implication of the evident stepwise developmental trajectory of strategies for warranting self-continuity displayed by the young participants in our research is that, in the usual course of their growing up, they ordinarily first subscribe to, and later reject, as many as three or four qualitatively different strategies for concluding in favour of self-sameness. As a result of this scalloped developmental pattern, it follows that, at selective moments in their adolescent lives, all these young persons regularly pass through a series of interim moments during which older and once serviceable methods for reasoning about personal persistence are rejected as childish and immature, sometimes before more mature replacement strategies are as yet comfortably in place. Caught in these awkward transitions, such individuals arguably lack the conceptual means necessary to negotiate a proper diachronic sense of selfhood and thus might be easily tripped up by what would ordinarily count as only minor adversities.

A part of what is potentially interesting about this on-again/off-again developmental picture of identity development is that it provides the interpretive means to make understandable a brace of otherwise perplexing findings. One of these paradoxes is that, more than any other age group, it is adolescents who most often attempt to take their own lives (Burd 1994). How, we wonder, could they – they with all of life's potential sweetness full on their lips – manage to act with such callous disregard for their own well-being? The second and equally puzzling matter turns on the fact that most young persons who try to kill themselves do not go on doing so relentlessly. Of course, some do, and for them the chances of their dying by suicide tend to mount with each successive attempt (Ennis, Barnes, and Spenser 1985). Still, much more often than not, suicidal youth who survive do not go on to become suicidal adults but tend to blend back in with the general population of young persons who end up choosing life over death. Among the many ways that things can and do go wrong, this is an unusual picture. More commonly, things that go wrong in adolescence simply go from bad to worse (Noam, Chandler, and Lalonde 1995). Because adolescent suicidal behaviour is not like that but peaks in the teenage and early adult years before falling back down to baseline, a developmental theory with its own peaks and troughs (a theory such as our own) seems just the ticket.

If, as our working model suggests, suicide becomes a serious option only when one's sense of connectedness to a hoped for future is lost, and *if,* as our own data indicate, a routine (if typically short-lived) part of growing up includes periodically abandoning old and outdated strategies for warranting self-continuity in favour of new and developmentally more appropriate working models, *then* the otherwise most perplexing aspects of youth suicide begin to make a new kind of sense. Young persons recurrently lose and typically regain faith in their own future as a predictable part of the usual identity-formation process, and these recurrent transitional moments leave them especially vulnerable – in ways that other age groups typically are not – to the risk of suicide.

If something like the above is true, the dramatic spiking of suicidal behaviours in adolescence becomes newly understandable, as does the fact that suicidality (at least among the young) is rarely a chronic condition. In addition, all that has just been said supports a fully testable hypothesis: adolescents who are currently actively suicidal should differ sharply from their nonsuicidal counterparts by showing themselves, at least for the transitional moment, to be entirely bereft of any workable means to understand their own personal persistence or self-continuity in time. Some of our earliest empirical efforts were designed as a direct test of this hypothesis.

This early work (Ball and Chandler 1989; Chandler and Ball 1990) involved individually administering an hour-long self-continuity interview to every young person admitted to a large adolescent in-patient psychiatric facility over an 18-month period. These young patients were then sorted into those who were and were not placed on active suicide precautions, and all were subsequently matched with an age-mate of the same sex and socioeconomic status drawn from the general community. All these adolescents completed a structured interview protocol that required them (1) to comment upon continuities in the lives of two *Classic Comics* characters (i.e., Jean Valjean from Victor Hugo's *Les Miserables* and Ebenezer Scrooge from Charles Dickens' *A Christmas Carol*) and (2) to speak to the question of their own self-continuity by attempting to warrant their own claims for personal persistence in the face of reminders about acknowledged changes in their own lives. The hospitalized participants also completed the Beck Depression Scale (Beck et al. 1974), and their medical records were carefully reviewed for evidence of recent suicidal behaviours.

The resulting interview protocols were then assigned to one of three scoring categories indicative of whether their responses to problems of personal persistence were (1) age-appropriate, (2) comparable to those of much younger children, or (3) uncountable as any solution to the problem of personal persistence at all. By these standards, psychiatrically hospitalized but nonsuicidal adolescents, although inclined to respond in more immature ways than their nonhospitalized counterparts, were nevertheless consistently committed to the same conviction that their own identities (like those of the story protagonists) persisted as self-same despite often dramatic personal changes. In sharp contrast – and this is the telling point – all but 2 (i.e., 85%) of the actively suicidal participants seriously tried, but consistently failed, to come up with what they or others might reasonably accept as a workable means to justify a sense of personal sameness in the face of change. They regularly came up empty-handed not because they were more depressed or because they had little or nothing to say but because, although their protocols were equally lengthy and complex, they simply tried and failed to understand how, given all of the changes they had experienced, they could either own their past or feel connected to their as yet unrealized future.

Taken together, the results of these studies make a strong case that, in contrast to their nonsuicidal age-mates (both in and out of the hospital), young persons who are at special risk of attempting to end their lives are characterized by having lost a workable sense of their personal persistence. These findings, because they are linked to a detailed account of the identity-formation process, are more than mere happenstance. Instead, because the rocky developmental course by means of which young persons ordinarily come to an increasingly mature understanding of themselves in time is at least now partially charted, the increase in suicidal behaviour found during adolescence is itself less perplexing, and there are now grounds for working out how best to get this process back on track when, as in the case of suicidal youth, it occasionally comes off the rails.

What was not made any clearer by this early work, however, is why it happens that suicides, especially youth suicides, are so tragically common in certain social or cultural or historical circumstances but not in others. Our approach to this critical problem has been to extend, to the level of whole communities, our working hypothesis that acts of suicide are best understood as the by-product of a fractured or disabled effort to secure a sense of identity in time. As already suggested in our brief introduction, if entire cultures are to be identified and re-identified as self-same, they must possess, like individual persons, some procedural means to warrant their claims for persistence despite all the changes inevitably wrought by time and circumstance. On this account, continuity (both self-continuity and cultural continuity) is constitutive of what it could possibly mean to be a self or to have a culture. Any serious disruption to those practices that serve to make a diachronic unity out of one's past, present, and future is likely to prove equally corrosive to well-being. More particularly, anything that serves to cost either individuals or whole cultures their ties to the past and their stake in the future will rob them of just those responsible commitments and hoped-for prospects that ordinarily make living seem better than dying.

On such prospects, some 10 years ago, we began a still ongoing cross-cultural study involving Aboriginal, or First Nations, communities on Canada's West Coast. Our working hypothesis was that the incidence of suicide – measured this time at the band or tribal-council level – would vary as a function of the degree to which these cultural communities already had in place practices or procedures or institutions that function to preserve a measure of cultural continuity in the face of change. The section that follows summarizes the current status of this unfolding project.

Cultural Continuity as a Hedge against Suicide in First Nations Communities

Suicides are ordinarily taken to be deeply private acts, so to attempt to reach beyond this singularity and to somehow understand them in the aggregate requires finding answers to a range of puzzling questions. What, for example, is a proper grouping factor, and when does it make sense to group together suicidal persons as a way to gain some better viewing distance on what might otherwise resolve into a mere conglomerate of anecdotes? Some of the commonly proposed answers to these questions start from much too far back. Computing the rate of Aboriginal suicide for the whole of Canada or for the whole of any province is a prime example of backing up too far. The differences that divide North America's Aboriginal communities account for upwards of 50% of all of the cultural diversity across the whole of the continent (Hodgkinson 1990) – far too much diversity,

MICHAEL J. CHANDLER AND CHRISTOPHER E. LALONDE

one might suppose, to safely overlook. In British Columbia alone, there are some 200 distinctive First Nations bands that collectively speak some 30 distinct languages, live in radically different ecological niches, subscribe to a panoply of largely incommensurable ontological, epistemological, and spiritual beliefs, and have dramatically different histories of interaction with their traditional neighbours and different experiences of colonization. Simply cramming all these unique peoples together into one catchall common denominator to compute some overall national or provincial suicide rate produces a figure that is effectively empty of meaning.

That said, it remains something of a puzzle to know how to respect such diversity without losing all prospects of generalizability. Our own solution to this problem with units of analysis was to undertake to calculate separately the suicide rate of each of British Columbia's 197 formally identified bands. Because they represent self-acknowledged cultural groups, the decision to focus on individual bands would have been both our first and our only choice if not for the fact that many of these communities are so small that just one or two acts of suicide automatically result in astronomically high suicide rates when reported in the usual manner of "suicides per 100,000." This difficulty can be moderated, although not entirely solved, by focusing attention on the province's 29 Aboriginal "tribal councils" – those sometimes natural and sometimes artificially aggregated collections of bands that have been assembled for various political and cultural purposes. The data summarized here – and reported in greater detail elsewhere (Chandler and Lalonde 1998; Chandler et al. 2003) – include, where possible, youth (and/or adult) suicide rates for both individual bands and tribal councils during the two periods: 1987-92 and 1993-2000.

Before we present these results, two further methodological details need to be clarified. First, all deaths counted here as Aboriginal suicides had been judged to be so by the BC Coroner's Office, following an inquiry that regularly involved consideration not only of the means and circumstances of the death but also interviews with relevant family members and acquaintances. There is no reason to doubt that this process is inherently conservative and that it seriously under-reports deaths that were in fact self-chosen but failed to meet what are understandably strict reporting standards. Aboriginal status and "band of origin" were similarly determined using information gathered as part of the coroner's inquest. Again, it can be assumed that not everyone who might have satisfied some common criteria of Aboriginality was correctly identified by these procedures or that one's "band of origin" was always accurately determined.

Finally, although the two epidemiological analyses reported here were undertaken at different times and despite the second's employment of a wider search pattern that included adults as well as children, the methods are sufficiently similar to allow the two data sets to be patched together to cover a single 14-year period for some variables. Nevertheless, for ease of presentation, the findings from our original 1998 study of suicide among Aboriginal youth are summarized here first.

The 1987-92 Data Set

The first and clearest finding to emerge from our 1998 study was that, although suicides among non-Aboriginal persons occur at roughly equal rates across the entire province, just the opposite is true for Aboriginal youth. As can be seen from an examination of Figures 10.1 and 10.2, the rate at which young Aboriginal persons took their own lives

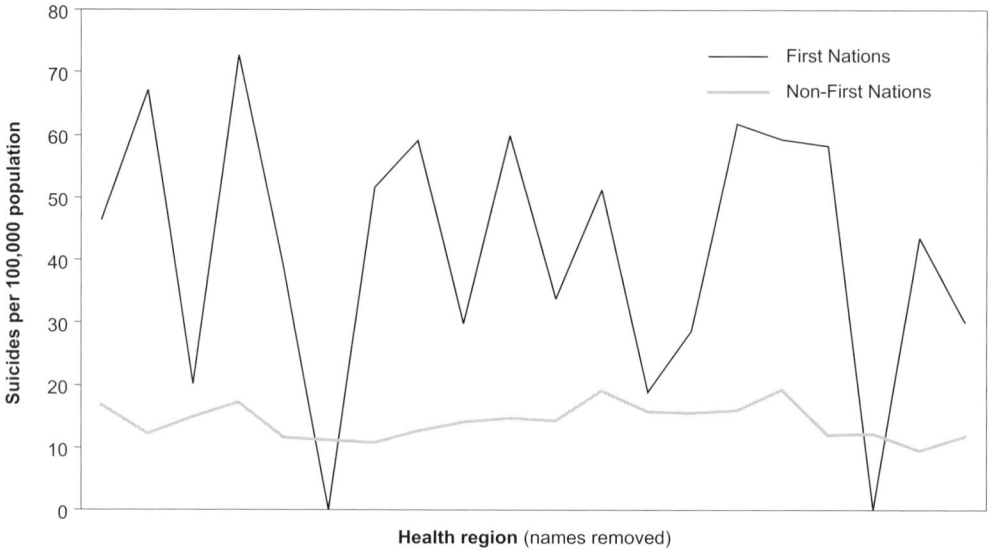

FIGURE 10.1   Youth suicide rate by health region (BC, 1987-92)

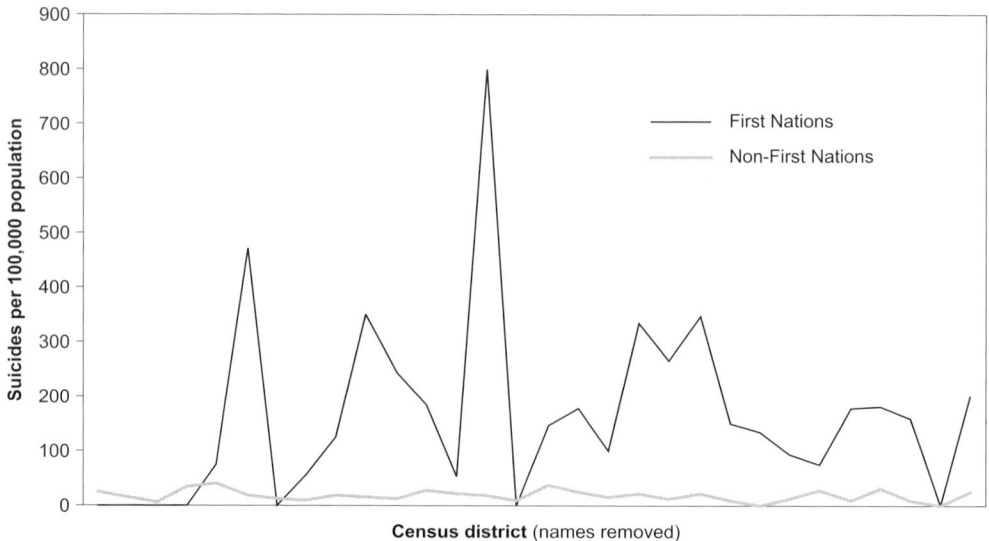

FIGURE 10.2   Youth suicide by census district (BC, 1987-92)

MICHAEL J. CHANDLER AND CHRISTOPHER E. LALONDE

is wildly saw-toothed, piling up dramatically in some locales and much less so in others. Some part of this variability is no doubt an artifact of the relatively small size of the over- all Aboriginal population (estimated to be about 3% by the provincial census) and of the dramatic way that an occasional death in small communities can radically impact such in- cidence rates. Still, there is little obvious difference across these various geographical re- gions that could account for the extreme variability observed – except that these different regions partially map onto territories occupied by specific Aboriginal bands and tribal councils.

Figures 10.3 and 10.4 more directly address the issue of differences between Aborig- inal communities by examining the youth suicide rates for individual bands and tribal councils. As can be seen from an inspection of these figures, community-by-community rates of Aboriginal youth suicide demonstrate in dramatic ways the differences that divide one cultural group from the next. When the rates are examined at the band level (Figure 10.3), for example, it becomes clear that more than half the province's Aboriginal com- munities suffered no youth suicides during this first 6-year study period. In other commun- ities the rate was as much as 800 times the provincial average. As can be seen in Figure 10.4, this same radically saw-toothed picture is again present when youth suicide rates are aggregated by tribal council. Here too, of course, distortions due to small group sizes are potentially at work, but one thing, at least, is clear. Although, when viewed as a col- lective, British Columbia's Aboriginal population does suffer heartbreakingly high rates of youth suicide, our data show that suicide does not occur in equal measure in all First Na- tions communities. Rather, whereas some First Nations communities in British Columbia

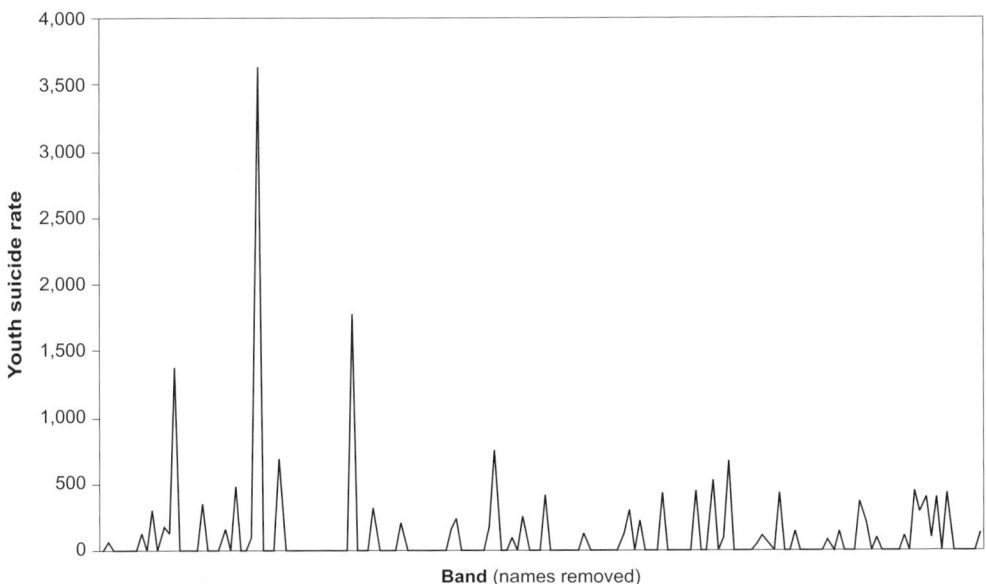

FIGURE 10.3   Youth suicide rate by band (BC, 1987-92)

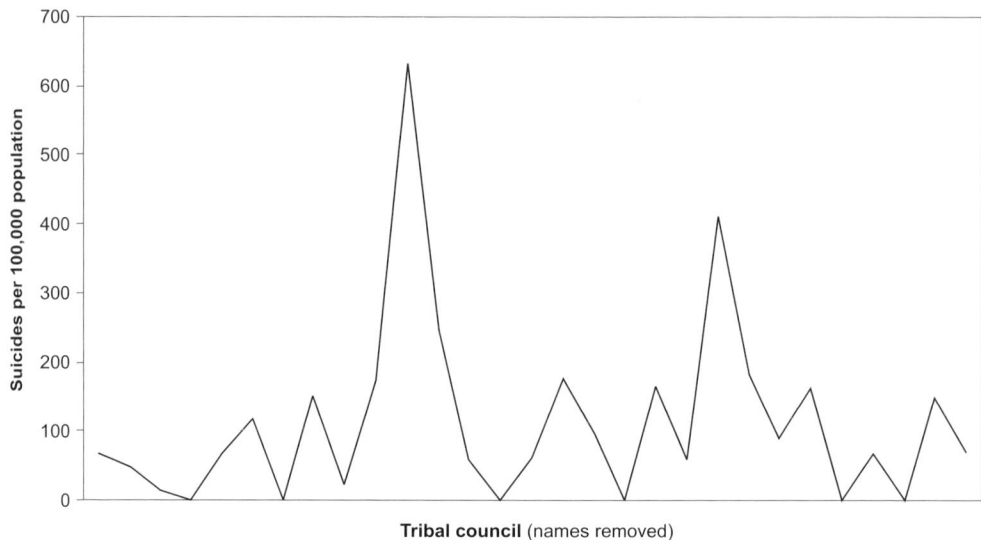

FIGURE 10.4   Youth suicide rate by tribal council (BC, 1987-92)

have experienced high rates of youth suicide, in other communities youth suicide remains unknown. These community-by-community differences make it clear that suicidality is not an attribute or defining feature of "Aboriginality" per se. With the "race card" removed from the deck, the interpretive task set by these data is to work out why youth suicide has so devastated some Aboriginal communities but not others.

The 1993-2000 Data Set

The epidemiological portion of our second study, especially as it applies to problems of youth suicide, amounts to a close replication of our 1998 work. Again the rate at which young Aboriginal persons took their own lives during this 8-year period varies not only as a function of geography (see Figures 10.5 and 10.6) but more particularly with band of origin. As was the case in our first data set, the incidence of youth suicide again varied dramatically from band to band (see Figure 10.7), and once again, the same communities generally proved either to be free of such deaths or to suffer them in elevated ways all out of keeping with the rest of the province. Again, roughly 90% of the suicides occurred in only 12% of the bands, and more than half of all First Nations communities suffered no youth suicides during this 8-year reporting period. As before, a similar picture emerged when individual band-level data were merged to calculate youth suicide rates for entire tribal councils (see Figure 10.8). In short, the 1993-2000 data amounted to a close copy of what was reported for the previous 6-year period.

New to our second study is the inclusion of comparable data dealing with the incidence of adult suicides. Although the model of identity formation we originally articulated was developed with an eye to the radical personal changes that largely define the adolescent

MICHAEL J. CHANDLER AND CHRISTOPHER E. LALONDE

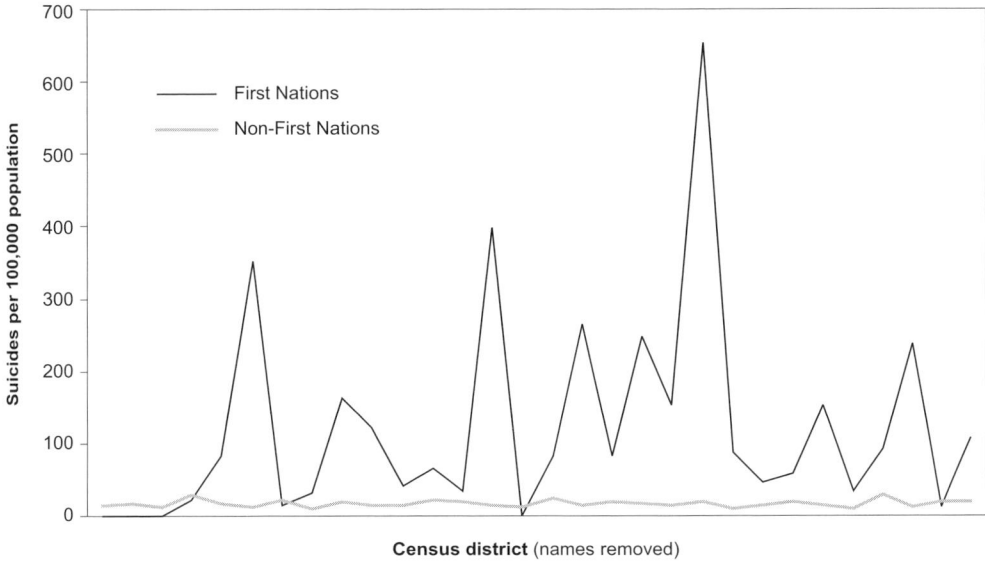

FIGURE 10.5   Youth suicide rate by census district (BC, 1993-2000)

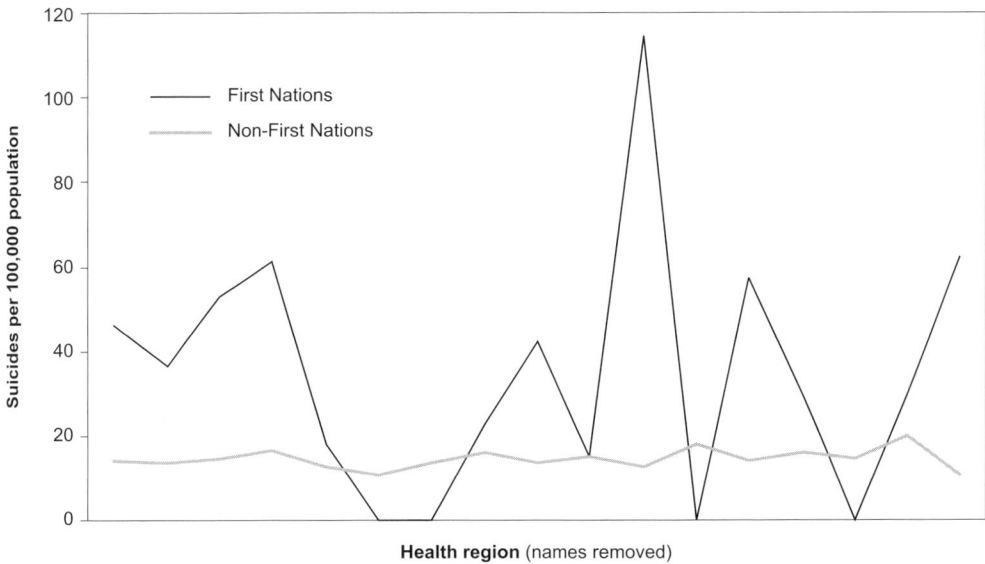

FIGURE 10.6   Youth suicide rate by health region (BC, 1993-2000)

years, there is no particular reason to imagine that older persons are immune to similar identity problems, especially as these manifest themselves in relation to large-scale cultural disruptions. This raises the likelihood that the community-level rates of adult suicides, like those of still younger people, will similarly vary as a function of the presence of

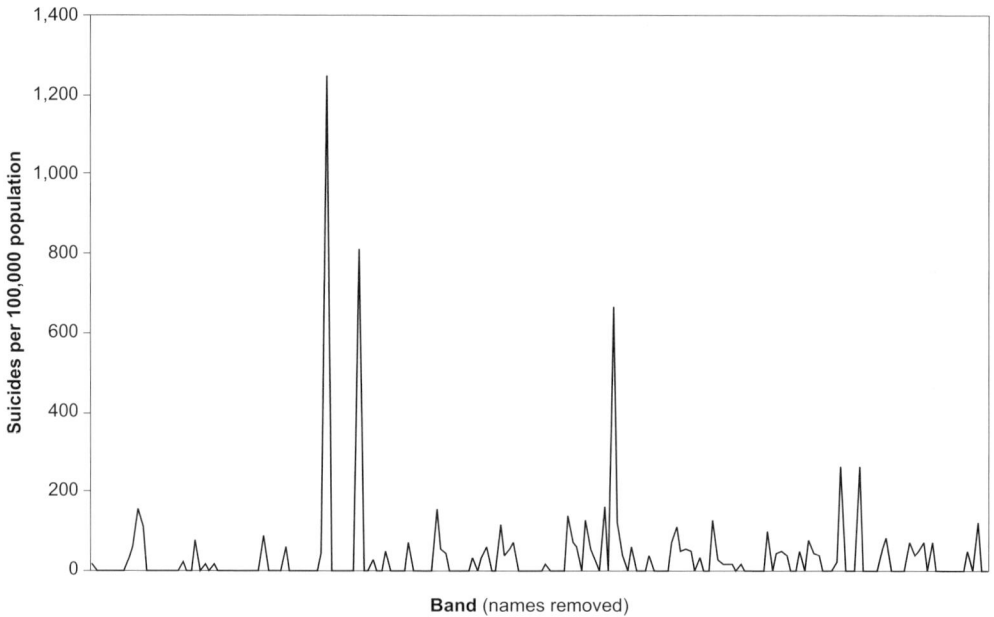

FIGURE 10.7   Youth suicide rate by band (BC, 1993-2000)

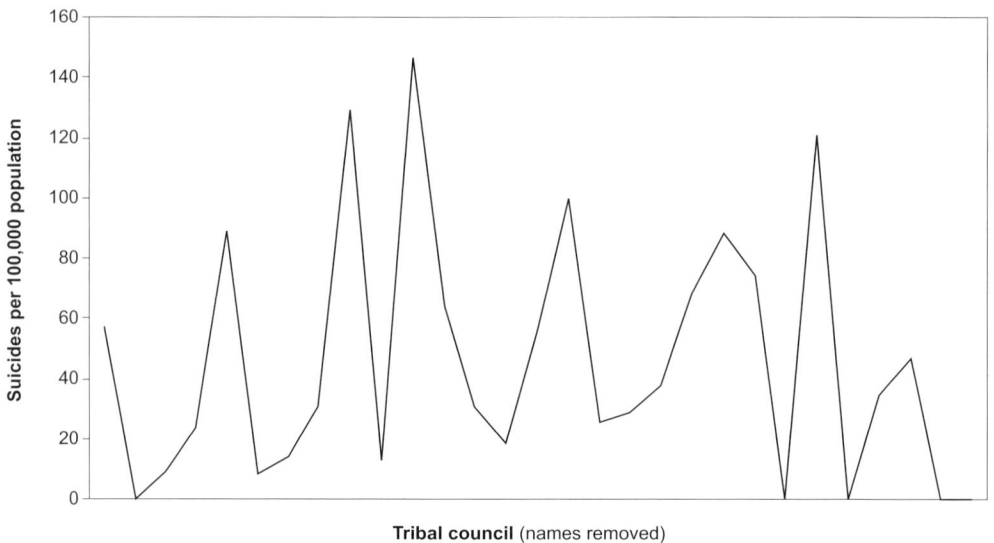

FIGURE 10.8   Youth suicide rate by tribal council (BC, 1993-2000)

sociohistorical conditions that either support or undermine cultural continuity. On the strength of such expectations, we hypothesized that much the same mix of circumstances associated with the dramatic band-by-band variability in Aboriginal youth suicide would also affect suicide rates among adult members of these same communities.

MICHAEL J. CHANDLER AND CHRISTOPHER E. LALONDE

Although, as our new data show, the community-level variation in rates of youth and adult suicides is not always identical, what is most evident from this analysis (see Figures 10.9 and 10.10) is that the band and tribal-council rates of adult suicide are both saw-toothed, with some communities evidencing no deaths by suicide, while others suffer suicide rates many times higher than the provincial average.

Predicting Community-Level Variations in Youth and Adult Suicide Rates

Given our documentation that Aboriginal youth and adult suicides are not at all evenly distributed across British Columbia's numerous bands, the compelling question is: What is it that especially characterizes bands and tribal councils marked by dramatically elevated suicide rates, and what distinguishes them from communities where suicide (both youth and adult) is effectively unknown?

As before, several guiding principles directed our search for answers to this question. Some of these were technical in nature, such as the need to restrict our search pattern to include only those variables for which band-level data are already available for all or most Aboriginal communities. Rather than trolling aimlessly through the mounting seas of Statistics Canada data in the blind hope of snagging something, we took our lead from available research (much of it our own) that supports the theoretical prospect that suicide (whether measured at the individual or community level) can be understood as an outcome of the collapse of those identity-preserving practices that serve to secure enduring

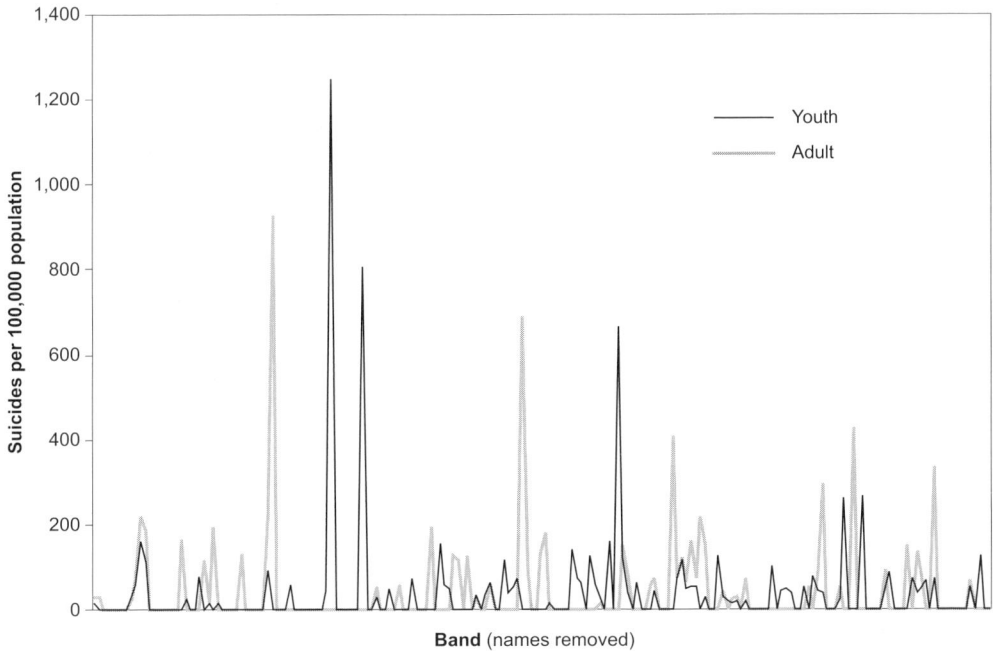

FIGURE 10.9   Suicide rates by band (BC, 1993-2000)

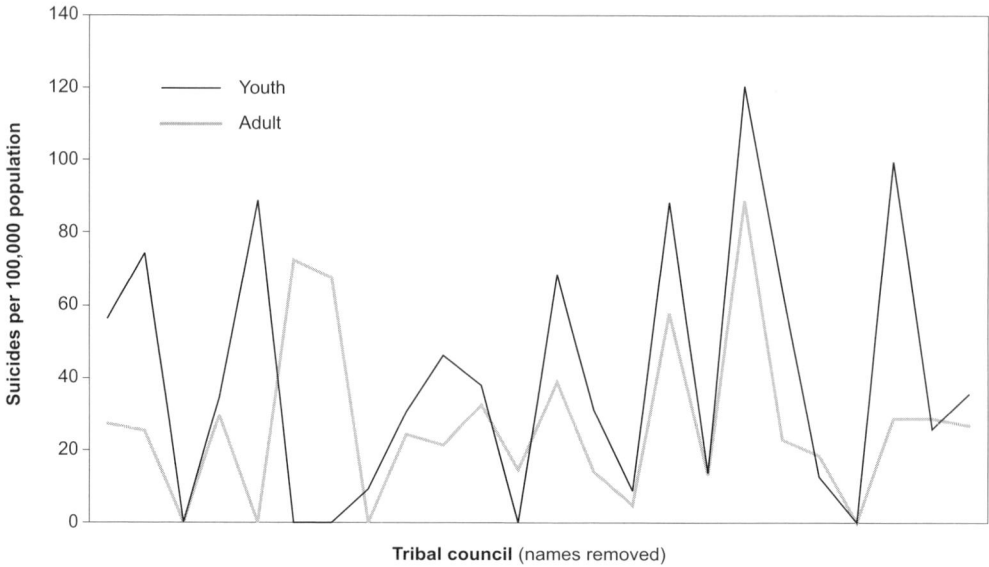

FIGURE 10.10   Suicide rates by tribal council (BC, 1993-2000)

connections to one's past and foreseeable future. However, because this prospect might well be seen as too roundabout, it was important to first consider the timeworn notion that high rates of Aboriginal suicide might be the direct consequence of some simpler and more straightforward social factor such as poverty or geographic isolation.

A well-recognized but frequently overlooked danger confronting all those concerned with identifying potential risk and protective factors in the lives of distinctive ethnic and racial groups is the possibility of conflating the negative impacts of poverty with whatever else might be involved in belonging to this as opposed to that culturally identifiable group (Clarke 1997). The burden of being poor, with its attendant lack of opportunities and frightening array of corrosive forces (e.g., deprivation, marginalization, isolation, discrimination, poor education, unemployment), is widely understood to both: (1) fall disproportionately on those living outside the cultural mainstream and (2) to condemn whole economic underclasses (whatever their racial or ethnic status) to a life that is often nasty, brutish, and short. However true this may be in the main, it is demonstrably true for indigenous groups in general and for Aboriginal groups in particular (see Durie, Milroy, and Hunter, Chapter 2). The Aboriginal population of North America is known to be the most poverty-stricken group on the continent, to have the highest unemployment rates, to be the most undereducated, to be the shortest lived, and to suffer the poorest health (Clarke 1997). Given all this, it is certainly possible that the high suicide rates of some Aboriginal populations might be assignable, in whole or in part, to the "tangle of pathology" (Wilson 1987, 21) produced by bone-grinding poverty.

MICHAEL J. CHANDLER AND CHRISTOPHER E. LALONDE

The evident spoiler to any such exclusively economic explanation, however, is that whereas almost every Aboriginal community is seriously impoverished, it is also true (as we have clearly demonstrated) that high rates of youth suicide characterize only some Aboriginal communities and not others. Still, some First Nations communities are necessarily poorer than others, so the prospect remains that responsibility for suicides, where they occur, might still be traced to the consequences of being the poorest of the poor. At least such a prospect is sufficiently plausible that it demands close consideration.

However, responding to this methodologic necessity is no easy task. Familiar measures of socioeconomic status (SES) are generally ill-suited for use in Aboriginal and especially reserve communities, and there are often few face-valid markers of economic well-being that are standardly recorded for each and every Aboriginal band – or at least this proved to be the case for the Province of British Columbia, where our research was conducted. These difficulties not withstanding, in the end we identified six proxy measures that were generally available and that provided some rough means to order British Columbia's approximately 200 bands in terms of their degree of impoverishment. These included the ratio of lone-parent to dual-parent households within the community, the population density per dwelling (a measure of crowding), the percentage of income derived from government (as opposed to other) sources, rates of unemployment and labour-force participation, labour-force skill levels, and rates of education completion.

As expected, some communities turn out to be considerably wealthier, better housed, more educated, more skilled, and more likely to contain working, dual-income parents than others. By conventional wisdom, these should be the communities with low to vanishing suicide rates. Surprisingly, this is not the case. Although suicide rates within Aboriginal communities do fall slightly with increasing wealth, the correlation is neither statistically nor socially significant. When taken as an omnibus measure – that is, when these measures are combined to produce an overall working index of the socioeconomic status of these communities – the correlation between SES and suicide is a modest $r = .11$, ns.

We came up similarly empty-handed when we examined "rurality" as an explanation for suicide. It might have been the case that the geographic variability we observed in suicide rates across First Nations communities was somehow associated with the distance of these communities from urban centres. That is, Aboriginal suicide rates might have been especially high in large urban centres, or conversely, perhaps suicide haunts those in more rural or remote areas of the province. To test this possibility, each of the communities under study was categorized as urban, rural, or remote (the latter includes communities that are not merely distant from urban centres but also reachable only by floatplane or by other extraordinary means). For both youth and adults (see Figure 10.11), suicide rates are highest in rural communities – and reach their highest levels in those rural communities that lie on the apron of the province's three largest urban centres. Although clearly of considerable interest, given that these are population data, the differences are not significant when subjected to inferential statistical tests commonly applied to sample data: $F_{(2,193)} = .50$, $p = .61$; $F_{(2,193)} = .91$, $p = .41$ for youth and adult rates, respectively.

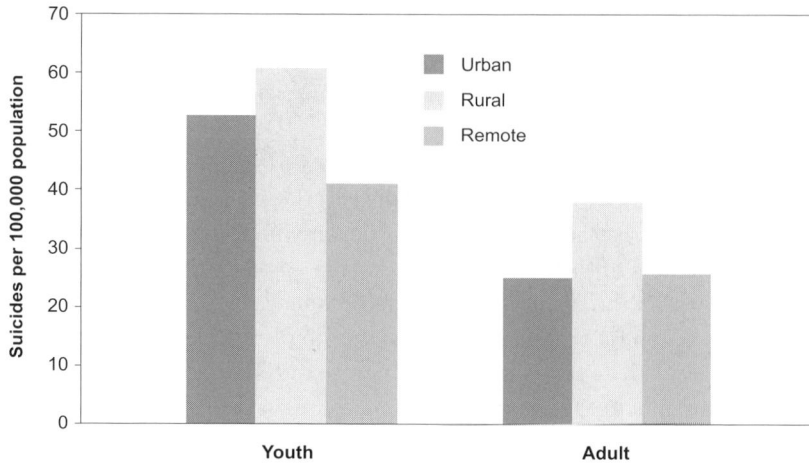

FIGURE 10.11   Suicide rates by band location (BC, 1993-2000)

Whereas suicide rates were largely unrelated to measures of poverty and isolation, they were strongly related to measures of cultural continuity, including efforts to regain legal title to traditional lands and to re-establish forms of self-government, to reassert control over education and other community and social services, and to preserve and promote traditional cultural practices. Finding ways to reliably capture the relative degrees of success that nearly 200 diverse communities have achieved in their efforts to maintain a sense of cultural continuity in the face of continued assimilative pressures and historical oppression has become a primary focus of our work over the past decade. As outlined in much greater detail in the published report of our first epidemiological study (Chandler and Lalonde 1998), the search for variables that act as reasonable proxy measures for the ability of whole communities to preserve their own cultural past and to create a shared vision of an anticipated common future is complicated not only by the sheer number and diversity of communities under study but also by the absence of any clear method for comparing one way of preserving culture to the next. We began with a set of six marker variables that met two essential criteria. The first of these, meant to ensure comparability, was that such variables could be measured accurately for each and every First Nations community in the province using data verified by local, provincial, or federal data stewards. The second criteria concerned the relevance of these variables to the cultural and political goals of these communities.

The half-dozen variables that met these criteria and formed our first set of cultural-continuity factors included (1) evidence that particular bands had taken steps to secure Aboriginal title to their traditional lands, (2) evidence of their having taken back from government agencies certain rights of self-government, (3) evidence of their having secured some degree of community control over educational services, police and fire services, and health-delivery services, and (4) evidence of their having established within their

MICHAEL J. CHANDLER AND CHRISTOPHER E. LALONDE

communities certain officially recognized "cultural facilities" to help preserve and enrich their cultural lives. The hypothesis supported in that initial epidemiological effort was that suicide rates would vary as a function of the presence or absence of these markers of collective efforts to preserve cultural continuity.

Round two of our epidemiological work has involved expanding this set of marker variables to include two additional binary variables: (1) the participation of women in local governance – a measure that is seen to be particularly important within the historically matrilineal First Nations of the West Coast of Canada – and (2) the provision of child and family services within the community. Among the many ways to quantify the level of participation of women in local band councils, the simplest was to count the number of council seats occupied by women in order to determine whether women constituted a majority of council members. Our child-services measure was constructed at the urging of Aboriginal leaders who were eager to assess the impact of their efforts to overcome what has become known as the "Sixties Scoop" – a period in the 1960s when large numbers of Aboriginal children were removed from parental care and placed, either temporarily or permanently, in the care of non-Aboriginal persons or institutions. Many communities have been labouring to gain control of child-custody and child-protection services from provincial child-welfare agencies. Our measure indexes the progress that communities have made in acquiring such control and in implementing these services at the local level. Finally, we supplemented this last variable with measures of the proportion of children within each community who had been removed from parental care. This continuous variable for children and youth in care served as a check against the possibility that control over child services was confounded with the relative size of the population of children in care. That is, the "devolution" of control over child and family services from provincial to local authorities might have proceeded not according to the actual capacity of the local community to undertake such services but according to government perceptions of the size of the problem.

As in our first study, the presence or absence of each factor within each First Nations community was assessed with reference to federal and provincial data sources and by contacting local community authorities. Suicide rates were calculated for each factor, and the number of factors present in each community was used to produce a measure of the cumulative impact of all these factors on suicide rates. In addition to replicating our earlier efforts to determine the ways that cultural continuity might affect youth suicide, we also collected data on all adult suicides.

Once again, each of our original set of six factors proved to be predictive of suicide rates. As shown in Figure 10.12, suicide rates are lower within communities that have succeeded in their efforts to attain self-government, or have a history of pursuing land claims, or have gained control over education, health, police, and fire services, or have marshalled the resources needed to construct cultural facilities within the community.

It was also the case, as shown in Figure 10.12, that communities in which women form the majority within local government are marked by lower suicide rates, as are

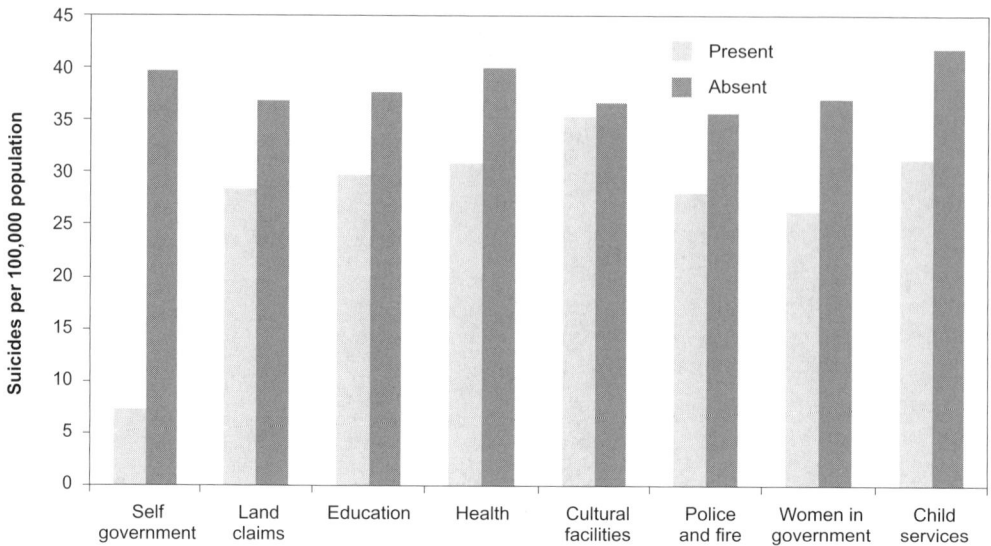

FIGURE 10.12   Suicide rates by cultural-continuity factor (BC, 1993-2000)

those who have managed to gain a considerable degree of control over child and family services.

Although there was a significant correlation between the suicide rate and the average proportion of children in care ($r = .18, p = .014$), communities in which the observed suicide rate was zero had reliably fewer children in care than did communities in which suicides had taken place. The mean percentage of children and youth in care was reliably higher in communities that experienced suicides (1.4%) than in communities that did not (1.1%) ($F_{(1,195)} = 5.15, p = .025$).

When communities were grouped according to the number of factors present – yielding a score that ranged from 0 to 8 – the cumulative effect of these variables on suicide rates became evident (see Figure 10.13). Once again, having more of these factors is better than having fewer, and attaining all eight reduces the suicide rate to zero. To gain a better purchase on the interrelations among the original set of six cultural continuity factors, we combined the two data sets to examine suicide rates across the full 14 years of our research efforts (i.e., 1987 to 2000 inclusive). The downside of this strategy is that it discards the new variables added in our second study, but this is more than offset by advantages that accrue from extending the time frame over which a low-incidence event such as suicide is calculated. The full details of this analytic approach are forthcoming, but, in short, here is what we found.

In relation to the other cultural-continuity factors, the attainment of self-government constitutes something of a capstone. Self-government is, for example, the only factor that never appears in isolation. Among the communities that have attained self-government, just two have fewer than five of the remaining factors. In overall statistical terms, the

MICHAEL J. CHANDLER AND CHRISTOPHER E. LALONDE

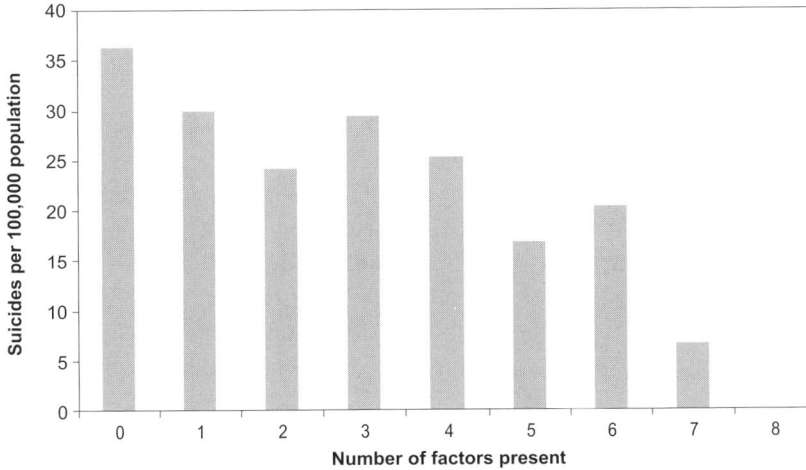

FIGURE 10.13   Suicide rate by number of factors present (BC, 1993-2000)

presence of self-government is strongly correlated with the total number of other factors present within the community (Kendall tau-b = .31, $p < .01$). More intriguing, perhaps, are the patterns that appear in the constellations of factors that characterize particular sets of communities – or rather in the hard choices that communities make regarding the allocation of scarce material and human resources across competing economic, political, and cultural goals.

As one might expect, within the select group of communities that have managed to wrest substantial independence from provincial and federal rule, all were also marked by a long history of land claims litigation. Given the general reluctance of governments to relinquish power, one could hardly imagine how things could be otherwise. Still, a history of land claims was no guarantee of self-government: communities that have not yet achieved self-government are evenly split between those that do (52%) and those that do not (48%) have a history of land claims. Similarly, all but one of the self-governing bands also contained cultural facilities (the remaining band had achieved all other factors), and all but one self-governing band also exercised control over health care provision (the remaining band had cultural facilities and control of local police and fire services). All but one controlled police and fire services (the remaining band having elected to concentrate on health care and cultural facilities).

By contrast, within the set of bands that have yet to achieve self-government, most (72%) have erected cultural facilities, while the majority (77%) has yet to gain control over education and health care services (58%). As noted above, these bands are roughly evenly split in their land claims history and in the provision of police and fire services (52% provide such services). Clearly, then, the attainment of self-government marks communities as having been especially successful in their efforts to strengthen their traditional culture and to re-establish local political control over a host of community services.

To further explore the interrelations among the factors, hierarchical loglinear analyses were conducted with the self-government variable removed. The simplest, best-fitting model (Likelihood Ratio π^2 (22) = 26.51, p = .23) contained a set of four two-way associations (all higher-order models were eliminated). The construction of cultural facilities is strongly paired with control over the provision of health care. Communities that have erected cultural facilities are more than twice as likely to have attained local control over health care services. Communities without cultural facilities are more than twice as likely also to lack control of police and fire services. The same relation holds for education and land claims: communities that either control the provision of education or have a history of land claims activity are twice as likely to control their own police and fire services and health care services.

What becomes readily apparent in these associations is that, in their quest for self-determination, communities elect to proceed in different ways. For many communities, success follows from the preservation or renewal of culture through the establishment of facilities dedicated to cultural purposes. Other benefits – in the form of increased control over local community services – appear to follow in due course. For other communities, land claims and education appear to be the primary goals. Here too success breeds success. The different constellations of factors that obtain as a result of these choices are reflected in the overall data pattern shown in Figure 10.14. Although having more factors present is evidently better than fewer, some combinations of factors offer more protective value than others. Whatever route is taken, as our numbers show, these communities clearly have their eyes trained on the prize of attaining self-government.

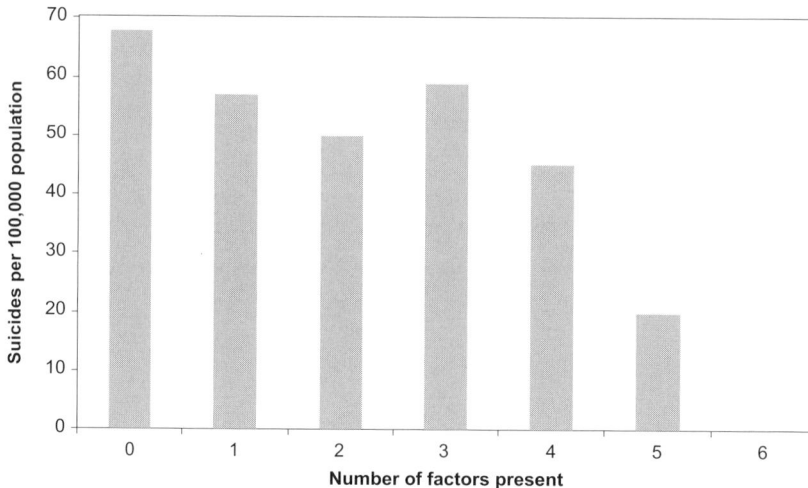

FIGURE 10.14   Suicide rate by number of factors present (BC, 1987-2000)

MICHAEL J. CHANDLER AND CHRISTOPHER E. LALONDE

Conclusion: From Data to Policy

Among the several action or policy implications that flow from the research just summarized, three in particular stand out. Two of these turn on the low to absent rates of suicide noted in many Aboriginal communities. The third grows out of advances in our knowledge of what specifically separates communities with high and low suicide rates.

The Myth of the Monolithic Indigene

The first of these implications is owed to our having exposed as false the mistaken idea that it is somehow possible, through the magic of long division, to capture generic truths about Aboriginal suicide in a single, totalizing, arithmetic gaze. It is, of course, technically possible to tally up suicide deaths, to divide through by the total of all Aboriginal persons, and to come up with a number indicating that "the" suicide rate among Aboriginal persons is somewhere between 3 and 7 times higher than the rate for the nation as a whole. Although who qualifies as Aboriginal and what counts as suicide are far from settled matters, the problem with such measures of "central tendency" is that the cross-community variability in suicide rates dwarfs anything else that might reasonably be said about these data. As a result, summary measures end up describing no one in particular and threaten to send us off in all the wrong directions. Clearly, if suicide rates across Aboriginal communities are as variable as we have shown them to be, then any summary statistic that represents Aboriginality as a seamless monolith is necessarily misleading and defamatory, and any "one size fits all" account or intervention strategy based on such summary figures cannot possibly be made to work. There is no monolithic indigene and no such thing as "the" suicidal Aboriginal. To imagine otherwise, and to invent uniform policies and procedures intended to serve Aboriginality in the large, needs to be seen as a mistake – one that represents, if anything, a kind of recoiling from "otherness" (Said 1978) and that threatens to squander scarce resources on preventing events that either do not happen or happen differently in different places (Duran and Duran 1995).

Whose Knowledge? Whose Best Practices?

A second set of implications contained in our research concerns matters of "indigenous knowledge" and arises not simply because suicide rates vary from one Aboriginal community to the next but because contained in this variable picture are so many bands for which suicide is essentially unknown. That is, it could have been, but was not, the case that British Columbia's tribal communities were still different, one from the other, in their respective suicide rates but that these differences simply ran from bad to worse. Instead, things were quite otherwise. As already mentioned, more than half the province's bands experienced no suicides during what is now a 14-year reporting period, and others enjoyed suicide rates equal to or lower than those found in the general population. The obvious implication of this finding is that, rather than simply being treated differently from their occasional counterparts whose suicide rates were found to be heart-stoppingly high, such communities should perhaps not be "treated" at all. Of course, some caution is required here; it could be that some Aboriginal communities without suicide are just those whose luck has not yet run out. It is, however, more likely that in Aboriginal communities that have no suicides, there must be sedimented knowledge about how to best avoid such tragedies – indigenous knowledge about how to create a life that is still worth living. This prospect not only runs counter to the widespread view that Aboriginal communities need to be saved from themselves but also invites a radical re-examination of two of government's most recently polished catchphrases: "knowledge transfer" and the "exchange of best practices."

These catchphrases are meant to prompt an audit of all the potential new knowledge that might be produced by a research program, along with some detailed strategy for ensuring that such information will be broadly shared. With rare exceptions, however, the only "best practices" one is likely to hear about are the positive findings to emerge from the reported research, and the words "transfer" or "exchange" are most often associated with plans to see that such findings are published in scholarly books or journals or otherwise communicated to one's academic peers. On rare occasions, plans are put in place also to deliver such information into the hands of communities, or at least those community leaders who can be counted on to put such "best practices" into action. Despite modest variations in such transfer schemes, knowledge exchange is invariably viewed as "top-down," and all that is required of lay people, end users, and community leaders is to quietly profit, as best they can, from the "trickle-down" of information produced by experts – information owned by the academy, promoted by government, and offered as largesse to those in need of being saved from themselves.

There are at least two sorts of practical reasons to recommend against an exclusive reliance on such top-down models of knowledge transfer and to entertain instead a much more horizontal, "lateral," or community-to-community form of information exchange, especially when such sharing concerns matters of Aboriginal suicide. One reason is that, because their efficacy is supported by at least some evidence, lateral transfers of information have some greater prospect of actually *working*. The other is that, in contrast to more trickle-down alternatives, efforts to promote sharing between Aboriginal communities – in this case, communities differently affected by suicide – could conceivably *be made to work*.

Working Out What Works

Simply knowing that some Aboriginal communities are free of suicide, while in others suicide is epidemic, is not the same thing as having adequately mapped suicide's epidemiologic causes and course. Nevertheless, it is a respectable empirical beginning, and in our own program of research, we have made some progress in sorting out what it is that distinguishes communities with especially high and low suicide rates. What we already know, at least in the case of British Columbia, is that those communities that have achieved a

MICHAEL J. CHANDLER AND CHRISTOPHER E. LALONDE

measure of self-government, that were quick off the mark to litigate for Aboriginal title to traditional lands, that promote women in positions of leadership, that have supported the construction of facilities for the preservation of culture, and that have worked to gain control over their own civic lives (i.e., control over health, education, policing, and child-welfare services) have no youth suicides and low to zero rates of adult suicide. This is not to say, of course, that anyone in communities without suicides necessarily has explicit or declarative knowledge of exactly what they are evidently doing right or that they chose to do the things they do for the reason that they might buffer against suicide. Nevertheless, such findings do provide some content for potentially productive community-level conversations about what to do next, and they will hopefully provide a beginning basis for the sharing of knowledge and practices between bands with low and high suicide rates.

Whatever their other merits, not every conceivable intervention strategy has the same prospects of being welcomed or endorsed by the communities they are meant to serve. Given the chronically subjugated status of Aboriginal peoples and the long history of "epistemic violence" (Spivack 1985, 126) directed against their traditional knowledge forms, it should come as no great surprise that they often show themselves to be mistrustful and less than welcoming of whatever appears next in the long train of government initiatives, all of which are alleged, in their turn, to be just what the doctor ordered. At least as analysts of postcolonial and colonial discourse would have it (e.g., Berkhoffer 1978; Duran and Duran 1995; Fanon 1965; Gandhi 1998; Nandy 1983; Said 1978), knowledge invented in Ottawa or elsewhere and then rudely transplanted root and branch into someone else's backyard is often and rightly understood to be just another flexing of the dominant culture's "technologies of power" (Foucault 1980) – another weapon wielded by those who have such power against those who must suffer it. A key plank in the platform of such accounts is that conquering cultures routinely work to brand "indigenes" as childlike, to label their indigenous knowledge as mere superstitions, and to reframe their own attempts to colonize the life-worlds of conquered peoples as well-intended educative or "civilizing missions" (Gandhi 1998, 13) aimed at dragging some otherwise "stone-aged" peoples kicking and screaming into the "modern" world. Such acts of epistemic violence, whatever else they may do, guarantee the positional inferiority of indigenous people, further marginalize their voices, and undermine any possibility that they might be seen to know best how to manage their own affairs. Instead, such fundamentally elitist views promote the idea that serious knowledge about how (in this case) suicide might be prevented all ends up being the exclusive province of experts.

Although it remains a matter for debate just how many of these postcolonial charges can be made to stick in the case of Aboriginal suicide, what is not in serious doubt is that something like such dynamics work to endorse what we have termed "top-down" models of knowledge transfer – models that imagine that all real knowledge is a product of the academy (Chandler and Lalonde 2004; Lalonde 2003). What is mistaken about such views is that, in addition to being frankly defamatory, they effectively rule out of court the very possibility that there might actually be indigenous knowledge and practices or that such information could be profitably put to use in some "lateral" or community-to-community intervention program aimed at promoting exchanges between groups that enjoy greater or lesser levels of success in addressing their own problem of suicide.

That many Aboriginal communities are effectively free of the problem of suicide is of course not the same thing as demonstrating that they already have explicit or declarative knowledge of why this is so. Consequently, a great deal obviously remains to be understood about (1) how social scientists might collaborate with Aboriginal communities to better access that knowledge and those practices that serve to insulate some, but not all, against the threat of suicide and (2) how this knowledge (or these "best practices") can be "transferred" or "exchanged" or, more simply, shared with other communities where such knowledge has not yet been accessed and where such practices continue to be left undone. Still, however short we may currently fall in knowing what needs to be done, the job of tackling all of this unfinished work seems altogether more promising than the alternative of simply clinging to that residue of lingering neo-colonialist thought that, as Fanon put it, continues to "want everything to come from itself" (1965, 63).

Note

1   That we have shown that some First Nations are operating in ways that work to reduce and even eliminate youth suicide has not gone unnoticed within the Aboriginal community and among government policymakers. In British Columbia the Office of the Provincial Health Officer and the BC Ministry of Health have adopted the methodology we developed as their de facto standard for surveillance of Aboriginal suicide. The findings from the latest study were featured prominently in the provincial health officer's 2001 report on *The health and well-being of Aboriginal people in British Columbia* (BC Provincial Health Officer 2002) and formed the basis for three of the six major policy recommendations contained in the report. At a national level, the work was presented by Indian and Northern Affairs Canada to the House of Commons Standing Committee on Aboriginal Affairs during the committee's deliberations on the proposed First Nations Governance Initiative, and it has been presented by representatives of the Aboriginal Healing Foundation to the Senate Committee on Aboriginal Peoples. This research was also extensively quoted in the final report of the Advisory Group on Suicide Prevention, *Acting on what we know: Preventing youth suicide in First Nations*, jointly commissioned by National Chief Matthew Coon Come of the Assembly of First Nations and the federal minister of health, Allan Rock. In particular, the research was used to underpin recommendations aimed at "supporting community-driven approaches; and creating strategies for building youth identity, resilience and culture" (Health Canada 2002, 7).

References

Ball, L., and M.J. Chandler. 1989. Identity formation in suicidal and non-suicidal youth: The role of self-continuity. *Development and Psychopathology* 1 (3): 257-75.

Beck, H., A. Weissman, D. Lester, and L. Trexler. 1974. The measurement of pessimism: The hopelessness scale. *Journal of Consulting and Clinical Psychology* 42 (6): 861-65.

Berkhoffer, R.F. 1978. *The white man's Indian.* New York: Vintage.

British Columbia Provincial Health Officer. 2002. *The health and well-being of Aboriginal people in British Columbia.* Victoria, BC: Ministry of Health Planning.

British Columbia Vital Statistics Agency. 2001. *Analysis of health statistics for status Indians in British Columbia, 1991-1999.* Vancouver, BC: British Columbia Vital Statistics Agency.

Burd, M. 1994. *Regional analysis of British Columbia's status Indian population: Birth-related and mortality statistics*. Victoria, BC: Division of Vital Statistics, British Columbia Ministry of Health and Ministry Responsible for Seniors.

Bynum, C.W. 2001. *Metamorphosis and identity*. Cambridge, MA: MIT Press.

Cassirer, E. 1923. *Substance and function*. Chicago: Open Court.

Chandler, M.J. 1994. Self-continuity in suicidal and nonsuicidal adolescents. In G. Noam and S. Borst, eds., *Children, youth and suicide: Developmental perspectives,* 55-70. San Francisco: Jossey-Bass.

–. 2000. Surviving time: The persistence of identity in this culture and that. *Culture and Psychology* 6 (2): 209-31.

–. 2001. The time of our lives: Self-continuity in Native and non-Native youth. In H.W. Reese, ed., *Advances in child development and behavior,* vol. 28, 175-221. New York: Academic Press.

–, M. Boyes, S. Ball, and S. Hala. 1987. The conservation of selfhood: Children's changing conceptions of self-continuity. In T. Honess and K. Yardley, eds., *Self and identity: Perspectives across the life-span,* 108-20. London: Routledge and Kegan Paul.

–, and L. Ball. 1990. Continuity and commitment: A developmental analysis of the identity formation process in suicidal and non-suicidal youth. In H. Bosma and S. Jackson, eds., *Coping and self-concept in adolescence,* 149-66. New York: Springer-Verlag.

–, and C.E. Lalonde. 1995. The problem of self-continuity in the context of rapid personal and cultural change. In A. Oosterwegel and R.A. Wicklund, eds., *The self in European and North American culture: Development and processes,* 45-63. Boston: Kluwer.

–, and C.E. Lalonde. 1998. Cultural continuity as a hedge against suicide in Canada's First Nations. *Transcultural Psychiatry* 35 (2): 191-219.

–, C.E. Lalonde, B.W. Sokol, and D. Hallett. 2003. Personal persistence, identity, and suicide: A study of Native and non-Native North American adolescents. *Monographs for the Society for Research in Child Development* 68 (2): 1-138.

–, and C.E. Lalonde. 2004. Transferring whose knowledge? Exchanging whose best practices? On knowing about indigenous knowledge and Aboriginal suicide. In J. White, P. Maxim, and D. Beavon, eds., *Aboriginal policy research: Setting the agenda for change,* vol. 2, 111-23. Toronto, ON: Thompson Educational Publishing.

Clarke, A.S. 1997. The American Indian child: Victims of the culture of poverty or cultural discontinuity? In R.W. Taylor and M.C. Wang, eds., *Social and emotional adjustment and family relations in ethnic minority families,* 63-81. Mahwah, NJ: Lawrence Erlbaum Associates.

Cooper, M., R. Corrado, A.M. Karlberg, and L. Pelletier Adams. 1992. Aboriginal suicide in British Columbia: An overview. *Canada's Mental Health* 40 (3): 19-23.

Duran, E., and B. Duran. 1995. *Native American postcolonial psychology.* Albany, NY: State University of New York Press.

Ennis, J., R. Barnes, and J. Spenser. 1985. Management of the repeatedly suicidal patient. *Canadian Journal of Psychiatry* 30 (7): 535-38.

Fanon, F. 1965. *A dying colonialism.* Trans. H. Chevaliar. New York: Grove.

Foucault, M. 1980. George Canguilhem: Philosopher of error. *Ideology and Consciousness* 7: 53-54.

Gandhi, L. 1998. *Postcolonial theory: A critical introduction.* New York: Columbia University Press.

Harré, R. 1979. Social being: A theory for social psychology. Oxford, UK: Blackwell.

Health Canada. 2002. *Acting on what we know: Preventing youth suicide in First Nations.* Final report of the Advisory Group on Suicide Prevention. http://www.hc-sc.gc.ca/fniah-spnia/alt_formats/fnihb-dgspni/pdf/pubs/suicide/prev_youth-jeunes-eng.pdf.

Hodgkinson, H.L. 1990. *The demographics of American Indians: One percent of the people, fifty percent of the diversity.* Washington, DC: Institute for Educational Leadership and Center for Demographic Policy.

James, W. 1891. *The principles of psychology.* London: Macmillan.

Lalonde, C.E. 2003. Counting the costs of failures of personal and cultural continuity. *Human Development* 46: 137-44.

–, and M.J. Chandler. 2004. Culture, selves, and time: Theories of personal persistence in Native and non-Native youth. In C. Lightfoot, C.E. Lalonde, and M.J. Chandler, eds., *Changing conceptions of psychological life,* 207-29. Mahwah, NJ: Laurence Erlbaum and Associates.

Locke, J. 1956 [1694]. *Essay concerning human understanding.* Oxford, UK: Clarendon Press.

MacIntyre, A. 1977. Epistemological crisis, dramatic narrative, and the philosophy of science. *The Monist* 60 (4): 453-72.

Nandy, A. 1983. The intimate enemy: Loss and recovery of self under colonialism. New Delhi, India: Oxford University Press.

Noam, G.G., M.J. Chandler, and C.E. Lalonde. 1995. Clinical-developmental psychology: Constructivism and social cognition in the study of psychological dysfunctions. In D. Cicchetti and D. Cohen, eds., *Handbook of developmental psychopathology,* vol. 1, 424-66. New York: John Wiley and Sons.

Parfit, D. 1971. Personal identity. *Philosophical Review* 80 (1): 3-27.

Said, E. 1978. *Orientalism.* New York: Pantheon Books.

Spivak, G. 1985. Can the subaltern speak? Speculations on widow sacrifice. *Wedge* 7 (8): 120-30.

Strawson, G. 1999. Self and body: Self, body, and experience. *Supplement to the Proceedings of Aristotelian Society* 73 (1): 307-32.

Taylor, C. 1988. The moral topography of the self. In S.B. Messer, L.A. Sass, and R. Woolfolk, eds., *Hermeneutics and psychological theory,* 298-320. New Brunswick, NJ: Princeton University Press.

Unger, R. 1975. *Knowledge and politics.* New York: Free Press.

Wiggins, D. 1980. *Sameness and substance.* Cambridge, MA: Harvard University Press.

Wilson, W.J. 1987. *The truly disadvantaged.* Chicago, IL: University of Chicago Press.

11

The Origins of Northern Aboriginal Social Pathologies and the Quebec Cree Healing Movement

ADRIAN TANNER

There is ample evidence that a large number of northern, relatively isolated Aboriginal communities have, over the past few decades, experienced an extraordinarily disturbing level of social pathologies. Individually, these problems each have labels, like substance abuse, child neglect, domestic violence, sexual abuse, petty crime, or suicide, but as yet there is no commonly accepted term that acknowledges that taken together these problems constitute a linked set. In the absence of such a general term, I will borrow the label of "social suffering" (Adelson 2000; Kleinman, Das, and Lock 1997).

Many different explanations, citing different causes and sometimes using mutually inconsistent kinds of logic, have been proposed to account for this widespread phenomenon. A cursory glance at the social-science literature reveals that this includes such factors as severe depression, stress, or trauma brought on by rapid social change, assimilation, and disempowerment (Abadian 1999; Chance 1968; Vallee 1968), the social impacts of poverty and industrialization (Niezen 1993), dispossession (Kulchyski 1988), forced settlement or relocation (Shkilnyk 1985), loss of cultural continuity (Chandler and Lalonde 1998), a lack of meaningful work (Elias 1996), and the impacts of residential schooling (Hodgeson 1990; Malloy 1999). Although we lack sufficient data to confirm or reject any of these explanations, perhaps we might ask a more fundamental question: What do these communities with social pathologies have in common?

Forty years ago there were still many northern indigenous people living most of the year in bush camps as self-reliant hunters and trappers. Around that time they were subjected to an accelerated policy of sedentarization, aimed to move them from these bush camps into government-built houses in crowded settlements. Several such cases of the negative impacts of what could be called "directed settlement" have been documented in the past few years (Busidor and Bilgen-Reinhart 1997; Driben and Trudeau 1983, 10; Samson 2003; Shkilnyk 1985; Stevenson 1968; Tester and Kulchyski 1994). York (1992), a journalist, mentions 10 cases of subarctic settlements that have faced epidemics of social problems. The conclusion that widespread social breakdown was caused by this settlement policy is sadly ironic, given that the move had an explicit social-welfare objective – that is, to extend public services, including public education and medicine, to the last Canadians to have access to them. Moreover, the resulting problems go beyond the tragic personal situations experienced by individuals or nuclear families; in several cases, a significantly large part of a local population periodically becomes so seriously affected that the normal functioning of the entire group is affected.

In this chapter, I look at what the Cree of northern Quebec experienced after they were subjected to this policy and moved into government-built houses. I focus on this particular case not because it stands as an especially tragic or extreme example of post-settlement Aboriginal social pathology, compared to other such cases in northern Canada, but to see what can be learned from a case in which local initiatives were taken to address the threat posed by the problem.

Social Theory

The sedentarization of the Quebec Cree, as with most other Canadian Indians, took place through the application of the reserve system, a set of legal and administrative provisions authorized by the Indian Act. One question that needs to be addressed at the outset is the degree to which the problems of social suffering resulted from the imposition of the reserve system as an administrative and social form. There has been a long debate within Canadian anthropology about the kind of social system that is characteristic of Indian reserves and whether these collectivities constitute real "communities" (Carstens 1991; Dunning 1964; Gerber 1979; Hawthorn 1966; Inglis 1969). We might note that some social scientists avoid the term "community" altogether on the grounds that it is ideological and culturally located and that it tends to imply unverified assumptions about how people in small face-to-face groups are supposed to interact (Brint 2001). In the debate about the social structure present on reserves, one common theme has been to suggest that this form of society (and by implication, the social problems of its members) has been strongly influenced by the government control found there, as well as by the generally corrosive influence of mainstream Canadian society, of which reserves seem to be on their way to becoming a marginalized component.

The debate was launched in a 1964 paper by Dunning, in which he proposed that we need to recognize a distinction between southern Canadian Indian bands, which had a considerable history of contact with mainstream society, and the more remote northern and isolated ones. Dunning felt that many of the latter had not yet been undermined by external influences and appeared "to be functioning with reference to ... indigenous social structures and norms" (3-4). We should hasten to add that this was written when the movement of these northern bands from hunting camps into settlements was only beginning to get under way. With respect to the southern bands, the thrust of Dunning's argument was to question whether, given their extensive contact with and acculturation toward mainstream Canadian society, they could be said to any longer constitute "real" social entities. Today, in light of the recent radical transformation of the northern groups, including the growth of government influence over them following their move into settlements, we may well ask whether Dunning's critical comments about the social structure of southern bands may not now also apply to them.

Inglis (1969) reviewed Dunning's and similar critiques of the social structure of Canadian Indian reserves and noted the contrast between reserves and non-Indian towns, in part due to the implications of the distinct legal and administrative status of the former. In particular, he noted the significance of the band membership of reserve residents, the distinctive relationship of these members to reserve land, and the form of political organization of the band, which are all based on quite different principles from anything that applies to non-Indian towns and which are also quite different from anything they experienced when living in bush camps. However, Inglis responded to the question of whether reserves are "real" social entities by arguing that they should not be seen as any more "artificial" than other aggregations of the Canadian population; instead, they are to be seen merely as hemmed in by a distinctive set of boundaries. Nevertheless, in the present context it is important to ask whether the special conditions of reserves play any part in contributing to the situation of social suffering.

In his study of a Canadian Indian reserve in the Okanagan region of British Columbia, Carstens (1991) takes for granted that those on the reserve constitute a "community," although he apparently uses the term only in the sense of a group of people with regular face-to-face interaction. He notes that the members of this Indian community are regarded as "insiders" by those outside their immediate group with whom they come into contact and have relations. However, although Carstens acknowledges the common notion that a rural community is a close-knit group with warm personal relations, he also notes that this description does not fit the majority of rural Indian reserves. Moreover, even for rural non-Indians, he asserts that such an image of the "community" is largely a romantic myth (1991, 139-40). Carstens sees group behaviour on reserves as reflective more of what he calls "reserve culture," a form that has been shaped more by "administrative determinism" than by the Aboriginal cultural tradition. This reserve culture is characterized by "a greater degree of conflict than in other Canadian communities," as people try to come to terms with their marginal position within Canadian society. In doing so, they adopt subtle but aggressive anti-white attitudes, expressed, for example, in their drinking behaviour (286-89).

The policy to settle northern Aboriginal people on reserves and hamlets can be seen as a case of social engineering. A recent study examines several examples of the twentieth century's disastrously failed grand schemes of "high modern" social engineering – large collective farms in the USSR, huge mechanized agricultural schemes in West Africa, totally planned cities erected virtually overnight in formerly rural locations in Brazil and India, and the compulsory "villagization" of dispersed subsistence farmers in Tanzania (Scott 1998). By comparison, the settlement of northern Canadian Aboriginal hunting peoples was less audacious but only due to its smaller scale and the apparent lack of overall planning. For the individuals subjected to this process, however, the results were sometimes equally unpleasant. In his study, Scott argues that what was overlooked in the cases of centralized social planning that he documents was any taking into account or use of local practical knowledge. One might suggest that this was also the case with the settlement of northern Aboriginal people in houses.

The Cree settlement process involved a major loss of both personal and residential group autonomy. The resulting anomie initially led to a dramatic increase in binge drinking and interpersonal violence. For the new Quebec Cree villages, this abuse of alcohol created a serious problem, with the result that affected individuals were sent to external alcohol- and drug-treatment programs. Local people, after moving into the first houses, found themselves marginalized by increasing government oversight, but eventually they began to take control of their new circumstances by applying local cultural knowledge to the new social problems. They did so by organizing social events and other initiatives, generally referred to as the "healing movement."[1] Today, this healing movement includes settlement-wide activities that exemplify local cultural themes and values. In my analysis of this movement, I show that the shift to settlement life challenged existing Cree values and practices and that the Cree have now set out to find a more satisfactory form of social life, one more in line with their values and cultural heritage but at the same time appropriate to their new circumstances.

By focusing attention on the group, rather than exclusively on the individuals with behavioural problems, as do the alcohol- and drug-treatment programs, the healing movement implicitly offers an account of the root of the problem that both complements and is distinct from that of the psychiatric approach. Without rejecting a concern for the particular difficulties faced by individuals suffering from behavioural problems, the healing movement takes the position that it is the local group that needs "healing." Later in this chapter, I argue that these local "healing" initiatives, by being directed at the whole settlement, are essentially forms of community building aimed at strengthening and renewing local social relations.

In retrospect, it would seem that much of the problem that northern Aboriginal people experienced in the move into houses arose, at least in part, because life in the new settlements had certain unintended consequences. With the institutionalized social controls of the hunting camp no longer operating, unrestrained settlement-wide binge drinking, which had previously occurred for only short summer periods at the trading posts, became relatively "normalized."[2] Although in the new Quebec Cree villages general public participation in, and even tolerance of, these settlement-wide drinking parties did not continue for many years, similar kinds of activity seem to have been a feature in many of the reported cases of social breakdown of some other northern Aboriginal groups following their move into houses. In some of these localities, moreover, this feature of settlement life continues, having recurred intermittently over the more than 30 years since people first moved into houses. In some of the more isolated northern localities, there is also a history of attempts (largely unsuccessful) to address the problem by limiting access to alcohol (O'Neil 1983; Smart 1979). But for most of the Quebec Cree villages, this option lost its potential effectiveness soon after settlement due to the opening of road access to nearby urban centres. Thus an important change that made way for the healing movement occurred in the mid-1970s, when settlement-wide public binge drinking became socially unacceptable. An important question to consider is why this rejection of public binge

ADRIAN TANNER

drinking happened in some settlements but not in all the new settlements across the North. In what follows, I examine the role of "healing" as a social movement in this process.

The East Cree

The healing movement among the East Cree arose within a unique local social and historical context, even though there was also some cross-fertilization with similar events occurring in other Aboriginal groups at around the same time. The immediate circumstance that gave rise both to the problem of social pathology among the East Cree and to the emergence of the healing movement was sedentarization. To understand the multiple impacts on the northern Cree caused by the change from living year-round in tents in the bush to living in houses in settlements, we need to understand something of the way of life that went before. Although this included some access to trade goods obtained by trading furs, it can be shown that throughout the fur-trade period, Cree hunting groups retained a significant degree of independence from the local monopoly trader, the Hudson's Bay Company (HBC) (Tanner 1979, ch. 1). Although some drinking occurred during trading visits, there is little evidence that it was a significant problem in the hunting camps. In the following account, I draw extensively on my own experience, particularly at Mistissini, Quebec, around the time the Cree moved into settlements.[3]

The Cree are one of the largest Aboriginal groups in Canada. Taken together, their local groups form a chain of peoples who speak dialects of the Algonquian language family, which extends across a major part of the boreal forest region, from Labrador to northern British Columbia. Other members of this language family include the Ojibwa, Blackfoot, and Mi'kmaq. Before European contact, the Cree of the northern forests were nomadic hunters who spent much of the year in small groups and assembled in larger gatherings only for brief periods at places of resource concentration to trade and to make marriage alliances. After European fur-trading contacts became established among them in the 1600s and 1700s, these gatherings became the basis of fluid bands, each associated with a particular trading post, where eventually contact was also made with Christian missionaries. However, in many ways life for the Cree probably continued much as before contact, with people living most of the year in small, family-based hunting groups.

The East Cree inhabit the area of Quebec east of James Bay. Prior to the time they were moved into settlements, they had remained largely independent of external control, living mainly from their own productive activities, which they organized in their own way and on their own land. Not only did most of their food come from their own hunting, fishing, and gathering efforts, but they also provided for most of their own cash needs, mainly from the fur they trapped, supplemented, by the 1950s, with a few social-welfare benefits (Tanner 1979, 61). While they were living in the bush, family groups were the units of production and consumption, independent of direction by others. Each shared food and supplies with other families in the co-residential hunting group, for which no specific return was required, although there was a moral obligation of reciprocity, meaning that when they were in need they could expect help from those able to provide it. These productive activities depended on each person's knowledge of the environment and on the groups' considerable survival skills. There were shortages, hunger, and in some rare cases starvation, as well as infant mortality, and life expectancy was less than it became after they had access to modern specialized medical care. But for the most part, the Cree had a better diet than today and took plenty of physical exercise, so most enjoyed good physical health.

Before sedentarization, the East Cree generally had living conditions that were consistent with their key cultural values, such as intimate knowledge of and involvement with their environment, use of manual skills, self-reliance, autonomy, generosity, and physical health. The move into settlements threatened all of these. Given the shortage of paid employment in the settlements and the increased monetary costs of settlement life, after the move most Cree found themselves increasingly economically dependent on the government. The built environment of the settlement's houses and machines was initially unfamiliar to most Cree, and few had the skills to effectively manage them. In many ways, people were increasingly under the authority of external agencies, so mature adults no longer felt in charge of or able to fully plan their own lives. Even those better off than others found they were unable to live up to cultural expectations of sharing their good fortune since they now found themselves living near more relatives than they could possibly assist. In the settlement, the cost and limited available range of store food resulted in a nutritionally inferior and culturally less valued diet, which, combined with the shortage of employment and consequent lack of exercise, resulted in an increase in health problems.

Despite all these factors, I consider the East Cree to have been relatively fortunate among subarctic Indians, given that in the early years of sedentarization most who wished to were able to continue to spend the winters in bush camps. Parents were not forced to live in the settlements to look after their school-age children because in the early years of settlement children could attend residential school. With the shift to local primary and secondary schooling through the 1970s, student residences were made available in some of the new settlements. Moreover, after 1975, Cree hunters had access to the Income Security Program (ISP), part of the James Bay and Northern Quebec Agreement, which also helped many of them to continue to live in the bush (Feit 1982). Because of residential schools and the ISP, the East Cree were able to make the transition to sedentary life more gradually and with fewer negative consequences than some other arctic and subarctic Aboriginal groups, even though they did not entirely avoid the associated problems.

In the hunting camps, the Cree were able to provide a good level of care for their children. The women and old people tended to remain close to camp, and older siblings were also expected to help with the care of younger ones. Consequently, there were usually several people who would share the responsibility of looking after all the children.

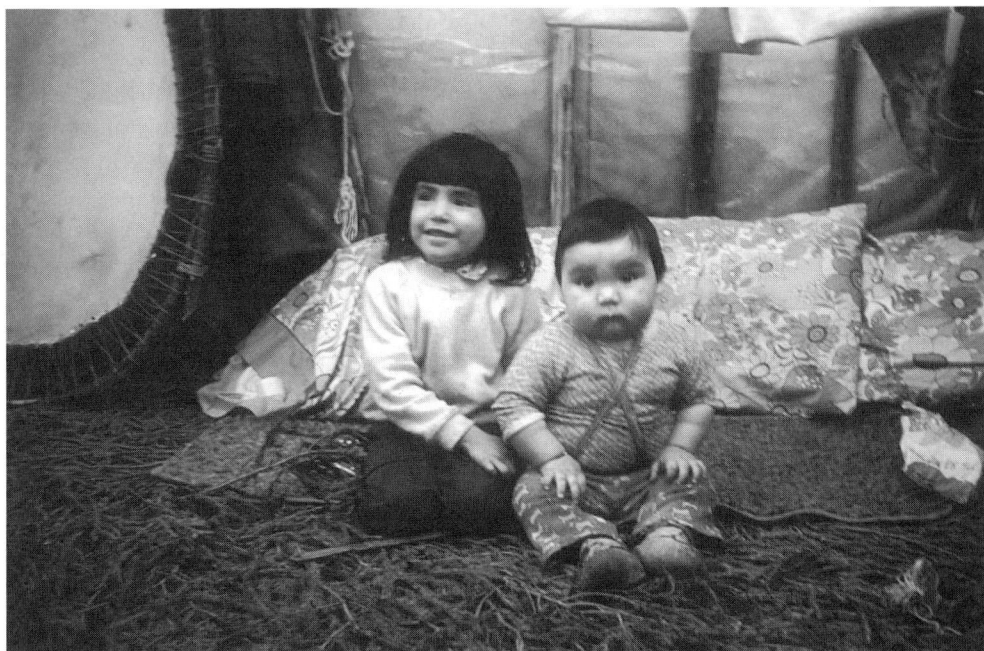

FIGURE 11.1   Older child caring for a younger one in a Mistissini hunting camp, early 1970s.
(Photo: A. Tanner)

Children were socialized and educated by affording them a considerable degree of freedom; they were encouraged to observe the activities of adults and eventually to attempt
small tasks, for which they were rewarded with praise. There were also many forms of
ceremonial recognition of their achievements. Apart from a few dangerous activities that
were forbidden to them, discipline was relaxed, and corporal punishment was both un-
necessary and repugnant. The individual autonomy of even relatively young children was
respected. But in the settlements these same childrearing values and practices proved inappropriate. Adults found it difficult to keep their eyes on their own or their relatives'
children all the time, and older siblings were less able to competently act in the increasingly challenging role of babysitters. Thus it became easier for children to get into trouble.

As noted, East Cree culture includes many values that people could regularly fulfil as
part of the hunting way of life. In the hunting camps, respect for Elders was not merely an
ideal; it was continually put into practice. This was based on the fact that group welfare
was highly dependent on the knowledge and experience of Elders, who were respected
for their practical experience and advice. Even those Elders who were no longer active
hunters remained at the centre of the group's everyday decision making. Men were made
to feel important every time they returned to the camp with game, and women were
acknowledged for their skills in the things that they made every day for the others. By

contrast, in the settlement the knowledge of the Elders, although it continued to be respected, had little relevance for day-to-day life. Many of the men could no longer command respect as the breadwinners, and women found it difficult to cope with the new and more complex issues of household management.

Sociologically, hunting groups were composed of a core family whose members had intimate knowledge of and historic attachments to their group's particular hunting territory. Others in the group generally had close kinship ties with this core family. Although the composition of many of these groups remained stable from one year to the next, if tensions arose between the families during a particular hunting season, there was a strong ethic to suppress hostility for the balance of the winter, with the understanding that the following summer it would always be possible for the antagonists to go their separate ways, reorganizing hunting-group membership for subsequent winters. The hunting groups were moral communities in the sense that during the winter season, the families, although highly independent, were nevertheless tied together by bonds of reciprocal exchange. The more fortunate hunters regularly made gifts of game meat to the less fortunate ones. The unity of the group was symbolically emphasized in frequent communal feasts and at other ceremonials. But as more time was spent in the settlements, separation of antagonistic individuals was not always possible. Moreover, the settlements were too

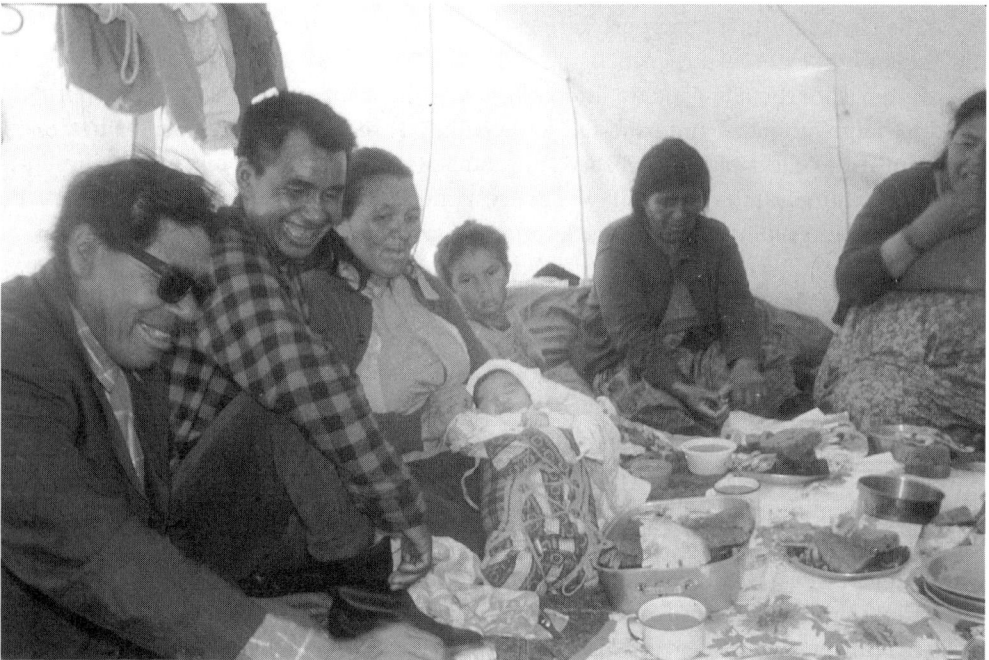

FIGURE 11.2   Multifamily communal feast in a Mistissini hunting camp, late 1960s. (Photo: A. Tanner)

ADRIAN TANNER

large to be effective moral communities in the same way that the hunting camps had been, so hostile schisms and factions sometimes emerged.

The religious traditions and practices of Cree hunting groups were directly relevant to their everyday existence. The environment was seen both in practical terms and as being infused with personalized spiritual powers. Individuals attributed their hunting success to powers rooted in each person's harmonious relations with the animals and the spiritual realm. Individual hunters communicated with the animal spirits by singing, playing the drum, and making offerings. A hunter's relations with the game were grounded in the principle that the animals were spiritual persons. The animals were believed to give themselves to hunters on condition that the hunters in turn treated the animals with respect. This belief system was used to account for any unusual hunting failures and for major declines in the population of certain animals. Most ordinary forms of sickness were explained in nonspiritual terms, and cures using material from the bush were known to most people; but illnesses that did not respond to these treatments were assumed to be due to some serious offence that the patient had given to an animal or spiritual entity or due to sorcery being practised against the person by someone with shamanistic powers. Although most Cree had been devout Anglicans for several generations, they saw no conflict between Christianity and continuing to receive communication from the spirit world. During the fur-trade period, a form of religious dualism was practised by the Cree – in winter, while they were in the bush, they practised the form of animistic religion outlined above, and, when they lived at the trading post during the summer, they practised Christianity under the guidance of external authority figures (Rousseau and Rousseau 1952). Many practices that were part of the animistic tradition of the hunting camps were held to be inappropriate behaviour within the context of the settlement. The sedentarization process threatened this animistic tradition and diminished the status of those who had previously enjoyed a respected reputation for their ability to process special power within the practices of the tradition. Moreover, many of the youth returning from residential school, not having experienced the animistic practices in the camps, acquired a distorted and overly negative view of them.

Before sedentarization, the short summer period at the trading posts was one of intense socialization. A ceremony was held when hunters first arrived at the post to initiate trading. Throughout the summer, marriages took place and there was regular church attendance as well as feasts and drinking parties. Some would leave with the canoe brigades to transport supplies to the trade post, and others would spend part of the time at camps near the post. Although alcohol had been introduced through the fur trade, this introduction does not by itself explain the later problems. By the 1960s, when the move to houses was under way, binge drinking and wild parties involving most of the band occurred. At these times, hostile feelings would sometimes come to the surface, and fights sometimes resulted. However, few long-term problems resulted from these fights since most people soon dispersed to bush camps for the long winter period. Sedentarization was in many ways an extension of these summer social conditions, which to some extent became the year-round state of affairs. But under these new circumstances, the pattern of binge drinking had far more serious consequences for the whole settlement.

Settlement

The move of the East Cree into settlement houses followed from the policy of extending "modernity" to isolated Aboriginal groups in the form of social services that other Canadians had come to accept as standard – mandatory local public education, public health services, and social welfare[4] – as well as from the policy of encouraging employment in the industrial economy. The process began in the 1950s and continued throughout the 1970s (Salisbury 1986). Houses, although at first meagre, as well as local schools and the prospect of jobs, attracted many Cree at the time, but as outlined above, these innovations had many implications that were apparently not understood by government planners, so no adequate preparations were made. Because of the legal and administrative basis of these settlements as Indian reserves, many aspects of daily life were established on the basis of external decisions.[5]

Once the sedentarization process was under way, the new settlements became much more accessible to outside contact than were the trading posts. For instance, as late as the 1960s, the community of Mistissini was still largely excluded from Canadian mainstream society. Although there were a few roads in the general area, until 1970 immediate access to Mistissini village generally involved a canoe or a snowmobile trip. Yet at that time, Mistissini was one of the more accessible East Cree settlements. Since then all but one of the East Cree settlements have acquired road access. One consequence for the Cree of the new increased accessibility was that some had their first experiences of overt racism in the nearby industrial towns.[6]

In the late 1960s and early 1970s, I was aware that many pressures were being placed on the Cree to abandon the hunting way of life. School children, in particular, were advised that hunting and trapping had no future (Asch 1995, 292; Ianzelo and Richardson 1974). During the 1960s, fur prices generally had been falling. At the same time, the HBC had adopted a general policy of eliminating credit to trappers, upon which the trapping economy was dependent. The need for cash to continue the hunting way of life was further increased by mechanization. This process had begun in a small way during the 1950s and had begun to make major changes to this way of life by the 1970s in the form of snowmobiles, outboard motors, trucks, and air transport. The consequent demand for cash for hunting was made worse by the sudden rise in the cost of oil in 1976.

In order to access government services that were available only in the settlements, people began spending longer periods of time there. Living together closely in permanent houses with several hundred other people was a new experience for northern Aboriginal people. The closest comparable occurrence during the preceding fur-trade period had been the summer gatherings at the post. The opening of the settlements to roads gave them access to new items that could be purchased and also provided the opportunity to visit other places, but both of these changes required further new sources of cash income.

ADRIAN TANNER

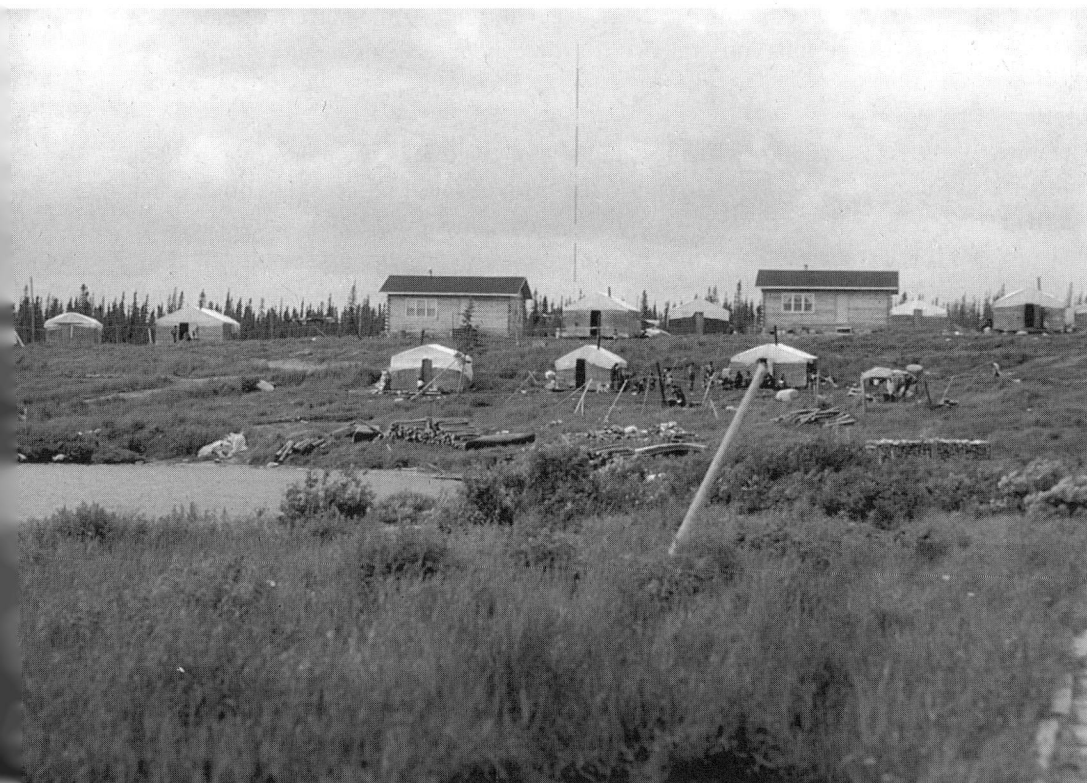

FIGURE 11.3   Some of the first government-built houses, alongside locally constructed tents, at Mistissini village, late 1960s. (Photo: A. Tanner)

Some administrative jobs became available in the community for the few with suitable education, and there were a few semiskilled jobs in house construction for a few months a year, but there was not enough work to support all families year-round. However, the government did little to prepare the Cree for this transition.

Although most northern Aboriginal groups at the time were under similar pressures to reduce their involvement in the hunting economy, to seek cash from other sources, and to spend longer periods in the settlement, in northern Quebec these factors would lead not to elimination of the Cree hunting economy but to its transformation. As there were no other viable economic alternatives for most people, some took advantage of government subsidies to continue hunting and trapping. A few school graduates found work, many of them taking over the types of jobs formerly held by Euro-Canadians in the increasingly complex local and regional form of governance of the Cree communities. Others found employment in resource industries and in construction, and still others took up jobs in the small local service sector. In little more than a generation, the Cree went

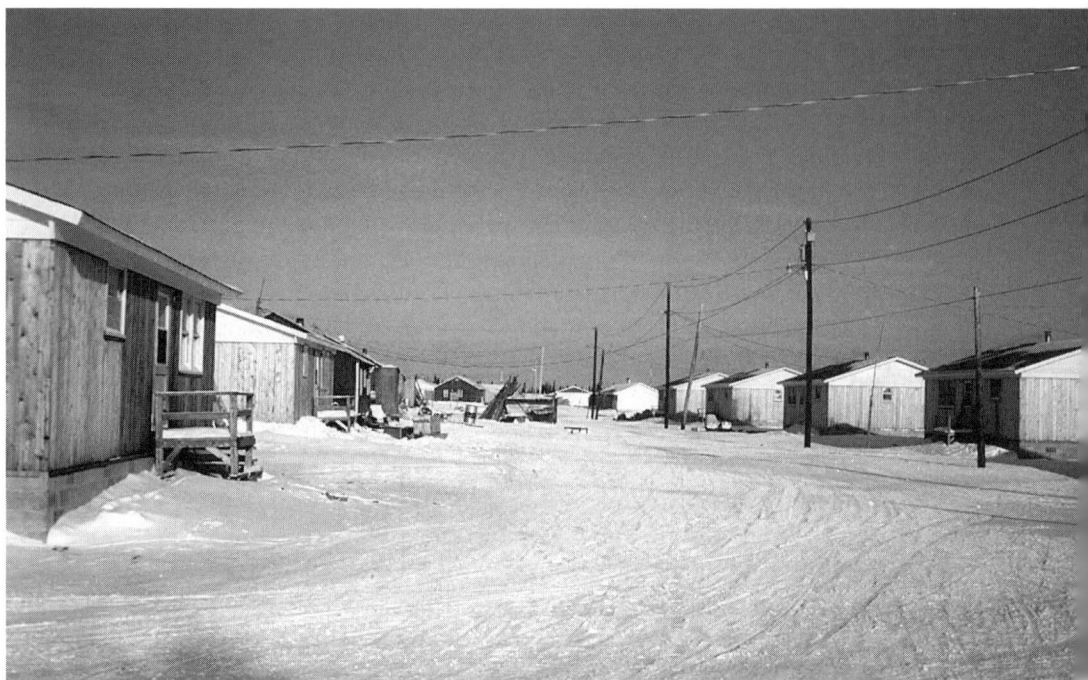

FIGURE 11.4 Newly built government housing at Eastmain village, 1976.
(Photo: Marguerite MacKenzie)

from a society in which all families had the same subsistence-oriented hunting/trapping economy and way of life to one with a complex division of labour and a consequent emerging class division.

Also during the 1970s, the Cree of the whole eastern James Bay region of Quebec began to assert themselves collectively within the political context of the Canadian state. Initially, this occurred mainly through the legal attempt to stop the James Bay Hydroelectric Project, which had been unilaterally announced by the Quebec government in 1971. After almost two years, the Cree achieved a significant legal victory against the project, but it proved too late to stop a project that was by then past a point of no return. However, the victory did make possible the subsequent negotiation of the 1975 land claims agreement. In these legal and political initiatives, the Cree found that, as a minority, they needed to become unified around a political ideology. They found such an ideology in their hunting legacy, with its central focus on their unique attachment to their land.

The signing of the James Bay Agreement introduced changes that, among other things, aided the Cree in their efforts to combat social breakdown. The Income Security Program (ISP) for hunters, already referred to, was a social program that was effectively a better alternative than social welfare: by subsidizing the continuation of the hunting way of life,

ADRIAN TANNER

it provided a socially and nutritionally preferable alternative to welfare recipients living idly in the village eating store food. Due to this program, more Quebec Cree are hunting than ever before, although given the overall population explosion, these hunters constitute a minority of the total population.[7] The school curriculum and the school calendar were also modified to provide for periods when children could spend time with their parents in the hunting camps, thereby improving proficiency in their own language and learning something of the bush way of life with their parents. Because of residential schools, and later the ISP and other benefits from the James Bay Agreement, the East Cree were able to maintain the hunting way of life and to make the transition to settlement life more satisfactorily than were many other arctic and subarctic Aboriginal groups.

The Healing Movement

Although alcohol was introduced to the Cree with the early fur trade, binge drinking became a significant social problem only in the 1960s, when people began to spend more lengthy periods in the settlement. In the early 1970s the Pentecostal Church became established in the region, effectively representing the first social movement in the Quebec Cree communities that directly addressed the problem of alcohol abuse. Not only did Crees who joined this church give up alcohol, they were also required by the church to abandon the practices of communication with the spirits, which had formerly been a major part of the hunting way of life. Pentecostal converts frequently burned the drums and other paraphernalia that they had formerly used when communicating with the spirits during the hunt.

Another reaction to problems like family breakdown caused by alcohol abuse was the formation of a local Aboriginal police force, also allowed for under the James Bay Agreement. Officers who came from the community were believed to be better able to deal sensitively with family disturbances than were strangers. Those Cree who had serious drinking problems were initially sent away to southern Aboriginal treatment programs, but later some of these alcohol programs were transferred to the community.

The first local community initiatives to address social breakdown had been instigated by returnees from the southern alcohol programs, who in these programs had been introduced to pan-Indian ceremonial practices, such as the sweat lodge, the peace pipe, sweet grass, and Pow-Wow drumming and dancing (Archambault 1996). Some tried to introduce these activities into their communities, but in many cases there was resistance to what were seen by others as non-Cree practices.

Some treated both Pentecostalism and pan-Indianism as outside influences, and these people complained that Cree local traditions ought to be utilized to deal with local social problems. They responded to these outside influences by initiating events based on local cultural practices, events that became known collectively as the "healing movement." One common feature of this movement is an annual "traditional" gathering, usually held in summer. The location, often at some distance from the settlement, represents a symbolic return to the bush and the hunting way of life, as well as to the past. In two communities,

Waswanipi and Nemeska, the gatherings are held at the site of the community's former trading post, long since abandoned. In these cases, the gathering is referred to by a Cree term, *ciiweydow,* which means "going back home." At Mistissini the location of the gathering is also highly symbolic. It is held part way up a lake on the canoe route that many hunters used on their way to the trading post in summer. During the fur-trade period, this camping site was the place where hunters and their families used to congregate, dress in their best clothes, and prepare themselves for their final entry to the trading post in a brigade of canoes.

Among the East Cree, these events are known as "gatherings," "culture camps," "cultural retreats," or "healing conferences." At these events, people self-consciously engage in traditional practices, living in the types of dwellings used in traditional hunting camps, eating traditional food cooked as it is in hunting camps, and engaging in ceremonies otherwise normally held only in the bush. In the evenings, traditional dances and feasts are held. These events are variously explained as efforts to overcome the disincentives to hunting, as forms of education for youth who otherwise experience discontinuities in their exposure to the traditional religion of hunting, or as forms of healing to address social pathologies.

On average, the gatherings last about a week. They depend to some degree on the financial support and organizational services of the band bureaucracy and also on the volunteer work of many community members. Game food that has been kept in family freezers is shared, and communal feasts are held. Elders have a special part to play, as they are called on to tell stories, prepare hides, demonstrate crafts, and prepare traditional medicines. Another focus is the children, who are intended to learn traditions from the Elders as well as to enjoy themselves. Stories are shared, and, at evening time, music is played and dances performed. Jokes, pranks, and good humour prevail.

A traditional gathering is often also the occasion to celebrate something in particular. For example, at one Mistissini gathering a re-enactment of a canoe brigade was held, complete with people dressed in old-fashioned clothes, with their canoes being towed one behind the other, as had been done in the past when families that were returning to the post in spring would arrive in a convoy, to be greeted with ceremonial gunfire. At another Mistissini gathering all those married 30 years or more were honoured with a feast that was a reconstruction of the kind of wedding feast the couples had enjoyed when they were first married. On a third occasion several young children were given a traditional communal "walking out" ceremony. This event, previously held in the hunting camps, marks the time when a child is first able to leave the dwelling on his or her own and symbolizes the gender-specific activity associated with the hunting way of life. A tree is set up in front of the door of the dwelling, and a path of boughs is laid between the door and the tree. The child is led to the tree dressed in traditional attire and carrying gender-appropriate implements – a gun or bow for males and an axe for girls. The child then takes a bundle from under the tree – a game animal like a beaver or goose in the case of boys and firewood or boughs in the case of girls. The child then returns to the house and presents the bundle to an Elder, often a grandparent, after which a feast is held.

Other traditional gatherings are organized to coincide with the climax of another separate event. One year at Waswanipi, the last day of the traditional gathering was arranged to coincide with the culmination of a 2-week long-distance canoe expedition by a group of young people. Another example of community recreation events being drawn into the healing movement involves communally organized long-distance snowshoeing, something that has become a popular part of the healing movement among the East Cree in the past few years (Nichols 2001; Wapachee 2001). These examples illustrate how healing-movement events incorporate other community forms of recreation. However, in contrast to other community sports events, those associated with the healing movement involve general community participation and are activities that have some symbolic connection to traditional Cree culture.

Sources of the Healing Movement

Although the East Cree have been in contact with Europeans for over 300 years, it was not until the advent of Western schooling that youth were subjected to prolonged contact with ways of thinking based on principles entirely different from those of their parents. Young East Cree people now finish high school having been intensively exposed to Western scientific notions about the natural world's being subject to physical laws as well as exposed to Christian-influenced moral philosophy. By contrast, most of them will have had relatively little exposure to their parents' forms of knowledge or to religious traditions concerning animals and the natural environment. This is because, apart from the activities of the healing movement, most of the time they spend with their families occurs in the settlement, while their parents generally bring animistic thinking into everyday life and practice only when they are living in the hunting camps.

The social breakdown that followed from the move to settlement life was marked by many personal tragedies, including suicides, homicides, and accidental deaths, events that have left their mark on whole communities. Not only did the resulting social dysfunction help add to the erosion of hunting, but there has also been some decline in the traditional rules of respect toward animals and the etiquette observed between hunters. Nevertheless, as the healing movement exemplifies, there has also been a general revitalization of certain traditional religious ideas. I see the development of this movement as having been fed by three distinct religious traditions, although in different proportions in each of the East Cree villages.

One of these influences is the pan-Indian religious ideology and its associated practices. These include several public ceremonies, including an annual "Pow-Wow" (an event principally involving drumming, dancing, and other traditional activities), the sweat lodge, and the pipe ceremony. The form of these rituals associated with the Pow-Wow has its origins among the Plains Indians, including the Plains Cree, who are located to the south and west of the forest-dwelling northern Cree. The pan-Indian ideology and associated activities were included in many Aboriginal-run treatment programs, particularly those of western Canada and Ontario.

Pan-Indian religious ideology and its associated practices have a greater focus on a single central entity, referred to as the "Creator" or "Great Spirit," compared to the local traditional animism practised by East Cree hunters, in which multiple spiritual entities are recognized. Although other animist entities are also recognized in pan-Indian ideology, there is little emphasis on the spiritual beings that, among the East Cree, are identified with specific animal species and forces of nature. In pan-Indian ideology more attention is paid to concepts and entities with multivocal and abstract symbolic referents, such as the "medicine wheel" (Archambault 1996). There is also a greater concern in pan-Indian ideology with curing than is the case with the East Cree animism, which is focused more on predicting and interpreting encounters with game animals. This theme of animal encounters does have a place in the pan-Indian religious ideology, however, particularly in the context of the "spirit quest." There are other features that are shared between pan-Indian and East Cree religious practice, like tobacco offerings, the sweat lodge, and the shaking tent ceremony, although each of these is used in a somewhat different way in each tradition. Other pan-Indian practices, like Pow-Wow costume dancing and the associated styles of drumming and singing as well as burning sweet grass for spiritual purification, are new to the present-day East Cree.

The second important, if less direct, influence on the development of the healing movement has been the Pentecostal Church. This denomination has gained a significant following over the past 20 years in some East Cree settlements, often effectively dividing settlements into two factions: converts and nonconverts. Although the religious ideology of Pentecostalism is totally incompatible with parts of the ideology of the healing movement, both focus attention on the prevalence of social pathologies. The arrival of Pentecostalism in a particular settlement had the effect of focusing public attention, among nonconverts as much as converts, on the symptoms of social pathology. It also caused some nonconverts to question the basis of their religious beliefs.

As noted above, before the advent of the healing movement, a form of "religious dualism" existed among the East Cree: traditional animism was largely confined to the hunting camp, whereas most Christian practices were largely confined to the settlement (Rousseau and Rousseau 1952). Whereas Pentecostalism openly sought to stamp out Cree animist practices, including those that remained relatively hidden from public view in the hunting camps, the healing movement has taken the opposite direction, bringing many aspects of the traditional animist religion of the camp into the settlement, effectively expanding their earlier social context. The effect of both these movements has been to break down the religious dualism of the past.

Despite its obvious conflicts with East Cree animism, Pentecostalism as practised by the Cree is not entirely opposed to an animist perspective. In fact, it actually entails a form of affirmation of the animist entities believed to control the forces of nature. When becoming a member of the Pentecostal Church, converts are required to publicly dissociate themselves from their former animist ritual practices. It was explained by the first Euro-Canadian Pentecostal ministers that the animist entities were actually forms of the Christian devil, meaning that rituals that involved communication with these entities had to be suppressed. However, the Pentecostal converts with whom I spoke some years later said they believed that only certain Cree animist practices, those involving sorcery and magic, actually constituted communication with the Christian devil. Although they had also stopped practising other animist rituals, including drumming and singing to animal spirits as well as hunting divination, they did this only as a sign of their new Christian status and also because they now considered it improper to use supernatural assistance in hunting. The issue for the Cree Pentecostals is thus not one of a Christian-animist ontological incompatibility. There is agreement between Pentecostals and animists over the existence and the power of the animist entities; the disagreement is over whether it is acceptable to have relations with them.

In contrast to those Cree who advocate either the Pentecostal or the pan-Indian approach to community healing, a third source of influence can be identified, involving people who reject both approaches because neither derives from their own local East Cree cultural traditions. However, in response to this complaint, some East Cree who do support pan-Indian events say that by participating in these events, they are now simply recovering former ritual practices. They assert that during the precontact period, these practices were shared by all the Cree, but after contact only the Plains Cree maintained them. But for some Quebec Cree, particularly some Elders, their reaction to pan-Indian ideologies and practices, as well as to those of the Pentecostal Church, has been to reject them as not stemming from their own local tradition. Instead, these people have organized a variety of events that incorporate local traditions, albeit in a new form. In some cases, these events were also a response to young people who complained that they knew nothing of their parents' own Aboriginal religious traditions.

Traditionally, East Cree religious practices were passed on without any formal apprenticeship; instead, the young were expected to acquire them in the hunting camps through silent observation of the activities of their Elders. Later, when living in hunting camps, the young Cree were expected to acquire religious knowledge through direct inspiration, in the form of dreams and visions, usually in connection with hunting. This whole learning process was completely disrupted by the introduction of formal education. Moreover, in the new settlement these methods of passing on knowledge were no longer adequate. The new organized events of the healing movement were effectively a "neo-traditional" way to pass on traditional knowledge.

At the same time, there has effectively been a reformulation of East Cree animist practice. Formerly, this had largely been focused on hunting. The organized gatherings and other events make animist ideas more appropriate to a settlement-based population. The neo-traditional events have also become the means for those adults whose jobs required them to live full-time in a settlement to spend time in a bush camp and to share some of the experience of bush living. Among the James Bay Cree, the experience of bush living is to some degree incorporated into modern life through the alteration of the school year to incorporate a break in the spring, which allows children to live with their parents at a camp, which for many is a goose-hunting camp. In some of the other programs, youth, including those undergoing treatment, are taken to live in a hunting camp in the bush.

A number of similarities can be seen among the above three religious influences on the modern healing movement. Pan-Indianism and neo-traditional animism are transformations of the animist concepts that were once followed by many northern Aboriginal people. Even Christian church services have begun to incorporate traditional animist elements; for example, the public declarations of personal salvation that characterize Pentecostal services sometimes include dream revelations, a basic component of the Algonkian animist religion.[8] Moreover, as noted above, acceptance of traditional spiritual entities may continue after conversion to Pentecostalism, although the position of these entities in the moral universe has changed, as they are now more likely to be seen as involved in sorcery and therefore bad, whereas before they were more often seen as good in terms of the assistance they provided to hunters.

To summarize, the healing movement, a new form that both draws on Aboriginal religious tradition and incorporates external influences, has certain key features. It sponsors settlement-wide communal rituals at formalized events, usually called "gatherings," which have the therapeutic goal of combating social pathology by bringing about a renewal and rehabilitation of personal pride and ethnic identity. At these events the knowledge, beliefs, and practices, both animist and nonreligious, which were until recently confined to bush camps as an adjunct to hunting, are reformulated and presented both to instruct the young and to make aspects of the hunting camp lifestyle accessible to those adults now largely confined to settlement life.

The Significance of the Healing Movement

Although many indigenous forms of therapies are identified with the contemporary Aboriginal "healing movement," this term also applies more broadly to other activities in which people engage as "communities" rather than focusing on the behaviour of problem individuals. I suggest that these group activities constitute local-level community-building initiatives that are intended to contribute to the general aim of collective support. Rather than being forms of treatment as such, these activities are intended to prevent problems from getting started, as well as to ensure that those who have completed treatment do not subsequently fall back into their former problematic ways.

These local-level community-building kinds of healing-movement activities embody certain characteristic principles that distinguish them from the therapeutic programs,

ADRIAN TANNER

whether or not the latter are explicitly considered part of the healing movement. One such principle is that the activities are based on an understanding that regardless of who is to blame for causing the problem of social pathology, it is those most directly concerned who must take responsibility for finding the solution. A second principle is that instead of dealing with the problem in the psyche of the individual patient, the activities address the problem within the collectivity. For this reason, "healing" is addressed at the level of the community as a whole, and the healing-movement activities are essentially exercises in community building. A third distinctive principle is that these kinds of healing-movement activities use local, culturally appropriate forms of action.

As already indicated, the healing movement can be seen as effectively in competition with Pentecostalism and pan-Indianism. Nonetheless, what must be stressed is that in contexts where these three paths cross, the Cree generally make every effort toward inclusion, consensus, and tolerance. The gatherings are arranged to involve as many of the community as possible. Thus, although the healing movement can be seen as stressing local, neo-traditional Cree ideology (in reaction to "external" Christian and pan-Indian influences), this aspect is distinctly muted at the traditional gatherings in deference to the feelings of others. Likewise, Pentecostals who do attend the gatherings no longer show offence if a traditional drum is brought out and played, although it is understood that some activities, such as the shaking tent performance, would be beyond acceptable bounds.

In my view, this tolerance between neo-traditional Cree, Pentecostalism, and pan-Indianism is based on a shared underlying animist ontology. Such ontology is non-Western, even though formal education and media have spread Western scientific and other conceptions of reality to the Cree, especially among the youth. Like other peoples, the Cree are capable of accommodating multiple ontologies. Although both Pentecostalism and pan-Indianism have a primary personified entity – the Christian God of the former and the Great Spirit of the latter – neither rejects the animist idea of "other-than-human persons" central to traditional Cree religion. When Pentecostals refuse to participate in ceremonial forms of communication with the spirit world, it is not because they do not believe in the existence or the power of these entities. On the contrary, they affirm them to be powerful forces but ones that are of such potential danger that they must be avoided. Similarly, pan-Indianism does not reject the local spiritual beliefs and practices. However, its practitioners believe in a more deep-seated reality behind the particular local practices and seek to find linkages between those of all North American Aboriginal peoples.

Unlike most alcohol-treatment programs, the healing movement does not generally single out and target individuals who exhibit problem behaviour, although neither does it exclude them. Where the sweat lodge and other healing ceremonies have been incorporated into the movement, they may be used to focus on such individuals, who in these ceremonies may experience profound emotional release. However, in most cases, the traditional gathering can be seen more in terms of addressing the problem of the collectivity. The solution to social breakdown is thus to build and heal the community, not to concentrate on the treatment of the problem individuals within it.

One focus in this community building is the youth, who may be felt to have lost their direction because they have lost their traditions; the gatherings represent an effort to reverse this trend by teaching. Another focus of the gatherings is to pay tribute and respect to the Elders of the community. There are few opportunities for this to occur in the settlement. Consequently, the Elders see the youth as not paying them the attention that is due to them, so they feel unable to pass on their knowledge. For the middle-aged, especially those who are employed and unable to live in the bush, the gatherings represent a recollection of childhood, a form of nostalgic pleasure.

The most salient general characteristic of the healing-movement activities described in this chapter, one that most clearly distinguishes them from the therapy programs, is that they are communal and open to everyone. Thus the focus of "healing" is the "community" rather than the healing needs of particular individuals or families that are undergoing problems. I believe it is significant that the underlying assumption of these healing-movement activities is that the cause of social pathology lies in the collectivity rather than in the psyches of problem individuals.

As noted, the term "community," which is widespread in Western social science, is a particularly difficult one to define. In its Western sense, it is a concept that is deeply based within European and American values and ideals about how people ought to behave toward each other when living in face-to-face groups. It harks back to agricultural origins in rural settlements. It suggests an altruistic attitude toward neighbourliness and communal co-operation. However, these ideals do not just appear equally in all human groupings but emerge from institutions that have given expression to certain ideals about collective life. We may thus understand the concept of "healthy community" as one that has the institutions and processes to allow residents to experience such ideals, although without imagining that the romantic image of community harmony is a permanent state of affairs that can be taken for granted.

The features of a "healthy community" do not just form naturally among all human residential groupings, which is what seems to have been the ethnocentric assumption made by government officials in planning and carrying out the public policies by which northern Aboriginal hunting peoples were moved into settlements. On the contrary, "community" must be seen as a culturally specific and situationally determined phenomenon. When one form of community, such as that of the Cree hunting group, is rapidly obliterated due to changed circumstances, a new form that is in keeping with the new circumstances of government-imposed settlement needs to be socially constructed if severe social problems are to be avoided. From the East Cree example, it appears that significant efforts and experimentation are required in order to construct this new form of community. In this case, the new community draws from the Crees' past but also reflects their present values. It seems to me that this kind of "community building" is what the healing movement, as here conceived, is all about.

ADRIAN TANNER

Notes

1 However, this term has also been applied to therapy programs that addressed the social problems of Aboriginal individuals and families with behavioural problems.

2 This kind of normalization of what would otherwise have been deviant, occurring under extreme circumstances, has been documented in other cases. Among some Brazilian slum dwellers, infant mortality rates became so high as to undermine the normal expression of maternal grief at the death of a child (Scheper-Hughes 1992). And among the dispossessed Ik of the Uganda-Kenya border region, who were undergoing forced settlement and starvation (Turnbull 1972), there was a suspension of normal interpersonal relations. However, these cases are to be distinguished from the settlement of northern Canadian Aboriginal groups in that the suspension of the normal in these cases was imposed by extreme material deprivation.

3 From 1969 to 1971 and in 1973, I lived in hunting camps of the Mistissini Cree (Tanner 1979). Previously, between 1957 and 1959, I observed Inuit camp life at Port Harrison (now Inukjuak), northern Quebec, some years before they were settled into houses. And in the Yukon, between 1964 and 1966, I lived with Tutchone hunters a few years after they had been settled into houses.

4 Apparently, no consideration was given to bringing education, health, and social services directly to the people in the bush camps by means of radio communication and direct visits, as was done, for instance, for the education of Australian children living on outback ranches.

5 Since that time this situation has begun to change under the influence of government policies to permit limited forms of self-government.

6 In 1967 one bar on the main street of Chibougamau, the nearest industrial town to Mistassini, had a sign above its main entrance: "No Indians."

7 In 1976 a total of 980 Cree families were registered in the Income Security Program. By 1995, this had risen to about 1,200 (Feit 1995, 122).

8 Elsewhere, I have detailed East Cree practices involving the interpretation of dreams in the context of hunting divination (Tanner 1979, 125-26).

References

Abadian, S. 1999. From wasteland to homeland: Trauma and the renewal of indigenous peoples and their communities. PhD diss., Harvard University.

Adelson, N. 2000. Re-imagining Aboriginality: An indigenous peoples' response to social suffering. *Transcultural Psychiatry* 37 (1): 11-34.

Archambault, J. 1996. Pan-Indian organizations. In F.E. Hoxie, ed., *Encyclopaedia of North American Indians,* 462-64. Boston: Houghton Mifflin.

Asch, M. 1995. The Slavey Indians: The Relevance of ethnohistory to development. In R.B. Morrison and C.R. Wilson, eds., *Native peoples: The Canadian experience,* 2nd ed., 260-85. Toronto, ON: McClelland and Stewart.

Brint, S. 2001. Gemeinschaft revisited: A critique and reconstruction of the community concept. *Sociological Theory* 19 (1): 1-23.

Busidor, I., and Ü. Bilgen-Reinhart. 1997. *Night spirits: The story of the relocation of the Sayisi Dene*. Winnipeg, MB: University of Manitoba Press.

Carstens, P. 1991. *The Queen's people. A study of hegemony, coercion, and accommodation among the Okanagan of Canada*. Toronto, ON: University of Toronto Press.

Chance, N.A. 1968. Implications for environmental stress for strategies of developmental change among the Cree. In N.A. Chance, ed., *Conflict in culture: Problems of developmental change among the Cree,* 11-32. Ottawa, ON: Canadian Research Centre for Anthropology, St. Paul University.

Chandler, M.J., and C. Lalonde. 1998. Cultural continuity as a hedge against suicide in Canada's First Nations. *Transcultural Psychiatry* 35 (2): 191-219.

Driben, P., and R.S. Trudeau. 1983. *When freedom is lost: The dark side of the relationship between government and the Fort Hope Band*. Toronto, ON: University of Toronto Press.

Dunning, R.W. 1964. Some problems of reserve Indian communities: A case study. *Anthropologica* 6 n.s.: 3-38.

Elias, P.D. 1996. Worklessness and social pathologies in Aboriginal communities. *Human Organization* 55 (1): 13-24.

Feit, H.A. 1982. The income security program for Cree hunters in Quebec: An experiment in increasing the autonomy of hunters in a developed nation sate. *Canadian Journal of Anthropology* 5 (1): 57-70.

–. 1995. Colonialism's northern cultures: Canadian institutions and the James Bay Cree. In B.W. Hodgins and K.A. Cannon, eds., *On the land: Confronting the challenges of Aboriginal self-determination,* 105-27. Toronto, ON: Betelgeuse Books.

Gerber, L. 1979. The development of Canadian Indian communities: A two-dimensional typology reflecting strategies of adaptation to the modern world. *Canadian Journal of Sociology and Anthropology* 16 (4): 404-24.

Hawthorn, H.B. 1966. *A survey of the contemporary Indians in Canada: Economic, political, educational needs and policies.* Vols. 1 and 2. Ottawa, ON: Canadian Department of Indian Affairs and Northern Development.

Hodgeson, M. 1990. *Impact of residential schools and other root causes of poor mental health*. Edmonton, AB: Necchi Institute.

Ianzelo, T., and B. Richardson. 1974. *Our land is our life.* Film. Montreal, QC: National Film Board of Canada.

Inglis, G.B. 1969. Canadian Indian reserve populations: Some problems of conceptualization. *Northwest Anthropological Research Notes* 5 (1): 23-36.

Kleinman, A., V. Das, and M. Lock, eds. 1997. *Social suffering*. Berkeley, CA: University of California Press.

Kulchyski, P. 1988. Towards a theory of dispossession: Native politics in Canada. PhD diss., York University.

Malloy, J. 1999. *A national crime*. Winnipeg, MB: University of Manitoba Press.

Nichols, W. 2001. Journeys. *The Nation* 8 (10): 3, 10-17.

Niezen, R. 1993. Power and dignity: The social consequences of hydro-electric development for the James Bay Cree. *Canadian Review of Sociology and Anthropology* 30 (4): 510-29.

O'Neil, J.D. 1983. Is it cool to be an Eskimo? A study of stress, identity, coping and health among Canadian Inuit young men. PhD diss., University of California.

Rousseau, M., and J. Rousseau. 1952. Le dualisme religieux des peuples de la forêt boréale. *Proceedings of the 29th International Congress of Americanists* 2: 118-26.

Salisbury, R.F. 1986. *A homeland for the Cree: Regional development in James Bay, 1971-1981*. Montreal, QC, and Kingston, ON: McGill-Queen's University Press.

Samson, C. 2003. *A way of life that does not exist: Canada and the extinguishment of the Innu*. St. John's, NL: ISER Books.

Scheper-Hughes, N. 1992. *Death without weeping: The violence of everyday life in Brazil*. Berkeley, CA: University of California Press.

Scott, J.C. 1998. *Seeing like a state: How certain schemes to improve the human condition have failed*. New Haven, CT: Yale University Press.

Shkilnyk, A. 1985. *A poison stronger than love*. New Haven, CT: Yale University Press.

Smart, R.G. 1979. A note on the effects of changes in alcohol control policies in the Canadian North. *Journal of Studies on Alcohol* 40 (9): 908-13.

Stevenson, D. 1968. *Problems of Eskimo relocation for industrial employment: A preliminary study*. Ottawa, ON: Northern Science Research Group, Indian and Northern Affairs.

ADRIAN TANNER

Tanner, A. 1979. *Bringing home animals: Religious ideology and mode of production of the Mistassini Cree hunters.* St. John's, NL: ISER Books.

Tester, F.J., and P. Kulchyski. 1994. *Tammarniit (mistakes): Inuit relocation in the eastern Arctic, 1939-63.* Vancouver, BC: UBC Press.

Turnbull, C.M. 1972. *The mountain people.* New York: Simon and Schuster.

Vallee, F.G. 1968. Stresses of change and mental health among the Canadian Eskimos. *Archives of Environmental Health* 17 (4): 565-70.

Wapachee, A. 2001. The journey: Journey of wellness. *The Nation* 8 (9): 23.

York, G. 1992. *The dispossessed: Life and death in Native Canada.* Toronto, ON: Little Brown.

12

Toward a Recuperation of Souls and Bodies: Community Healing and the Complex Interplay of Faith and History

NAOMI ADELSON

The missionaries have tremendous difficulty converting the savages when they listen to these "conjurers." When the last embrace the Christian religion, they will disabuse their compatriots, explain to them the means they use to fool them and facilitate their adherence to Christianity.

– ATTRIBUTED TO FATHER LACOMBE, 1874

I am sorry, more than I can say, that we tried to remake you in our image.

– ARCHBISHOP MICHAEL PEERS, PRIMATE, ANGLICAN CHURCH
OF CANADA, 6 AUGUST 1993

Spiritual Colonization and the Legacy of Social Suffering

In 1997, while sitting deep in the bowels of Washington's Smithsonian Institution and immersed in the 1950s world of anthropologist John Honigmann's Great Whale River, a pleasantly helpful archivist gently touched my shoulder and asked whether I would be interested in seeing a document written in French, apparently (as she could not speak the language) related to the same region of Canada that I was researching. Dusting off my hands and shaking myself free from images and field notes from a more recent past, I accepted what I quickly realized could only be part of a missionary's diary and began to read. The excerpt, tellingly titled "La Médecine chez les Sauvages de l'Amérique du Nord" and dated 1874, was attributed to a Father Lacombe and consisted of detailed accounts of the shamanic and herbal healing practices of a western Cree population. Its contents revealed not only a host of successful indigenous therapies but also an author with keen observational and writing skills. Despite admitting all along his own surprise at the extent to which the treatments he observed were successful, he nonetheless ends his accounts with the following passage:

In this backward country, the missionary priest is the doctor of souls as well as bodies. These poor savages place their confidence in him and it is impossible to persuade them that the missionary cannot cure their sicknesses. This last procurement often alleviates their sadness by the confidence inspired and this is a means towards their conversion. Sometimes just a few words of encouragement is enough to put them at ease [leur mettre l'esprit en repos] and help them heal. Nonetheless the missionary is sometimes obliged to improvise the medicine. That is how Father Lacombe, by healing the son-in-law of a chief, who was diagnosed with an acute infection on his arm followed by the amputation of the hand, got the whole tribe to convert. (My translation)

This passage, gleaned from a diary serendipitously acquired, remains the impetus for this exploration into the relationship between faith, bodies, time, and healing. It is not simply the arrogance of the missionary's words that still shake me but also the apparent ease by which he simultaneously ministered to and, in effect, attempted to colonize peoples' bodies *and* souls. Yet this missionary's actions were far from unusual. So many priests' journals from this era attest both to their seemingly wilful blindness to the rich and vital belief system long in place throughout Aboriginal Canada and to their own conviction of the fundamental links between medicine and salvation (Kelm 1998). Bringing what they believed to be a "healing civilization" (Comaroff 1993; Kelm 1998) to the North, the missionaries attempted to systematically eradicate what they viewed as heathen beliefs and practices.

Despite being just one segment of the colonial enterprise, missionization remains to this day one of the most contentious domains of the history of contact and the key symbolic site of cultural slaughter and disenfranchisement. It is for this reason that, for many indigenous peoples, organized religion is emblematic of the entire enterprise of colonization. For others, however, Christian doctrine is a vital element of, and seamlessly incorporated into, a much older spiritual belief system. In this chapter, I examine the complex configuration of faith in people's lives as part of the contemporary effects of a history of both contact and conflict. In particular, I consider the reconfiguration of healing and recuperation in a small Cree community of northern Quebec.

We are all too aware of the high numbers of mental health issues in First Nations communities today, including interpersonal and intergenerational violence, substance abuse, and related accidental deaths and suicides (Adelson 2005; Kirmayer, Brass, and Tait 2000; Waldram, Herring, and Young 1995). To a large extent, these personal problems are individual expressions of social suffering. By "social suffering," I mean the embodied expression of damaging and often long-term and systemic asymmetrical social and political relations. In this instance, the social suffering of many Aboriginal persons is rooted in, but not limited to, the destructive legacy of colonization. In this postcolonial era, we are seeing communities actively grapple with, and attempt to expunge, the emotional, physical, and cultural effects of that colonial process. This is a period of *recuperation,* a time both of "taking back" (not simply retrieving) a lost or damaged past and of regaining individual and community health and strength in the process.

Many Aboriginal people speak about this recuperative process in terms of healing, and for many part and parcel of that process is a (re)awakening or renewal of indigenous spirituality (Harper 1995). Both healing and spirituality are potent and multilayered concepts, textured as much by what people are healing *from* as what they are healing *toward.* They are made even more complex by the fact that there are often varying interpretations of what constitutes a proper course of recuperation. Indeed, some First Nations communities are divided by exactly this process, imbued as it is with all the contemporary realities of diversity and difference that inform interpretations and valuations of spirituality, culture, tradition, and belief (for examples from Australia, see Rowse 1996; Kolig 2003). It is increasingly difficult, in other words, to navigate a course through customary practices, new interpretations of these practices, a barrage of media images and ideas about what it is supposed to mean to "be Native," and the stresses and strains of daily life, regardless of whether one lives in an urban, rural, or remote community. The recuperative process is equally complex, mediated as it is by a similar range of cultural, social, and political influences.

Mental health programs address the individual expressions of social suffering (e.g., depression, substance abuse, suicidal ideation), and many are looking for ways to develop appropriate, culturally sensitive models of care for First Nations populations (see Tanner, Chapter 11). There is an important and growing body of literature that addresses the ways that spiritual therapeutics (such as sweat lodges, pipe ceremonies, and other specific herbal or spiritual treatments) are being incorporated into the standard care of Aboriginal people in psychiatric as well as general medical practice (Waldram 1998; Waldram, Herring, and Young 1995). Increasingly, however, there is a shift toward a model of health care for indigenous peoples that relies on a far too static notion of tradition and culture, removing them entirely from lived contexts (see Calabrese 1997; Tolman and Reedy 1998). This sort of wholesale incorporation of "tradition" or "culture," however, may not adequately acknowledge the individual, community, social, and political contingencies or the range of locally based beliefs and practices that are not circumscribed within a set of predetermined boundaries of what constitutes either tradition or culture (see Grim 1996). More specifically, we cannot presume that any one form of Aboriginal spirituality, or healing for that matter, is commonly and equally shared by all members of any given community (Brady 1995; Rowse 1996; Waldram, Herring, and Young 1995; Tanner, Chapter 11). Nor can we assume that there is any one program of recuperation that would transcend these differences. With a view of culture as "contingent, negotiated and dynamic" (Adelson 2002, 292; Linnekin 1992; Rowse 1996), I will now move to an analysis of the scope and density of valuations of faith, spirituality, and healing in one small northern Cree community.

NAOMI ADELSON

Healing and Spirituality

Healing is never simply a personal, physical phenomenon. Although it implies a process of recuperation and recovery from personal or social traumas, healing always, by definition, takes place in a particular historical and social context. It must be understood, after all, that there would be nothing to recuperate *from* if the travesties associated with loss of land, resources, culture, or community were not at the heart of the personal traumas faced by so many First Nations people today. Political foot-dragging on issues of Aboriginal rights, land, and resources, inattention to the legacy of racist policies, and ignorance of the personal and cultural losses incurred through those policies and through practices such as residential school programs are the framework, context, and reason for healing. The social and political action now being taken by indigenous people across Canada attempts to actively address the decades of silence or inaction on these issues. The past decade's efforts of reconciliation by both government and religious communities have been important early steps in the recuperative process.[1] The 1993 apology by the Anglican Church of Canada is significant in that it was the first outright admission of guilt by a national church for the tremendous wrongs practised in the name of forced conversion (Peers 1993). Additionally, Elijah Harper's Sacred Assembly (Harper 1995),[2] the Royal Commission on Aboriginal Peoples, and, as one outcome of that, the federally funded Aboriginal Healing Foundation and its initiatives to redress the traumas inflicted through residential schools are all significant examples of the initial efforts to address some of the wrongs of the past. Inseparable from these broader political processes are the personal and community acts of recuperation, as people attempt to reconcile the embodied legacy of colonization. Healing thus connotes both a dynamic process of recuperation from an extensive burden of social, cultural, spiritual, political, and economic losses as well as the physical recuperation of bodies and minds.

What does spirituality mean in the context of healing, and how is it currently defined and practised? For many northern Quebec Cree (*Iiyiyu'ch,* pl.; *Ilyiyu,* sing.), for example, one's sense of spirituality is inseparable from one's sense of being. Fundamental to Cree life for many is a spiritual awareness and belief that is rooted in a hunting and land-based culture that simultaneously permeates everyday social relations and practices (Adelson 2000a; Feit 1986; Tanner 1979). This kind of spiritual belief is not, as the Elders explain later in this chapter, necessarily incongruent with Christian doctrine and, for many, has long been enmeshed with Christian belief (Preston 1981; Tanner, Chapter 11).

When we speak about Native spirituality today, however, many associate the term with particular beliefs that transcend – but do not exclude – specific, local practices. While not immediately connected to locally held beliefs, that form of spirituality is also based on the relationship between people living on earth and their spiritual ancestors. While we may associate Native spirituality with particular practices, such as the sweat lodge, healing circles, and pipe ceremonies, these are only the more highly visible elements of a far more complex, integrated, and holistic spiritual belief system.

Given that this belief system encompasses all aspects of life, it also includes a complete range of healing practices. Spiritual Elders are those who are recognized for their ability to communicate with or to act as an intermediary for spirit ancestors. These gifts may include medical knowledge, as spirit ancestors guide an Elder's actions in this world. As Samson succinctly explains, "[Elders] do not claim expertise over the physiological workings of the body. Rather, their power lies in an understanding, often intuitive, of the ways in which the cosmos connects with individual people" (1999, 77).

There has been a tremendous growth of Native spirituality across indigenous Canada, and this growth has occurred, significantly, in tandem with the larger, more overt political recuperative process. In Whapmagoostui, for example, both Mi'qmaq and eastern and western Cree Elders (pipe carriers, spiritual advisors, healers) have regularly been invited into the community over the past decade as guests of the community's cultural program. These Elders offer spiritual guidance, perform a variety of healing practices and ceremonies, lead sweat lodges, and train local members of the community to perform similar ceremonies. They have brought what is commonly referred to as "Native spirituality" into Whapmagoostui, to the delight of many but also to the dismay of others.

For many individuals, Native spirituality is viewed as an essential part of the recuperative process and, for them, replaces the imposed, organized religion brought by missionaries, which is more closely associated with the annihilation of indigenous spiritual belief and practice. As well, healing and Native spirituality are often inseparable, either because one turns to Native spirituality in order to heal or because healing, by definition, implies an adherence to the beliefs and practices of spirituality. Healing thus often connotes a recuperation of Aboriginal awareness, which is becoming increasingly synonymous with Native spirituality. For others in the same community, however, this form of spirituality is not only abhorrent but also anathema to their fundamental Christian beliefs. Indeed, fundamentalist (Pentecostal) Christianity is on the rise in some Cree communities (as outlined by Tanner in Chapter 11), while others continue to adhere to the older, more established churches (Church of England, Catholicism). Yet others are attempting – or continuing – long-practised forms of syncretic religious conduct, incorporating both Christian and Native spiritual norms. Thus, although there is a growing adherence to Native spirituality in Cree communities, there is simultaneously a range of Christian belief (including Pentecostalism, Anglicanism, and Catholicism) and concomitant enthusiastic involvement in the church. In sum, and as I will demonstrate below, at the community level one finds a tremendous diversity of spiritual practices and beliefs in this era of recuperation.

Healing and Spirituality in Whapmagoostui: In Conversation with Church Elders

I began to take particular interest in the complexity of spirituality, faith, and healing as I watched a small community debate exactly this issue. Although there was consensus around a reinvigoration of Aboriginal cultural values and practices, there was less agreement about what constituted those values and practices (Adelson 2000b, 2002). Divisions started to emerge, particularly around interpretations of faith. Of course, kin and social ties, political affiliations, and economic concerns (which programs get funded, which do not) all played a role in the alliances of thought on this subject. And, even though some people remained indifferent and others quietly chose from the range of options available, there seemed to be an almost palpable line dividing two particular camps of opinion in one very small community: those who are ardent (Anglican) church adherents and those who are actively and avidly turning to Native spirituality. It seemed as though the debate was growing more fractious with each passing year. Indeed, with rumours of a Biblical rationale to kill one of the guest spiritual Elders, the vocal and sometimes bitter debate seemed to have reached new heights.[3] It was not long after this particular rumour circulated that I began to discuss the subject directly with particular members of the community, namely the church Elders.[4] Having been born and raised on the land, yet being strong and long-time adherents to the church, these Elders represent a unique and valuable voice on this subject. I was not disappointed. The Elders all had passionate yet, for the most part, tempered and extremely thoughtful perspectives on an issue that is often all too fractious.

The political rhetoric that I consciously make use of as an anthropologist is of course absent from the voices of the Elders. They employ their own political nuance, however, allowing the listener (and reader) to contemplate a range of meanings behind their words. Regardless of where the Elders situate themselves, it is clear that they, along with the rest of this small community – and like so many other communities across Canada – are negotiating their sense of faith and of history in this era of recuperation. What follows are excerpts from my interviews with the Elders, selected in order to represent a spectrum of positions on Cree religious syncretism, Christianity, Native spirituality, and the recuperative process. Let me first, however, present a brief history and description of the community of Whapmagoostui.

The Community of Whapmagoostui

Whapmagoostui First Nation, one of the nine communities that make up the James Bay Cree (Iiyiyu'ch) First Nation, is located on a small spit of land on the Hudson Bay coast at the mouth of the Great Whale River. The permanent village that now exists at this site is but a few decades old and only a fraction of the land that is considered home to the northern Iiyiyu'ch. Nonetheless, the village is where people live most of the year, with more houses being built annually as the young population continues to grow. Also located in the village are the elementary and high schools, the local-government (band) offices, the church, clinic, stores, and hockey arena. This is, in other words, the main residence for most of the Iiyiyu population, although it is not the only residence, as the entire community spends at least a portion of the year on the land and engaged in hunting practices or the preparation and cooking of the hunted game.[5]

Although the Whapmagoostui Iiyiyu'ch (Cree) have lived and travelled in the northeastern region of present-day Quebec for well over 1,000 years, prospectors and fur traders arrived in the region less than 300 years ago, and missionaries arrived only about

150 years after that. The Iiyiyu'ch of present-day north-eastern Quebec continue to maintain strong links to the land and animals of this region (Adelson 2000a; Tanner 1979). The missionaries, however, saw Aboriginal spiritual life as abominable and worked very hard to eradicate what they viewed as inappropriate beliefs (Long 1985; Waldram, Herring, and Young 1995).

Indeed, much to the frustration of the missionaries, the Cree were far more willing to accept their material offerings than their religious doctrine. Reverend Edwin Watkins, who was the first missionary stationed at Fort George (1852-57) and who travelled out to the farther reaches of Cree lands (including the Little and Great Whale rivers), could never reconcile the reluctance the Cree felt toward Christianity. Watkins conveys some of his frustration with the Cree in his personal diaries, lamenting that whereas the people "felt little need for assistance for the soul, they readily applied for help for the *body*" (quoted in Long 1985, 94, original emphasis). If only, he later bemoans, they were as interested in the church as the "food, clothing and the blessings of the present life ... If Jesus had come into the world to give them flour, and oatmeal and tea they would have loved ... him and easily have remembered his name" (quoted in Long 1985, 105).

Later missionaries had more influence on the northern Cree than Watkins, in part because they were stationed at trading posts in these more northern reaches of Cree lands. In particular, Rev. Edmund Peck, who in 1876 became the first missionary to live among the northern Iiyiyu'ch, and Rev. W.G. Walton, who followed, are to this day remembered as having had the most influence in the missionization process (Adelson 2000a; Francis and Morantz 1983; Leith and Leith 1912). Even Walton, who had a truly profound effect, still never fully "converted" the Cree to the Church of England. Some argue that the reason the Cree never wholly incorporated Christianity was because they did not spend a long time at any given mission site or because, despite being in agreement with the teachings, there was little interest in the formal doctrine (Long 1985). This was very likely true, but aside from the practical limitations associated with a hunting lifestyle, one cannot downplay the independence of mind of the northern Cree (Morantz 1983; Francis and Morantz 1983). Indeed, Watkins despaired that even after four years of instruction, he was continually "confronted by the strong hold of what he referred to as 'superstitions'" (quoted in Long 1985, 102).

Regardless of why it was so, it is clear that, although deeply influenced by the church teachings, the northern Cree never accepted Christianity to the exclusion of Cree spiritual belief. This was confirmed by Bishop Caleb Lawrence, who, when interviewed in 1995, admitted that he realized that the Cree church Elders had always interspersed Cree and Christian spiritual beliefs as soon as he could speak their language.[6] Indeed, he feels very strongly that from the very earliest entry of Christianity into Cree belief, it was always as a modified form of Cree spirituality.

With the regular presence of Watkins, then Edmund Peck, and finally Rev. W.G. Walton, and with the growth of the village of Whapmagoostui as a more and more permanent settlement (with a permanent church and missionary in situ), the people increasingly incorporated the teachings of the Old and New Testaments. Although some individuals shunned or stopped practising some of what the church historically referred to as "heathen" acts (particularly the shaking tent ceremony), there was nonetheless a regular and unproblematic melding of Christianity and the vital animistic belief system. Preston (1981) refers to a "Cree Anglicanism" practised in the Hudson Bay coastal region, and this term aptly describes the religious practices of many of the Whapmagoostui Cree. The Cree Anglicanism that is practised is by no means a "folk" religion but a syncretic integration of two forms of religious belief and practice that has fused Cree and Christian beliefs in the interpretation of supernatural forces within Cree orthodoxy. The Christian God, for example, has traditionally been viewed as the omnipotent being in the hierarchy of spirits within Cree cosmology (Adelson 2000a; Feit 1983; Long 1985; Tanner 1979). The following excerpts from discussions with Whapmagoostui church Elders explain this cosmology:

> As soon as it is daylight, I look all around outside, at the mountains and the trees, and these things remind me that God has given us this town and all that we see on the land that grows. God has made everything that we see on earth. It is these times when we remember this that we must give thanks to God for these gifts and the land. The land is like a living person, that is alive. The food of the animals is growing on the land; everything is there to sustain them. In turn, the animals reproduce every year. That is what God had intended for the land to be like, everything that he had deemed for the Iiyiyu to survive on earth. When I look at the plan of God, which has been going for a long time, what He had given us Iiyiyu on the land, including the medicines from the land, He put everything on earth for us to live ... Everything that is beneath the land [implying the spirit world] is also always available. A person can be helped by these things if they want to know about *iiyiyu pmatisiiuun* [way of life]. (Interview 1)

> [Cree spirituality and Christianity] is the same thing. The *ntuhun* [wildlife] also has a *i'chaakw* [spirit]. The spirit of the ntuhun was the thing that told the Iiyiyu where to go to find the ntuhun when he is searching for them. The spirit of the Iiyiyu was the one that interpreted what the spirit of the animal has told him. His understanding of it came from his own spiritual life. That is how it was. When I mention the *ntuhun i'chaakw* [animal spirit], this spirit could not communicate to the Iiyiyu directly, but the spirit of the Iiyiyu was the interpreter of the animal spirit and told what this spirit had said. As it is told in the story, we are told that when someone conducts a *kusapichikin* [shaking tent ceremony], it was his *mistapaau* that told him things.[7] This is what I meant. The mistapaau understood everything and all language. The Holy Spirit understands

everything. All the languages come from this Spirit. It was like when the Holy Spirit came upon the Apostles when Jesus sent them the Holy Spirit. When the Holy Spirit came upon them, the Apostles were able to speak all kinds of languages. (Interview 2)

You must have heard when they talked about the geese and that people are supposed to watch how many geese they kill. Some people think differently about this. I have heard some Iiyiyu's opinions about this on the radio. I am only talking about the nine Cree communities. These are the only Iiyiyu that I can understand when they speak. Some Iiyiyu think that the geese are not available because it may be God's will that the geese are not growing in numbers, but there may be a reason for this. Some Iiyiyu make sure that the feathers of the geese are not blowing all over the place, and they gather them in one place. Some people pluck outside, and then the feathers blow all over the place. Some Iiyiyu saw some geese where the "whiteman" hunted where they only took the breasts and left the rest to rot. When these things happen, we are continually being watched from heaven. If we do too many bad things, we are shown in some way our wrongs. That is what the old man I heard talking said. Sometimes we are shown that we have not shown respect to a certain animal, and that is why it does not grow in abundance. Some others think about it differently. We cannot all think the same. (Interview 3)

These statements attest to the ease of transition between animistic and Christian spiritual beliefs, which together form a congruous whole, a particular form of Christianity permeated and enhanced by the inherent power of animals and higher spirit beings (Preston 1981; for a comprehensive discussion of spirit hierarchies and power, see Feit 1983, 1986).

These animistic beliefs, however, are far more relevant to those who spend, or have spent, a considerable part of their lives on the land. The spirituality that so richly imbues both hunting and the land with meaning is, for the most part, lost in the village context and, for some, even in the context of current hunting practices. All the Elders with whom I spoke agree that, of course, the way of life today is very different from what it was when they were younger men and women. Despite a frustration with what constitutes Iiyiyu ways, there has, over recent years, been a surge of interest in the community to maintain and revive Cree practices and traditions through school programs, culture camps, and annual summer gatherings (Adelson 2000a; Tanner, Chapter 11). This revival, however, as one Elder comments, does not supercede Biblical teachings. Nor, for that matter, does an adherence to Christianity necessarily diminish Cree beliefs or practices:

Right now even the ministers are trying very hard to understand how they have wronged the Iiyiyu, and they are now seeing the wrong that they have

NAOMI ADELSON

done to the Iiyiyu. They see that it was wrong of them to tell the Iiyiyu to completely abandon their ways. In the community, too, the Iiyiyu'ch are trying to get back and are searching for what the Iiyiyu'ch had and are trying it.

... I am trying my best to help out where I can with maintaining and reviving the Iiyiyu way of life because I know I was meant to be an Iiyiyu, and this is where we were put to live as Iiyiyu ... I also tell what I have seen from the Bible because I have gotten much from the Bible as it is written why I should be respectful to creation and to all people that come my way. I know that whatever talents or gifts people have, they come from God and were given by God ... I know that some people do not like some of the teachings of the iiyiyu pmatisiiuun that are being taught these days. I do not see which part of the iiyiyu pmatisiiuun I should be unhappy about because I was put here as an Iiyiyu. These are my own thoughts about these things, but I cannot tell things that I think about. All I know is that I am trying to think of people equally and feel love for them for the love they feel for their own ways ...

There are a lot of things under the earth [at a different dimension or level] that are there that can help us and will come to us if we seek to know the Iiyiyu wisdom. It is because we have abandoned the past Iiyiyu way of life that it has left us, too. If we want to go back to the Iiyiyu wisdom, then it will come to us, that which can help us. (Interview 1)

Thus the Elders agree, for the most part, that the revival of past Cree beliefs and practices is a positive development for the community. Some, however, reject specific past practices that were banned by the early missionaries and emphatically refuse to accept their return. This became clear in my discussions with the church Elders as we broached the topic of the relatively recent incorporation of Native spirituality in this community.

The reason why Moses was able to do this was because he was doing what God wanted of him. As for the pharaoh, he was leaning more towards the will of the evil one. The evil one also has great works to show people here on earth. You must have heard what happened here this past summer [referring to the shaking tent ceremony]. That was one thing that the Iiyiyu was stopped completely from knowing and practising. This kind of knowledge comes from the evil one. The *mitauun* [shamanic power] comes from the evil one. The reason why the Iiyiyu did not continue to practice the mitauun is because when the missionaries first came here and talked to them, they told the Iiyiyu to forget about this and to pray all the time instead. A lot of anger resulted from this kind of knowledge when the Iiyiyu still were practising the *mituchisaan* [sweat lodge] and kusapichikin [shaking tent]. A lot of anger came from this.

The way that I look at it and the way I believe it is that our salvation comes from the message that Jesus brought personally to earth with him ... But before He came, some of the things that happened were not very good. It is those things that I am not very interested in knowing – what happened in the past. These things will not lead to salvation, only the path that Jesus made is the only thing that will bring me salvation. (Interview 4)

In the following quotation, the same church Elder not only reflects on the importance of church in his life but also offers a tempered, if firm, view on the recent changes in Whapmagoostui:

I personally think that the church is more important than anything that could possibly happen. But no one is forced to go to church. No one is told, "tell your relatives to go to church." It is up to each person to decide when they will go to church. It is known that the only thing that will be saved is the words and the message spoken in church. That is the only thing that will be saved and everything else will be destroyed on earth and in the sky. That is the reason why it is said that the church is very important, because of the message given there. I personally deem it very important, the religion that the "whiteman" brought to me ... As soon as the Iiyiyu'ch were told about religion, they abandoned everything that they did: sweat lodges and conducting shaking tent ceremonies and dancing with the drum and singing with the drum. They abandoned all these things. I have a cassette recording of an old man who died six years ago, when he was singing with a drum. He said, before he started singing, "I am singing this way because this is the way the old men of the past used to sing. This is the only thing they would do before the religion [Christianity] was made known to them." This was the only thing they did, only before the religion was made known to them, when they wanted to find something out. As for myself ... when you want to find something out, you may turn to the written words [i.e., the Bible], that is exactly what I do ... More and more different things are happening around us. Even the Iiyiyu'ch think that they will hold onto what they know [of the religion that they now practise]. There are many things from the south [i.e., Native spirituality] that are being introduced into our village. Some people do not like it, but it is brought here because some people do like it. Some people do not agree that these things should be brought in. These new things are trying to break or push the religion that we have aside. As for myself, as long as there is the church, I will not think in other terms. I can only look after myself. (Interview 4)

As this Elder describes, Native spirituality is not only different from Cree spiritual belief but is also an "introduced," or foreign, and potentially incompatible form of religious belief. Although others are somewhat less intransigent about the degree to which Native spirituality can be incorporated into other local belief systems, there remains for this Elder a sense that it is still coming from outside the community itself and is not necessarily an ingredient in the local effort toward cultural recuperation.

> We were given different ways to worship. There are different religions in Canada. We use different religions. Even we who are called Iiyiyu have different knowledge [than] the Iiyiyu of the south. They have a different knowledge that we do not have. What they have and if we wanted to mix it with what we have, it will not work. What will happen is that one of these practices, if combined, will cripple the other. Each person was given their own mind and one kind of religion; therefore, it is not right for another to bother the other about their religious practices and say, "here, have this." It is not right to do this. I have heard the minister and the bishop saying that no one should be bothered and just have the religion that they want to have. For example, if you were to say to me, "I will be with the Pentecostals ... I will no longer be with you," it would not be right of me if I were to bother you about your decision. I am just talking about you and me. Same thing goes for me if I were to tell you, "I will do this when I hold a church service." You should not bother me, either. It is not right to bother each other. You would do what you want to do.
>
> It has been three years that community members have had different views about what you are asking about. We all have different opinions about what you are asking about. Some people make a great effort to educate themselves about it. Some of them really want to have knowledge about this, and some do not even want to know about it. There is a reason why people do not even want to know about it. Soon after people are born, like myself, their parents take them to the church ... to get baptized ... When they come into consciousness [i.e., get older] and understand things, their parents tell them about the time they and others made vows on their behalf. Some people make decisions to forget about this. Some people think that when the *waamstikuushiiu* [whiteman] first came to bring this religion, the one that we are using, he was not doing a good thing when he brought them the religion. But we do not know how he did this. I imagine that he was given the power to do this. He could not have been able to do this if he was not given the power to do so.
>
> What is happening here in our town, it is not always the "whiteman" that brings new things into our village. It is the Iiyiyu'ch themselves who bring these new things. If there are many Iiyiyu who will be swayed to follow a

different path [from the present, existing religion] by what they are being told and what they see, things will be very different from what they were before. I personally believe that if we don't fight against what is being shown in our community, if the Iiyiyu do not fight it, many children will be led astray and go the wrong way. (Interview 4)

Recuperation, Faith, and History

The last quotation is, without doubt, tremendously difficult for some in Whapmagoostui to reconcile with their own position. Although some may agree with the Elder who spoke these words, there are others for whom a more pan-Native spirituality is a vital element of self-identity today. The church Elders whom I interviewed are a small segment of the community's population, but these excerpts do reflect a range of perspectives shared by their generation and point to an important debate that is taking place in this small community. This debate – as difficult as it is for some of its participants – is part and parcel of the recuperative process in the contemporary context. Indeed, it is exactly this heady mix of perspectives and voices that signals an assertion of identity in all of its fullness and diversity, emerging, as it has, out of a complex past and equally complex present (O'Neil and Postl 1994; Voyle and Simmons 1999; Warry 1998).

I began with a quotation from a nineteenth-century journal, detailing the way that a missionary ministered at once to both souls and bodies. The colonization of First Nations peoples did not begin with the church, yet that institution's fervent interest in the process remains one of the most potent symbols of penetration into and eradication of the cultural and spiritual core of indigenous communities. Despite that history, however, and paradoxically for some, Christianity today is an important and basic aspect of spirituality for many of the Elders whom I interviewed. Their words speak directly to the complex interplay of faith and history in the contemporary recuperative process as individuals and communities find ways to repair the damage of the colonial process.

The effects of the early Christian missionization resonate loudly in the postcolonial context. Indeed, the struggle to assert and maintain cultural and spiritual identity against the sometimes overwhelming influences of the church to a large extent define this period. Too often, however, when we discuss this postcolonial period, we assume clearly delineated divisions between those who colonized and those who were colonized. As indicated here, however, we cannot simply draw a line dividing the two. Regardless of its history of penetration, Christianity today is as important and fundamental an aspect of spirituality for some as Native spirituality is for others. The recuperative process, in other words, is not occurring (nor should it occur) in any sort of neat or readily defined fashion. The process is as complex and varied as the individuals and histories that make up First Nations communities today, and it is this complexity of faith at this particular moment in history that we must more fully understand if we are to appreciate the extent and vitality of a community's process of recuperation.

Increasingly, this debate and this process are shifting to a new generation as a growing number of youth interpret and enact local practices through their own experiences and education. With increased travel outside of the community and with ready access to a variety of media, satellite television, and the Internet, the youth see themselves as different again from their Elders. Many of the community's youth are increasingly aware of and showing interest in a wide range of pan-Native spiritual practices. This more abstracted form of spirituality, removed from the immediacy of Cree bush life, is readily accessible to a generation as familiar with hockey arenas and the Internet as with bush living. Although I have focused here on the reactions of church Elders to the newly invigorated practices of Native spirituality, it is crucial to remember that new ideas are already beginning to shape another generation. Thus, although the Elders speak passionately about their own Christian beliefs and even though some may fear this new turn to spirituality, there is also a generation growing up whose experiences are very different from those of the Elders. The Elders today spent, and continue to spend, a significant portion of their lives in the bush. The young men and women of today, although skilled at bush living and hunting, do not share to the same extent the kind of lived practice of spirituality or bush life that their Elders did when they were growing up. Perhaps for these young adults the new spirituality offers a less land-based but more tangible option for an expression of their faith and belief.

Extending now beyond the bleakest years of the colonial project, the recuperation process is far more complex than a recovery or discovery of a series of spiritual practices. Recuperation – in terms both of healing and of taking back – is imbued with myriad meanings. These meanings, in turn, will continue to change as new generations contemplate and navigate their own history and their own faith.

Acknowledgments

I acknowledge, with gratitude, the research funding provided by the Native Mental Health Team and the Fonds de recherche en Santé du Québec (FRSQ). I thank the members of the Whapmagoostui community who took the time to discuss these issues with me; Emily Masty for her superb assistance and translation skills; Monique Skidmore, Martha Macintyre, and Dr. Ian Anderson at the Center for the Study of Health and Society at the University of Melbourne; as well as Jacquelyne Luce, Emily Masty, Robert Auclair, and the late Arthur Cheechoo for the many lively debates and discussions, which were invaluable in shaping this chapter. Any shortcomings are mine alone.

Notes

1 More recently, the Government of Canada has apologized for its direct role in the residential school mistreatment of generations of Aboriginal youth through, in particular, the national apology of 11 June 2008 and the initiation of a truth and reconciliation process.

2 Elijah Harper, a member of the provincial Parliament and a former Cree chief, organized a Sacred Assembly in 1995 that brought together Aboriginal peoples from across Canada with religious leaders, politicians,

and the general public in order to kick-start a reconciliation process. One significant outcome of this process was the institution of National Aboriginal Day. This first Sacred Assembly was followed by a less successful 1997 event.

3 The shaking tent ceremony, viewed as a heathen practice by the missionaries, was chosen as the clearest representation of forbidden acts and thus was introduced into the Cree-language Bible. Versions of this Bible are still used, and the implication, according to rumour, was that there was a Biblical directive to remove anyone caught practising these particular "heathen" acts. The shaking tent ceremony was used primarily to communicate with the animal spirits and, in particular, to guide the hunters to the animals as part of the respectful interconnection between humans and the animal world.

4 I address this topic because it is an ongoing concern in the Iiyiyu (Cree) village of Whapmagoostui, where I conducted this research. The people whom I interviewed – church Elders – do not speak for the entire community. I specifically chose to speak with these Elders because I wanted to hear their opinions, thoughts, and concerns about the growing friction in the community around questions of faith. There are, of course, numerous other positions and opinions on this oftentimes contentious subject.

5 For a more extensive discussion of the village of Whapmagoostui and its contiguous neighbour, the Inuit village of Kuujjuarapik, as well as the distinctions made between village and bush life, see Adelson (2000a) and Barger (1981). The Cree travelled to this site long before the arrival of any non-Natives in the region as part of the annual cycle, following both the seasons and the animals. With the burgeoning whaling industry in the late eighteenth century and well into the nineteenth century, both the Cree and the more northern-dwelling Inuit travelled to this site in order to participate in the whaling industry. The outpost grew into a village in the early twentieth century and was entrenched at the end of the Second World War with the construction of a mid-line radar station and army base at this site. Today, the Cree and Inuit find themselves living as two separate municipalities on such a small spit of land as a result of the James Bay and Northern Quebec Agreement, in which both the Cree and Inuit are allocated communities through separate regional governments.

6 Bishop Lawrence lived and worked with the Whapmagoostui Cree (and Inuit of Kuujjuarapik) for 11 years. He became fluent in both Cree and Inuktitut during this time and took it upon himself to press the lay ministry to have peoples' Cree names written on their birth records. After 6 months of deliberation, the ministry agreed. While sick in bed with pneumonia, Lawrence added everyone's Cree name to his or her birth record. In addition, he charted a family tree for each individual on the reverse side of his or her birth record.

7 The shaking tent ceremony was conducted in the past for a variety of reasons. In particular, however, the ceremony was used when game was scarce and had to be sought out by whatever means were available to the Iiyiyu'ch. The *mistapaau* is a person's spirit intermediary, who is called upon to search for the spirit of the animals (and ultimately lead the hunters to the game). The tent would shake upon the presence of one's mistapaau.

References

Adelson, N. 2000a. *Being alive well: Health and politics of Cree well-being*. Toronto, ON: University of Toronto Press.

–. 2000b. Re-imagining Aboriginality: An indigenous peoples' response to social suffering. *Transcultural Psychiatry* 37 (1): 11-34.

–. 2002. Gathering knowledge: Reflections on the anthropology of identity, Aboriginality, and the annual gatherings in Whapmagoostui, Quebec. In C. Scott, ed., *Aboriginal autonomy and development in northern Quebec and Labrador*, 289-303. Vancouver, BC: UBC Press.

–. 2005. The embodiment of inequity: Health disparities in Aboriginal Canada. *Canadian Journal of Public Health* 96 (suppl. 2): S45-S60.

Barger, W.K. 1981. Great Whale River, Quebec. In J. Helm, ed., *Handbook of North American Indians*, vol. 6, *Subarctic*, 673-82. Washington, DC: Smithsonian Institute.

NAOMI ADELSON

Brady, M. 1995. Culture in treatment, culture as treatment: A critical appraisal of developments in addictions programs for indigenous North Americans and Australians. *Social Science and Medicine* 41 (11): 1487-98.

Calabrese, J.D. 1997. Spiritual healing and human development in the Native American Church: Toward a cultural psychiatry of peyote. *Psychoanalytic Review* 84 (2): 237-55.

Comaroff, J. 1993. The diseased heart of Africa: Medicine, colonialism and the black body. In S. Lindenbaum and M. Lock, eds., *Knowledge, power and practice: The anthropology of medicine and everyday life*, 305-29. Berkeley, CA: University of California Press.

Feit, H. 1983. The power to "see" and the power to hunt: The shaking tent ceremony in relation to experience, explanation, action and interpretation in the Waswanipi hunters' world. Unpublished manuscript.

–. 1986. Hunting and the quest for power: The James Bay Cree and white men in the twentieth century. In R.B. Morrison and C.R. Wilson, eds., *Native peoples: The Canadian experience,* 1st ed., 171-207. Toronto, ON: McLelland and Stewart.

Francis, D., and Morantz, T. 1983. *Partners in furs: A history of the fur trade in eastern James Bay, 1600-1870.* Montreal, QC, and Kingston, ON: McGill-Queen's University Press.

Grim, J. 1996. Cultural identity, authenticity, and community survival: The politics of recognition in the study of Native American religions. *The American Indian Quarterly* 20 (3-4): 353-77.

Harper, E. 1995. Excerpts from the first day's addresses of the Sacred Assembly '95. http://www.ottawa.net/~peaceweb/pnsacred.html.

Kelm, M.E. 1998. *Colonizing bodies: Aboriginal health and healing in British Columbia, 1900-1950*. Vancouver, BC: UBC Press.

Kirmayer, L.J., G.M. Brass, and C.L. Tait. 2000. The mental health of Aboriginal peoples: Transformations of identity and community. *Canadian Journal of Psychiatry* 45 (7): 607-16.

Kolig, E. 2003. Legitimising belief: Identity, politics, utility, strategies of concealment, and rationalisation in Australian Aboriginal religion. *Australian Journal of Anthropology* 14 (2): 209-28.

Leith, C.K., and A.T. Leith. 1912. *A summer and winter in Hudson Bay*. Madison, WI: Cantwell.

Linnekin, J. 1992. On the theory and politics of cultural construction in the Pacific. *Oceania* 62 (4): 249-63.

Long, J.S. 1985. Rev. Edwin Watkins: Missionary to the Cree, 1852-1857. In W. Cowan, ed., *Papers of the 16th Algonkian Conference*, 91-117. Ottawa, ON: Carleton University Press.

Morantz, T. 1983. Not annuall [sic] visitors: The drawing in to trade of northern Algonquian caribou hunters. In W. Cowan, ed., *Actes du quatorzieme congrès des Algonquinistes*, 57-73. Ottawa, ON: Carleton University Press.

O'Neil, J.D., and B.D. Postl. 1994. Community healing and Aboriginal self-government: Is the circle closing? In J.H. Hylton, ed., *Aboriginal self-government in Canada: Current trends and issues*, 67-89. Saskatoon, SK: Purich.

Peers, Archbishop M. 1993. Anglican Church of Canada's apology to Native people, 6 August 1993, http://www.anglican.ca/Residential-Schools/resources/apology.htm (accessed 13 May 2008).

Preston, R. 1981. Eastmain Cree. In J. Helm, ed., *Handbook of North American Indians*, vol. 6, *Subarctic,* 196-207. Washington, DC: Smithsonian Institution.

Rowse, T. 1996. *Traditions for health: Studies in Aboriginal reconstruction*. Casuarina, NT: North Australia Research Unit.

Samson, C. 1999. *Health studies: A critical and cross-cultural reader*. London: Blackwell.

Tanner, A. 1979. *Bringing home animals: Religious ideology and mode of production of the Mistassini Cree hunters*. St. John's, NL: ISER Books.

Tolman, A., and R. Reedy. 1998. Implementation of a culture-specific intervention for a Native American community. *Journal of Clinical Psychology in Medical Settings* 5 (3): 381-92.

Unknown. 1874. La Médecine chez les Sauvages de l'Amérique du Nord. Smithsonian Institution National Archives Document #1091.

Voyle, J.A., and D. Simmons. 1999. Community development through partnership: Promoting health in an urban indigenous community in New Zealand. *Social Science and Medicine* 49 (8): 1035-51.

Waldram, J. 1998. *The way of the pipe: Aboriginal spirituality and symbolic healing in Canadian prisons*. Peterborough, ON: Broadview Press.

–, A. Herring, and T.K. Young. 1995. *Aboriginal health in Canada*. Toronto, ON: University of Toronto Press.

Warry, W. 1998. *Unfinished dreams: Community healing and the reality of Aboriginal self-government*. Toronto, ON: University of Toronto Press.

NAOMI ADELSON

13

Locating the Ecocentric Self: Inuit Concepts of Mental Health and Illness

LAURENCE J. KIRMAYER, CHRISTOPHER FLETCHER, AND ROBERT WATT

I can still see my father drum dancing. He danced with great joy to my mother's singing, chanting loud cries and reaching innermost insights and outermost spirits – making a connection to the past and to the land. The land is about stories. Inuit simply means "the people," those who live here. We are the place.

– PETER IRNIQ, "FOREWORD," IN ROBERT SEMENIUK,
AMONG THE INUIT (2007)

In this chapter, we present some reflections on Inuit concepts of mental health based on ethnographic research and clinical consultations in Nunavik, Quebec. Our aim is to identify cultural knowledge and practices relevant to mental health services, promotion, and planning. At the same time, we hope to show how contemporary knowledge of mental health and illness is a complex and shifting outcome of cultural models of affliction, familiarity with a variety of contemporary forms of counselling and healing practices, popular theories spread through mass media, and the exigencies of a rapidly changing way of life.

More than 50,000 people in Canada identify themselves as Inuit (Statistics Canada 2008). Most live above the 50th parallel in the territories of Nunavut and Nunavik (northern Quebec), although increasing numbers make their lives in the major cities of Canada (see Figure 13.1). The Inuit have been among the most intensively studied peoples in the world since their long history of survival in the stark environment of the Arctic has captured the imagination of explorers and anthropologists. In recent years, with increasing control over their land and systematic efforts to record their history and traditional knowledge, Inuit across Canada have become concerned with how to maintain or recuperate the vital elements and values of their tradition while advancing the well-being of their people as equal citizens within a modern multicultural nation.

This challenge is especially acute because of the recency and intensity of cultural, social, and economic change in Inuit communities, which has led to radical disjunctures between the experience of the generations (Brody 1975). Many Elders in the communities

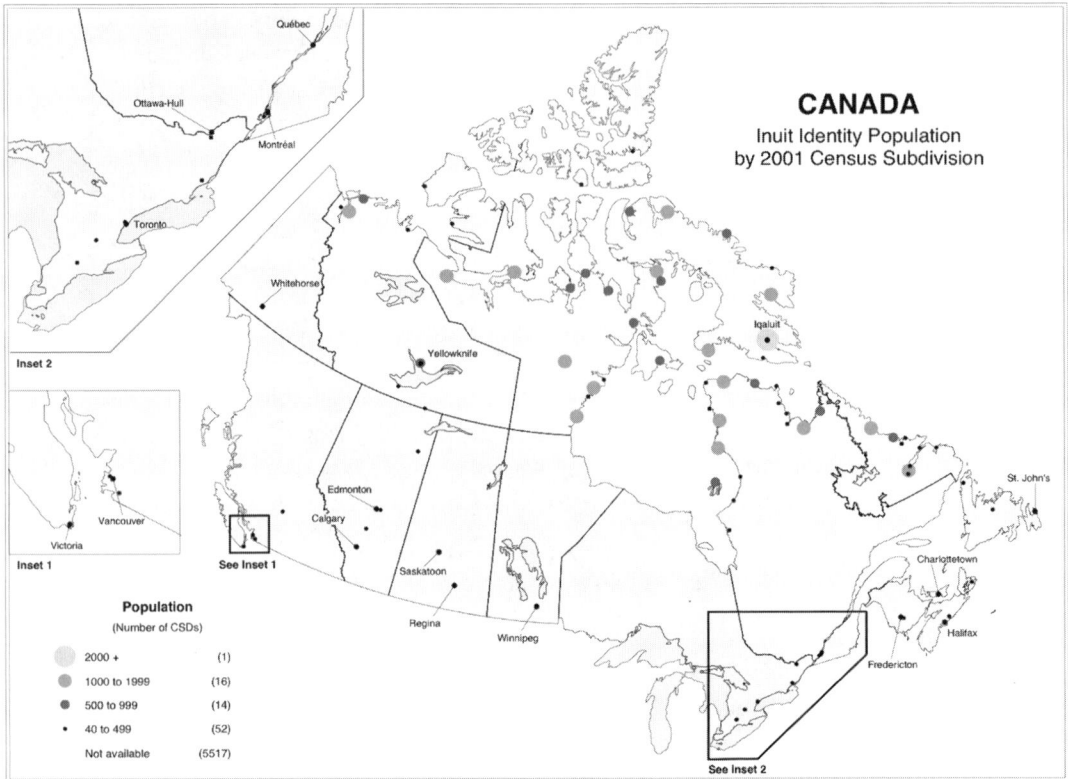

FIGURE 13.1 This map shows the distribution of the Inuit population in Canada based on data from the 2001 Census. The population is represented by symbols of varying size and tints, 40-499, 500-999, 1,000-1,999, 2,000+. *Source:* Statistics Canada, 2001 Population Census, Natural Resources Canada, GeoAccess Division.

were brought up in circumstances profoundly different from those of their children and grandchildren. With few exceptions, the communities that dot the North today were small commercial and administrative outposts with no permanent housing as recently as the early 1960s. People lived almost exclusively on the food species available in the North, following the animals' seasonal cycles and capturing them by employing detailed knowledge of their behaviours (Brody 1987). Many in the generation that is currently middle-aged were displaced at a young age from the lifestyle of their parents and experienced the hardships of prolonged hospitalization for tuberculosis or attended residential schools that aimed to suppress and transform their cultural identity. The younger generation is being educated within the communities, in school systems that now acknowledge Inuit tradition and that are under Inuit control through completed land claims agreements. This generation is the most self-consciously "global" in that, through mass media, its members have been saturated with the sights and sounds of an international youth culture that

LAURENCE J. KIRMAYER, CHRISTOPHER FLETCHER, AND ROBERT WATT

celebrates a fast-paced urban life that is hard to realize in their small, remote communities. This sketch of generational differences suggests some of the many influences on individual concepts and experiences of self, community, and place that co-exist within the current population.[1]

Although for convenience we will refer to Inuit as a group (as in "Inuit culture" or "Inuit concepts"), it is important to recognize that this way of speaking creates a sense of homogeneity and consensus that does not reflect the diversity of viewpoints, and sometimes disagreements, among individuals within any community. Contemporary cultures are not closed, homogeneous societies but open systems cross-cut by diverse flows of information that allow individuals to adopt different perspectives and to position themselves in many different ways (see Waldram, Chapter 3). Nevertheless, most Inuit share a common language, historical tradition, ethnocultural identity, family and community structures, and social predicament. This makes it meaningful to consider how the shared elements of their background contribute to individual and collective knowledge of illness and well-being.

Every culture has explicit notions of how people "work" that could be termed an "ethnopsychology," and all individuals navigate these ideas in their own ways to make sense of their own and others' behaviour. These notions include what the sociologist Marcel Mauss (1979) called the "cultural concept of the person," which characterizes what it is to be a socially valued and well-functioning human being. The mental health disciplines, including psychiatry, psychology, and social work are underwritten by specific cultural concepts of personhood that include an emphasis on the autonomy of individuals, the value of open expression of feelings, and the centrality of rationality, self-direction, and internal conflict in determining behaviour (Kirmayer 2007; Rose 1996). These concepts are woven into academic research and training in mental health and are also expressed in popular culture, so they have been widely exported along with the mental health professions. However, the assumptions of conventional mental health practices do not always fit with local cultural understandings of the person. There is increasing recognition that mental health practices must be rethought and adapted to local social and cultural realities if they are to be effective and not undermine core cultural values.

The impact of local social and cultural realities on models of mental health and illness became clear to the first author (LJK) during the period 1988-93, when he served as a psychiatric consultant to the Inuit communities on the east coast of Hudson Bay. To explore understandings of mental health and illness in Inuit communities, he conducted an ethnographic study in Nunavik in the early 1990s (Kirmayer et al. 1994). The study involved interviews with 80 key informants in four communities to identify the symptoms, signs, and meanings of behaviours and experiences likely to be related to conventional psychiatric disorders and to a broad range of social problems. Interviews also explored local knowledge of the causes and appropriate treatment of mental health problems, the impact of culture change, and models of childrearing.[2] This ethnographic work was interpreted against the backdrop of clinical experience. The second author (CF) took part in this study and also conducted participant-observation research annually for varying amounts of time toward a general ethnography of contemporary Inuit life-ways in communities in Nunavik between 1990 and 2000. The third author (RW) was raised in Nunavik, participated in the study, and has subsequently served as an educator, administrator, and advocate for Inuit health. Because the social world of the Inuit population continues to change rapidly, it is likely that knowledge and practice have changed since these studies. Contemporary Inuit understandings of mental health and illness reflect both traditional knowledge and ongoing influences of educational institutions, mental health services, and mass media. As with any population, there is enormous variation in the experience and perspectives of individuals. However, we believe that the basic issues we outline remain relevant to the delivery of mental health services and to broader considerations of health promotion.

The Ecocentric Self

The Inuit concept of the person has been called "ecocentric" in that it gives a central role to connections among individuals and to place in the health and well-being of the person (Stairs 1992; Stairs and Wenzel 1992). Inuit notions of the person view the individual as in constant transaction with the physical environment. This occurs both through subsistence activities, like hunting and fishing, and through the act of eating, in which the substance of animals is incorporated into the body and the person. This accounts for the importance given to eating traditional "country foods," including raw meat and fish, and directs attention to the central role that the land *(nuna)* takes in Inuit culture, thought, and experience. The northern landscape has many kinds of significance in this context. People frequently point to the land and its food resources as reassuring evidence that Inuit have always been able to support themselves and can continue to do so, even if at present one can survive comfortably within a cash economy. The land presents a constant reminder of cultural history in that places, topographical features, and travel routes constitute an Inuit memoryscape (Nuttall 1992).[3] Conversely, from the vantage point of the new challenges and constraints of community life, the land may signify how much has changed and perhaps the distance that now exists between the people and some aspects of their cultural history. Nevertheless, for most Inuit with whom we spoke, the landscape continues to provide a healthy space that can bring calm to troubled individuals and joy to families camping out on the land; more than that, skills in living on the land are viewed as a source of strength and resilience relevant to surviving in the modern world. As Inuit activist Sheila Watt-Cloutier put it in a recent interview: "Young people are prepared for life through the hunt, how to be patient, to be bold under pressure, to withstand stress, to focus, be tenacious, how not to be impulsive, to be courageous, to exercise sound judgments and ultimately, how to be wise" (McIlroy 2006, A3).

The land continues to be a source of real sustenance for most Inuit. In conversations with Inuit of Nunavik, the consumption of country foods was closely associated with generalized feelings of health and well-being. When food from the land was not available, people reported that they had feelings of weakness, lassitude, and tiredness, and these extended to emotional states of irritability, uncooperativeness, lack of interest in daily events, indifference toward children, and generalized depression. For example, a man in his mid-thirties, who was not a regular hunter and expressed a lack of interest in the hunting lifestyle, explained that the only times he went out hunting were when he was feeling depressed and lazy because of the lack of country food in his system. (He referred to his "system" in general but rubbed the veins on his forearm while talking, implying his circulatory system.) At these times, he would go seal hunting to replenish himself and would always feel much better for some time afterward.

Borré found similar sentiments among Inuit of Clyde River, Northwest Territories. She describes the case of a woman who was experiencing depressed mood, nausea, and headaches. She declared that she needed seal meat to feel better, and upon receiving some, "the next day her headache and nausea were gone, and she was working as usual. She explained that her blood had become weak from the lack of seal meat and that she needed seal meat for the next few days to be sure she was well" (1991, 56).

Other Inuit in Borré's study reported that depression was a common occurrence when they were unable to consume seal meat for extended periods of time. In Nunavik elderly Inuit reported a need for beluga whale skin (a highly valued food) with a similar rationale. Eating beluga could also alleviate the feelings of depression experienced by some elderly people when they were no longer able to participate in camp life or in hunting. Consuming beluga rejuvenated them through its effect on the blood and hence on both body and mind.

The beluga whale is an important animal on a symbolic level to many Inuit in Nunavik. Beluga travel in family groups, are highly social, follow a leader, are intelligent, and, like Inuit, can carry their young on their backs (amaut).[4] The capture and consumption of beluga are charged events. Eating beluga blood, skin, and fat (maktak) reconstitutes the human physically and mentally and imparts some of the animal's intelligence and social qualities to the person. To be without beluga as food is to be slowly drained of an essential element of health and well-being. One person stated:

> There is something you should know, it is the blood that is very important for
> the health and Inuit eat mainly meat because it has blood in it and that helps
> the individual very much, more than meat with little blood ... and the person
> will be in better health, his blood will be more ... stronger. Its visible even on
> the cheeks, the cheeks were redder we say (in the past). (Salluit, 1 November
> 1992)[5]

The late Taamusi Qumaq of Puvirnituq, a noted Inuit linguist, author, and intellectual, stated:

When I am sick, I think perhaps I could be helped by the nurses and that I could take some medication. I say especially that if I eat the food that I like I will get better faster. I also say that if my family is with me I will get better. It happened to me that I was sick at a time when my family was away. I said *qailaurli, qailaurli, qailaurli* [come back]. I am not in the habit of taking medication that the nurses and doctors give. I prefer to use the fat from marine mammals and plants. (Quoted in Therrien 1995, 81, translated from French by CF)

In addition to the notion of food as the most basic medicine, Qumaq explicitly linked the curative powers of northern foods to the importance of the company of family in the healing process – a connection that points to the inseparability of sociality and physical healing in Inuit models of health maintenance. Of course, the actual capture and consumption of food species engages social, physical, and intellectual activities that are

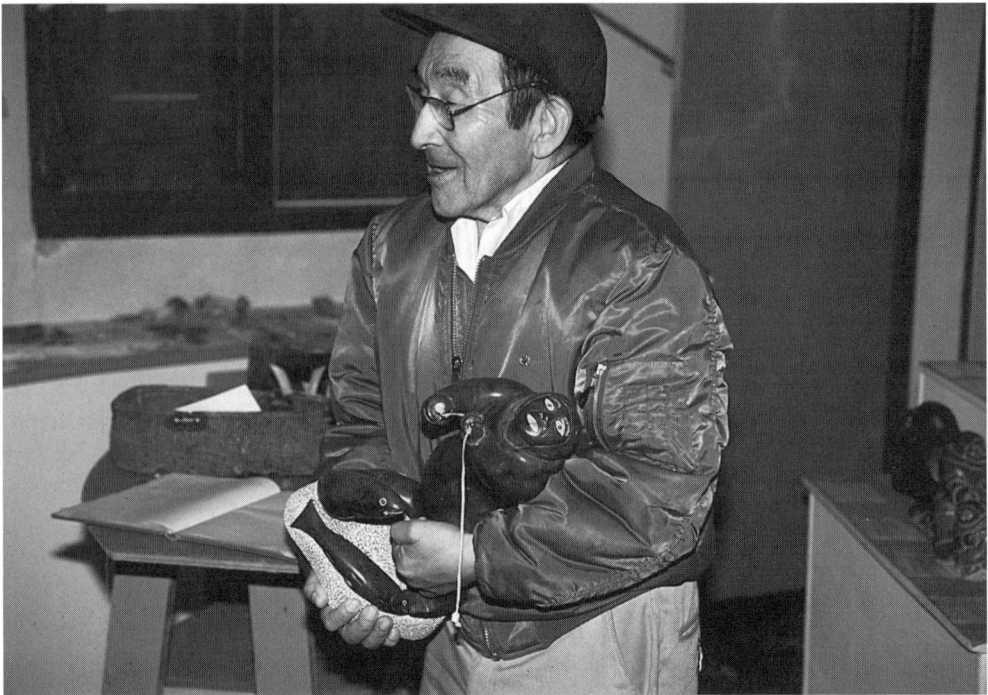

FIGURE 13.2   In the 1980s, Taamusi Qumaq, Inuit activist, historian, linguist, and one of the founders of the co-operative movement in northern Quebec, converted an abandoned building in Inukjuak into a cultural museum. "He appealed to the community and went around collecting material items that were no longer in use and mementos of past members of the community. He said time was like a vast river carrying everything in their culture out to sea to be lost forever. So he built a *saputik*, a weir, to catch all these things before they were lost" (Graburn 2006, 145). (Photo: L.J. Kirmayer)

fundamental to healthful life for Inuit. Finally, the Inuit diet is also a self-conscious marker and conveyor of Inuit identity, and parents are concerned to get their children to learn to eat and enjoy such foods as *maktak* (whale skin and blubber) or *qisaruaq* (stomach of a caribou or other grazing animal) (Graburn 2006).

Inuit recognize a close link between food, blood, and mental well-being, and this counters the tendency in Western biomedical views to separate mind and body in health and illness (Kirmayer 1988). The brain is considered the seat of consciousness and, like other organs, is nourished by blood, which transports healthy materials throughout the body. The quality of blood is directly affected by the quality of food consumed. Weakness associated with the impoverishment of blood quality or quantity is best remedied by consuming raw meat containing a lot of blood (seal, ptarmigan) or blood itself. It is for this reason, according to people who spoke with us, that when Inuit must leave their communities for hospital treatment in the south, they may become weak and depressed over time, for they are being fed essentially bloodless southern food. At the same time, they are far removed from the support of family and friends, which they would otherwise experience, in part, through convivial activities of food sharing and consumption.

Several participants in the research mentioned environmental factors as causes of mental health and illness. Participant-observation research, as with previous ethnography, emphasizes the central role of the physical environment in Inuit concepts of the normal functioning of the person. For example, in Salluit several people attributed the perceived higher prevalence of mental disorders to the fact that the settlement was ringed by mountains on three sides. This setting could make people feel "closed in" and uncomfortable. It was considered more natural for people to live with wide-open spaces over which they can range freely. Indeed, being cooped up in an office might make people ill. This is particularly a problem among men for whom being outside and moving across large territories while hunting has been an important element of experience and identity buttressed by cultural, linguistic, and cosmological principles (Therrien 1987). Women were more accustomed to confined spaces since they would spend much time together at the family camp.

There is broad agreement today that being out of the community on the land has a rejuvenating effect on the mind and the body, and people use camping, hunting, and fishing as ways to regain a sense of well-being. This way of interacting with the environment also persists in prescriptions for men to control anger or to deal with other difficult feelings by going out on the land. The various constraints on mobility and access to the land that characterize community life today – tied to the availability of time, equipment, and cash – may then contribute to the exacerbation of illness. For many people, the sense of well-being is tied to the visual experience of open vistas of tundra and ocean. Lack of access to this sort of visual expanse may provoke feelings of distress, disorientation, and anxiety.

In Inuit accounts, the environment is not an impersonal, inanimate landscape but is alive and closely linked to personal memories. Looking out the window from an airplane landing at a settlement, a young man remarked, "I know that coast line like the back of my hand." His eyes filled with tears of emotion at returning home. The sense of place is

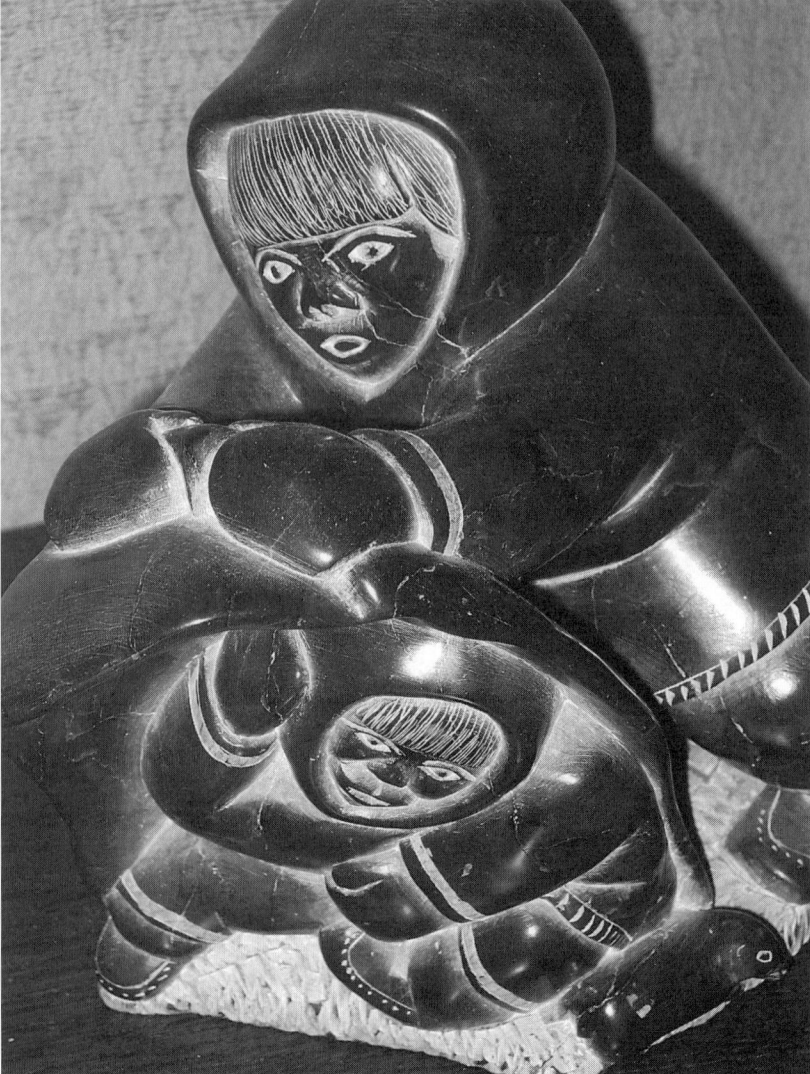

FIGURE 13.3   The shaman makes a sealskin blanket magically appear in order to warm a young boy he has rescued from a fall through the ice. The shaman's spirit helper, a lemming, appears at his foot. (Sculpture: Pauloosie Kasudluak, Inukjuak, 1999) (Photo: L.J. Kirmayer)

very strong and tied to highly valued activities like hunting that are the basic sources of self-esteem for many men. Animals, in particular, have held a central place not just in Inuit subsistence patterns but also in traditional religious belief, mythology, and artistic expression. Animals were viewed as nonhuman persons who had their own autonomy

LAURENCE J. KIRMAYER, CHRISTOPHER FLETCHER, AND ROBERT WATT

and agency and were deserving of respect (Stairs and Wenzel 1992; see also Fienup-Riordan 1990). There are many legends that describe the close ties between animals and people and that tell of transformations of people into animals and vice versa. The shaman *(angakok)* drew his power from animal helpers. Although traditional notions of the links between people and animals were displaced by Christian doctrines and have been largely supplanted by more purely utilitarian views, many Inuit retain a strong sense of admiration and respect for animal life.

Concepts of Mental Health and Illness: The Transition to Community Living

There is relatively little historical or ethnographic material that directly addresses Inuit ideas about mental health. Vallee's (1966) report, based on interviews and case studies collected in Inuit communities on the Hudson coast in 1963, remains unique in the literature and is close to the concerns of the present study. His observations are probably indicative of cultural knowledge in the first half of this century since, at the time of his survey, only about 10% of Inuit could read and write in English, although most were literate in Inuktitut syllabics.

Finding no general indigenous concept of mental or psychiatric disorder,[6] Vallee chose as his basic criterion of mental breakdown: "incapacity of the person to perform some or all of his normal roles accompanied by behavioral oddity, as defined by the interviewees, and where the incapacity and oddity are attributable to the head rather than to some other body organ" (1966, 57). He thus requested that his informants talk about "happenings in which people were rendered incapable of performing in their everyday capacities and where there was no obvious physical cause for this inability, and where the individuals behaved in an unusual, although not necessarily unpatterned, manner" (57). From these open-ended ethnographic interviews, Vallee identified four distinct patterns of emotional/behavioural illness, which corresponded roughly to epilepsy, "simple hysteria" (i.e., isolated episodes of conversion or dissociation), withdrawal with acute melancholy, and a state of agitated, accelerated, and incoherent behaviour called *quajimaillituq,* a term applied to rabid dogs and, in this context, conveying the sense "he does foolish things and does not know what he does" (61). All of the Inuktitut terms were attached to states, not discrete entities or categories of persons. After the condition had passed, the person was no longer in that state and was not labelled sick. However, persistence or chronicity of the condition could be denoted by an infix meaning "usually."

While Vallee's findings might be taken as indicative of "traditional" knowledge, it is important to recognize that the period from the late 1950s through the 1960s was a time of major social and economic upheaval and profound disempowerment for Inuit across Canada. Throughout the North, people were emerging from a period when epidemic disease killed many, evacuations to southern sanitoria for tuberculosis were frequent, and community living with mandatory primary schooling was being implemented. All of this had a destabilizing effect on Inuit society. Families were fragmented, and traditional so-cialization and social control norms were undermined. In a very real sense, powerlessness reached its apogee in the 1960s and is today exemplified by the story of the High Arctic relocation (Tester and Kulchyski 1994) and by ongoing efforts among Inuit organizations to have the slaughter of sled dogs by the Royal Canadian Mounted Police (RCMP) – a high-ly contested historical event – redressed through political and legal mechanisms.[7] Without dogs, Inuit were effectively immobilized in the new communities and highly dependant on local administrators to supply them with the basic needs of life. It is interesting to note that one of the cases of qaujimaillituq that Vallee describes involves a man who was coerced by non-Inuit into shooting a number of seemingly rabid dogs, actions that were contested by people in his community. He contracted influenza in the "annual epidemic" (1966, 70) and subsequently felt that people were trying to harm him. He dressed in mock military style and went about shooting at imaginary dogs and ultimately developed a full-blown state of qaujimaillituq. While speculative, it is possible to interpret this episode as a reaction to the highly stressful events of the transition period grounded in the cultural alienation of the times – stresses that were particularly concentrated on individuals who mediated between the Qallunaat (non-Inuit) and Inuit populations' expectations and ideologies.[8]

Contemporary Views of Mental Illness

In our fieldwork in the early 1990s in northern Quebec, participants in the study recog-nized four broad classes of causes of mental health problems: (1) physical or organic, (2) emotional or psychological, (3) spirit possession, and (4) the impact of rapid social and cultural change. Similar frameworks for thinking about illness have also been document-ed in collaborative work with Elders at Arctic College in Iqaluit, Nunavut (Therrien and Laugrand 2001).

Physical or Organic Causes of Mental Illness
Organic mental health problems were generally recognized to be those with which a per-son was born. Epilepsy, mental retardation, Down syndrome, and other problems evident at birth or from a young age were considered by most people to be organic in origin. They can be caused by environmental factors, the mother's behaviour during pregnancy (par-ticularly drug and alcohol use), trauma encountered during pregnancy, problems encoun-tered during parturition, accidental trauma at a young age, and biological variability among individuals. One person in Kuujjuarapik explained that just as some animals are born with birth defects, so too can human children be born with a variety of defects, including defects in the brain, which may cause the individual to behave in an unusual manner. In another community, an individual who had experienced lifelong seizures, per-sonality problems, and intermittent extreme antisocial behaviour was known to have been born that way, although her condition was aggravated by physical abuse suffered during

childhood. Despite the disruptive personality and extensive hardship suffered, it should be noted that this individual was not adrift in the community. In times of familial crisis, people would house and care for her with great tenderness. The possibility that a seriously ill person would simply be cast aside and ignored – as seems to many Inuit to be the case for the mentally ill in southern cities – is anathema to the ethos of shared responsibility that permeates Inuit society.

In our interviews, a great variety of problems were attributed to the mother's use of drugs during the pregnancy. This often carried a degree of moral censure of the mother. The implication of this prenatal vulnerability is that pregnant mothers must take special care to ensure their children turn out normal.

> When you're pregnant, I think it's very important that you take care of yourself. Sleep well and have a lot of rest, and get consultations from one of the older people. Then your baby can be very healthy in mind and in physical. When I was pregnant my mother was preparing me for it. I had to do certain things: get up early, get a good sleep, get good rest, try to do things rapidly so that they will not linger on in your mind all the time, try to get things done fast. (Puvirnituq, 16 July 1992)

> Before birth, I guess if the woman is involved with drugs or alcohol that is mostly likely that a person or a child will be like that in her life. Mostly today it would happen. More often than in past because in the past we didn't have anything, eh? Today, there's everything. Maybe in the future we will see lots of people are like that – you know, they could be like handicapped or they would have a mental illness caused by these drugs. Other than that, if the mother is healthy and she doesn't fool around with these other things I think a child would be very normal. (Puvirnituq, 27 August 1992)

Difficult and prolonged labour can also cause behavioural problems in children related to developmental disabilities: "In your labor, it might take a long time to for the baby to get out. I did not believe that for a little while but then I told myself it can be true because it can follow your personality and everything. It might have a personality that's not very likable, who's not saying, who's not listening to other people" (Puvirnituq, 16 July 1992).

Among the physical reasons for mental illness that research participants mentioned were drug use, sleep deprivation, or some other bodily problem. People could also experience a wide range of mental health problems as a result of head trauma at any age.

Psychological Causes of Mental Illness

Many participants expressed the notion that mental health problems could follow from too much thinking *(isumaaluttuq)* or being completely unable to think because of "having no mind" *(isumaqanngituq)*. This points to an ethnopsychological model of the workings

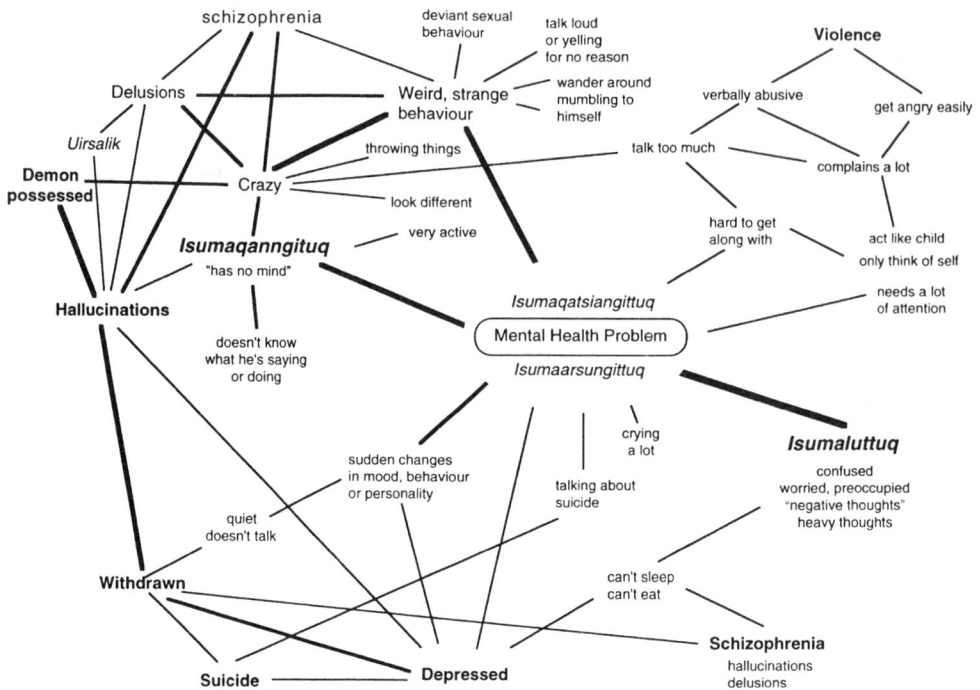

FIGURE 13.4 Signs and symptoms of mental disorder and Inuktitut terms according to Inuit respondents in Nunavik, 1989-91. The thickness of each line is a rough representation of the frequency of the association in 80 interviews (Kirmayer et al. 1994, 35).

of the mind and capacity for thought (*isuma*) as the cause of emotional and behavioural problems.

Isumaaluttuq is a term glossed as "having heavy thoughts," "having a lot on one's mind," "thinking too much," "being worried," or "being anxiously preoccupied." It covers a very broad range of problems and situations, ranging from ordinary worry and preoccupation to profound depression, withdrawal, and behaviour clinically consistent with psychosis. One informant explicitly noted it could be applied to people either with depression or with schizophrenia, although the two groups clearly had different problems. At the mild end of the spectrum, one informant stated that a hunter concerned about where the caribou are located might experience "isumaaluttuq." More serious anxiety was implied in the following account: "Isumaaluttuq would be, if someone is lost, out in the tundra. The mind, the thought that the person keeps coming back to ... in a way that doesn't give you peace. It worries you. So ... something that keeps coming back to you, that makes you worry. Or that doesn't, doesn't imply being well, mentally well" (Puvirnituq, 29 January 1992).

As well as describing normal states of preoccupation, isumaaluttuq covers mild to moderate forms of depressed or anxious mood. It was offered as a label for behaviour manifested by worried facial expression, distractibility or difficulty concentrating, confusion, dysphoric mood, and other difficulties in everyday functioning: "When a person has a mental health problem, what I see is ... the person cannot think very well, very well. The way he acts, the way he does things, and they get confused, he has ... the word for Inuktitut can, we can say that it's isumaaluttuq. Which means doesn't think positive things" (Puvirnituq, 30 January 1992).

The severity of isumaaluttuq can usually be judged directly from the person's account of what is troubling them, from bodily posture, from attentiveness to the world around them, and from the quality of eye contact. Other indications of isumaaluttuq include trouble sleeping "because the person is disturbed." Isumaaluttuq is essentially a psychological concept since it implies difficulty with thought processes. As such, it can be used as an explanation of mental health problems as well as a label of specific symptoms. Since it names a state of mind rather than a characteristic of a person, isumaaluttuq in itself has no expected course or prognosis (Kirmayer, Fletcher, and Boothroyd 1997). It can change as rapidly as the person's mental state and experience change.

The second term offered by many informants as having broad applicability for mental health problems, *isumaqanngituq,* implied more severe problems. Isumaqanngituq was glossed as "he has no mind/brain," "crazy," "doesn't know what's going on around him," "doesn't know what he's doing," "acting strange." A literal translation in English is "she/ he is without thoughts" and suggests an inability to act normally because of incoherent thoughts.

> We usually call them not very bright with mind ... isumaqanngituq ... They will probably think that this person has no mind to think ... they will do things that a normal person wouldn't do. Like facing other people with madness. They have to be different ... They talk to themselves or they blame other people for absolutely no reason and they are very isolated from other people and actually some of them are quiet and one or what would you say, a pain in the neck. (Puvirnituq, 7 July 1992)

This same term can be used for someone who is profoundly intellectually disabled or demented. An alternative term used by some informants as a more accurate translation of "mental illness" was *isumaqatsiangittuq*, which they glossed as "losing their mind," "going crazy," "having a mental illness." Both isumaqanngituq and isumaqatsiangittuq tended to imply a persisting condition or permanent state of affairs. A temporary mental illness was denoted with a change of infix as *isumarsungittuq.*

Isumaaluttuq implies thinking too much, whereas isumaqanngituq is not thinking at all. Both terms can be applied to similar behaviours but carry different implications about the underlying process. For example, both can be used to explain violent behaviour, but isumaaluttuq would imply that the violence is not totally irrational but stems from brooding, anxiety, depression, or nonpsychotic jealousy. In contrast, isumaqanngituq would imply the violent person was literally "out of his mind" and was acting destructively for completely irrational reasons or without any self-awareness or reflection. The distinction meets a grey zone in explanations of delusions and hallucinations, which were more often understood as "thinking too much" rather than "having no mind."

Another common theme concerned the interpersonal determinants of mental health. Most people had clear notions of the positive effects of kindness and open communication among parents and children and recognized the negative effects of criticism and rejection. One Elder in particular – who spoke only Inuktitut and hence might be expected to have had less direct influence of current "pop" psychology and Euro-American ideals of childrearing – eloquently described her vision of healthy childrearing through an interpreter:

> What she thinks, she's not sure, but what she thinks is that parents who always treat their children, or make them feel low, are those who don't really care about their children. And she thinks that they don't think about their future. Like they're young, they're growing up and their mother is taking care of them. Even as they grow, a parent should care. Even if the kid is an adult, that they should care and be willing to help their child. But she thinks that they parents who, they take care of their children, but when it comes to doing something bad, they criticize them because they don't really care about them. (Puvirnituq, 13 February 1992)

The negative effects of troubled family relationships, harsh words, and abuse were even more emphatically stated. Family conflict was regularly described as the major cause of the complete range of mental health problems – with the partial exception of conditions that were viewed as predominately organic, like mental deficiency or seizures, although even here the family's response was recognized as an important determinant of the course of the illness.

Physical and sexual abuse and neglect of children, rape, and spousal abuse have become more evident in Nunavik in recent years, and informants were unequivocal about the harmful consequences of these forms of violence. Emotional trauma suffered as a result of abuse, particularly sexual abuse, is an important cause of mental health problems according to many informants. People interviewed suggested that the cycle of abuse from victim to perpetrator was an important factor in the abuse occurring throughout the North.[9]

Some older informants suggested that, for many, the abuse cycle started at the hands of non-Inuit. In the 1940s and early 1950s, Inuit suffered severe hardship as a result of disease, poverty, government policies, and game shortages. Their desperate situation was taken advantage of by several non-Inuit, who were becoming more numerous in the region at the time. There are stories of school administrators, priests, and other people who

LAURENCE J. KIRMAYER, CHRISTOPHER FLETCHER, AND ROBERT WATT

abused women and children with impunity. These people had control over the allocation of goods, the few available jobs, and relations with the outside world – all of which gave them a great deal of power over the lives of the Inuit and led to many instances of coercive, violent, and exploitative sexual relationships. Some of these victims, abused at the hands of powerful non-Inuit, went on to abuse others. Social, political, and legal avenues for dealing with these cycles of abuse are only now becoming more widely available, and in most communities resources are still not adequate to address the emotional problems suffered by many people.

Other sources of emotional trauma, which put the individual at risk for mental health problems, come from the sphere of interpersonal conflict and communication. Several study participants described the importance of forgiveness in maintaining personal emotional health. In these instances, forgiveness may be viewed as a healing act that allows the victim to reorganize traumatic life experience into both a constructive social event and a coherent personal experience. Equally important, particularly when the abuser is a community member, is the potential for the victimizer to be recognized and offered a chance to acknowledge the pain he or she has caused. This provides an opportunity for victim and victimizer to create a new social context and maintain a measure of continuity in family and community. A number of people with whom we spoke discussed the futility of incarceration for many abusers who where themselves the victims of abuse. A socially grounded accounting and resolution is a preferable alternative in some instances (see Drummond 1997). The possibility of personal transformation and reconciliation through acknowledgment of wrongdoing, contrition, and forgiveness fits with the Christian values embraced by many Inuit as well as with the notion that behaviour is determined largely by changeable psychological states or patterns of thinking rather than by obdurate character traits.

In addition to the psychological and interpersonal factors described above, social factors such as isolation, unemployment, and poverty were also very commonly offered as explanations for such problems as drug abuse, depression, suicide, and violence among adults.

> It's hard to answer you this question. I think it would have – a person who is isolated or drinks too much, takes drugs too much – it could easily turn to have these kinds of problems. A person who doesn't have a job, who doesn't have anything, or who don't have any equipment to hunt. I guess it goes to these people to feel get tired of life. I guess that's mostly the causes. (Puvirnituq, 27 August 1992)

Although some individuals recognized larger social and historical determinants of health, for many these social circumstances were viewed as difficult to change or implacable, so an emphasis on personal, psychological, moral, and religious factors may have seemed to lead to more possibilities for positive change or healing.

Spirit Possession

Accounts of traditional Inuit culture note that some illnesses were considered to be caused by the interaction between the soul of a person, place, or thing and the individual affected by the illness (Merkur 1991). In Inuit cosmology, humans were considered to be the amalgamation of three types of souls: the name-soul *atiq*, the life-breath *anirniq,* and the shadow-soul *tarniq* (Saladin d'Anglure 1984, 2001, 2006; Guemple 1965). Each type of soul was subject to manipulation by *angakuit* (shamans), who could exert constructive or destructive forces on individuals and groups. Shamanic healing practices involved spirit journeys to confront the hostile evil spirits and placate or defeat them with the shaman's own spirit allies. Many individuals had some shamanic experiences and powers, and a wide range of unusual experiences and behaviours were tolerated and interpreted as the result of spirit communications. Spirits *(mitilit)* might pay brief visits or live for an extended time with individuals, who, if they were not impaired in their social functioning, were not viewed as deviant or afflicted.

Although these traditional explanations of affliction now are generally downplayed in favour of psychological or physical explanations, in our ethnographic interviews and participant-observation work in Nunavik in the early 1990s, spirit possession or attack was offered as a potential cause in many cases of bizarre and aberrant behaviour.[10] There was no single criterion or method for determining whether someone had become possessed, although it tended to be considered a possibility when a person's attitude and behaviour changed suddenly, with no warning and no previous occurrences. People who were known to have been possessed in the past and began again to exhibit bizarre behaviour were presumed to be possessed again. Some informants stated that the symptoms of mental illness could be essentially identical to those of possession. These explanations were not mutually exclusive, and in many cases a person could be viewed as having a mental illness and also as suffering from possession. Such possessions could result in a wide range of symptoms and behaviours of varying severity, including substance abuse, argumentativeness, violence, and florid psychotic states.

Three forms of interaction with spirits or demons were identified (Fletcher and Kirmayer 1997). *Utuuluttaq* involved disembodied spirits attacking individuals when they were vulnerable. The spirit was experienced as a force, as feelings of the uncanny, or through its symptomatic effects. It could be dispelled by refusing to traffic with it or by acceding to its influence. This form of "possession" is probably related to traditional notions of spirit intrusion or attack, although no natural agency or malevolent shaman was identified as being behind utuuluttaq. It may be linked to experiences of sleep paralysis, which give rise to unusual and compelling bodily experiences that fit explanations in spiritual terms (Law and Kirmayer 2005).

A second form of possession, which also seems to derive from traditional beliefs, involves the acquisition of a spirit husband or wife, called *uirsalik* or *nuliatsalik,* respectively. This can occur when individuals have intense longing for an idealized mate and constantly think, daydream, or obsess about him or her. In response to this concentration

LAURENCE J. KIRMAYER, CHRISTOPHER FLETCHER, AND ROBERT WATT

of thinking, a free spirit may be attracted to the individual's thoughts and come to inhabit him or her. The person can see and interact with this spirit partner. This accounts for such phenomena as hallucinations and otherwise senseless or delusional actions, like knitting clothing for nonexistent children. People may live peacefully with a uirsalik or nuliatsalik for many years, and this does not, in itself, constitute an illness. However, since most affected individuals are withdrawn, "strange," hallucinating, or have other interpersonal difficulties, it often constitutes a social problem.

The model of uirsalik/nuliatsalik possession makes it clear how close the link is between psychological processes (desiring, longing, obsessing) and the spirit world. Just as psychological processes have an obvious moral dimension referring to the individual's harmful or selfish actions, so the activity of spirits is mediated through psychological processes.

The third form of possession closely followed the prototype of Christianized demonic possession found around the world (Goodman 1988). Although it is tempting to view this as simply an importation of southern Pentecostal Christian practices, it is probably more accurate to see all three forms of possession as syncretic belief systems in which traditional forms of possession are integrated with Christian beliefs to provide a credible explanation for aberrant behaviour. Conviction in the possession diagnosis is grounded in bodily experiences of the uncanny and the interpretive authority of individuals aligned with the church or evincing personal power and charisma. The possession model is appealing because it leads to specific treatments in which many community members can participate. The rise of evangelism is perhaps the most significant, and poorly understood, social movement in Inuit communities today. It is explicitly oriented to "healing" psychological trauma and victimization of various origins. However, its long-term impacts on mental health and social cohesion are unknown.

Finally, although spirit possession was a common theme in many interviews, it should be noted that several people did not believe in demon possession in any form:

> Yeah, demon – this I do not believe. Maybe it's the people that get things long enough to disturb their mind, that their mind is playing tricks on them because they're left feeling alone. Or they have difficulty in life and they have family problems. They cannot talk to each other. That's what I think, because I never had this kind of thing happening to me. (Puvirnituq, 10 February 1992)

Skeptics tended to have had more formal education and were less closely affiliated with the church. For the most part, however, even skeptics kept open the possibility that possession was a real phenomenon, perhaps because of the compelling nature of stories in wide circulation in the early 1990s.

Impact of Rapid Culture Change on Childrearing and Mental Health

Many people with whom we spoke introduced historical awareness of recent social and cultural changes as important causes of mental health problems, especially substance abuse, suicide, family violence, and child abuse and neglect. The Inuit of Nunavik have experienced profound changes in their life-ways in just two to three generations. This sort of rapid culture change, and the specific demands that have come with it, was widely recognized by informants as a contributor to the range of mental health problems. This did not take the form of a vague nostalgia for times past but involved explicit links between mental health, childrearing, life circumstances, and changes in the scale and configuration of the community, the family, and the economic and educational systems.

Before the implementation of mandatory schooling and social housing regimes, Inuit lived in small migratory bands composed of one or a few extended families. In winter people tended to congregate in larger camps, whereas in summer extended family groups fractured and people spent much time in relative isolation. Larger gatherings were times of celebration, and any conflicts that arose would be solved by Elders' mediation (Minor 1992).

In camp life, parents' activities were captivating for children, who would naturally gravitate to watch and learn by modelling and imitation. Hence, except in situations of immanent danger, traditional childrearing did not involve explicit teaching but patient modelling and waiting for the child to catch on. Education occurred through the continual testing of the physical and intellectual limits of children by their elders so that they knew both the certainties and vagaries of their world (Briggs 1970, 1985, 2000). For example, Jean Briggs (1998) eloquently describes how a young girl comes to know herself, her kin, and her culture through a series of dramas enacted by adults to destabilize knowledge of her world only to reaffirm it through a learning exercise. The stable and reassuring social world of the child is thus constructed with her participation even while the cautionary lesson is instilled that things can change precipitously.

Education prior to the advent of formal schooling was achieved through close interactions within the family that also served to comfort and reassure parents and children:

> All she can remember about her childhood is that when she was a little girl, as she was growing, they always used to go camping – either a few nights, or really go camping in the summer. She was always there with her parents, with her mother, and she feels she was never separated from them. When she had her mother and she was living with her mother when she was still a young person, she had nothing to worry about. But as an adult with growing children, she started to worry about things. Worry about her children. (Puvirnituq, 13 February 1992)

Many adults report joyful memories of time spent in close association with parents and grandparents while on the land. This satisfaction continues to be enacted for many, particularly in spring and summer camps located away from the communities. Camp life still allows families to regain some of the comfort and harmony of traditional life by providing a context commensurate with ideas about relationships.

Well, when you're away on your own, personally speaking, when I am out camping, I let my kids go and do whatever they like. There's nothing really they can do wrong. There's nobody else there. There's no property to damage. There's no other kids to fight with. Nothing to steal. And, well, it's harder to keep them outside at the camp. It's as hard to keep them outside at the camp as it is to keep them inside at the village. Do you know what I mean? They tend to stay inside to see what you're going to cook up next, or what kind of neat thing you're going to do. What their mother's going to do. [In the settlement] they see other kids horsing around outside, they want to take part. And when it's time to come in it's harder to bring them in ... in the past ... and that maybe some of the traditional ways of childrearing fit that situation very well. (Salluit, 19 August 1992)

Methods of childrearing and social control of inappropriate or troublesome behaviour that were effective in the traditional context are often found not to work in the current communities (Matthiasson 1992). These communities have created new forms of social segmentation and stratification by age and economic level. To some extent, they have eroded the central importance of the family and the authority of family heads in particular. In current communities, children are sent to school – which parents expect to replace much of their own socialization efforts – or else they wander about the community freely, in continuation of the laissez faire approach that fit camp life but that now seems to some community members to border on neglect.

The kids went to school. They were out of their parents' sight from 9 to 3 in the afternoon, 3:30 or 4 in the afternoon. And parents didn't have to deal with that anger any more. I mean the parents didn't want to take the time to teach their child any more. They were told that the teacher would teach the child everything. How to live, how to earn money, how to grow up, how to be, everything. They trust that all these books are, the kids are learning all that, how to be a human being. They don't understand that they've lost control of their position. That's why they get angry. They can't understand why there are so many dropouts. Why the school system is failing. They don't want to deal with that anger any more. (Puvirnituq, 29 January 1992)

In the absence of traditions that fit the current social context, people have to fall back on their own devices in childrearing, thinking through the alternatives they are exposed to by popular media, church, school, and health services or by their own experiences in residential schools or in other southern institutions.

Well, I'm kind of caught between being a strict disciplinarian and being a lenient father who advises his children against things that are wrong. The lenient approach is, on the extreme, allowing your child to do whatever he wants, up to a certain point. Not allowing him, or her, to be outside past a certain hour at night. And expecting him to be there when it's time to go home. But if he's not, saying "well don't let it happen again." Whereas, a strict approach, using the same example, would be to preach to your child, in a fire and brimstone way, as to how not to behave. And if you catch your child behaving like that, or hear that your child has behaved that way, administering corporal punishment, as it's termed in the schools, with physical punishment. Personally I try not to, punish my kids every time with the flat of my hand. If I feel they deserve it, I'll yell at them but then if they've been exceptionally bad I won't think twice about putting them over my knee and spanking them. (Salluit, 19 August 1992)

Corporal punishment was little used in the past except as a way to curb immediately dangerous behaviour (like slapping the hand of a child who was reaching toward something that might burn him or her), with adults relying on the strong attachments and moral authority intrinsic to family life. Some adults who were sent to residential schools or who endured prolonged hospitalizations for tuberculosis may have experienced or witnessed corporal punishment and other harsh sanctions and thus have incorporated notions of strict discipline into their ideas about "ideal" childrearing.

When a child was caught stealing something, without realizing they were actually stealing, they were just taking something they wanted. Nothing really belonged to anybody, speaking of food, for example. A hunter's harpoon is more or less sacrosanct. You didn't touch that, it belongs to that guy. It's taboo to take that away. It's taking away food from his family. But, let's say I had a full meal just a few hours before, and this family had nothing to eat all that day. And their parents, my friend's parents brought home a small piece of dried meat from another household. And I took that small piece that was intended for my friend. Well, my parents would most likely reprimand me. "You already had something to eat – it's that child's turn. We'll get something else for you to eat tomorrow." That kind of thing. (Salluit, 19 August 1992)

Teasing has been described as an important part of traditional childrearing aimed at establishing interpersonal control and preparing children for uncertainty (Briggs 1970, 1998). In the present study, when asked about it explicitly, however, most informants did not report teasing as an intentional or conscious aspect of childrearing, and many mentioned the emotionally damaging effects of unfair or excessive teasing.

The change in the nature of youth culture was a concern to many people, who viewed it as an intrusion of non-Inuit values through the various media and as a source of suffering for young people and their parents alike. The discrepancy between the lifestyle depicted in mass media and the roles available in Inuit communities is especially stark for young men. The shift from hunting and a subsistence-based economy to a status hierarchy based on wage earning and the ability to successfully negotiate with local and distant bureaucracies has left many men, young and old, feeling marginalized and ineffective.

> For people in the North, there isn't much work. Only a good person, or posi-
> tive people who can work well, because we don't have higher education. We
> don't have diplomas. We don't have certificates. We didn't have long-term
> schooling. Because there was no high school in the North. Even though we
> tried to go to high school down south. People get homesick. People get tired
> of living down south. Where the drugs and the alcohol are. We miss the nature
> of our home. But when we get home there's hardly anything to work for. We
> try to apply for good jobs, but only the good person can be hired. (Puvirnituq,
> 30 January 1992)

Conclusion

As a hunting people living in rugged conditions, intimate knowledge of the land, weather, and wildlife was essential to Inuit survival. Despite exposure to Euro-American ideas of individualism and images of the urban landscape, the central importance of the land and animals in Inuit concepts of the person and well-being persist. This is expressed in an ecocentric concept of the person that goes beyond connection to other human persons to include relationships with the land. Health, including mental health, is maintained by opportunities to live on the land and, especially, to eat country food. The association of positive childhood experience, individual autonomy, good food, and cultural continuity with access to the land lends a logic to the ecocentric model of the self and to the healing strategies often employed individually and collectively, whether formally or informally, within Inuit communities today.

In our ethnographic interviews in Nunavik in the 1990s, mental health problems were attributed to four broad classes of causes: (1) physical or organic effects of the environ-ment or human behaviour; (2) psychological or emotional factors related to childrearing, interpersonal relations, and mental functioning; (3) various forms of spirit possession, intrusion, or attack; and (4) rapid culture change and social disadvantage. People readily employed multiple explanations for complex or severe mental health problems. The choice of explanations and their relative emphasis reflected the area of concern: the personal, familial, sociomoral, or political significance of the individual's condition.

Congenital problems were widely interpreted as physical disorders linked to accident, to environmental or hereditary influences, and especially to the prenatal care taken by the mother. Maternal drug abuse was most often mentioned as a cause of problems through physical effects prenatally. For childhood problems, the emphasis in causal explanations shifted to the quality of parenting and the atmosphere in family life. Children who were treated harshly or neglected were seen to grow into adults with mental health problems. There was much diversity, uncertainty, and conflict of opinion over appropriate child-rearing, reflecting the dramatic changes in Inuit lifestyle in recent decades that have rendered traditional methods difficult to apply or sometimes ineffective.

Among adolescents, rapid culture change, lack of educational success and vocational opportunities, drug abuse, and the "youth subculture" were all invoked as explanations for the widely recognized increased prevalence of suicide, depression, and related mental health problems (Kirmayer, Fletcher, and Boothroyd 1998). Depression in adults was more likely to be attributed to loss of parents or significant others, marital conflict and abuse, and childhood emotional neglect and abuse. Verbal and physical abuse was noted as having an especially strong negative impact on children and adults.

Most informants were very "psychologically minded" by the standards of mental health practitioners. In fact, some of the most traditional, least acculturated individuals, who spoke only Inuktitut, offered sensitive accounts of psychological processes underlying emotional suffering and advocated models of childrearing based on the importance of clear communication, expression of love, and empathy for another's feelings. There was a clear concept of the role of mental processes in well-being and in suffering, articulated in terms of the functions of *isuma* – mind, thought, or rationality. Psychological explanations overlap the moral domain. Bad actions within the family give rise to painful thoughts and feelings that, in turn, may lead to further bad actions in subsequent generations.

A series of ruptures of the order and coherence of traditional life amplified through time have fostered a substrate of social and emotional difficulties today. Whereas in the past the people we now see as mentally ill would have lived their lives within a largely supportive extended family, today they have lost much of the positive support they enjoyed. But they also have recourse to a wide range of healing systems, including bio-medicine, and these have been incorporated into common ways of understanding mental health and illness.

Clearly, there are connections between this intercultural dynamic and mental health issues today. For example, Tester and McNicoll (2004) locate the high prevalence of suicide in Inuit communities today within this colonial dynamic and its effects on self-esteem. However, it is simplistic and potentially disempowering to reduce the entirety of abuse, suicide, and suffering to a problem brought by outsiders. Certainly, current dilemmas were set in motion by contact and colonization and were maintained by political policies, economic forces, and bureaucratic and professional practices that have undermined au-tonomy and fostered dependency. Exclusive focus on these extrinsic forces, however, ignores the ways that communities have become caught in their own self-perpetuating cycles of social suffering. To address these internal problems, communities must take hold of their own direction and work together to create a healthy social environment. To some extent, this requires new ways of thinking about community and collective action. Despite the frequency and severity of mental health problems, there is an ongoing social ethos of caring, empathy, and concern for others that can provide a solid basis for building social cohesion, collective efficacy, and well-being (Fletcher 2004).

The events of the community-transition period have created conditions far removed from the ethnographically imagined "traditional" Inuit lifestyle. Although we have juxtaposed traditional knowledge and practice and the current confluence of ideas, the dynamic between local and global knowledge demands much closer examination. Current mental health theory and practice have focused mainly on the psychological dynamics of the individual. Even the smaller fields of community psychology and social psychiatry have tended to focus on individuals and communities in urban settings. This suggests two crucial areas in need of further study in the mental health of Inuit and other indigenous peoples. The first concerns the effects of collective disempowerment on social cohesion, on individual and collective distress, and on subsequent social suffering. Within the literature of mental health and cultural psychology, culture change usually has been depicted as an impersonal or purely psychological process, which ignores the issues of power and violence that drive it. The second issue concerns the effects of dislocating people from a highly mobile land-based way of life to a sedentary community-based society. The contribution of sense of place to individual and collective identity, health, and well-being is poorly understood. This is an area where work with Inuit scholars and communities can contribute much, both to the development of effective methods of promoting well-being and to the broader project of advancing an ecological psychology and psychiatry that take seriously our relationship to the environment, viewing the landscape not simply as a backdrop to our lives or as something to be exploited but as the webs of connectedness that constitute our very being.

Acknowledgments

The research reported in this chapter was supported by grants to the first author from the Conseil québécois pour la recherche sociale (CQRS), the Fonds de recherche en Santé du Québec (FRSQ), and the Nunavik Regional Board of Health and Social Services. This chapter is based on an earlier unpublished report by Kirmayer and colleagues (1994).

Notes

1 For more on the history of the Inuit of Nunavik see Saladin d'Anglure (1984), Graburn (1969), and Dorais (1997). See also the discussions of similar changes in Nunavut in Duffy (1988), Matthiasson (1992), Damas (2002), and Kral and Idlout (Chapter 14).
2 The study involved both qualitative ethnographic methods and quantitative analysis of questionnaire data. The research was conducted with full attention to the ethics guidelines available at the time, including those of the Association of Canadian Universities for Northern Studies (1990). In particular, community residents and agencies were involved in the planning and development of the project. The research protocol was approved by the Kativik Regional Board of Health and Social Services, the Council of Physicians, Dentists, Pharmacists and Midwives of the Inuulitsivik Health Center, and the Research Ethics Committee of the Sir Mortimer B. Davis – Jewish General Hospital in Montreal. In addition to this institutional evaluation, the proposal was presented to representatives of the communities' health committees for their evaluation and approval.

3 Collignon (2006) describes how Inuit place names are part of cultural and historical knowledge and wisdom about the land ("geosophy") that provide both geographic emplacement and narrative emplotment to individual identities and experiences.

4 *Amautik* is the term for the large hooded parkas that Inuit women use to carry their infants.

5 Unless otherwise noted, all quotations are drawn from interviews with key informats conducted by the authors in Nunavik.

6 According to Vallee, there were no precise terms for mental disorders in Inuktitut. A variety of idiomatic expressions described "relatively benign, commonplace behavior" that was odd, silly, or evidence of stupidity. The nearest word translating "mental illness" is *niaqureriyuq:* "he has an illness of the head" (from *niaquq* = head of man or animal). See Schneider (1985): *niaqulirivuq* = to have an illness in the head (that causes one to lose one's balance); *niaqunguvuq* = he has a headache, which applied to any organic malfunctioning of the head. A related term is *quajimaillituq* (he does not know what he is doing), which however has a more restricted application.

7 Along with other Inuit leaders, Pita Aatami, president of the Makivik Corporation (the Inuit holding company for the James Bay and Northen Quebec Agreement), has commented on the RCMP investigation of the issue frequently. See for example http://www.cbc.ca/north/story/atami-dogslaughter-11052005.html (accessed 3 June 2008).

8 This interpretation would be consistent with Dick's (1995; 2002) re-analysis of episodes of *pibloktoq,* a prototypical "culture-bound syndrome," which occurred in association with Robert Peary's expeditions to Greenland (1895-1909). Peary employed the Greenlandic Inuit men to map the land, while their wives served as something akin to "comfort women" for his sailors. Seen in this context, pibloktoq seems less a distinctive culture-bound syndrome than a response to exploitation and abuse (see also Waldram 2004, 195-99).

9 There has been a popularization of the notion that people who have been abused are more likely than others to become victimizers. In some cases, this view has stigmatized the abused as potentially dangerous and has led some victims to fear their own future behaviour. This mistrust of one's self may exacerbate the emotional and social difficulties faced by victims of abuse.

10 It is possible that "possession" was used metaphorically in some instances, in much the same way that "crazy" is used in English. However, there is a widely known and accepted etiology of possession linked to behavioural states with clear antecedence in Vallee's (1966) ethnographic description and in well-documented historical episodes of religious movements (Grant 1997).

References

Association of Canadian Universities for Northern Studies. 1990. Ethical principles for the conduct of research in the North. *Northern Health Research Bulletin* 2: 13-14.

Borré, K. 1991. Seal blood, Inuit blood, and diet: A biocultural model of physiology and cultural identity. *Medical Anthropology* 5 (1): 48-62.

Briggs, J.L. 1970. *Never in anger: Portrait of an Eskimo family*. Cambridge, MA: Harvard University Press.

–. 1985. Socialization, family conflicts and responses to culture change among Canadian Inuit. *Arctic Medical Research* 40: 40-52.

–. 1998. *Inuit morality play: The emotional education of a three year old*. New Haven, CT: Yale University Press.

–. 2000. *Childrearing practices*. Iqaluit: Nunavut Arctic College Language and Culture Program.

Brody, H. 1975. *The people's land: Eskimos and whites in the eastern Arctic*. Middlesex: Penguin.

–. 1987. *Living Arctic: Hunters of the Canadian North*. Vancouver, BC: Douglas and McIntyre.

Collignon, B. 2006. Inuit place names and sense of place. In P. Stern and L. Stevenson, eds., *Critical Inuit studies: An anthology of contemporary Arctic ethnography,* 187-205. Lincoln, NE: University of Nebraska Press.

Damas, D. 2002. *Arctic migrants/Arctic villagers: The transformation of Inuit settlement in the central Arctic*. Montreal, QC, and Kingston, ON: McGill-Queen's University Press.

Dick, L. 1995. "Pibloktoq" (Arctic hysteria): A construction of European-Inuit relations? *Arctic Anthropology* 32 (2): 1-42.

–. 2002. Aboriginal-European relations during the great age of north polar exploration. *Polar Geography* 26 (1): 66-86.

Dorais, L.-J. 1997. *Quaqtaq: Modernity and identity in an Inuit community.* Toronto, ON: University of Toronto Press.

Drummond, S.G. 1997. *Incorporating the familiar: An investigation into legal sensibilities in Nunavik.* Montreal, QC, and Kingston, ON: McGill-Queen's University Press.

Duffy, R.Q. 1988. *The road to Nunavut: The progress of the eastern Arctic Inuit since the Second World War.* Montreal, QC, and Kingston, ON: McGill-Queen's University Press.

Fienup-Riordan, A. 1990. *Eskimo essays: Yup'ik lives and how we see them.* New Brunswick, NJ: Rutgers University Press.

Fletcher, C. 2004. Continuity and change in Inuit society. In B.R. Morrison and R.C. Wilson, eds., *Native peoples: The Canadian experience,* 3rd ed., 52-73. Don Mills, ON: Oxford University Press.

–, and L.J. Kirmayer. 1997. Spirit work: Nunavimmiut experiences of affliction and healing. *Études Inuit Studies* 21 (1-2): 189-208.

Goodman, F.D. 1988. *How about demons? Possession and exorcism in the modern world.* Bloomington, IN: Indiana University Press.

Graburn, N.H.H. 1969. *Eskimos without igloos: Social and economic development in Sugluk.* Boston: Little, Brown.

–. 2006. Culture as narrative. In P. Stern and L. Stevenson, eds., *Critical Inuit studies: An anthology of contemporary Arctic ethnography,* 139-54. Lincoln, NE: University of Nebraska Press.

Grant, S.D. 1997. Religious fanaticism at Leaf River, Ungava, 1931. *Études Inuit Studies* 21 (1-2): 159-88.

Guemple, D.L. 1965. *Saunik*: Name sharing as a factor governing Eskimo kinship terms. *Ethnology* 4: 323-35.

Kirmayer, L.J. 1988. Mind and body as metaphors: Hidden values in biomedicine. In M. Lock and D. Gordon, eds., *Biomedicine examined*, 57-92. Dordrecht: Kluwer.

–. 2007. Psychotherapy and the cultural concept of the person. *Transcultural Psychiatry* 44 (2): 232-57.

–, C. Fletcher, E. Corin, and L.J. Boothroyd. 1994. Inuit concepts of mental health and illness: An ethnographic study. Working paper no. 4. Montreal, QC: Culture and Mental Health Research Unit, Department of Psychiatry, Sir Mortimer B. Davis – Jewish General Hospital.

–, C. Fletcher, and L.J. Boothroyd. 1997. Inuit attitudes toward deviant behavior: A vignette study. *Journal of Nervous and Mental Disease* 185 (2): 78-86.

–, C. Fletcher, and L.J. Boothroyd. 1998. Suicide among the Inuit of Canada. In A. Leenars, S. Wenckstern, I. Sakinofsky, R.J. Dyck, M.J. Kral, and R. Bland, eds., *Suicide in Canada,* 189-211. Toronto, ON: University of Toronto Press.

Law, S., and L.J. Kirmayer. 2005. Inuit interpretations of sleep paralysis. *Transcultural Psychiatry* 42 (1): 93-122.

Matthiasson, J.S. 1992. *Living on the land: Change among the Inuit of Baffin Island.* Peterborough, ON: Broadview Press.

Mauss, M. 1979. *Sociology and psychology: Essays.* London: Routledge and Kegan Paul.

McIlroy, A. 29 December 2006. A global crusade to save the Great White North. *Globe and Mail,* A3.

Merkur, D. 1991. *Powers which we do not know: The gods and spirits of the Inuit.* Moscow, ID: University of Idaho Press.

Minor, K. 1992. *Issumatuq: Learning from the traditional healing wisdom of the Canadian Inuit.* Halifax, NS: Fernwood.

Nuttal, M. 1992. *Arctic homeland: Kinship, community and development in Northwest Greenland.* Toronto, ON: University of Toronto Press.

Rose, N.S. 1996. *Inventing our selves: Psychology, power, and personhood.* Cambridge: Cambridge University Press.

Saladin d'Anglure, B. 1984. Inuit of Québec. In D. Damas, ed., *Handbook of North American Indians,* vol. 5, *Arctic,* 476-507. Washington, DC: Smithsonian Institution.

–. 2006. The construction of shamanic identity among the Inuit of Nunavut and Nunavik. In G. Christie, ed., *Aboriginality and governance: A multidisciplinary perspective,* 141-65. Penticton, BC: Theytus Books.

–, ed. 2001. *Cosmology and shamanism.* Iqaluit, NU: Nunavut Arctic College.

Schneider, L. 1985. *Ulirnaisigutiit: An Inuktitut-English dictionary of northern Quebec, Labrador and eastern Arctic dialects.* Laval, QC: Les Presses de l'Université Laval.

Semeniuk, Robert. 2007. *Among the Inuit.* Vancouver, BC: Raincoast Books.

Stairs, A. 1992. Self-image, world-image: Speculations on identity from experiences with Inuit. *Ethos* 20 (1): 116-26.

–, and G. Wenzel. 1992. "I am I and the environment": Inuit hunting, community and identity. *Journal of Indigenous Studies* 3 (2): 1-12.

Statistics Canada. 2008. *Aboriginal peoples in Canada in 2006: Inuit, Métis and First Nations, 2006 Census.* Ottawa, ON: Ministry of Industry.

Tester, F.J., and P. Kulchyski. 1994. *Tammarniit (Mistakes): Inuit relocation in the eastern Arctic, 1939-63.* Vancouver, BC: UBC Press.

–, and P. McNicoll. 2004. *Isumagijaksaq:* Mindful of the state: Social constructions of Inuit suicide. *Social Science and Medicine* 58 (12): 2625-36.

Therrien, M. 1987. *Le corps Inuit.* Paris: SELAF.

–. 1995. Corps sain, corps malade chez les Inuit, une tension entre l'intérieur et l'extérieur: Entretiens avec Taamusi Qumaq. *Recherches Amérindiennes au Québec* 25 (1): 71-84.

–, and F. Laugrand, eds., 2001. *Perspectives on traditional health.* Iqaluit, NU: Language and Culture Program, Nunavut Arctic College.

Vallee, F. 1966. Eskimo theories of mental illness in the Hudson Bay region. *Anthropologica* 8: 53-83.

Waldram, J. 2004. *Revenge of the Windigo: The construction of the mind and mental health of North American Aboriginal peoples.* Toronto, ON: University of Toronto Press.

14

Community Wellness and Social Action in the Canadian Arctic: Collective Agency as Subjective Well-Being

MICHAEL J. KRAL AND LORI IDLOUT

In the 1970s, following decades of outside influence and intrusion, Inuit in Canada began a social movement toward reclaiming their land and forming an independent political territory. In 1993 an Inuit land claim agreement was established, and 1999 saw the creation of a new territorial government in the eastern Canadian Arctic called Nunavut, or "our land" in Inuktitut. Nunavut residents chose to use the public style of governance as opposed to an Aboriginal government. The effects of colonialism run deep, however, and social problems continue to take a toll on Inuit well-being. These problems include poverty, drug and alcohol abuse, domestic violence, and suicide (Bjerregaard and Young 1998; Burkhardt 2004; Griffiths et al. 1995; Haggarty et al. 2000; Kirmayer, Fletcher, and Boothroyd 1998). Injuries accounted for about 30% of all deaths in Nunavut in the 1990s, and most of these deaths were by suicide (Injury Surveillance On-line 2004). The suicide rate among young Inuit between the ages of 15 and 24 has been increasing dramatically in Nunavut since the 1980s, bringing the total rate across all ages to 122.5 per 100,000 for the period 1999-2003 (Nunavut Bureau of Statistics 2003) – 10 times the rate for Canada. In Nunavik of northern Quebec this rate is even higher (Boothroyd et al. 2001).

These social problems are a sad pattern existing among many indigenous peoples who have been colonized and have experienced much upheaval in their lives in recent decades. In some countries, such as Canada, governments have made efforts to ameliorate this suffering. Although well intentioned, many such efforts take the form and function of the dominant, colonizing society and enable little substantive involvement in their development by the indigenous communities so served. In this chapter, we review community wellness programs, policies, and actions among the Inuit in Nunavut. We examine in particular differences between approaches to wellness and mental health from outside versus inside Inuit communities and argue for an urgent need to continue support for the latter.

A Brief Colonial History

Nunavut has had humans living on the land for over 4,000 years. The Inuit stem from the Thule people (about 1,000 years ago), who replaced or absorbed the Dorset (about 2,500 to 1,200 years ago), who followed the pre-Dorset (about 4,500 years ago). Inuit oral history describes finding a people they call the Tuniit, who were the late Dorset people (McGee 1981). Today, the population of Nunavut is about 27,000, and, save for its capital, Iqaluit, where half the population may now be non-Inuit, (or Qallunaat), the typical community of between 350 and 1,200 people is about 95% Inuit.

Nunavut, like much of the circumpolar North, has been a more recent colonial frontier of the twentieth century. Yet the Inuit had earlier visitors. The Inuit had encountered Nordic occupants between AD 1000 and 1400; however, the first contact with Qallunaat of Western written and Inuit oral historical note began in the sixteenth century, when Inuit fought with and were captured by English, first by Sebastian Cabot in 1501 or 1502 and then by Martin Frobisher between 1576 and 1578. Visits by Danish-Norwegian and Dutch ships between 1605 and 1660 resulted in about 30 Inuit being captured, most of them for exhibition in Europe. Inuit captives were occasionally brought to Europe over a period of a few centuries (Idiens 1989; Sturtevant and Quinn 1989). The eighteenth century saw some trade but also increasing hostilities between Inuit and European explorers seeking a Northwest passage, minerals, and fur (Fossett 2001; Williams 2003). The eighteenth century also saw fighting between Inuit and French off the southern Labrador coast (Taylor 1984), with Inuit taken as slaves in New France (Trudel 1994). Scottish and American whalers began to have some effect on Inuit lives between approximately 1860 and 1915, as many Inuit relocated near their ships and worked in exchange for food and some European material goods (Damas 2002). This adaptation to European and American ways continued when the Inuit began trading fox furs with the Hudson's Bay Company, beginning in the early twentieth century. The first Royal Canadian Mounted Police (RCMP) began to arrive in the 1920s. Christian missionaries began the conversion of Inuit in Greenland in the eighteenth century; however, they were not in Nunavut until, primarily, the 1920s and 1930s. Although much of the Inuit traditional lifestyle remained, religious conversion was relatively swift in the context of epidemic diseases that took many lives; some estimate that most Inuit were killed by disease by the early twentieth century (Crowe 1991). Missionaries forbade shamans, or *angakuit,* to continue their public spiritual practices. After 1941 and into the Cold War, Canadian and US soldiers established meteorological and radar stations throughout the Arctic, and the government era began (Wenzel 1991). Social change was massive following the establishment of the Department of Northern Affairs and Natural Resources in 1953.

The Canadian government became involved in the creation of settlements, including relocations of families in the 1950s and 1960s in the midst of a severe tuberculosis epidemic (Grygier 1994). This relocation and migration is of concern given that place has had a critically important function for indigenous peoples' identities, including Inuit (Basso 1996; Dorais and Searles 2001; Rasing 1999). Inuit lived primarily in extended-family camps on the land until the government era. The government's aggregation of many unrelated extended families in one location, often different from the place where they had been living, had a disruptive effect on kinship and social organization (Condon 1988; Graburn 1969). Mandatory schooling began for Inuit children with the introduction of residential and federal day schools (Milloy 1999). Residential schools were opened in five communities in the Northwest Territories between 1955 and 1971, and day schools began in 1957 (Crandall 2000; King 1999). By 1964 three-quarters of Inuit children between the ages of 6 and 15 were enrolled in school (Duffy 1988). Rhoda Kaukjak Katsak recalled her experience:

> When I went to school, when I came off the land, everything changed for me all at once ... When I came off the land, the people with any type of authority were Qallunaat. The teachers were Qallunaat, the principals were Qallunaat, the RCMP were Qallunaat, the administrators were Qallunaat, the nurses were Qallunaat, it was them who told us what to do ... It was difficult for me to learn when I was a child that there are other races, like the Qallunaat, who have the power, who have the authority. It was difficult for me. (Wachowich et al. 2004, 208)

Municipal governments were established by the federal government and were run by Qallunaat for many years, further disrupting and changing Inuit social patterns and taking away Inuit control over their decision making (Brody 1991; McElroy 1975, 1979; O'Neil 1983). The new wage economy began to show some growth with the seal industry of the 1970s, but its collapse in the early 1980s following the European boycott and antisealing campaigns turned Nunavummuit (Inuit of Nunavut) into poor welfare recipients (see Wenzel 1991). The last half of the twentieth century saw the most profound and rapid social change in Inuit history.

Community Wellness

In April 1995 the Government of the Northwest Territories (GNWT), Canada, released a document entitled *Working together for community wellness: A directions document* (Northwest Territories 1995). Developed with input from Inuit communities and several government departments, the document was a proposal for a "new vision" of healthier communities across the Canadian Arctic, a region at that time called the Northwest Territories. In 1998 the GNWT developed a Mental Health Framework to begin planning for integration of mental health services. Since the creation of the government of Nunavut in 1999, discussion surrounding community wellness has been taken more seriously.

Although there is evidence that some nationally known determinants of health are also valid for Native peoples in Canada (Wilson and Rosenberg 2002), it is vital to understand mental health and well-being from local and indigenous perspectives. The Bathurst Mandate (Nunavut 1999a) appears to have defined the Inuit perspective on mental health as

Inuuqatigiitiarniq, "the healthy interconnection of mind, body, spirit, [people], and the environment." Studies of suicide among Native North Americans have shown a relationship between community ties to traditional values and practices and attenuated suicide rates (Berlin 1987), as well as between fewer suicides and community/tribal control related to education, health services, police and fire services, self-government, and cultural facilities (Chandler and Lalonde 1998; Chapter 10). In a review of suicide prevention programs for Native American and Alaskan Native communities, Middlebrook and colleagues (2001) concluded that programs work best if they are both culturally relevant and developed with major community input. Community involvement in and control of policies and programs, commonly referred to as community empowerment, have thus been shown to make a significant difference in subjective well-being. Below, we will try to show that it is community control and collective agency that are the determining factors in successful suicide prevention and mental health outcomes in indigenous communities.

Well-being among Inuit in the Canadian Arctic has been moving in the direction of local control. The devolution or transfer of power of health services from the federal government to the Northwest Territories began in the 1980s, culminating with the transfer of responsibility for health care from the federal government to the GNWT in 1988. Little impact of this change, however, was felt at the community level (O'Neil 1990). The bureaucracy was not working, and new ideas were needed (Waldrum, Herring, and Young 1995). The 1995 GNWT report on community wellness, referred to earlier, resulted from concern over the continuing rise of social problems within Inuit communities. These problems have included intergenerational segregation, leading to the weakening of traditionally strong bonds of affection, respect, and teaching roles across generations; family and interpersonal violence; alcohol and drug abuse; child abuse and neglect; suicide; fetal alcohol syndrome; high rates of teen pregnancy; and sexually transmitted diseases, including HIV/AIDS. The programs and services addressing mental health were not working, and there was a lack of co-ordination across the relevant government departments. By 1993 a GNWT working group had been established to develop a community wellness strategy for Inuit communities. It was resolved that communities would be responsible for their own healing and wellness strategies and that the government would assist and support as was seen fit by the communities. It was a strategy of community empowerment and shared responsibility, replacing one of external control and authority by a largely Qallunaat government. The seat of the northern government was still in the western Arctic, or Denedeh, while many of these problems were significantly worse in the central and eastern Arctic, or Nunavut. For example, although the population of the western Canadian Arctic is almost twice that of Nunavut, over 70% of suicides were taking place in Nunavut by 1997. The western Arctic comprises mostly the Dene First Nation, while the east is almost all Inuit.

In two important community-based workshops and numerous meetings organized by the GNWT in 1994, the first order of business in the development of a community wellness

MICHAEL J. KRAL AND LORI IDLOUT

strategy was agreement on a definition of a healthy community. It is noteworthy that the Inuit "community" before the government era was the extended-family camp, whereas the settlements that are now called communities are of a very different order. They are a mixture of multiple extended Inuit families and Canadian bureaucracy. Several GNWT departments jointly sponsored these 1994 meetings in Yellowknife and Rankin Inlet, and Aboriginal and community participants attended them. The departments included Education, Health and Social Services, Culture and Employment, Justice, Municipal and Community Affairs, and the NWT Housing Corporation. The following characteristics of a "healthy community" were agreed upon: having a strong sense of community; having a strong sense of family life; an emphasis on personal dignity; a state of well-being; a strong sense of culture and tradition; zero tolerance for violence, substance abuse, and child abuse/neglect; and integrated services. Attention was then directed toward four areas of planned change: (1) prevention, healing, and treatment, (2) education and training, (3) interagency collaboration, and (4) community empowerment. Government money was spent, action was taken. Three crisis lines were established or further supported, women's shelters were set up in a number of communities, an alcohol/drug-rehabilitation clinic was opened in Iqaluit, suicide-prevention training workshops were held over a 3-year period for selected representatives of communities, and additional training programs were established or further supported, some within Nunavut Arctic College. These programs were to provide training in nursing, community health, social services and social work, teacher education, general counselling, and drug/alcohol counselling. Front-line health and social-service workers began to receive additional training. In spite of such intervention, suicide in Nunavut has continued to rise.

Top-Down Training Opportunities

Community empowerment meant significant involvement in the planning and administration of members' own health and social services based on these guidelines. Youth committees were established or further supported in each community, beginning in the Baffin region. Each community in Nunavut had, in addition to a Hamlet Council with elected representatives, an education committee, housing committee, Elders' society, hunters-trappers' organization, and numerous other committees or groups overseeing the broad spectrum of health and well-being. Controlled drinking communities, ones where a limited amount of alcohol can be ordered every month, had active alcohol committees whose members reviewed all orders for alcohol and the people doing the ordering. The members of these committees were exclusively or almost exclusively Inuit. Health remains, however, in the control of the territorial government, as do social services in most Inuit communities.

The new Nunavut government has since 1999 incorporated the administrative and service models of the previous GNWT and the federal government; however, it has declared as its mandate the incorporation of traditional knowledge, or *Inuit Qaujimajatuqangiit* (IQ), into this model (Nunavut 1999a). Forms of this incorporation have begun to take place in education, corrections, health, social services, and the Departments of Sustainable Development and Environment, including the 2003 Nunavut Wildlife Act, for example. Yet this blending of Inuit and Euro-Canadian philosophy and social organization remains a major challenge. Western health services that are individually focused, including mental health services, can be at odds with the family's being at the centre of Inuit well-being (Kral 2003). Inuit knowledge emphasizes the particular and personal, the practical and functional, and the relational and reciprocal, while scientific Western knowledge is general, abstract, and hierarchically authoritative (Kublu, Laugrand, and Oosten 2004). The challenge stems, in part, from what kind of community is imagined and by whom.

Health and wellness remains, however, in the control of the territorial government, as do social services in most Inuit communities. Communities are still given programs by the government whose content they have virtually no opportunity to determine or contribute to. Furthermore, these programs continue to create some divisions between Inuit communities and government, and within communities, because they are usually administered by community-based government workers. Knowledge from Elders, the traditional teachers of life-ways, is usually taken as advice in a superficial manner. The Government of Nunavut has "IQ Committees," which conduct advisory meetings, but the information provided to the Elders is usually restricted.

The Canadian government has been making an effort to improve the well-being of indigenous peoples in this country. One example is the blending of Western and indigenous wellness approaches under a program called Brighter Futures (2006). Brighter Futures was initiated in 1992-93 to develop culturally sensitive, community-based health programs for First Nations and Inuit in Canada. These programs are directed primarily at young children but are designed to foster health and wellness within the family and community. Based in the First Nations and Inuit Health Branch of Health Canada, Brighter Futures has been a financial resource for communities seeking funding for projects directed toward the improvement of "physical, mental and social well-being." Program elements have included community mental health (e.g., hiring counsellors, suicide- or violence-prevention workshops, healing), child development (e.g., preschool programs, youth programs), solvent abuse (e.g., peer counselling, education), injury prevention (e.g., first aid or safety courses), healthy babies (e.g., workshops to promote awareness of fetal alcohol syndrome), and parenting skills (e.g., workshops on parenting and communication).

Brighter Futures in the Nunavut government is administered through the Department of Health and Social Services, and in keeping with the original goal of the program, it is strongly community-based. By 2000 most of the projects funded in Nunavut were in community mental health (107), followed by child development (76), parenting skills (12), injury prevention (7), and solvent abuse (3) (see Brighter Futures 2006). Separate funding has been available for solvent abuse through the federal government's National Native

Alcohol and Drug Abuse Program (NNADAP). Project examples have included the hiring of community wellness co-ordinators, teaching youth traditional hunting and language skills, providing breakfast to schoolchildren, holding a youth-Elder conference, healing sessions for sexual-abuse survivors, a Bible-study camp, drug/alcohol healing sessions, hockey-skills development, student filmmaking, mathematics and language tutoring, a men's self-help group, suicide-prevention training, and recording oral histories from Elders. It is important to note that these projects were designed and/or managed within the communities. Other programs funded though the same branch of Health Canada are the Building Healthy Communities Initiative, directed at increasing community services in mental health, homecare nursing, and solvent abuse; Non-Insured Health Benefits funding, mainly for dental, vision, and prescription coverage, which also provides some coverage for one-on-one professional mental health treatment; and the NNADAP, which supports community-based prevention programs and residential treatment centres.

Although the concept is well intentioned, Brighter Futures faces many administrative challenges. Funding is allocated to a community project for 1 year starting 1 April, yet it can take up to 6 months before a community is able to receive the money. Then, in order to continue receiving funding, communities must submit an evaluation report, which itself takes much time. This means that communities might have only 3 to 4 months, instead of 1 year, to actually run their programs. Unused money must be returned at yearend, with often insufficient time to spend it. Brighter Futures can thus become administratively complex at both government and community levels. Yet Inuit communities in Nunavut are increasingly taking wellness into their own hands, and it is here where we are seeing the first significantly positive outcomes. Recent examples can be found in many Inuit communities, but given space constraints we will mention only two concerning suicide prevention.

Mental Health from the Inside

Community empowerment can become personal empowerment through community discourse on healing, argues Catherine Degnen (2001). She points to the importance of Aboriginal communities initiating their own healing, one way they are regaining control over their lives. Many communities have begun to address the problem of suicide through such local discourse. Suicide has continued to increase among youth in Nunavut, although with wide variation in suicide rates across communities. We will briefly describe activities that began in two Nunavut communities just before each experienced a decrease in suicide, activities that community members attributed to the saving of lives.

The first community is Qikiqtarjuaq, formerly called Broughton Island, with a population of about 500. It is an island off the eastern coast of Baffin Island, above the Arctic Circle. In 1994 it had the highest suicide rate of any community in the Canadian Arctic, with 12 youth suicides taking place between 1986 and 1993. Then the suicides stopped for several years. Inuit in other communities were saying that the people of Qikiqtarjuaq did something "from within" that had worked. In 1998 one of us was conducting field-work in that community and inquired about what had been done (Kral 2003). Inuit there, including a few who had helped to organize local suicide-prevention activities, reported that two related events had taken place. One was the gathering of community members, regularly over a period of time, in the gymnasium located in the basement of the Hamlet Council building. The council brought people of all ages together there. The local Youth Committee also gathered youth under the age of 24 to meet independently in the same place but at different times. These groups talked about suicide and about wanting the suicides to stop. Suggestions were made, including having people stop and speak to any-one they saw who appeared sad, worried, or whose behaviour had changed (e.g., social withdrawal). The local Anglican minister in this highly Christianized community also had people meet in the church to discuss suicide. The first event thus centred on talking. This talking may have been cathartic, but its purpose was one of synchrony – identifying shared feelings, ideas, concerns, and motivations about suicide and its prevention in the community.

A second activity related to suicide prevention in this community was organized by the local Housing Committee. All houses were publicly funded rather than privately owned, so this committee removed from each house the primary method of suicide in Nunavut: the closet rod. The most common suicide script here is hanging oneself from this rod in the bedroom at night when the family is asleep, usually facing the wall on the left side of the closet. Every closet rod was removed from every house, and locks were removed from bedroom doors. It was their version of "means restriction," analogous to gun control, which has had an effect of decreasing suicide where shooting oneself is the primary method for death by suicide (Carrington and Moyer 1994; Lester and Murrell 1982). This effect has been found for the restriction of any suicide method that is a culturally popular choice (Clarke and Lester 1989). Individuals do not tend to change the suicide method when the script for it is broken, suggesting that imitation and the internalization of cul-tural norms play a significant role in suicide (Kral 1994, 1998).

The second community example comes from Igloolik, an island in Foxe Basin above Hudson Bay and also above the Arctic Circle, with a population at this time of about 1,300. Up to 1994 this community had one of the lowest suicide rates in the Arctic. There had been only 1 suicide in the previous 10 years. Within the next 4 years, Igloolik had a large number of suicides: eight youth and one Elder. Yet this community recently celebrated the occasion of not having had a suicide for an entire year. Two events had taken place that community members talk about in relation to suicide prevention. The first was that Igloolik's Youth Committee had taken a major proactive step. The Youth Committee, about eight or nine young Inuit, held meetings every 2 weeks in response to the large number of recent suicides. Young people came together at these meetings to discuss what they viewed as important, including ways to improve community life and what young people can do to help Elders. This committee developed, together with the Igloolik film company, Isuma, a drop-in Youth Centre. During the day, two Elders were there to teach youth about traditional ways of life, and in the evenings youth had a place to be with other youth. Elders provided separate group-counselling sessions for young women and men. The Youth Committee also developed a local crisis helpline and had six youth serving as peer counsellors, who received training through the community-controlled Department of Social Services. The Youth Committee also organized two spring camping trips with Elders and youth through the Youth Centre, something they had begun prior to its development. The Youth Committee also produced a video on suicide prevention with Isuma. Another video was made of a play they produced on the subject of suicide prevention. Older Inuit became further involved in the Youth Centre when it organized weekly board games, such as chess and Scrabble. Finally, the centre was actively promoting the learning of Inuktitut and its dialects. The financial picture, unfortunately, became problematic, and these services and activities stopped for a number of years. Indeed, a lack of continued funding and financial management, in addition to problems with the building itself, was the major reason for the closing of the Youth Centre after only one and a half years of operation.

The other event related to suicide prevention in Igloolik was more indirect: the making of a film by Inuit filmmakers and actors, all from Igloolik and centred in the Inuit film company in this community, Isuma Productions. The film was *Atanarjuat: The Fast Runner,* which was released in Canada in 2001 and the United States in 2002, and which has won numerous international awards, including the Caméra d'Or at Cannes. It was Canada's official selection for the 2003 foreign-language Oscar. The film is about an ancient Inuit legend, and the story takes place before contact with Qallunaat (see Apak Angilirq, Cohn, and Saladin D'Anglure 2002). A shaman disrupts the stability of two families, and conflict ensues across a vast landscape and across time. It is the story of Atanarjuat, a man on a journey of tremendous spiritual importance in the restoration of harmony for his family. Inuit of Igloolik were involved in the making of this film, from writing, directing, acting, and filming to sewing caribou parkas and designing and making the traditional *kamutiq,* or sledges, from whalebone and sealskin. Inuit of Igloolik have prided themselves for upholding their traditional culture.

Inuit youth spoke during the film's initial stages of the importance of their involvement in its production. In discussing his sense of belonging, of feeling a part of the community, or *ilagiijttiarniq,* one 19-year-old Inuk talked about the importance of young people working together with adults and Elders on the making of this film. This young man told of how being involved in making the film made him feel good about himself "because it tells me how my ancestors used to live, and I see it with my own eyes and I see the environment how it was before." Lucy Tulugardjuk, of the Youth Committee, was ecstatic when she learned that she had been given a lead role in the film. She soon helped youth to develop theatre in Igloolik, while another Igloolik actor from *Atanarjuat*, Natar Ungalaq, helped youth to develop film and video productions.

During the filming of a second major film production, *The Journals of Knud Rasmussen,* which finished shooting in 2005, Isuma involved Inuit youth in an apprenticeship program. Participants received on-the-job training in filmmaking, television, and website design. One of these youth, Jason Kunnuk, spoke about how being on the sets and working with Inuit filmmakers and actors strengthened his sense of belonging and had a profound and positive effect on him. "I can't find the words to express how I really felt looking at the people, my history, and how they worked so hard for us to be here." He reported feeling encouraged and motivated to "maintain my culture." He added that the experience made him aware that suicide "is not the Inuit way." Meeting the challenge of blending two cultural worlds together was made more clear to him, Jason said, and he shared a metaphor he has found helpful through the image of the kamutiq, or sled. The sled, historically, was made of "organic material. Right now it's [made of] wood, plastic, rope ... [yet] it still has the same purpose. We know where we came from. We know pretty much where we're going. But sometimes when you get lost, you could look back, behind your tracks, to see which mistakes you did. And mainly to look forward, to going on forward ... it always goes forward."

Youth were also hired by Isuma to help Elder women experts to make fur clothing for the actors, which allowed the youth to learn this important traditional skill. One young woman learned to prepare and sew caribou skin for the first time, and with a smile she said that she and her mother were now spending a lot of time talking about this. It was something her mother had done throughout her life but a skill they were never able to share with each other until then. Here was an important bolstering of family ties. Leah Angutimarik, who at age 21 played a lead role in the new film, talked about the positive impact this experience had on her shortly after the shooting was completed. She learned, hands-on, various traditional Inuit practices such as lighting the *kulliq,* or oil lamp, and spoke of the older Inuit in the film as role models. She came away from the film with a better sense of herself, saying "I want to be me more. I want to be myself more." She said that she was a stronger person because of it. It created a desire in her to learn even more about her culture and to help other young Inuit like herself learn the same. "We're losing our history," Leah indicated, adding that she believed that this loss of history and identity is related to current problems of suicide and anger among Inuit youth.

The director of these two films, Zacharias Kunuk, is committed to bringing his people back in touch with who they are and have always been (personal communication, October 2002). There is good evidence that learning about one's culture enhances self-esteem (Phinney 1991). The film *Atanarjuat* sings of reclamation and recovery. The concurrent activities of the community and Youth Committee, and the production of the two films, were initiated within the community; they were home-grown. Isuma received funds to open a Youth Centre and to make an initial film/video project with youth. Thus it was directly tied to the larger project of community youth wellness. Suicides stopped for a noticeable period of time in a community that had been beset by too-frequent suicides. The "tipping point," as the saying now goes (see Gladwell 2000), for the reduction of suicide

MICHAEL J. KRAL AND LORI IDLOUT

was not likely any one factor in the two communities discussed here but a spread of wellness that coincided with and, we believe, is directly related to community control.

Programs bringing youth and Elders together are being developed in many northern communities in response to the increasing intergenerational segregation mentioned earlier and the centrality of family and community to Aboriginal life. One such program took place in the Kitikmeot region of Nunavut in the central Arctic (Eyegetok, Thorpe, and Iqaluktuuttiaq Elders 1998; Thorpe 1998). A small group of youth and Elders spent time on the land in the summer, with the Elders teaching traditional skills and knowledge in the context of storytelling and practice. "The elders gave skills, culture, experience and knowledge as gifts. The youth showed enthusiasm, cooperation and an eagerness to learn which was noticeable in their attempts, attitudes and morale ... Together, these positive elder-youth experiences and Inuit knowledge recordings will provide a legacy of memories that will last well beyond the camp" (Eyegetok et al. 1998). A similar "culture camp" took place among the Yup'ik in south-western Alaska, where Elders passed on their stories to youth, "teaching nothing less than how to learn" (Fienup-Riordan 2002, 173). Youth themselves are involved in and often organize these activities across communities. Intergenerational experiences of trauma and loss are well known in Aboriginal country, and this form of negative mimesis or transmission can be countered by today's young people (LeVine 2000).

The Statewide Suicide Prevention Council of Alaska (2002, 2003) has implemented a strategy that appears to be working. A set of general principles for suicide prevention was produced, such as having a crisis team in each village, yet each participating community developed its own program. This was based in a shared belief across the council and Alaska Native communities that imported suicide-prevention programs could not address local place and culture. The council, which includes youth and Elders, conducted "listening sessions" where it learned from community members, including survivors and professionals, while local tribal councils were involved in training their own suicide-prevention co-ordinators. It is important to note that these were not training sessions but listening sessions. Several villages with suicide rates higher than the Alaska average established their own prevention projects and between 1990 and 1997 showed a decrease in these rates, while villages without their own projects saw an increase in suicide rates. One of the plans of the council is to have communities share their particular projects with each other. The essential feature of these successful prevention projects is that they are community-owned to their core.

Warry (1998) has pointed out that Aboriginal community control over health and mental health activities and programs has been central to their success. This can also be seen in Australia's National Aboriginal Community Controlled Health Organization (NACCHO). Established in the 1970s, the philosophy behind NACCHO is for each Aboriginal community to control its own delivery of health and mental health services, including the initiation of such services. An increase has been seen not only in a wide variety of needed services being provided across communities but also in an increase in member utilization of these services (OATSIH-NACCHO 2003). The Health Transfer Agreements being signed between Canadian Aboriginal communities and Health Canada of the federal government, begun in 1989, are similar to the Australian model, as they are designed to allow communities to determine their own health priorities and to establish culturally appropriate programs. In Canada this is further supported by the government's 1995 Inherent Right to Self-Government Policy for First Nations and Inuit, recognizing their constitutional right to self-governance. It should be noted that once community action begins, it can be catching. The opportunity to develop programs and activities toward well-being within a community can itself lead to further solidarity and commitment to these goals by its members, as it has been shown that social action itself is a determinant of such commitment (Kelly and Kaplan 2001; Passy 2003).

Nunalingni Silatuningit – Community Wisdom

We would like to go beyond possible remedies for Durkheim's *anomic suicide,* which include the restoration of social regulation, the meeting of expectations, the feeling of normative belonging, and the stabilizing of runaway social change (Durkheim 1951), and also beyond the idea of *social capital,* the newer term used to describe social membership and exchange, trust, and "collective action for mutual benefit" (Galea, Karpati, and Kennedy 2002, 1374). Although these constructs address the important benefits of solidarity for individuals and groups, they do not focus strongly on the idea of social action, of collective agency and control, as producing such social well-being. Personal control has been identified as an important factor in mental health across cultures (Grob 2000; Vaillant 2003). Among Inuit, as for other Aboriginal peoples, decision making was taken away from individuals, families, and communities. There is good reason to believe that collective control is important for collective mental health, and Bellah and colleagues (1991) have argued that decentralized power is necessary for communities to thrive. As noted above, such control appears to be the critical feature in suicide prevention in Aboriginal communities (e.g., Chandler and Lalonde 1998; Chapter 10).

We are here discussing the idea of community or collective agency. The term "agency" in its modern sense refers to the individual and is founded in Protestantism, capitalism, and liberalism (Asad 1996). Indeed, it has been traditionally pitted against the collective (Bakan 1966; Fuller 1998). Collective agency, however, can be viewed as an internal locus of control felt by individuals that is at once shared around both activity and identity – the two being interdependent. Collective agency takes place when members of a group or community participate in an activity that they have created themselves, is "theirs" over time, and is recognized as positive. Agency is here seen as a quality of action, a process, rather than as a bounded, internal force. Yet knowing and believing that one can execute a particular action is the self-efficacy tied to mental health. Much has been written on the beneficial psychological effects of both internal locus of control and self-efficacy on individual well-being (Grob 2000), and we extend these concepts to the community. Collective efficacy – "a group's shared belief in its conjoint capabilities to organize and execute the courses of action required to produce given levels of attainments" – is predictive of such attainments (Bandura 1997, 477). It is here that the personal/subjective and the collective share a common ground. Collective agency becomes directly tied to personal agency. It is ownership, control, and engagement tied to the human need to belong (Baumeister and Leary 1995). This may be especially relevant to indigenous peoples, who have historically formed kinship-based cultures (DeMallie 1998; Miller 2002). Family-centred interdependence may be one type of collectivism that is relevant to Inuit within the multidimensionality of the idea of collectivism (see Ashmore, Deaux, and McLaughlin-Volpe 2004). Although individual autonomy has always been highly respected among Inuit, kinship and interdependence have historically been the basis of their social organization.

Consensus without Coercion

Inuit communities today comprise multiple families and are increasingly mobile, which presents an organizational challenge. Yet a community can become a social network whose members work toward collective goals, even as co-operative smaller social networks within the community (e.g., Wetherell, Plakans, and Wellman 1994). Community action becomes the route to collective ownership and responsibility.

Personal agency and collective agency do not need to be contradictory. Sampson (1988) adds a dimension to power and control that is on the other side of the internal, self-contained individualism common in Western society, which he refers to as field control. Here, power and control are located in "a field of forces that includes but goes well beyond the person" (16). It is a control within what he calls "ensembled individualism," an inclusive indigenous psychology that captures a more fluid self-other boundary. Autonomous selves are experienced as such even in collectivist cultures like that of Hindu India (Raval and Kral 2004), and in the ensembled individualism of Aboriginal societies the locus of control is both personal and collective. Indigenous community control is a kind of field control that integrates personal and social responsibility.

Yet cultures and communities that have lost much control over their lives (e.g., via colonialism and state control) manifest significant social problems. It is a basic collective human need to have self-determination, and we have learned much about this from world history when this need has been taken away from a people. Peter Penashue, the president of the Labrador Innu Nation, writes about the need for control based at the community level: "I think that we have learned now that when people are oppressed, when people are not involved in determining the direction of their lives, they are deeply damaged" (2001, 29). Perceived control is especially important to well-being when the domain under control is highly salient (Grob 2000). It is important to understand and explore what domains are salient for different peoples, generations, contexts, and communities. Community control over mental health resources thus becomes an efficacious route that focuses on local salience. Services, programs, and activities become tailored by and for the people, who most understand themselves.

Mason Durie (1998) has highlighted that for the Mäori of New Zealand, *mana,* or sovereignty, has become salient in the context of colonialism and is now directly related to the well-being of his people. These are the types of narratives and histories that help to locate the meaning of agency in the plural. The reclamation of collective self-determination is never a smooth process. The Innu, Mäori, Inuit, First Nations, and other indigenous and Tribal peoples have struggled, even staggered, but they have not fallen (Amagoalik 2000).

Returning to our critique of unidirectional, top-down knowledge transfer from governments and agencies to communities, we hope that we have made clear an awareness of the importance of knowledge transfer going in the other direction. The most important knowledge is already in the community. Chandler and Lalonde (2004) have recently made this same argument, adding that lateral knowledge transfer *between* communities is another important route. This is beginning to take place in Nunavut. The Isaksimagit Inuusirmi Katujjiqatigiit, or Embrace Life Council, an organization in Nunavut dedicated to suicide prevention and community wellness, organized its first conference in early 2005, which was attended by 59 representatives of every Nunavut community. The conference was titled Avamut Iqajuktigiit Katimavikjjuanignat – Conference of Helping One Another – and among its objectives, the central feature was the sharing between communities of their own wellness activities and programs, ones believed locally to be directly responsible for youth well-being and suicide prevention. A primary theme that emerged from the meeting was that Inuit communities need to be in control of their own wellness strategies (Embrace Life Council 2005). This is one form of lateral knowledge transfer that becomes a larger collectivity of social action toward well-being, a widening of the circle of sharing.

Although the examples of local, community-based suicide prevention and mental health presented in this chapter are brief and few, they speak to something much more important than a well-intentioned mental health program being passed on to or imported for Inuit and other indigenous communities. The Inuit communities mentioned here did something unique. From our knowledge of the communities, it seems likely that these actions fit with a deeper and very local sensibility of how things work and of what remedies are most effective. They did something that came from within, something that they created. The success of the suicide-prevention projects initiated by Inuit communities in Canada and Alaska is likely due to the fact that *it does not appear to matter so much what the project is as much as that the program or initiative is the community's own*. This is in line with the move toward community empowerment of the GNWT in the mid-1990s, and it fits with the Nunavut government's mandate to have each community develop its own plans for wellness (Nunavut 1999b). We are suggesting that internal community control, or collective agency, is responsible for the positive outcomes discussed above, however short-lived

MICHAEL J. KRAL AND LORI IDLOUT

they may be so far. This is a critically important point. Joseph Gone (2004; Chapter 19) has argued that Western clinical mental health practices can incur an invisible cultural proselytization, replacing local knowledge about wellness and healing with models that are not based on the cosmology of the people living there. The new knowledge is historically and experientially incongruent. It is a form of the state's standard grid of top-down legibility that excludes local knowledge (Scott 1998). Top-down, outside-in approaches to substance-abuse prevention still appear to be the norm for Native American communities, for example (Hawkins, Cummins, and Marlatt 2004), and these approaches continue to collide with local culture (Prussing, forthcoming). O'Neil (1988) referred to this as a form of colonization by Western medicine, complicit with the larger colonial subordination of indigenous values and practices. In Chapter 17 of this volume, Mary Ellen Macdonald shows that culture has yet to find a place in Canadian federal health care policy. Yet we know that community is an essential cultural concept for Aboriginal mental health (Manson 2000; Waldram 2002). Culture can become realized in mental health initiatives through community power and control.

Inuit Elder Mariano Aupilardjuk stated recently: "We need to implement the Inuit counseling and healing practices with Inuit approaches" (Nunavut Social Development Council 2001). These practices must start with local control and local planning if they are to be Inuit. There is a crucial difference between a community deciding how to implement and control a program of the government and a community *designing its own plans*. The latter engages and empowers the community in ways that remedies applied from the outside cannot. On suicide prevention, an Inuit woman Elder from Igloolik stated: "We have to look at what the community wants." And a 17-old Inuk from the same community emphasized: "Just a whole community working together can make a difference" (Kral 2003). Writing about hunting societies, including Inuit, Hugh Brody emphasizes: "Elders in many indigenous societies are clear about the benefits of their way of life ... Their argument is that the 'traditional' system secured important benefits and could continue to do so. Change, they say, is for the most part a result of pressure and invasion rather than an expression of preference. Of course they want to be modern – but on their own terms" (2000, 148).

Philip McMichael (2000) has argued that the broader development and globalization projects have not included the empowerment of local cultures. He believes that those designing such projects need to rethink priorities toward long-term improvement of the human and environmental condition. These priorities will include, at their base, what Arturo Escobar (1995) was told by the Organization of Black Communities of the Pacific Coast of Columbia: a people's own "life projects." The Mental Health Working Group of the Assembly of First Nations/Inuit Tapirisat of Canada has made it clear that "the most important thing about mental wellness is that it must be well defined in terms of the values and beliefs of First Nations and Inuit communities" (2001, i).

Self-determination at the community level is not simple. Rather, new levels of complexity arise, as some indigenous communities have experienced internally regarding, for example, disagreements about specific goals, people, and methods. The local also cannot always or even easily be independent of the regional, territorial, or federal in Nunavut in terms of activities and programs related to health, education, and social services, even if these activities and programs are created by the community. Not at this time. What we are writing about in this chapter is a form of indigenous anarchism in co-operation with the state – a contradiction but one that is currently developing, although not without struggle, in Canada (see Graeber 2004). In addition to community control, and just as important, is a focus on sustaining community-developed action over time. Suicides resumed in the two Inuit communities discussed above after the activities/programs begun by each community came to an end. A major reason for the cessation of programs in at least one of the communities was a lack of sustained funding. Program continuity must also incorporate flexibility at the community level, where changes in personnel are common. A topic beyond the scope of this chapter, the continuity of truly community-based actions and programs toward well-being and mental health, is in need of serious attention. This new complexity of community self-management is, we believe, worth the effort of time and money.

Local conceptions of indigenous mental health must be made clear and utilized. This will likely be some form of blending between Aboriginal and Western approaches. Such a convergence needs critical attention and dialogue. Yet this also needs to be in the context of the further identification and sustaining of local endeavours toward and control of psychological and community wellness at the site of the community itself. The tool for community wellness is a respect for and listening to *nunalingni silatuningit,* or collective wisdom, of a community.

Acknowledgments

Appreciation is extended to Laurence Kirmayer and Theresa O'Nell for comments on earlier versions of this chapter and to Edward Tapardjuk, Leappi Akoomalik, Natar Ungalaq, Lucy Uyarak Tulugardjuk, and Norman Cohn for valuable ideas and information. The writing of this chapter was supported by a Doctoral Fellowship from the Social Sciences and Humanities Research Council (SSHRC), a Canadian Polar Commission Scholarship, and the Canadian Bicentennial Professorship Endowment, Yale Center for International and Area Studies, awarded to Michael Kral, who also thanks the Department of Anthropology, Yale University, for providing him with a wonderful environment during that time. Some of the research discussed in this chapter was funded by a grant from the National Health Research and Development Program, Health Canada.

References

Amagoalik, J. 2000. Wasteland of nobodies. In J. Dahl, J. Hicks, and P. Jull, eds., *Nunavut: Inuit regain control of their lands and their lives,* 138-39. Copenhagen, DK: International Work Group for Indigenous Affairs, doc. no. 102.

Apak Angilirq, P., N. Cohn, and B. Saladin D'Anglure. 2002. *Atanarjuat: The fast runner.* Toronto, ON: Coach House Books; Montreal, QC: Isuma Publishing.

Asad, T. 1996. Comments on conversion. In P. van der Veer, ed., *Conversion to modernities: The globalization of Christianity,* 263-73. New York: Routledge.

Ashmore, R.D., K. Deaux, and T. McLaughlin-Volpe. 2004. An organizing framework for collective identity: Articulation and significance of multidimensionality. *Psychological Bulletin* 130 (1): 80-114.

Bakan, D. 1966. *The duality of human existence*. Chicago, IL: Rand McNally.

Bandura, A. 1997. *Self-efficacy: The exercise of control*. New York: W.H. Freeman.

Basso, K.H. 1996. *Wisdom sits in places: Landscapes and language among the Apache*. Albuquerque, NM: University of New Mexico Press.

Baumeister, R.F., and M.R. Leary. 1995. The need to belong: Desire for interpersonal attachments as a fundamental human motivation. *Psychological Bulletin* 117 (3): 497-529.

Bellah, R.N., R. Madsen, W. Sullivan, A. Swidler, and S. Tipton. 1991. *The good society*. New York: Knopf.

Berlin, I.N. 1987. Suicide among American Indian adolescents: An overview. *Suicide and Life-Threatening Behavior* 17 (3): 218-32.

Bjerregaard, P., and T.K. Young. 1998. *The circumpolar Inuit: Health of a population in transition*. Copenhagen, DK: Munksgaard.

Boothroyd, L.J., L.J. Kirmayer, S. Spreng, M. Malus, and S. Hodgins. 2001. Completed suicides among the Inuit of northern Quebec: A case control study. *Canadian Medical Association Journal* 165 (6): 749-55.

Brighter Futures. 2006. *Building brighter futures: 2006 and 2007*. Ohsweken, ON: National Aboriginal Achievement Foundation. http://www.gov.nu.ca/nsssite/nssmain.shtml.

Brody, H. 1991 [1975]. *The people's land: Inuit, whites, and the eastern Arctic*. Vancouver, BC: Douglas and McIntyre.

–. 2000. *The other side of Eden: Hunters, farmers and the shaping of the world*. Vancouver, BC: Douglas and McIntyre.

Burkhardt, K.J. 2004. Crime, cultural reintegration and community healing: Narratives of an Inuit community. PhD diss., University of Windsor.

Carrington, P., and S. Moyer. 1994. Gun control and suicide in Ontario. *American Journal of Psychiatry* 151 (4): 606-8.

Chandler, M.J., and C.E. Lalonde. 1998. Cultural continuity as a hedge against suicide in Canada's First Nations. *Transcultural Psychiatry* 35 (2): 221-20.

–, and C.E. Lalonde. 2004. Transferring whose knowledge? Exchanging whose best practices? On knowing about indigenous knowledge and Aboriginal suicide. In J. White, P. Maxim, and D. Beavon, eds., *Aboriginal policy research: Setting the agenda for change*, vol. 2, 111-23. Toronto, ON: Thompson.

Clarke, R., and D. Lester. 1989. *Suicide: Closing the exits*. New York: Springer-Verlag.

Condon, R.G. 1988. *Inuit youth: Growth and change in the Canadian Arctic*. New Brunswick, NJ: Rutgers University Press.

Crandall, R.C. 2000. *Inuit art: A history*. Jefferson, NC: McFarland.

Crowe, K.J. 1991. *A history of original peoples of northern Canada*. Rev. ed. Montreal, QC, and Kingston, ON: McGill-Queen's University Press.

Damas, D. 2002. *Arctic migrants, Arctic villagers: The transformation of Inuit settlement in the central Arctic*. Montreal, QC, and Kingston, ON: McGill-Queen's University Press.

Degnen, C. 2001. Country space as a healing place: Community healing at Sheshatshiu. In C.H. Scott, ed., *Aboriginal autonomy and development in northern Quebec and Labrador*, 356-78. Vancouver, BC: UBC Press.

DeMallie, R.J. 1998. Kinship: The foundation for Native American society. In R. Thornton, ed., *Studying Native America: Problems and prospects*, 306-56. Madison, WI: University of Wisconsin Press.

Dorais, L.-J., and E. Searles. 2001. Inuit identities. *Études/Inuit/Studies* 25 (1-2): 17-35.

Duffy, R.Q. 1988. *The road to Nunavut*. Montreal, QC, and Kingston, ON: McGill-Queen's University Press.

Durie, M. 1998. *Te mana, te kâwanatanga: The politics of Maori self-determination*. Auckland, NZ: Oxford University Press.

Durkheim, É. 1951 [1897]. *Suicide: A study in sociology*. Glencoe, IL: Free Press.

Embrace Life Council. 17-18 February 2005. *Report of the Conference of Helping One Another*. Iqaluit, NU: Akhaliak.

Escobar, A. 1995. *Encountering development: The making and unmaking of the Third World*. Princeton, NJ: Princeton University Press.

Eyegetok, S., N. Thorpe, and Iqaluktuuttiaq Elders. 1998. *The Hiukitaak River Elder-youth camp report*. Tuktu and Nogak Project: http://www3.telus.net/tuktu/main.html.

Fienup-Riordan, A. 2002. "We talk to you because we love you": Learning from Elders at culture camp. *Anthropology and Humanism* 26 (2): 173-87.

Fossett, R. 2001. *In order to live untroubled: Inuit of the central Arctic, 1550 to 1940*. Winnipeg, MB: University of Manitoba Press.

Fuller, S. 1998. From content to context: A social epistemology of the structure-agency craze. In *What is social theory? The philosophical debates,* 92-117. Malden, MA: Blackwell.

Galea, S., A. Karpati, and B. Kennedy. 2002. Social capital and violence in the United States, 1974-1993. *Social Science and Medicine* 55 (8): 1373-83.

Gladwell, M. 2000. *The tipping point: How little things can make a big difference*. Boston, MA: Little, Brown.

Gone, J. 2004. Keeping culture in mind: Transforming academic training in professional psychology for Indian country. In D.A. Mihesuah and A.C. Wilson, eds., *Indigenizing the academy: Transforming scholarship and empowering communities,* 124-46. Lincoln, NE: University of Nebraska Press.

Graburn, N.H.H. 1969. *Eskimos without igloos: Social and economic development in Sugluk*. Boston, MA: Little, Brown.

Graeber, D. 2004. *Fragments of an anarchist anthropology*. Chicago, IL: Prickly Paradigm.

Griffiths, C.T., D. Wood, E. Zellerer, and G. Saville. 1995. Crime, law, and justice in the Baffin region: Preliminary findings from a multi-year study. In K.M. Hazlehurst, ed., *Legal pluralism and the colonial legacy: Indigenous experiences of justice in Canada, Australia, and New Zealand,* 130-58. Aldershot, UK: Avebury.

Grob, A. 2000. Perceived control and subjective well-being across nations and across the life span. In E. Deiner and E.M. Suh, eds., *Culture and subjective well-being,* 319-39. Cambridge, MA: MIT Press.

Grygier, P.S. 1994. *A long way from home: The tuberculosis epidemic among the Inuit*. Montreal, QC, and Kingston, ON: McGill-Queen's University Press.

Haggarty, J., Z. Cernovsky, P. Kermeen, and H. Merskey. 2000. Psychiatric disorders in an Arctic community. *Canadian Journal of Psychiatry* 45 (4): 357-62.

Hawkins, E.H., L.H. Cummins, and G.A. Marlatt. 2004. Preventing substance abuse in American Indian and Alaska Native youth: Promising strategies for healthier communities. *Psychological Bulletin* 130 (2): 304-23.

Idiens, D. 1989. Eskimos in Scotland, c. 1682-1924. In C.F. Feest, ed., *Indians and Europe: An interdisciplinary collection of essays,* 161-74. Lincoln, NE: University of Nebraska Press.

Injury Surveillance On-line. 2004. *Injury deaths*. Ottawa, ON: Health Surveillance and Epidemiology Division, Centre for Health Human Development, Health Canada. http://dsol-smed.hc-sc.gc.ca/dsol-smed/is-sb/c_quik_e.html.

Kelly, J.D., and M. Kaplan. 2001. *Represented communities: Fiji and world decolonization*. Chicago, IL: University of Chicago Press.

King, D.P. 1999. The history of the federal residential schools for the Inuit located in Chesterfield Inlet, Yellowknife, Inuvik, and Churchill, 1955-1970. MA thesis, Trent University.

Kirmayer, L.J., C. Fletcher, and L. Boothroyd. 1998. Suicide among the Inuit of Canada. In A.A. Leenaars, S. Wenckstern, I. Sakinofsky, M.J. Kral, R.J. Dyck, and R. Bland, eds., *Suicide in Canada,* 189-211. Toronto, ON: University of Toronto Press.

Kral, M.J. 1994. Suicide as social logic. *Suicide and Life-Threatening Behavior* 24 (3): 245-55.

–. 1998. Suicide and the internalization of culture: Three questions. *Transcultural Psychiatry* 35 (2): 221-33.

–. 2003. *Unikkaartuit: Meanings of well-being, sadness, suicide, and change in two Inuit communities*. Report submitted to National Health Research and Development Programs, Health Canada.

Kublu, A., F. Laugrand, and J. Oosten. 2004 [1999]. The nature of Inuit knowledge. In G. Robinson, ed., *Isuma Inuit studies reader,* 122-25. Montreal, QC: Isuma Publishing.

MICHAEL J. KRAL AND LORI IDLOUT

Lester, D., and M.E. Murrell. 1982. The preventive effect of strict gun control laws on suicide and homicide. *Suicide and Life-Threatening Behavior* 12 (3): 131-40.

LeVine, R.A. 2000. Epilogue. In A.C.G.M. Robben and M.M. Suárez-Orozco, eds., *Cultures under siege: Collective violence and trauma,* 272-75. Cambridge: Cambridge University Press.

Manson, S. 2000. Mental health services for American Indians and Alaska Natives: Need, use, and barriers to effective care. *Canadian Journal of Psychiatry* 45 (7): 617-27.

McElroy, A. 1975. Canadian Arctic modernization and change in female Inuit role identification. *American Ethnologist* 2 (4): 662-86.

–. 1979. The negotiation of sex-role identity in eastern Arctic culture change. In A. McElroy and C. Matthiasson, eds., *Sex-roles in changing cultures: Occasional papers in anthropology no. 1,* 49-60. Buffalo, NY: Department of Anthropology, State University of New York at Buffalo.

McGee, R. 1981. *The/Les Tuniit.* Ottawa, ON: National Museums of Canada.

McMichael, P. 2000. *Development and social change: A global perspective.* 2nd ed. Thousand Oaks, CA: Pine Forge Press and Sage.

Mental Health Working Group. 2001. *Comprehensive culturally appropriate mental wellness framework: First Nations and Inuit health and wellness discussion document.* Ottawa, ON: Assembly of First Nations – Inuit Tapirisat of Canada.

Middlebrook, D.L., P.L. LeMaster, J. Beals, D.K. Novins, and S. Manson. 2001. Suicide prevention in American Indian and Alaska Native communities: A critical review of programs. *Suicide and Life-Threatening Behavior* 31 (suppl.): S132-S49.

Miller, J. 2002. Kinship, family kindreds, and community. In P.J. Deloria and N. Salisbury, eds., *A companion to American Indian history,* 139-53. Malsen, MA: Blackwell.

Milloy, J.S. 1999. *A national crime: The Canadian government and the residential school system, 1879 to 1976.* Winnipeg, MB: University of Manitoba Press.

Northwest Territories. 1995. *Working together for community wellness: A directions document.* Yellowknife, NWT: Government of the Northwest Territories.

Nunavut. 1999a. *The Bathurst mandate.* Iqaluit, NU: Government of Nunavut.

–. 1999b. *Report from the September Inuit Qaujimajatuqangit workshop.* Iqaluit, NU: Department of Culture, Elders, Language and Youth, Government of Nunavut.

Nunavut Bureau of Statistics. 2003. *Statistics on death by suicide in Nunavut.* Iqaluit, NU: Government of Nunavut.

Nunavut Social Development Council. 2001. *Ihumaliurhimajaptingnik/On our own terms: The state of Inuit culture and society.* Iqaluit, NU: Nunavut Social Development Council.

OATSIH-NACCHO. 2003. *Service activity reporting 2000-2001 key results: A national profile of Australian government funded Aboriginal and Torres Strait Islander primary health care services.* Canberra, AU: Office for Aboriginal and Torres Strait Islander Health and National Aboriginal Community Controlled Health Organisation.

O'Neil, J.D. 1983. Is it cool to be an Eskimo? A study of stress, identity, coping and health among Canadian Inuit young adult men. PhD diss., University of California.

–. 1988. Self-determination, medical ideology and health services in Inuit communities. In G. Dacks and K. Coates, eds., *Northern communities: The prospects for empowerment,* 33-50. Edmonton, AB: Boreal Institute for Northern Studies, University of Alberta.

–. 1990. The impact of devolution on health services in the Baffin region. In G. Dacks, ed., *Devolution and constitutional development in the Canadian North,* 157-93. Ottawa, ON: Carleton University Press.

Passy, F. 2003. Social networks matter. But how? In M. Diani and D. McAdam, eds., *Social movements and networks: Relational approaches to collective action,* 21-48. Oxford, UK: Oxford University Press.

Penashue, P. 2001. Healing the past, meeting the future. In C.H. Scott, ed., *Aboriginal autonomy and development in northern Quebec and Labrador,* 21-29. Vancouver, BC: UBC Press.

Phinney, J. 1991. Ethnic identity and self-esteem: A review and integration. *Hispanic Journal of Behavioral Sciences* 13 (2): 193-208.

Prussing, E. Forthcoming. Sobriety and its cultural politics: An ethnographer's perspective on "culturally appropriate" addiction services in Native North America. *Ethos*.

Rasing, W. 1999. Hunting for identity: Thoughts on the practice of hunting and its significance for Iglulingmiut identity. In J. Oosten and C. Remie, eds., *Arctic identities: Continuity and change in Inuit and Saami societies,* 79-108. Leiden, Netherlands: CNWS Publications, Leiden University.

Raval, V.V., and M.J. Kral. 2004. Core versus periphery: Dynamics of personhood over the life-course for a Gujarati Hindu woman. *Culture and Psychology* 10 (2): 162-94.

Sampson, E.E. 1988. The debate on individualism: Indigenous psychologies of the individual and their role in personal and societal functioning. *American Psychologist* 43: 15-22.

Scott, J.C. 1998. *Seeing like a state: How certain schemes to improve the human condition have failed.* New Haven, CT: Yale University Press.

Statewide Suicide Prevention Council. 2002. *FY 2002 annual report.* Anchorage, AK: State of Alaska.

–. 2003. *FY 2003 annual report.* Anchorage, AK: State of Alaska.

Sturtevant, W.C., and D.B. Quinn. 1989. This new prey: Eskimos in Europe in 1567, 1576, and 1577. In C.F. Feest, ed., *Indians and Europe: An interdisciplinary collection of essays,* 61-140. Lincoln, NE: University of Nebraska Press.

Taylor, J.G. 1984. Historical ethnography of the Labrador coast. In D. Damas, ed., *Handbook of North American Indians,* vol. 5, *Arctic,* 508-21. Washington, DC: Smithsonian Institution.

Thorpe, N.L. 1998. The Hiukitak school of Tuktu: Collecting Inuit ecological knowledge of caribou and calving areas through an Elder-youth camp. *Arctic* 51 (4): 403-8.

Trudel, M. 1994. *Dictionnaire des esclaves et leurs propriétaires au Canada français.* 2nd ed. LaSalle, QC: Éditions Hurtubise.

Vaillant, G.E. 2003. Mental health. *American Journal of Psychiatry* 160 (8): 1373-84.

Wachowich, N., A. Agalakti Awa, R. Kaukjak Katsak, and S. Pikujak Katsak. 2004 [2001]. Saqiyuq: Stories from the lives of three Inuit women. G. Robinson, ed., *Isuma Inuit studies reader,* 183-213. Montreal, QC: Isuma Publishing.

Waldram, J.B. 2002. Everybody's healing, but what does that mean? A critical examination of "traditional" approaches in Aboriginal mental health treatment. Paper presented at the Annual Meeting of the American Anthropological Association, New Orleans, LA.

–, D.A. Herring, and T.K. Young. 1995. *Aboriginal health in Canada: Historical, cultural, and epidemiological perspectives.* Toronto, ON: University of Toronto Press.

Warry, W. 1998. *Unfinished dreams: Community healing and the reality of Aboriginal self-government.* Toronto, ON: University of Toronto Press.

Wenzel, G. 1991. *Animal rights, human rights: Ecology, economy and ideology in the Canadian Arctic.* Toronto, ON: University of Toronto Press.

Wetherell, C., A. Plakans, and B. Wellman. 1994. Social networks, kinship, and community in eastern Europe. *Journal of Interdisciplinary History* 24 (4): 639-63.

Williams, G. 2003 [2002]. *Voyages of delusion: The quest for the Northwest Passage.* New Haven, CT: Yale University Press.

Wilson, K., and M.W. Rosenberg. 2002. Exploring the determinants of health for First Nations peoples in Canada: Can existing frameworks accommodate traditional activities? *Social Science and Medicine* 55 (11): 2017-31.

PART 4

Healing and Mental Health Services

15
Aboriginal Approaches to Counselling

ROD McCORMICK

It is an exciting time to write a chapter on Aboriginal counselling approaches, as this ancient yet new profession is experiencing a period of rapid growth and development. To be clear, the profession of counselling is ancient because Aboriginal people have sought out guidance and "counselling" from expert helpers in their communities and on their lands for a long, long time. The counselling field is also new and emerging because re-sourceful healers and counsellors have recently started combining mainstream psycho-logical approaches and traditional healing approaches in a complementary fashion, thereby creating new and increasingly effective ways to help others. Some clients will always pre-fer the traditional approaches to healing and will seek out traditional healers, whereas others will opt for treatment via mainstream psychological therapies. Aboriginal people seeking help now have a third option: to see a therapist/healer who is able to use and combine aspects of both teachings in a complementary way.

In this chapter I will describe a few of these innovative approaches and in doing so provide a brief overview of Aboriginal counselling. The chapter will first examine aspects of Aboriginal worldviews that are relevant to counselling, such as balance, connectedness, spirituality, nature, ceremony, and culture. An overview of mainstream and traditional approaches that facilitate healing for Aboriginal people will then be provided as a back-ground to what happens when it is possible to combine the best of both. Research results describing the general theme of facilitation of healing will be described. Following that, examples of Aboriginal counselling and healing approaches will be provided for a broad range of counselling concerns, including counselling victims of physical and sexual abuse, career and vocational counselling, suicide prevention, and substance-abuse counselling. It should be noted that much of the information in this chapter is presented in the form of results from research performed by the author and other specialists in the field of Aborig-inal counselling. This reliance on research findings is not accidental but represents a per-sonal and professional bias of the author that practice must be based on sound research. Note that I use the term "Aboriginal" but sometimes refer to "First Nations" or "indigen-ous" peoples; in such cases, I am referring to the same peoples. As noted elsewhere in this volume, there is great diversity among Aboriginal peoples, and although it is therefore improper to generalize, there are also great similarities between Aboriginal peoples. Thus I use some generalizations to distinguish between Aboriginal and non-Aboriginal cultures.

Aboriginal Worldviews

Counselling and psychotherapy cannot take place without communication, and we cannot communicate with someone unless we have a shared language and worldview (Torrey 1986). To communicate with and provide counselling services to Aboriginal people, providers must understand the traditional worldview of Aboriginal people. Worldview inevitably affects our belief systems, decision making, assumptions, and modes of problem solving (Ibrahim 1984). LaFromboise, Trimble, and Mohatt summarize this concept clearly when they state: "Knowledge of and respect for an Aboriginal worldview and value system – which varies according to the client's tribe, level of acculturation, and other personal characteristics – is fundamental not only for creating the trusting counsellor-client relationship vital to the helping process but also for defining the counselling style or approach most appropriate for each client" (1990, 629).

Balance

The Aboriginal medicine wheel is perhaps the best representation of an Aboriginal worldview related to healing. The medicine wheel describes the separate dimensions of the self – mental, physical, emotional, and spiritual – as equal and as parts of a larger whole. The medicine wheel represents the balance that exists between all things. Traditional Aboriginal healing incorporates the physical, social, psychological, and spiritual being. It is difficult to isolate any one aspect (Primeaux 1977). It is thought that people become ill when they live in an unbalanced way (Medicine Eagle 1989). Balance, then, is essential for the Aboriginal person because the world itself is seen as a balance of transcendental forces, human beings, and the natural environment (Hammerschlag 1988). Counsellors must therefore realize that Aboriginal clients expect their counsellor to address their problems in a holistic way that incorporates the mental, physical, emotional, and spiritual dimensions of experience. It is also very important that the counsellor be balanced and centred when working with Aboriginal clients (Hart 2002).

Connectedness

The individual's connection to the world outside the self plays a significant role in Aboriginal healing. This theme of interconnectedness is prevalent throughout most Aboriginal cultures and has been aptly described as a series of relationships, starting with the family, that reaches further and further out so that it encompasses the universe (Epes-Brown 1989). Traditional Aboriginal therapeutic approaches, unlike many Western approaches, usually involve more than just the therapist and client. Relatives and community members are often asked to be part of the healing process. Healing is often in the form of a community-sanctioned and community-run cleansing ceremony that involves the whole community (Ross 1992; Torrey 1986). For problems that arise within the Aboriginal community, it is thought that the best place to develop and initiate programs to deal with such problems is in the community itself (Nelson and McCoy 1992). Even in the case of individual problems, connections with family, community, and the larger environment often hold the keys to understanding the problems and facilitating healing. The one-on-one interaction characteristic of many Western counselling approaches is isolated outside the context of the community and family; therefore, it must be questioned as a valid means of dealing with Aboriginal client problems (Dauphinais, Dauphinais, and Rowe 1981).

Spirituality

For Aboriginal people, spirit plays as large a role in sickness and wellness as do the functioning of mind and body (Hammerschlag 1988). For many Aboriginal people, spirit means being connected with all of creation. Many different Aboriginal healing ceremonies and healing programs stress the need for reconnection with one's spirituality in order to heal. In the vision quest ceremony, for example, the Aboriginal person makes contact with his or her spiritual identity (Hodgson and Kothare 1990). Although the vision quest ceremony itself varied from nation to nation, there were many aspects common to all. The following description of the vision quest therefore attempts to be generic:

> About the time of puberty a boy was encouraged to go into the forest or
> the hills for several days at a time, fast during the day, and dream at night.
> To stay out for four days at a time was highly desirable. The fast was either
> a complete one or one with very little water and almost no food. The intent
> was to clear the mind so that they would be able to see the vision. Embark-
> ing on the Vision Quest, the youth would first enter a sweat lodge and go
> through a body purification. Then clutching sage grass in his hand, he would
> climb to an elevated site, either on a hilltop or in a perch in a tree, high above
> the world. There the youth would pray and fast waiting on the Great Spirit.
> Eventually, he would make contact and commune with his spirit, symbolic
> of his spiritual identity. Through this vision he would come to terms with
> his innermost self and accept his strengths and weaknesses. (Hodgson and
> Kothare 1990, 112)

Regardless of the ceremonies or practices used to connect with, strengthen, or cleanse the spirit, there exists a close association between illness and the spirit for most indigenous people around the world (Torrey 1986).

Nature

Nature, in the sense of the natural world outside cities and human habitations, is an important source of healing for many Aboriginal people, whereas mainstream psychological theory and practice reinforce the separation of healing practices from nature. This often leads to people disregarding nature as a means of healing. For many Aboriginal people there is a spiritual connection that exists between nature and humans because humans are seen as part of nature. All of creation is seen as being equal and part of the whole and is therefore equal in the eyes of the Creator. Connection to nature – which may be experienced by going out on the land and engaging in traditional land-based activities – often helps Aboriginal people who are seeking help to feel part of something much larger as well as to feel less lonely, stronger, more grounded, and more secure. The following comment by a young woman from a West Coast tribe who worked with the author illustrates one of the principles of connection with nature: "Learning to open up my heart to nature helped. The Elders have a name for that in my language – 'kan dalfta.' This means heart opened up. When I opened up my heart to the beauty and peace of nature, it made me feel good. Problems aren't that great that you can't solve them once you have reached that level where you can go with the flow of nature."

Ceremony

Ritual and ceremony are tried and true ways for many Aboriginal people to give expression to personal experience while at the same time connecting with others in their community (Hammerschlag 1993). Ceremonies such as the spirit dances, the sweat lodge, and the pipe ceremonies are tools to maintain and deepen the individual's sense of connectedness to all things (Ross 1992). Although there has not been empirical research conducted on the efficacy of traditional healing ceremonies such as those mentioned, anecdotal evidence exists within the literature to attest to their effectiveness in healing (Hammerschlag 1988; Jilek 1982; Torrey 1986).

Tradition/Culture

One of the major roles of therapy and healing for traditional Aboriginal people is to reaffirm cultural values (LaFromboise et al. 1990). In a study examining Aboriginal drug and

ROD McCORMICK

alcohol counselling in British Columbia, a suggested culturally sensitive counselling framework for Aboriginal people included the theme of importance of personal and cultural identity (Anderson 1993). In a study conducted to determine the characteristics of recovery of personal meaning for Aboriginal people, one of the major themes or characteristics that emerged was that individuals valued knowledge of traditional Aboriginal culture (More 1985). Another characteristic of personal recovery in that same study was that the Aboriginal language was maintained or relearned. It is not surprising that the teaching of traditional culture has been found to be a successful way to facilitate healing in Aboriginal people. In one Aboriginal community, it was possible to reduce dramatically the teen suicide rate by having tribal Elders teach traditional culture to the teens in a group setting (Neligh 1990). By providing Aboriginal people with culture through stories and shared cultural activities, Elders were able to provide community members with guidance, direction, and self-understanding (Halfe 1993). This incorporation of self, or identity, with traditional ideology also provides Aboriginal people with strength for coping in the mainstream environment (Axelson 1985). This movement toward reconnecting with cultural beliefs, tradition, and ceremony as a way to overcome problems has been referred to as "retraditionalization" (LaFromboise et al. 1990).

What Facilitates Healing for Aboriginal People?

The major part of the literature that examines healing for Aboriginal people tends to be based on opinion and conjecture, not on research. In the field of counselling, the literature often provides advice to counsellors so that they can be more effective with Aboriginal clients, but it does not provide empirical evidence to support such advice. Several researchers (Dauphinais et al. 1981; Wohl 1989) refer to the lack of empirical studies that examine the effectiveness of specific counselling approaches with Aboriginal people. Having noted the lack of research in this field, this chapter will briefly examine some of the research and writing that does exist in an effort to identify effective counselling strategies and the key factors that facilitate healing for Aboriginal people.

Effective Mainstream Counselling Approaches with Aboriginal Clients

Western, or mainstream, healing approaches have been only partially successful in assisting Aboriginal people with their healing (LaFromboise et al. 1990; Sue and Sue 1990). There are several reasons for this. First, mental health programs and interventions that have been designed from a mainstream biomedical perspective do not recognize or meet the health needs of Aboriginal people, for they ignore the cultural, historical, and sociopolitical context (Smye and Mussell 2001). The traditions, values, and health belief systems of Aboriginal people are poorly understood by mental health providers and often not respected or even considered (Smye and Mussell 2001). Aboriginal clients have sometimes complained that mainstream therapy tries to shape their behaviour in a way that conflicts with Aboriginal lifestyle orientations and preferences (LaFromboise et al. 1990). Aboriginal clients may also fear that the mainstream therapist may try to change their cultural values and thereby alienate them from their own people and traditions (LaFromboise et al. 1990). In a discussion paper for the Royal Commission on Aboriginal Peoples entitled "The development of Aboriginal counselling," Peavy (1993) identifies several faulty assumptions and negative consequences that arise when mainstream counselling practices are imposed on Aboriginal people. These include cultural misconceptions of what is normal; an emphasis on individualism; fragmentation of the mental, physical, emotional, and spiritual dimensions of the person; neglect of Aboriginal history; and neglect of the client's social-support system. Nevertheless, and despite widespread difficulties in access, many Aboriginal people have turned to psychotherapy and counselling, although it may take considerable time and experience in talking with a therapist before they can begin to establish an effective working relationship with that therapist (Wing and Crow 1995). In one of the only reviews of the use of mainstream therapies with Aboriginal clients, LaFromboise and colleagues (1990) found that social-learning therapy and behavioural therapy had the most to offer Aboriginal people. Social-learning theory has strengths in terms of its use with Aboriginal clients, as it extensively uses role modelling (LaFromboise et al. 1990). Behavioural therapy can be effective because of its action-oriented focus on the present rather than the past. Both behavioural and social-learning therapies may be misused, however, when the therapist adopts a narrow or inappropriate focus that does not represent the client's goals (LaFromboise et al. 1990). Behaviour therapy, with its focus on behaviour rather than on feelings, is compatible with Aboriginal culture as long as counsellors help their clients to assess the possible consequences of making behavioural change. Cognitive therapy can also be popular, as its cognitive focus may downplay the expression of feelings. Each form of therapy is based on tacit models of the person and associated cultural values (Kirmayer 2007). Although the dominant theories of counselling emphasize individualism, for many Aboriginal peoples, relational notions of the self that connect the person to others (sociocentric), to the natural world, and to the spirit world are important. The danger is that without adequate understanding and respect for Aboriginal cultural values, the therapist may mistakenly try to change core cultural values of their Aboriginal clients.

In addition to individual approaches to therapy, some group approaches have seen successfully used with Aboriginal people. The attraction of group approaches to therapy is that they are similar to Aboriginal healing approaches such as the sweat lodge (Garrett and Osborne 1995). Family-systems therapy may be especially appropriate because of the importance many Aboriginal people place on the extended family. Indeed, the field of family therapy itself has been influenced by Aboriginal perspectives, notably in the development of family-network therapy (France, McCormick, and Rodriguez 2004; Speck and Attneave 1973). The danger here again, however, is that the values of mainstream counselling, such as individuation, self-actualization, independence, and self-expression, may not be embraced by many Aboriginal clients.

The Role of the Family and Community in Counselling Aboriginal People

A key factor in healing for Aboriginal people is the process of dealing with problems with the assistance of others rather than by oneself. Assistance can be obtained from friends, the family, and the community as well as in the context of group counselling or on a social basis. According to traditional Aboriginal views, a person's psychological welfare must be considered in the context of the community (Trimble and Hayes 1984). Similarly, therapy for Aboriginal people should encourage the client to transcend him or herself by conceptualizing the self as being embedded in and expressive of community (Katz and Rolde 1981). Traditional healing methods often prove effective because they include the participation of family and community members, which increases the social support of the individual (Renfrey 1992). In a study with a Washington Tribe, Guilmet and Whited (1987) also found that the extended family was essential to most Aboriginal clients in terms of emotional support.

Should Western and Traditional Approaches to Healing be Combined?

In one review of successful healing strategies utilized by 50 Aboriginal people in British Columbia, it was found that the successful programs stressed traditional values, spirituality, and activities that enhanced self-esteem (McCormick 1995). Although most successful Aboriginal healing programs have been run using Aboriginal values and approaches, it is recommended by some that they could be enhanced by a fusion with mainstream psychological techniques (Anderson 1993). In an article considering the vision quest ceremony from an attachment-theory perspective, McCormick (1997) demonstrates how this traditional Aboriginal ceremony and a well-known mainstream psychological theory provide very similar teachings. According to attachment theory, a therapist must attempt to provide a secure base in order to help the client to reconstruct his or her faulty childhood parental attachment in a positive way. A traditional healing approach aims to foster re-attachment not to a therapist but to the Great Spirit as manifested in nature (i.e., to the individual's spirituality). The reattachment process could be in the form of a vision quest ceremony in which the child or adult could attach him or herself to "Father Sky" or "Mother Earth" as metaphors of a spiritual bonding with nature and all of creation.

Integration is often not the easiest or best solution, however, as there exists a power differential between Western medicine and traditional healing. Western medicine has the power of the government, the law, and the medical system behind it and is therefore likely simply to overwhelm and assimilate traditional medicine in any attempt at integration. A more balanced and appropriate form of partnership may be a complementary one in which both systems collaborate, working side by side.

Facilitation of Healing

A study was conducted in the field of counselling psychology by McCormick (1995) to examine what facilitates healing for Aboriginal people. By asking Aboriginal people what actually worked for them in their own healing journeys, it was possible to obtain important information from the "real experts." The participants in this study were Aboriginal people ranging in age from the early twenties to the early fifties. The mean age was 35. Geographically, the 50 participants came from approximately 40 different communities in British Columbia. The location of these communities ranged from the interior of the province to the west coast of Vancouver Island and from as far north as Fort Nelson to as far south as the Musqueam reserve in Vancouver. Fifteen of the participants were male and 35 were female. Four of the participants originally came from another province but had been living in British Columbia for at least 5 years. Nineteen of the participants were university students, while 31 were employed in a wide variety of occupations such as housewife, administrator, secretary, and labourer. Through interviews with the 50 participants, 437 critical incidents or healing events were obtained that described what facilitated healing for the participants. The 437 events were placed into 14 categories that were found to be reasonably reliable. These categories are participation in ceremony, expression of emotion, learning from a role model, establishing a connection with nature, exercise, involvement in challenging activities, establishing a social connection, gaining an understanding of the problem, establishing a spiritual connection, obtaining help/support from others, self-care, setting goals, anchoring self in tradition, and helping others. These categories were then organized into 4 divisions that reflect the path of healing: separating from an unhealthy life, obtaining social support and resources, experiencing a healthy life, and living a healthy life.

This initial analysis of the healing path was not intended to represent a fixed sequence of steps or stages, as it is theorized that individuals may follow different paths and sequences. It is interesting to note, however, that these tentative stages parallel the three stages of ritual identified by van Gennep (1960). Based on an extensive analysis of ceremonies and the content and order of the activities associated with these ceremonies, van Gennep was able to discern three phases of transition: separation, transition, and incorporation. Separation involves detachment from the present life or way of being. Transition requires the dying of the old life and the birth of a new one. Incorporation means that the individual is incorporated or reincorporated into the community in his or her new state, role, and way of being.

A preliminary examination of the healing outcomes for Aboriginal people in the study found five main outcomes: empowerment, cleansing, balance, discipline, and belonging. Distinct themes in Aboriginal healing were also developed as a result of analyzing narrative accounts of participants. These themes are as follows: a broad spectrum of healing resources are available to Aboriginal people; Aboriginal people have a different way of seeing the world, which has to be understood before effective counselling services can be provided; Aboriginal people expect that whatever is healing should help them to attain and/or maintain balance; self-transcendence followed by connectedness is a common route to healing for Aboriginal people; and Aboriginal people act as agents for their own healing. Similar healing themes and goals are described by Michael Hart (2002) in his account of social-work practice based on Cree values. According to Hart, the goal of attaining *mino-pimatisiwin* (the good life) involves a lifelong healing journey in which one grows toward centredness, which includes balance, harmony, connection, and wholeness.

Counselling Victims of Physical and Sexual Abuse

Aboriginal peoples in Canada are currently engaged in mediation, negotiation, and legal battles with the Canadian government and Canadian churches for reparation to all those Aboriginal children (now adults) who were physically and sexually abused in the residential schools. For approximately 120 years, Aboriginal children in Canada were forced to attend church- and government-operated residential schools. The Government of Canada and the Assembly of First Nations have only recently agreed to a settlement whereby all who attended these schools will receive a cash payment for their suffering. Many of the children who attended these schools experienced physical and sexual abuse by the nuns and priests. It is thought that many of the mental health problems plaguing Aboriginal peoples today can also be traced to that legacy of abuse (Royal Commission on Aboriginal Peoples 1996).

A few years ago, the author was fortunate to supervise a study for the Association of BC First Nations Treatment Programs (2002) that examined the successful healing journeys of two groups: approximately 100 residential school survivors who were victims of physical and sexual abuse and those affected on an intergenerational level. The results of this study confirm and extend the research concerning the facilitation of healing for Aboriginal people. Previous scholars have stressed a number of factors that they believe have facilitated healing for Aboriginal survivors of physical and sexual abuse. These factors were empirically supported in this research, which confirmed the following categories: participation in ceremony, traditional healer/medicine person, cleansing, cultural connection, changing thinking, identifying and expressing emotions, therapist/counsellor, shared experiences, forgiveness, Elders, role model/mentor, group psychotherapy, connection with nature, spiritual connection, treatment/healing centres, support groups, seeing intergenerational patterns, self-acceptance, workshops/programs, family support, personal identity, peer support, helping others, community connection, apologized to, and self-care. This research went beyond these 23 previously identified categories by providing evidence for the importance of additional categories of facilitating factors: self-knowledge, sobriety, humour, Aboriginal identity, dreams and visions, training, accepting responsibility, bodywork, learning, family role, self-expression, telling your story, and knowledge of residential school history. All of these categories represent potential ways to facilitate healing for Aboriginal survivors of physical and sexual abuse.

Career and Vocational Counselling

Another area that has seen considerable development for the Aboriginal population is career and vocational counselling. The failure of mainstream models of career counselling for Aboriginal clients has led to efforts to develop more culturally appropriate models (Dolan 1995; Herring 1990). As stated by Ahia, "whenever alien psychologies are applied to different cultures without modification or contextualization – the result is professional discouragement and stagnation" (1984, 340). Currently, there are very few career-counselling models for Aboriginal people and a general lack of research on Aboriginal career development (Herring 1990). Most contemporary career-development models are based on generalizations taken from white, middle-class, male populations (Axelson 1993; Osipow and Littlejohn 1995); and it is the generally held opinion that these approaches reflect Western cultural values. Counselling services provided to Aboriginal people in the past have been based on adherence to these contemporary approaches despite a mismatch between mainstream career-development models and an Aboriginal worldview (McCormick and Amundson 1997). For example, research has shown that in career counselling with Aboriginal clients, it is culturally appropriate and desirable for clients' family and community members to have input into clients' career decisions (McCormick and France 1995; McCormick and Amundson 1997). Family and community members can help clients to identify their interests, aptitudes, needs, values, and temperament.

The Aboriginal Career-Life Planning Model, developed by McCormick and Amundson (1997), was designed to respect an Aboriginal worldview and its values. Aboriginal culture does not emphasize a philosophy of individualism but reflects a collective orientation. Lee (1984) found that compared to their non-Aboriginal counterparts, Aboriginal students' career choices were more influenced by parents. By involving family and community members in the career-counselling process for young people, the Aboriginal Career-Life Planning Model focuses on individual potential in the context of family and community roles and responsibilities. *Guiding circles,* an Aboriginal workbook for career self-exploration developed by McCormick, Amundson, and Poehnell (2002), continues with the tradition of involving family and community input in a process of client self-exploration. At present, it is the most widely used career-exploration tool for Aboriginal people.[1]

ROD McCORMICK

Counselling Suicidal Youth

Another crucial area that is demanding attention from counsellors and other providers and researchers of mental health services concerns how best to help Aboriginal youth who are suicidal. A preliminary study conducted by McCormick and Arvay (forthcoming), points to some of the factors that can help suicidal youth. Further research such as this study needs to be conducted on a national level in order to inform counselling practitioners and other mental health providers about how best to assist Aboriginal people who are suicidal. In this study, the critical-incident technique was also utilized, as it was important to hear from the real experts: Aboriginal people who had successfully recovered from being suicidal. Through interviews with 25 participants, 280 critical incidents were elicited that facilitated healing and recovery for Aboriginal youth who were suicidal. The 280 critical incidents were then grouped into 22 categories. Listed in order from most significant to least significant, the categories that facilitated healing and recovery for Aboriginal youth were: self-esteem/self-acceptance, obtaining help from others, changing thinking, connection with culture/tradition, expressing emotions/cleansing, spiritual connection, responsibility to others, future goals/hope, learning from others/role models, participation in ceremonies, connection to nature, guiding visions/dreams, understanding the problem, helping others, keeping occupied, recognizing/identifying emotions, exercise/sports, shutting down emotions, humour/perspective, learning problem-solving/communication skills, removing self from bad environment, and eliminating drugs and alcohol.

Substance-Abuse Counselling

One of the best-known applications of Aboriginal approaches to counselling is in the field of substance-abuse treatment for Aboriginal people. For over a quarter-century, Aboriginal people have been developing culturally appropriate ways to help clients who suffer from addictions. Attempts made by mainstream health-service providers to assist Aboriginal people in recovering from alcohol and substance abuse have led to only minimal success (Wing and Crow 1995). Ross (1992) argues that assistance measures taken by the majority culture to assist Aboriginal people have been, and continue to be, misguided and counterproductive. For various reasons, Aboriginal people tend not to use the services provided by the majority culture, and of those who do, approximately half drop out after the first session (Sue and Sue 1990). Differences in value orientations between Aboriginal people and mainstream health-service providers may lead to different beliefs concerning the causes and solutions of mental health problems (Darou 1987; McCormick 1996; Trimble 1981; Wohl 1989). An obstacle to utilization of mainstream services by Aboriginal people concerns differences in help-seeking behaviour. Wing and Crow (1995) describe two common cultural barriers to obtaining help. One obstacle is that for traditional Aboriginal people, it can be very shameful and embarrassing to admit to having problems of drug and alcohol abuse. This embarrassment is aggravated by common stereotypes in Canadian society that portray Aboriginal people as prone to alcohol and substance abuse and related problems (see Samson, Chapter 5; Culhane, Chapter 7; Tait, Chapter 9). This stigma and embarrassment can prevent individuals from seeking help. A second common barrier reflects the distinction between family and community members and outsiders. It may take Aboriginal people considerable time with a therapist before they can begin to establish an effective working relationship. Trust and intimacy are not things that are freely shared with strangers. This may be especially true with non-Aboriginal therapists because the history of colonialism, misunderstanding, and oppressive relationships may influence the development of the therapeutic relationship. These examples illustrate some of the reasons why alcohol-treatment programs based on the medical model favoured by many mainstream service providers often fail in their efforts with Aboriginal people.

Aboriginal Conceptualization of Substance Abuse

The Aboriginal conceptualization of alcohol abuse and its treatment encompasses more than the biological and psychological explanations emphasized by mainstream medicine. To understand Aboriginal traditions in the treatment of substance abuse, health professionals must also have an understanding of the spiritual component of substance abuse. Duran and Duran put this as follows: "Traditional Native people have a way to describe alcohol and the conceptualization of alcohol that differs from non-Natives. Alcohol is perceived as a spiritual entity that has been destructive of Native American ways of life. The alcohol 'spirits' continually wage war within the spiritual arena and it is in the spiritual arena that the struggle continues" (1995, 139).

For Aboriginal people, spirituality can be described in terms of "getting beyond the self." It is only through getting beyond the self that humans are able to connect with the rest of creation. Creation is described in terms of family, community, culture, the natural world, and the spiritual world. Traditional cultural values provide Aboriginal people with teachings on how to attain and maintain connection with creation. Many of the mental health problems experienced by Aboriginal people can be attributed to a disconnection from their culture. Inducing this disconnection was a "deliberate" strategy utilized by various churches and the Government of Canada in an attempt to assimilate Aboriginal people into Euro-Western culture. For many Aboriginal people, consumption of alcohol has been their attempt to deal with the state of powerlessness and hopelessness that has arisen due to the devastation of traditional cultural values. Research has demonstrated that cultural breakdown is strongly linked with alcohol abuse (Duran and Duran 1995; York 1990). The degeneration of traditional culture experienced by Aboriginal people has led to the taking of desperate measures. From this perspective, "alcohol use and even suicide may be functional behavioral adaptations within a hostile and hopeless social environment" (Duran and Duran 1995, 193).

An Existential Conceptualization

Many Aboriginal Elders and healers believe that reconnection to culture, community, and spirituality is healing for Aboriginal people. This belief makes perfect sense when one realizes that, for many individuals and communities, it was disconnection from these sources of meaning and support that made Aboriginal people unhealthy in the first place. A Euro-Western theory of psychotherapy that approximates this way of thinking is logotherapy (Frankl 1962). As an existential-humanistic approach, logotherapy is based on the claim that the primary motivation for people is to obtain meaning in their lives. According to the theory, meaning can be obtained through sources such as spirituality, work, significant relationships with others, and contributing to one's community. Values are described as collective sources of meaning (Fabry 1968). Values are the activities that provide meaning to families, communities, and whole cultures. A collectively oriented culture, such as Aboriginal culture, is more likely to provide sources of meaning to its members through family, community, and cultural values than is an individually oriented culture. To be disconnected from those values is to be disconnected from potential sources of meaning. In an individually oriented society such as mainstream Canada or the United States, meaning tends to be derived from individual activities and generally not from collective sources. This is because the individual is less likely to be influenced by family, community, or cultural values. Due to the increasing trend toward individualism, the extended family, the church, and the state no longer have the influence on North American people that they once enjoyed (Fabry 1968). Individuals must seek out meaning on their own. Failure to find meaning can result in existential anxiety. According to logotherapy, existential anxiety can be dealt with constructively if it is used as a means to motivate and enable people to take actions that will connect them to those activities that provide them with meaning.

Unfortunately, not everyone deals with anxiety in a constructive way. Existential anxiety can cause some people to feel sad and hopeless. Alcohol use is one of the ways that people seek to replace this sad and anxious feeling with an artificial state of happiness. For Aboriginal people, this alternative became all too easy when faced with the abundance of alcohol provided by the early traders and others who wanted to take their land. The artificial "spirit" found in alcohol has been used as a poor substitute for the real "spirit" possessed by Aboriginal people who are connected to their culture and to creation. In research on effective health care practices for treating alcohol abuse among the Muscogee (Creek) Indians of the south-eastern United States, Wing and Crow (1995) found that traditional Aboriginal people believe that alcoholism is caused by a lack of spirituality. Hammerschlag (1993) writes of the effects of disconnection from spirit, culture, and creation in his book *Theft of the spirit*. Although he initially describes the effects that this "theft" has had on Aboriginal people, Hammerschlag suggests that other cultures, including Euro-American culture, have also experienced the effects of a loss of spirit. Aboriginal people of Canada are perhaps more aware of the effects of disconnection from cultural values because their loss has been the result of a transparent, relatively recent, and purposeful attempt at assimilation. The devastating effects of these attempts at cultural genocide have revealed to Aboriginal people the strong link between cultural dislocation and sickness. Alcohol abuse has simply been one symptom of this sickness. The path to wellness has also been revealed to Aboriginal people in this same link. Quite simply, this path is reconnection to one's "spirit" and "culture" and to one's inherent sources of meaning. Connection to traditional Aboriginal culture and values means that a person must become connected to extended family, community, the natural world, and the spirit world – in essence, to all of creation.

Strategies That Work

Although information on the prevalence of alcohol abuse among Aboriginal people and the various attempts at treatment can be readily found in the research literature, what is much less evident are studies of successful substance-abuse treatment strategies used by Aboriginal people. Aboriginal people have a rich heritage of healing strategies in dealing with substance abuse. For Aboriginal people, the most effective solution is based on cultural and spiritual survival and renewal (Maracle 1993). For example, cultural and spiritual revival has been the strategy used by the Aboriginal community of Alkali Lake, located in central British Columbia. This community employed traditional Aboriginal healers to help its members revive traditional dances, ceremonies, and spiritual practices. Community members were introduced to cultural activities such as Pow-Wow dancing, sweet-grass and sweat-lodge ceremonies, and drumming. The treatment strategy used by the people of Alkali Lake has been copied by other Aboriginal treatment programs, such as those at Poundmaker Lodge and Round Lake. The guiding philosophy of these treatment programs has been: "Culture is treatment, and all healing is spiritual" (York 1990). The outcomes of programs using this philosophy/strategy have been very promising (Guillory, Willie, and Duran 1988).

Community and Family Ownership

Counselling interventions in Aboriginal communities can complement the political movement toward self-determination by encouraging local initiatives in substance-abuse treatment and intervention. Considerable commitments have been made by many Aboriginal communities toward the treatment and prevention of substance abuse. This community involvement is essential if strategies are to work (Edwards and Edwards 1988). The community must acknowledge that a substance-abuse problem exists and must be committed to and involved in addressing the problem. The substance abuser's family also plays an important role in effective treatment and prevention. For Aboriginal people, the extended family is important in determining positive and negative behaviours (Trotter and Rolf 1997). In response to the devastating impact of alcohol on their community, leaders in Alkali Lake mobilized their community toward a goal of sobriety (Johnson and Johnson 1993). Based on a historical study of the interventions used in this program between 1972 and 1993 as well as on the data gathered in a research study, Johnson and Johnson (1993) found that the family was described by community members as the second most effective intervention after spiritual support. When participants were asked, "What significant event or thing caused you to commit to be sober?" almost half (48%) of the respondents identified family as the cause. It can be argued that the extended family is still the central institution in Aboriginal cultures, even for urban dwellers. Inside the family, norms of sharing and mutual support traditionally provided a safety net for every individual. These norms were severely disrupted by assimilationist policies such as residential schools and the forcible removal of Aboriginal children from their families through foster placement and adoption. Testimony given to the Royal Commission on Aboriginal Peoples (1996) continuously stressed the importance of family in Aboriginal society. Many Aboriginal people told the commission that the future they wish for is impossible unless the bonds of the family that give individuals and communities their stability are reclaimed and strengthened. Graveline refers to this reclamation or revival as "spiritual resistance which flourishes through treasuring our children and honouring the visions and words of our ancestors" (1998, 45).

Many types of connection have been stressed in this discussion of substance-abuse counselling, including connection to meaning, family, spirituality, and identity. One connection that cannot be emphasized enough is the connection to culture. The understanding of this connection is the reason why Round Lake Treatment Centre in British Columbia uses the motto "Culture is treatment" on all of its correspondence. It is essential that both researchers and practitioners recognize this connection and incorporate culture into the field of Aboriginal substance-abuse treatment. Because substance abuse conflicts with traditional Aboriginal cultural beliefs about courage, humility, generosity, and family honour, cultural wholeness can serve as both a preventative and a curative agent in substance-abuse treatment.

Aboriginal people are currently developing strategies to deal with the pain of cultural dislocation and the resultant problem of substance abuse. These strategies utilize the community and family to provide culturally appropriate alternatives to the abuse of alcohol and drugs. Traditional cultural values, ceremonies, and healing techniques have been known to provide substance abusers with the knowledge and skills to attain and maintain a meaningful connection with creation. It is to these values and teachings that Aboriginal people are now turning in an effort to let the "good spirits" guide them.

Conclusion

In this chapter I have attempted to provide a brief overview of the basic values and perspectives of Aboriginal counselling while describing some of the innovative approaches being developed by Aboriginal counsellors and mental health professionals. Respect for Aboriginal worldviews is essential if counselling is to establish the therapeutic relationship and to engage cultural resources for healing. Concepts of balance, connectedness, spirituality, nature, ceremony, and culture are all important aspects of healing for Aboriginal people. Uniquely Aboriginal perspectives on counselling and healing are being developed in several areas, including counselling for victims of physical and sexual abuse, career and vocational counselling, suicide prevention, and substance-abuse counselling. The future will undoubtedly bring important new efforts to integrate Aboriginal and mainstream counselling perspectives as well as new modes of collaboration between the different helping and healing traditions. Emerging research in this field is addressing some of the gaps in the literature. There is a need for empirical research to validate the effectiveness of different counselling and healing approaches. Research is also needed to explore the link between the level of individual psychological problems and the larger issues of politics and identity. Finally, work is needed on ways to understand the differences and to promote collaboration between traditional and mainstream helping professionals.

Note

1 The workbook is currently marketed and distributed by the Aboriginal Human Resources Development Council of Canada (AHRDCC).

References

Ahia, C.E. 1984. Cross-cultural counseling concerns. *The Personnel and Guidance Journal* 62: 339-41.

Anderson, B.M. 1993. Aboriginal counselling and healing processes. MA thesis, University of British Columbia.

Association of BC First Nations Treatment Programs. 2002. *Report on therapeutic safety in healing: Facilitation of healing for Aboriginal school survivors*. Vernon, BC: Association of BC First Nations Treatment Programs.

Axelson, J. 1985. *Counseling and development in a multicultural society*. Monterey, CA: Brooks Cole.

–. 1993. *Counseling and development in a multicultural society*. 2nd ed. Pacific Grove, CA: Brooks Cole.

Darou, W.G. 1987. Counselling the northern Native. *Canadian Journal of Counselling* 21 (1): 33-41.

Dauphinais, P., L. Dauphinais, and W. Rowe. 1981. Effect of race and communication style on Indian perceptions of counselor effectiveness. *Counselor Education and Supervision* 21 (1): 72-80.

Dolan, C.A. 1995. A study of the mismatch between Native students' counselling needs and available services. *Canadian Journal of Counselling* 29 (3): 234-43.

Duran, E., and B. Duran. 1995. *Native American postcolonial psychology*. New York: SUNY Press.

Edwards, E.D., and M.E. Edwards. 1988. Alcoholism prevention/treatment and Native American youth: A community approach. *Journal of Drug Issues* 18 (1): 103-14.

Epes-Brown, J. 1989. Becoming part of it. In D.M. Dooling and P. Jordan-Smith, eds., *I became part of it: Sacred dimensions in Native American life,* 9-20. San Francisco, CA: Harper.

Fabry, J.B. 1968. *The pursuit of meaning.* Boston, MA: Beacon Press.

France, M.H., R. McCormick, and M. Rodriguez. 2004. Issues in counselling for the First Nations community. In M.H. France, M. Rodriguez, and G. Hett, eds., *Diversity, culture, and counselling,* 59-75. Calgary: Detselig.

Frankl, V. 1962. *Man's search for meaning: An introduction to logotherapy.* Boston, MA: Beacon Press.

Garrett, M.W., and W.L. Osborne. 1995. The Native American sweat lodge as a metaphor for group work. *The Journal for Specialists in Group Work* 20 (1): 33-39.

Graveline, F.J. 1998. *Circle works: Transforming Eurocentric consciousness.* Halifax, NS: Fernwood.

Guillory, B.M., E. Willie, and E.F. Duran. 1988. Analysis of a community organizing case study: Alkali Lake. *Journal of Rural Community Psychology* 9 (1): 27-36.

Guilmet, G.M., and D.L. Whited. 1987. Cultural lessons for clinical mental health practice: The Puyallup tribal community. *American Indian and Alaskan Native Mental Health Research* 1 (2): 1-141.

Halfe, L. 1993. Native healing. *Cognica* 26 (1): 21-27.

Hammerschlag, C.A. 1988. *The dancing healers: A doctor's journey of healing with Native Americans.* San Francisco, CA: Harper and Rowe.

–. 1993. *The theft of the spirit: A journey to spiritual healing with Native Americans.* New York: Simon and Schuster.

Hart, M.A. 2002. *Seeking mino-pimatisiwin: An Aboriginal approach to helping.* Halifax, NS: Fernwood.

Herring, R.D. 1990. Attacking career myths among Native Americans: Implications for counseling. *School Counselor* 38 (1): 13-18.

Hodgson, J., and J. Kothare. 1990 *Native spirituality and the church in Canada.* Toronto, ON: Anglican Book Centre.

Ibrahim, F.A. 1984. Cross-cultural counseling and psychotherapy: An existential psychological perspective. *International Journal for the Advancement of Counseling* 7: 159-69.

Jilek, W. 1982. *Indian healing: Shamanic ceremonialism in the Pacific Northwest today.* Surrey, BC: Hancock House.

Johnson, J., and F. Johnson. 1993. Community development sobriety and after-care at Alkali Lake Band. In *The path to healing: Report of the National Round Table on Aboriginal Health and Social Issues,* 227-30. Ottawa, ON: Royal Commission on Aboriginal Peoples.

Katz, R., and E. Rolde. 1981. Community alternatives to psychotherapy. *Psychotherapy, Theory, Research and Practice* 18: 365-74.

Kirmayer, L.J. 2007. Psychotherapy and the cultural concept of the person. *Transcultural Psychiatry* 44 (2): 232-57.

LaFromboise, T., J. Trimble, and G. Mohatt. 1990. Counseling intervention and American Indian tradition: An integrative approach. *The Counseling Psychologist* 18 (4): 628-54.

Lee, C. 1984. Predicting the career choice attitudes of rural black, white, and American Indian high school students. *Vocational Guidance Quarterly* 32: 177-84.

Maracle, B. 1993. *Crazy water: Native voices on addiction and recovery.* Toronto, ON: Penguin.

McCormick, R.M. 1995. The facilitation of healing for the First Nations people of British Columbia. *Canadian Journal of Native Education* 21 (2): 251-319.

–. 1996. Culturally appropriate means and ends of counselling as described by the First Nations people of British Columbia. *International Journal for the Advancement of Counselling* 18 (3): 163-72.

–. 1997. An integration of healing wisdom: The vision quest ceremony from an attachment theory perspective. *Guidance and Counselling* 12 (2): 18-22.

–, and M.H. France. 1995. Counselling First Nations students on career issues: Implications for the school counsellor. *Journal of Guidance and Counselling* 10: 27-31.

–, and N.E. Amundson. 1997. A career/life planning model for First Nations people. *Journal of Employment Counselling* 34: 171-79.

–, N.E. Amundson, and G. Poehnell. 2002. *Guiding circles: An Aboriginal guide to self-discovery*. Saskatoon, SK: Aboriginal Human Resources Development Council of Canada.

–, and M. Arvay. Forthcoming. The facilitation of healing for Candian Aboriginal youth who are suicidal.

Medicine Eagle, B. 1989. The circle of healing. In R. Carlson and J. Brugh, eds., *Healers on healing,* 58-62. New York: J.P. Tarcher/Putnam.

More, J.M. 1985. Cultural foundations of personal meaning: Their loss and recovery. MA thesis, University of British Columbia.

Neligh, G. 1990. Mental health programs for American Indians: Their logic, structure and function. *American Indian and Alaskan Native Mental Health Research* 3 (3): 1-280.

Nelson, S.H., and G.F. McCoy. 1992. An overview of mental health services for American Indians and Alaskan Natives in the 1990s. *Hospital and Community Psychiatry* 43 (3): 257-61.

Osipow, S.H., and E.M. Littlejohn. 1995. Toward a multicultural theory of career development: Prospects and dilemmas. In F.T. Leong, ed., *Career development and vocational behavior of racial and ethnic minorities,* 251-61. Mahwah, NJ: Lawrence Erlbaum Associates.

Peavy, R.V. 1993. Development of Aboriginal counselling. Brief submitted to the Royal Commission for Aboriginal Peoples.

Primeaux, M.H. 1977. American Indian health care practices: A cross-cultural perspective. *Nursing Clinics of North America* 12 (1): 55-65.

Renfrey, G.S. 1992. Cognitive behaviour therapy and the Native American client. *Behaviour Therapy* 23 (3): 321-40.

Ross, R. 1992. *Dancing with a ghost: Exploring Indian reality*. Markham, ON: Octopus.

Royal Commission on Aboriginal Peoples. 1996. *People to people, Nation to nation: Highlights from the report of the Royal Commission on Aboriginal Peoples*. Ottawa, ON: Canadian Ministry of Supply and Services.

Smye, V., and B. Mussell. 2001. Aboriginal mental health: What works best. Unpublished discussion paper.

Speck, R.V., and C.L. Attneave. 1973. *Family networks: Retribalization and healing*. New York: Pantheon.

Sue, D.W., and D. Sue. 1990. *Counselling the culturally different: Theory and practice*. 2nd ed. Toronto, ON: John Wiley and Sons.

Torrey, E.F. 1986. *Witchdoctors and psychiatrists: The common roots of psychotherapy and its future*. New York: Harper Row.

Trimble, J.E. 1981. Value differentials and their importance in counseling American Indians. In P. Pederson, J. Draguns, W. Lonner, and J.E. Trimble, eds., *Counseling across cultures,* 3rd ed., 177-204. Honolulu, HI: University of Hawaii Press.

–, and S. Hayes. 1984. Mental health intervention in the psychosocial contexts of American Indian communities. In W. O'Conner and B. Lubin, eds., *Ecological approaches to clinical and community psychology,* 293-321. New York: Wiley.

Trotter, R.T., and J.E. Rolf. 1997. Cultural models of inhalant use among Navajo youth. *Drugs and Society* 10 (2): 39-59.

van Gennep, A. 1960. *The rites of passage*. Chicago, IL: University of Chicago Press.

Wing, D.M., and S.S. Crow. 1995. An ethnonursing study of Muscogee (Creek) Indians and effective health care practices for treating alcohol abuse. *Family and Community Health* 18 (2): 52-64.

Wohl, J. 1989. Cross-cultural psychotherapy. In P.B. Pederson, J.G. Draguns, W.J. Lonner, and J.E. Trimble, eds., *Counseling across cultures,* 3rd ed., 177-204. Honolulu, HI: University of Hawaii Press.

York, G. 1990. *The dispossessed: Life and death in Native Canada*. London, ON: Vintage.

16
Respecting the Medicines:
Narrating an Aboriginal Identity

GREGORY M. BRASS

Medicines could even be powerful words. Words that move you. Words that make you feel something. Those are powerful. That's medicine.

– JACOB, SAULTEAUX, 10 OCTOBER 1997

Actually, all my life I ask myself, "When will, when am I going to feel better? When am I going to heal? When am I going to stop feeling like this?" I asked those questions all my life – waiting for myself to heal when it is not coming. 'Cause we just sit around – do nothing. If you don't try to create yourself into something it's not going to come. You have to try to make it happen. When you sit around smoking [dope], you go deeper and deeper and make yourself a hell of your life – that's all you do if you don't try to help yourself. But when you help yourself, you could start to understand that somewhere along the line in the future – or in the future I can be better, if you do things in better ways. But you have to make that happen; it doesn't happen like candy in a machine. You have to work for it. You have to sweat. You have to even cry sometimes in order to make yourself free. This pain inside you it's like ... cysts and swollen things ... that make your skin hurt and you have a needle or sharp knife to get that pus out. And even when you take out that pus with a needle or a sharp knife, it doesn't heal right away; it usually starts to get better with time. When that pus goes out and your body, your skin starts to heal slowly. Same way with your soul – you have to talk about it; cry about it so this pain will go away. Not just like that [snaps his fingers]. Slowly but surely starting to feel more at ease – do I make sense? That's how I see it – life itself. You have to talk about it.

– D.W., INUK, 9 OCTOBER 1997

In this chapter, I discuss the dynamics of healing among formerly incarcerated Aboriginal men through the use of narrative reconstructions of identity, or re-presentations of self, based on "pan-Indian" spirituality. The quotations above, which come from my interviews with clients at Medicine House,[1] a halfway house for Aboriginal men, point to the intense struggle each encountered as part of the process of healing. Although each person must find his or her own healing path, the activity of healing oneself at Medicine House is grounded in the reliving of painful memories in the presence of others in a group setting. This form of group intervention is complicated by the unique make-up of the house, which includes Aboriginal men from many different backgrounds.[2] This diversity gives rise to complex dynamics around issues of identity, authenticity, and belonging.

As an ethnic term, "Aboriginal" denotes a definable segment of the Canadian population: peoples who are culturally, historically, and legally distinct from the general national population by virtue of their indigenous origins. But in day-to-day conversation, and in the specific case of bureaucratic and clinical practice addressed in this chapter, the term has more profound implications. Here, denoting "Aboriginality," it has connotations that can homogenize diverse and competing notions of local as well as personal senses of identity (see Waldram, Chapter 3). The following offers a critique of the clinical deployment of Aboriginality as a discursive practice within Medicine House, which provides exclusive residential and intensive psychotherapeutic services for men of Aboriginal ancestry. At Medicine House, being Aboriginal is both a rhetorical means to therapeutic ends and a way to reconcile a bureaucratic policy that does not acknowledge local indigenous identities in the first place.

This discussion will focus on the experiences of three residents, Jacob and Samson (and to a lesser extent, Thomas), whom I got to know through group therapy and interviews over the course of my ethnographic fieldwork at Medicine House. In talking about their lives, both of these residents drew on the clinical rhetoric enacted by the counselling staff to reconfigure their past experiences in terms of pan-Indian spirituality.[3] The individuals I have chosen to focus on illustrate the power of this therapeutic discourse. However, not all their fellow residents bought into the clinical rhetoric as readily as did Jacob and Samson, either actively resisting or passively humouring the efforts of clinical staff. Although all residents had stories to tell about themselves to themselves, to counsellors, to fellow residents, and to myself, some clearly avoided filtering their narratives through the models and metaphors provided by the counsellors. The reasons for this resistance to clinical rhetoric will be discussed in a later section of this chapter.

The Incarcerated Aboriginal

That Medicine House exists at all is due to the particular niche it fills within the mandate of the federal and provincial correctional systems. The house provides a psychotherapeutic service for Aboriginal men, who constitute a disproportionate number of incarcerated persons in Canada's federal and provincial prisons. The house opened in 1988, the same year a government task force, assigned to investigate this problem, released its findings (Canada 1988).[4] Many of the issues and themes raised in this report foreshadowed the restorative-justice movement, aimed at finding alternatives to incarceration, as poignantly described by assistant Crown attorney Rupert Ross (1992, 1996). The clinical staff of Medicine House were familiar with Ross' writing and supportive of this broad movement in the Canadian justice system; the house's therapeutic practices and value system clearly reflected the values and aspirations of this movement.

The overrepresentation of men of Aboriginal ancestry in Canada's criminal justice system has been a well-documented fact for over a decade. Although approximately 3% of the national population is composed of Aboriginal peoples, in 2001 they constituted 18% of all offenders under federal jurisdiction (Correctional Services of Canada 2006). Correctional institutions under provincial jurisdiction have similarly elevated rates of incarceration of Aboriginal peoples in most provinces, although the number of offenders of Aboriginal ancestry in prisons varies considerably across the country. The disproportionate number of Aboriginal offenders is highest in federal and provincial institutions on the Prairies. In the provincial institutions of Manitoba, Saskatchewan, and Alberta, Aboriginal men constitute fully 59%, 76%, and 38% of prison populations respectively, while in the federal institutions they represent 36% of the incarcerated population from the Prairie region. In British Columbia, Aboriginal men represent 20% of the provincial population and 19% of those in federally run institutions. Interestingly, Quebec does not have elevated rates of incarceration for Aboriginal men in either its federal or provincial institutions – a trend that appears consistent with the eastern provinces as well. The reasons for this remain unclear, but the trend likely reflects differences in the geographic location of communities, differences in urban migration, and historical differences in relationships between Aboriginal populations and the larger society.

In its day-to-day bureaucratic policies and practices, the Canadian state generally does not fully distinguish among or recognize the wide spectrum of cultural and social identities of its indigenous populations. When it does make distinctions, it is within a specific geographic, historical, or legal domain – for example, Inuit and Métis populations or "status" versus "nonstatus" Indians. This lack of differentiation applies to the criminal justice system as well. As a consequence, in its day-to-day relationship with Corrections Canada and other agencies, Medicine House is required to accept men whose backgrounds encompass considerable cultural, historical, geographic, legal, linguistic, political, and socioeconomic diversity. As well, there is a pervasive and powerful notion among European Canadians (and among many Aboriginal peoples as well) that all Aboriginal peoples share some sort of essential commonality with each other, often in terms of their religious systems and spirituality. Given these premises upon which the house operates, it is perhaps not surprising that the counselling staff have developed and now use a therapeutic ideology and set of practices that further homogenize the diverse cultural identities of its Aboriginal residents. Clearly, the policies of the Canadian state that concern and directly affect indigenous peoples and their communities have, to a large extent, already created this homogenous category. These practices are historically rooted in colonial encounters with the indigenous "other." Thus Medicine House is simply acting within a pre-established discursive framework that is inseparable from its bureaucratic state context.

Field Research and Methods

From June to August 1997 I conducted fieldwork research at Medicine House.[5] In the fall of 1997 and spring of 1998 in-depth interviews were undertaken with 8 residents and 2 members of the clinical staff of the house. Much of the fieldwork concentrated on the group-psychotherapy program, referred to in this chapter as the Medicine Community Circle.[6] These group-therapy sessions normally occurred 3 times a week, with each session lasting about 2 to 3 hours. In July 1997 I also participated in a 1-week intensive-therapy session at a camp retreat off the Island of Montreal. For the most part, my interaction with residents and staff was limited to the setting and activities sponsored by the house. On one occasion, however, I escorted a resident to his community; unfortunately, no follow-up interviews with this resident were possible since his stay at the house was brief and tenuous.[7] At the time of the research, the house was located in the City of Montreal and had been in operation for 10 years. The house accepts Aboriginal men who have been paroled from federal and provincial institutions. It also accepts men awaiting sentence who have a sentencing requirement to undergo psychotherapy or who have been referred by their community social services. During my fieldwork, there were at any given time from five to seven different cultural groups represented at the house, including Algonquin, Cree, Inuit, Mi'kmaq, Mohawk, and Naskapi. It was not uncommon for each resident to have come from a different indigenous people. As well, residents spoke English, French, and/or their own indigenous languages. About 1 in 4 of the residents were Inuit from Nunavik (northern Quebec). As well, although most residents had resided in or were strongly affiliated with their indigenous communities, some had been raised in urban centres, either because of adoption or because of their families' migration to the city.

Diversity was the rule, not the exception, at Medicine House. My interest in the house centres on the link between what I view as an inclusive but vague bureaucratic and "ethnic" category – Aboriginal peoples – and the Medicine House clinical staff's conscious and strategic deployment of a set of generic beliefs, ideas, and themes within its therapeutic ideology and practices – what I refer to as "Aboriginality" or as a clinical rhetoric of "pan-Indianism." The challenge was how to make sense of the relationship between the house's therapeutic ideology of "pan-Indian" spirituality and the marked cultural diversity of the residents.

Pan-Indian identity, or pan-Indianism, refers to "a supratribal ideology" (Snipp 1996, 654) and projection of a generalized sense of indigenous identity;[8] it can be "defined as cultural patterns that cut across traditional tribal boundaries to unite people in a wider, regional or national identity" (Lerch and Bullers 1996, 390). Pow-Wows are a primary example of pan-Indianism, along with national or international political movements such as the American Indian Movement, a militant Aboriginal political movement that emerged in the late 1960s. Pan-Indian spiritual healing can be described as a culturally generalized representation of indigenous identity, particularly in terms of religious beliefs and spiritual practices; it lacks a specific reference or boundedness to any one Aboriginal cultural tradition. For the most part, pan-Indianism borrows heavily from the cultural imagery and traditions of Plains societies, utilizing the practices of the sweat lodge, smudging, deference to and honouring of the wisdom and authority of Native Elders, and the expression of the spiritual teachings of Lakota or other Plains societies. Some practices are drawn from other cultural traditions, including Navajo, Hopi, Cree, South American Tribes, and many other Aboriginal nations. The use of pan-Indian spiritual healing as a therapeutic approach has been discussed in an international context by Brady (1995), who documents the history of professional exchanges between Australian and Canadian indigenous groups and the attempt to export some of the therapeutic models and practices. These cultural approaches were often rooted in 12-step alcohol-recovery programs and in pan-Indian spiritual healing and were developed and used within Aboriginal-run treatment centres across North America.

In his study of symbolic healing practices among Native inmates in a Saskatchewan penitentiary, Waldram (1993, 1997) discusses the use of rhetoric in healing. Referring to Csordas' (1983) study of Catholic Pentecostal healing, Waldram argues that the religious community is essential to the process of transformation: "Through the use of symbols, the interchange of language and other forms of communication between healer and patient is essential, leading to a transformation in the patient's understanding of the problem. Such a conception presupposes that the language and symbols used are meaningful for both the healer and the patient. The religious community plays a crucial role in this interchange. Both the definitions of the problem and the cure 'conform to the agenda of the religious community,' and 'healing is understood to occur in terms of integration of the healed person into the religious community'" (1997, 72).

Given the staff's reliance on symbolic healing approaches, there was strong evidence in the house of the rhetoric of healing, the integration of the sufferer within a therapeutic community, and the transformation of one's problems from a source of despair and suffering into a source of revitalization and strength. For many residents who desired to transform their negative experiences in life and the pain and sadness that goes with these experiences, the house's therapeutic language of community and healing had positive effects while they were in the "care" (as opposed to the custody) of the house.

An important finding by Waldram was that this cultural brand of spiritual healing is made problematic by the involvement of a culturally heterogeneous Aboriginal population. In Waldram's study, inmates had widely differing orientations to Aboriginal and Euro-Canadian cultures, and these differences affected their receptivity to the pan-Indian spiritual healing. To foster greater therapeutic responsiveness, inmates had to be taught the symbols of pan-Indian spiritual healing. Similarly, not all residents at Medicine House responded to the clinical rhetoric in the same way, and although they were encouraged to adopt the language and symbols of pan-Indian healing over the course of treatment, for some clients, these did not resonate with their experience.

Respecting "the Medicines"

The basis and relevance of my critique can be understood through examples from in-depth interviews with two residents of Medicine House. The first resident is Jacob, a man in his early twenties who came to the house from the provincial correctional system. The other is Thomas, a man in his forties from a Mohawk community who came from a federal institution. The interviews revealed divergent understandings of the meaning and role of a central therapeutic metaphor, "the medicines":

> GB: When they talk about "the medicines," what do they talk about? When they say, "Respect 'the medicines.'"
> Jacob: I don't know, traditional medicines. They talk about when you're smudging and – I don't know – medicines could be even powerful words.
> GB: How do you mean powerful words could be medicines?
> Jacob: Words that move you. Words that make you feel something. Those are powerful. That's medicine. It's all symbolic of everything.
> GB: These things we just talked about, are they important to you?
> Jacob: The medicines? They have, they are important to me. I don't know about if they actually have a physical effect on me. But they do have an emotional feeling to them. They belong to the way things been done for centuries. A long time ago this is how things were done. And now they're still being done; it's part of our past. It's the relationship with earth. (Jacob, Saulteaux, 10 October 1997)

Jacob offered this answer in response to my question about the meaning of "the medicines" during a session of group psychotherapy called the Medicine Community Circle. This group therapy aimed to provide a means for residents to help each other through the (often intense) sharing of confessional personal narratives. The counselling staff relied on pan-Indian rhetoric to foster a sense of community among residents. It was hoped that, in the process, residents might see aspects of themselves in each other and learn to reflect more deeply on the problems they faced in their lives. Ideally, those residents who responded positively to this process would learn to control their addictions, stop their criminal behaviour, and leave the revolving door of the correctional system.

"The medicines" were also a critical part in this process. In the Medicine Community Circle "the medicines" generally referred to the cedar, sage, sweet grass, tobacco, and other organic material used in smudging, a form of ritual cleansing with smoke. The rhetoric surrounding "the medicines" was a way to cultivate an ancestral spiritual presence in the "group," and it taught the residents the precepts that, according to the counselling staff, are fundamental to every Aboriginal community: sharing, caring, honesty, and respect. In essence, to "respect the medicines" meant to respect their sacredness and spiritual potential to heal. And by extension, it meant to respect the group and, most important, the healing of fellow residents. For some of those residents, as evidenced by Jacob's deeply felt articulation, "the medicines" did not just imply a tradition; they *were* the tradition.

But not all residents heard the counselling rhetoric in the same way. For some, it appeared to be vague and largely meaningless. This was especially true for Thomas, the Mohawk resident. He provided a comparison of "the medicines" used at the house with those he had learned about from a culturally knowledgeable mentor.

> Thomas: When I go [home to my community] – when I work with my Elder – he'll give me medicines. Like, we'll go out and he'll help me. He'll pick it for me and he'll explain it to me – what it's for and when to use it. Like, if it's for something when you're sick, he'll tell you everything about it. But over here [the counsellors] don't tell you nothing about it.
>
> GB: So, generally, when they're talking about "medicines," what do you think they're talking about?
>
> Thomas: I don't know. Sometimes I think they don't even know what they're talking about. (Thomas, Mohawk, 18 October 1997)

For Thomas, the meaning of "medicines" was linked to a specific context of tutelage – a set of personal memories of exploring the country with another community member who had more knowledge than he did about medicinal plants in the environment. Real medicines are inseparable from particular knowledge of a local world or landscape. Jacob, the resident mentioned earlier, did not have such personal memories. He had been adopted out of his family and separated from his community at an early age. This early rupture was a source of despair and had created a persistent sense of loss. For Jacob, the house provided a surrogate Aboriginal community, giving him a place to belong. It is not surprising, then, that he was more receptive to the pan-Indian rhetoric of healing. As a whole, Jacob seemed to respond well to group psychotherapy and had a good relationship with his counsellor. In contrast, Thomas was more resistant to the therapy. He did not trust the counselling staff and was quite cynical about the house, even suggesting that it was simply an extension of the prison system. According to his own account and those of the counselling staff, Thomas rarely shared any personal stories during group or even in his individual counselling sessions. The divergent views of "the medicines" by these two residents raise important questions about how individuals are socialized to accept therapeutic interventions, and, central to the concern of this chapter, they highlight the importance of the rhetorical content of therapy.

Medicine House is located within a continuum of supports and services for men trying to exit the correctional systems. The therapeutic program aims to respond to the challenge of providing psychotherapy to former inmates, many of whom have personal issues with addictions and substance abuse, who remain distrustful of authority, and who may subvert attempts to help them change patterns of negative social behaviour. The rhetorical content of the therapeutic interventions was a distinctive feature of the house's therapeutic program: the use of pan-Indian notions about collective and personal identity as a means to healing, recovery, and reintegration for formerly incarcerated men of indigenous ancestry. These notions were part of a persuasive and powerful discourse of Aboriginality. This clinical rhetoric offered residents (and probably some counsellors as well) a generic and selective representation of what it means to be an indigenous person in contemporary Canadian society. The resistance to therapy on the part of some clients reflected a conscious choice about how they wished to narrate their identities and an explicit rejection of the clinical rhetoric of what it means to be an Aboriginal person in terms of a pan-Indian ideology.

Aboriginality

Ethnographies are stories about cultural others, and as Bruner (1986) tells us, they are always products of their discursive epochs and historical times. Bruner demonstrates this point by showing how ethnographies of Native Americans changed over a span of decades. Specifically, the stories these ethnographies tell about the fate of Native Americans differ dramatically between the pre- and post-Second World War epochs. For example, Bruner writes, "in the 1930s narrative it was the past that pervaded the present; in the 1970s narrative it is the future" (1986, 140). Anthropological writings on Native American peoples in earlier decades reflected a sense of doom in regard to their cultural distinctiveness and the supposed inevitability of their gradual assimilation into dominant North American society. In contrast, in later decades ethnographic writing portrayed Native American communities and peoples as resisting this process of assimilation and even demonstrating a remarkable cultural resilience in the face of North American hegemonic forces.

Bruner's article also underscores the point that colonial history and anthropological writings about Native American cultures and peoples have had a powerful effect on their representation in popular imagination and political process. Since anthropological investigations of Native Americans began in the nineteenth century, they have become the objects of a Euro-American cultural gaze that first constructed and then regulated or policed their cultural identities. Of course, as James Clifford (1988) has pointed out, anthropological writing has also contributed to the subjugation of other world populations. In the case of indigenous peoples, Aboriginality implies that there exists an internally homogenous category of peoples in the world distinguished by having been collectively "othered" or sociopolitically marginalized from nation-state populations. In drawing attention to this social construction of Aboriginality, the aim is not to deny that Aboriginal peoples exist or that Aboriginality is an inauthentic source of identity. Rather, the aim is to point out how the locally constructed cultural identities of some of the world's human populations have been historically subsumed within a larger discourse. In other words, "Aboriginal" and "Aboriginality" are historical social constructions and need to be understood as such. More important, the effects of this historical process must be critically appreciated and carefully examined.

Aboriginality is a socially constructed body of knowledge that serves as a "dividing practice," one that has separated (and then marginalized) some members of the world's populations. Aboriginality, then, is a way to conceive indigenous peoples as cultural "others." As a discursive practice it has been well studied in Australian anthropology (Archer 1991; Beckett 1988; Hollinsworth 1992; Lattas 1991). Lattas (1993), in particular, uses a Foucauldian approach to look at the discourse of Aboriginality among white intellectuals as a type of knowledgeable "gaze" that polices the cultural and political expression of Australian Aboriginal populations. Lattas argues that this form of white liberal surveillance defines and delimits the construction of identity among a black underclass and cultivates modes of resistance among this marginalized population.

Over the centuries of contact, colonialism, and then neo-colonialism, knowledge has served as a way for expansionist and industrial societies to subsume those human populations whose lands were conquered and who appear to be opposed to the cultural values, economic practices, and political systems of European colonizers. Present-day North American society must contend with the devastating historical, political, and social legacies of this period. Consequently, Aboriginality remains the dominant form of knowledge of many developed "First World" nation-states in their relations with these "historically residual" indigenous populations.

This history can be appreciated by considering the impact of the popular image of the Indian, which has been well documented, especially in comparative literature studies. For example, in *The Whiteman's Indian*, Berkhofer (1979) demonstrates that the knowledge that developed around North American indigenous populations came from a number of competing sources: diplomats, missionaries, military men, and men of science. The historical images Berkhofer presents of Native Americans demonstrate that the relationship between the colonizer and colonized was at times deeply ambivalent and contradictory. Yet these images played a powerful role in shaping the identity of North American indigenous peoples. In an epilogue, Berkhofer writes: "From this survey of the idea of the Indian over time, two dramatic historic trends emerge. What began as a reality for the Europeans ended as image and stereotype for Whites, and what began as an image alien to Native Americans became a reality for them. For Native Americans the power of the whites all too often forced them to be the Indians Whites said they were regardless of their original social and cultural diversity" (1979, 195).

The effect of these Euro-American representations of Native Americans was to homogenize the wide cultural and social diversity of indigenous populations. This has been the case not just in North America but, arguably, also throughout the world wherever indigenous populations were conquered and then subjected to economic marginalization, intense political control, and state-sponsored cultural oppression, if not outright attempts at genocide. Ironically, this oppression has often been coupled with romantic valorization of Aboriginal peoples as holders of natural, ecological, or spiritual wisdom. In the words of the anthropologist Alice Kehoe:

> Thousands of Americans and Europeans believe ... that American Indians retain a primordial wisdom that could heal our troubled world. American Indians are supposed to be Naturvolker (natural peoples), in contrast to the civilized nations alienated from Nature. Personified as Mother Earth, Nature is the embodiment of life and thus hope of a future ... Lovejoy and Boas called this "cultural primitivism ... the discontent of the civilized with civilization." That discontent gives rise to one of the strangest, most potent, and most persistent factors in western thought – the use of the term "nature" to express the standard of human values, the identification of the good with that which is natural. (1990, 194)

The dialogic/therapeutic practices of the counsellors at Medicine House represent a local clinical strategy that constitutes one vein within this broader discourse of Aboriginality. Among other elements, this perspective appears to uphold the romantic notion that Aboriginal peoples embody a natural and pure source of spiritual or ecological wisdom. In the context of the therapeutic program of Medicine House, this view of indigenous peoples as "in touch with nature" and as possessing a special wisdom is expressed through the rhetoric of a pan-Indian Native spirituality. Elements of this spirituality that were invoked regularly in conversations with staff and residents at the house included discussing encounters or the expectation of encounters with "Little People" (i.e., small, mystical humans said to occasionally appear and/or cause mischief, such as borrowing and misplacing personal effects); a tendency to seek explanations of seemingly inexplicable occurrences as mystical or spiritual in nature; interpreting one's dreams, especially those involving animals and creatures, as signs and symbols of an ancestral spiritual encounter with significant personal meaning; the assumption that one should be able to intuitively feel the power and presence of various "medicines" (e.g., smudging with cedar, sage, or sweet grass); and most important, the notion that the healing circle contained an ancestral spiritual presence that was invoked and empowered by honest and open conversation (or offended by dishonesty and disrespect) among those in the circle. All these elements and symbolic imagery, aided by visual cues in the form of Aboriginal emblems placed on a central pillar in the room, flowed in and out of the talk of counsellors and residents while the lingering smoke from smudging wafted in the air, providing attendees with a constant sensate reminder throughout the session that this was a special time and place. These sessions were often deeply moving experiences, especially when some residents effectively articulated their painful memories and triggered cathartic expressions of emotion among fellow residents.

Pan-Indian spiritual healing represents a cultural idiom that is quite new in its current form and function, and it evokes a romanticized portrait of indigenous cultures as inherently more spiritual than other world cultures. Medicine House, as a treatment centre for Native people, shares many therapeutic commonalities with other Native-run treatment centres where pan-Indian spirituality, the "Red Road," or healing circles are enthusiastically embraced as standard healing practices. And like these other Native-run treatment programs, the house employs a therapeutic approach assembled from various indigenous traditions and from a variety of standard psychotherapeutic methods – some borrowed from mainstream, academic, and popular psychology as well as from other helping professions – that do not engage a critical understanding of the collective identities of past and contemporary Aboriginal peoples. Instead, this pan-Indian healing tends to promote a generic representation of essentialized and universalistic Aboriginal values. This point is driven home most clearly by Waldram (2004, 239-70), who argues that this representation within mainstream academic psychology, which has spilled over to the wider society, has a long history and remains largely unchallenged (269).

As pointed out earlier, on a daily basis the staff of Medicine House must confront a significant degree of cultural, geographic, and linguistic pluralism among residents, which makes the delivery of effective and culturally sensitive (or relevant and specific) therapeutic interventions and programs difficult. As part of their therapeutic approach, the staff homogenize the cultural identities of residents and construct a sense of (Aboriginal) community among residents. Residency at the house implies that one is and desires to act as a temporary member of the medicine community. This surrogate Aboriginal community is founded on the principles of caring, sharing, honesty, and respect. To sustain this community, clinical staff deploy a series of metaphors – "the circle," "the community," "the medicines," "the medicine wheel," "the sacred fire" – to impart a moral imperative to the therapeutic interventions as well as to invoke a common spiritual purpose among residents. It is these generic themes of collective identity that some residents use as points of reference to ground their individual narratives of suffering, recovery, and healing, thereby projecting a recuperated Aboriginal self.

Narrating an Aboriginal Self: The Young Warrior and the Prodigal Son

Narrative is a way to situate the self in the world (Kirby 1991; Ricoeur 1984). The human impulse to narrate one's experiences is a fundamental, possibly universal characteristic of all cultures (White 1980; Mink 1981). Narrative brings a sense of temporal order and coherence to human experience. But the act of narration never occurs in a political or social vacuum (Bruner 1986).

Both the audience and context influence the direction, intention, and substance of narratives. As Mattingly (1998) argues, the rituals of the therapeutic encounter offer a dramaturgical context that helps to create the aesthetics of the story told. Shafer (1980) makes a similar point in reviewing the Freudian psychoanalytic exercise as a form of inter-pretation jointly crafted between analyst and analysand. He argues that the dialogic ex-change between reliable (analyst) and unreliable (analysand) narrators serves to construct the meaning of personal narratives within a therapeutic milieu. Likewise, Kirmayer shows how the therapeutic encounter as a dialogic interchange of give and take between patient and therapist can lead to clinical impasses that "reveal structural problems and ideological conflicts in medical care" (2000, 157). The understanding that emerges from these studies is clear: narratives are fundamental to our conception of the world and to our sense of place within it, yet all narratives are shaped by the social interactions and discursive for-mations within which they are located. All narratives, especially those of illness and suf-fering, are informed by and express the unique exigencies of a cultural world (Garro 2000).

The interaction between therapeutic language and larger discursive formations of Ab-originality is illustrated by the stories of two residents, Jacob and Samson.

Jacob

Among the residents whom I interviewed, Jacob was one of the most responsive to Medi-cine House's therapeutic program. As mentioned earlier, Jacob had been adopted out of his family, and there had been little or no contact with his First Nations community or with his adoptive family. Jacob's life before he came to the house was marked by periods of alcohol and drug abuse, criminal activity, and transience. Jacob spoke of searching for a Native identity, and he would occasionally travel and live with other Native people. He was admitted to the house after being told about it by a person within the correctional system. For the most part, Jacob demonstrated a deep commitment to the therapy and had a great deal of respect for the staff. When I met Jacob, he was in the process of changing his adopted last name – what he referred to as a "slave name" – to his birth name. Jacob was interested in Native issues, very politically active, and committed to social change. He was involved in the Oka Crisis of 1990 and felt that it was among the most significant events in his life.[9]

Jacob's political sympathies for militant Native social movements became the source of a conflict between a number of residents and the staff of the house. At issue was the flying of the "Mohawk Warrior" flag (also called the "Aboriginal Solidarity" flag) on a pole at the intensive-therapy camp outside Montreal.[10] Staff reacted very strongly and swiftly to its presence at the camp. According to the staff, several years previously a resident had worn a jacket with this same image when visiting a nearby summer cottage town. A local newspaper had sensationalized its sighting, claiming that members of the Hells Angels and the Mohawk Warrior Society were occupying the local church-owned camp where Medicine House holds its summer healing retreats. The house's board members and staff were forced to meet with mayors from the surrounding towns to respond to the public outcry that resulted from this ludicrous media coverage. Following a group meeting, Jacob and the residents who had put the flag up reluctantly took it down. He related to me his feelings about the incident:

> Jacob: Yeah, I got mad at that. Because, people view it as a bad thing ... and they didn't know what it was about. It's just typical. It's like looking at ... some bum on the street. You don't know where he's been. You don't know what he's done. But you can classify him. You can make a judgment and say well he's nothing because he doesn't have a fucking job. He's a bum; that's all he'll be and that's all he'll ever be. But it's not that way. If you at least stop and ask that person how he is, what happened to him and how come he's that way, and you'll get a whole different view. But no one will take the time to understand and appreciate that flag and what it's about.
>
> GB: For you, what is that flag about?
>
> Jacob: It's about a pride. It's about a way, a dream that's been going on for a long time: an interconnection through you to others – uniting everybody. Uniting everybody; it's a great dream. It's a great thing to accomplish. I'll stand by it regardless of whatever may happen. (Jacob, Saulteaux, 3 October 1997)

Jacob's own journey is woven across a broad tapestry of Aboriginality; his narrative incorporates seemingly incompatible statements of militancy and resistance with statements of healing and spirituality. Further, he recounted that through his late teens and early twenties he sought out the company of other Native people and travelled to different Native communities. He was trying to acquire an authentic source of a Native identity – something he felt was severely lacking in his own life. As both of us were of Saulteaux ancestry, he was appreciative of what minimal cultural and historical knowledge I could share with him.

During the camp retreat, the counsellors conducted a ceremony they said was a Cree Indian mourning ceremony. According to them, the ceremony was used to help people who were having difficulty in overcoming grief for a lost loved one. A boulder – or gravestone – was suspended on a rope and pulled between two competing parties in a tug of war. The object was to bring the stone to the gravesite of the loved one against the wishes of those who could not overcome the death. In Jacob's case the counsellors wanted him to address the loss of his mother and confront his sense of failure and worthlessness. The counsellors constructed a mock gravesite with a cross and plastic skull and pulled Jacob away from it. When it did not seem to have the desired effect – Jacob was resisting the therapy – they reversed it so he pulled the stone toward the grave. While he battled the counsellors, they mocked and humiliated him. Eventually, Jacob became engrossed in the action of pulling and was visibly angry. When the counsellors saw that Jacob was tiring and becoming too upset, they stopped and began to console him. Jacob buried his face in the ground and cried for a very long time over the loss of his mother, the desertion of his adopted family, and his insatiable thirst to be accepted and loved.

> I remember crawling on the floor when I did ... that ceremony. I was crawling and I can't remember why I was crawling, but I knew I was crawling. I don't know where I was going. I was crying and just letting go. I don't know why I was doing that. Some people gave me an idea: maybe it was shame; maybe it's part of that or something else. That's why it's important why I find out. Maybe something happened before I was five. Maybe that's what made me cry – something when I was a little baby, looking for something, somewhere to go, maybe go and hide, maybe to go towards somebody. I can't figure it out. Maybe if I do it again I'll figure it out. I was thinking of doing it again. (Jacob, Saulteaux, 17 October 1997)

This passage illustrates Jacobs' uncertainty about the meaning of these events and his tentative use of psychological idioms to describe his experience. The process of "figuring it out" is the preliminary stage in narrative emplotment, in which the narrator tries to join the disparate elements of experience into a coherent and workable framework. In struggling to make sense of his experience during the therapeutic ritual, Jacob is trying to establish a sequence of memories of the past that will account for his life in the present and provide meanings upon which to draw for the future. Jacob's narrative of personal healing is unfolding within a pan-Indian spiritual healing that borrows, configures, and modifies cultural practices from a broad spectrum of local indigenous populations and popular psychology.

Samson

> *It was meet that we should make merry, and be glad: for this brother was dead, and is alive again; and was lost, and is found.*
>
> – LUKE 15:32

Samson is a Naskapi man in his late forties whom I first met at the intensive-therapy camp. He arrived at Medicine House near the end of my fieldwork. He had come to the house from a provincial institution after serving a short sentence for charges related to impaired driving and resisting arrest. He was experiencing prolonged withdrawal symptoms from drug addiction. One afternoon, during a break in programs, I was sitting in the main room of the dilapidated clubhouse where "group" was held. Samson walked up to

GREGORY M. BRASS

where I was sitting and introduced himself. He had heard I was an anthropology graduate student and wanted to talk with me. In his youth, he had some encounters with anthropologists conducting research in his community, and he enjoyed the experiences. Samson told me he spoke his language and was raised on the land but educated in the south at a Canadian university. He claimed he had a good upbringing by strict parents and was exposed to many wonderful learning experiences as a child. While studying in the south, he became politically active and was involved with the American Indian Movement. Also, he began to experiment with drugs, including LSD and cocaine, with the latter substance becoming a recurring lifelong addiction. He found the stress of working in the south and yearning to be back on the land too difficult for him. Samson suggested to me that he was suffering from what he called "PCSS – postcultural stress syndrome" – an emotionally fatiguing experience of trying to manage oneself across two cultural divides; this strain eventually wore him down and made him more vulnerable to drug use and self-destructive behaviour. His drug habit took its toll not just on him but on his marriage and family as well. At the time, a former love had re-entered his life, and his affection for her was apparent throughout our dialogue. Like himself, she had gone through recovery and was highly supportive of his effort to heal himself.

Samson related his personal notions of healing, which in many ways paralleled the cultural eclecticism of the therapeutic dialogues of the house. He was also interested in the house's Native spirituality. His own cultural background and upbringing in Naskapi bush life predisposed him to the search for spiritual meaning. He related an experience as an adolescent when he had his first hunting vision:

> Yeah, my first time I visioned ... I was in camp. I was with an Elder. It happened through that time growing up. I had to leave [university] just to hunt 'cause the [drug] culture I was caught up in. And this happened in October 1970 at the end of September. We were in a camp and I had this – a vision in my sleep. I dreamt I was carrying on a backpack, a yearling, a Caribou, a one-year-old caribou. And I was, that day before the dream, I was with this Elder. The other men were out [hunting] on the land and they came back that evening. They were on a freighter, a boat. And the next morning we were having breakfast. During the dream – the dream I had was very clear. So I told them I had this dream and I told them what I had saw. And they didn't say anything. So after breakfast we moved out and we had to walk. We took the boat, a freighter. And we got off after about an hour – out of the freighter. And we walked about ten miles and we came to this place in the bush. And in the clearing there was a yearling. And one of the men said, "There's your vision." They had killed a caribou the day before and they didn't tell us – when they were out. So I can say that – I consider that as a vision. Like they had shot a yearling too. (Samson, Naskapi, 1 November 1997)

This narrative of a hunting vision corresponds to the ethnographic work of Adrian Tanner (1979; Chapter 11), who has shown that hunting among some northern peoples serves as a form of spiritual questing. Samson's own hunting vision was culturally consistent with local Naskapi practices. Yet Samson drew upon alternative sources to account for his present-day emotional pain and need for spiritual redemption. For instance, Samson informed me that during the 1970s he first understood he had a problem with drugs after listening to The Eagles' song "Hotel California."[11] He also related that he had recently been having dreams that he felt were forms of spiritual instruction. During one of our conversations at camp, he asked me whether I knew about a song called "Prodigal Son" by Neil Young.[12] He then proceeded to tell me about a dream in which he recalled seeing an old woman and looking at a CD by Neil Young. On its cover was an eagle. One of the songs on the CD was called "Prodigal Son." He asked me whether I knew what the song "Prodigal Son" was about. He interpreted this dream to mean that he needed to understand the lyrics to the song. Further, he believed that the eagle on the CD cover, as well as the rock band that first made him aware of his addiction, implied that this animal might be his spiritual totem. In constructing his narratives of recovery and renewal, Samson drew from a diverse set of sources: Naskapi hunting culture, Christian Biblical parables, and popular rock music.

Not unexpectedly, Samson was very receptive to Medicine House's pan-Indian spiritualism. He was deeply committed to "the medicines." And like Jacob, he was disturbed by the behaviour of fellow residents who did not show appropriate respect toward others' expressions of suffering. Samson discussed a circle ceremony he attended outside the house that demonstrated his genuine interest in pan-Indian spirituality.[13]

> Samson: And I managed to bring in my medicine wheel to the circle. At that
> time ... there was a sweat-lodge conductor there in the circle. And
> she told the circle, when it was her turn to speak, that I had brought
> in my medicine wheel there ... first I brought in the grandfathers and
> grandmothers ... and then the medicine wheel came in there.
> GB: What do you mean you brought your medicine wheel in there?
> Samson: I don't know. When I was talking something came into the circle.
> This sweat-lodge conductor, I guess, saw it and sensed it through
> her power. And she told me what I had in the four directions: in the
> east, golden eagle; and in the south, snake; and to the west, an owl;
> and to the north, a weasel; and that I'm bear clan. I never knew I had
> these things. (Samson, Naskapi, 1 November 1997)

Samson presented these images as though they had been invoked from within him. The sweat-lodge conductor is portrayed as a person gifted with spiritual powers that allowed her to draw these internalized beings out of him. Samson demonstrates his receptivity to pan-Indian spirituality and incorporates its models and metaphors to help

GREGORY M. BRASS

construct a path toward personal healing. Yet at the end of the quotation he adds, "I never knew I had these things." This comment points to a paradox: on the one hand, pan-Indian spirituality is part of the construction of Aboriginality; on the other hand, it partially reconstructs the world of its Aboriginal subjects – an ephemeral state of being in the world is experienced as "always" and eternally existing. Above all, it is the profound sense of the (re)discovery of an enduring or sacred truth within these experiences that gives credence to the message of healing and sets a meaningful course for him to follow into the future.

In terms of narrative, Samson later related to me how this same sweat-lodge conductor, or medicine woman, suggested to him that the troubles in his life might be related to "bad medicine" – that is, he may have been living his life under a curse willed by an envious person. He referred to this curse as a "bear walk," in which his spirit was under the influence of malevolent forces. Although he was aware that there was free will in his life choices (i.e., who he married, the drugs he used, the decision to leave his wife), this curse meant that danger and trouble always seemed able to find him. In one instance, he told me a story of a time when he went hunting during the winter. He and his hunting party split up to find an animal. After a long period of no luck, he went back to their truck. He decided to shorten the journey by climbing down a bluff and in doing so nearly fell to his death. On another occasion, when he and his wife had split up, he was working as a consultant for other Native communities. He used his truck to sleep in, often on the outskirts of the communities where he was consulting. One night, as he was sleeping, he was confronted by a group of men from the community who accused him of chasing their women and threatened to beat him up. He managed to escape. He claimed their accusations were false and that he had not been looking to create any problems for himself. But he wondered why these men went after him and how they found him. He gave many instances in his life where trouble just seemed to find him. Locating these tales within a larger spiritual framework of meaning served partially to explain them.

In summary, throughout the time I knew Samson at the house, he demonstrated a consistent and strong commitment to the therapeutic program and immersed himself in its rhetoric of healing. Since his late adolescence and early twenties, pan-Indian ideas and themes had been a pervasive influence in his life, both through the counterculture of the early 1970s and through the American Indian Movement. Arguably, the house's therapeutic program was an extension of the romantic aspirations of the social movements to which Samson was already sympathetic. At the same time, he articulated a deep resolve to overcome his personal tribulations. This resolve became the narrative centre of his journey of personal healing, ordering his past trials and future projects along a trajectory that made sense and offered hope.

As we have seen, both Jacob and Samson reconfigured past experiences into narratives of healing through the use of the models and metaphors of pan-Indian clinical rhetoric. For Jacob, the house served to ground him in a generic sense of Aboriginal community that was compatible with his own present venture – an opportunity to articulate and give coherence to his emotional pain as well as to gain a sense of belonging. Although his identification with militant political activism was contentious and challenged by the staff, the house affirmed its importance and relevance.

For Samson, the house represented a return to an earlier, more exciting and romantic time of his youth in the early 1970s, when he was actively involved with the American Indian Movement. A significant feature of the idioms of healing on which he relied was their eclecticism. He expressed his suffering and recovery through a creative and wide assemblage of therapeutic mediums – the musical lyrics of The Eagles and Neil Young, an insightful mystic healer, and a speculative referencing of numerous religious sources. His narrative offered a syncretic spiritual cadence of Biblical allegory, pan-Indian religious imagery, a culturally grounded vision of the Naskapi hunter, and that old-time rock 'n' roll.

Other Narrative Commitments

As pointed out earlier, not all residents subscribed to the clinical rhetoric offered by the staff of Medicine House as readily as Jacob and Samson. There were a number of reasons for this distancing or rejection of the therapeutic dialogue. Here, I will focus on two possible explanations: one concerns the therapeutic context, the other the content of therapy itself.

In the former case, resistance to therapy could be attributed to the socializing context: a therapeutic setting for men. Many of them were coping with addiction issues and leaving the correctional system, and they often held a deep distrust for authority and remained emotionally guarded. All the residents whom I interviewed had done time in prison and were accustomed to the curtailment of personal freedoms that incarceration involves. For the house to operate effectively as a therapeutic service, the staff had to maintain an alcohol- and drug-free environment in which residents could begin to recover. Furthermore, for the house to retain its licence to operate as a halfway house and remain credible to its funding sources and the surrounding community, it was essential to avoid any presence of street drugs in the house. For their part, residents were normally required to abstain from the use of drugs and alcohol while on parole. Still, not all the residents came to the house to recover, and some either simply did not or could not take the therapy seriously. These residents frequently and knowingly breached the rules of the house, becoming both the consumers and the purveyors of illegal substances, undermining the therapeutic efforts of clinical staff and distracting those residents genuinely trying to recover. Administrative and clinical staff knew this was a fact of life in the house and acted accordingly. From time to time, the house was locked down, personal freedoms were curtailed, rooms were searched, and, when warranted, some residents were sent back to prison and might even be charged with possession of narcotics or breach of parole. In short, the house periodically oscillated between healing and disciplining, and, in the latter mode, it became much like an extension of the system of incarceration that Thomas, the Mohawk resident, suggested it was. For residents like Thomas and others who had spent years in the penal system, it was natural to revert to what was learned in prison: emotional guardedness and suspicion of others, along with resistance to and subversion of all forms of authority. In a sense, some residents never really left prison. That is, in the face of social actions that resemble imprisonment, residents like Thomas re-implemented a narrative of self that referenced and reinforced a symbolic code of behaviour common among prison inmates.

In his narrative, however, Thomas represented an interesting combination of reasons for resistance to the therapeutic interventions of clinical staff. His resistance was influenced by the context of therapy as well as by its rhetorical content. We should recall that he dismissed a core therapeutic device, "the medicines," as meaningless gabble expressed by therapists who did not know, on a cultural level at least, what they were talking about. For Thomas, who was raised in his community and maintained a continuous connection with a cultural mentor there, the house's generic presentation of what constituted authentic Aboriginal cultural traditions seemed lacking in substance and authenticity compared to the richness of his localized Haudonosaunee cultural and spiritual practices.

Based on my interviews with other residents, Thomas' skepticism was shared by several of them. This was especially true of two Inuit residents I interviewed, who both found that the pan-Indian rhetoric of therapy rang hollow. From the perspective of Inuit culture, pan-Indianism appears as something distinctly foreign. When I asked both of these residents about "the medicines," neither expressed a clear understanding nor showed much interest in the clinical rhetoric. In fact, one Inuk resident admitted that his motivation to learn about the medicines was simply to get along with residents and staff.

> Medicines, actually, for being an Inuk, I'm not really – how would you call it? Well, there's a lot of names for medicines. I really can't say what they're called. I would have to hear it again in order to call it. To me, that's how it is; I don't know very much about Indian things – but to tell myself to respect how it works around here. I have to get along with, with fairly strange things for an Inuk, strange things. At first they were very strange 'cause in my life I never prayed to God. Like they call Him, Creator, and with this smoke [the medicines]. I never prayed like this before in my life before I came here. But I have to respect other cultures – how they pray and try to understand that. I mean try to see them just the same way as I would pray. I respect believers in what they believe like myself. I am a believer to something greater to myself. So I have to respect people when they pray to this Creator, they call him. And myself, I just call him God. (D.W., Inuk, 9 October 1997)

For this Inuk resident, the pan-Indian spirituality of Medicine House is an "other culture" foreign to the cultural practices of his own communities, where Christianity has maintained a strong presence for many decades (Dorais 1999). For most Inuit, pan-Indian spirituality is conceived of as distinctively "Indian and southern." Although the Inuit residents I interviewed seemed to be motivated by a desire to respect the beliefs and practices of southern residents more committed to "the medicines" and "Indian things," they nevertheless did commit themselves to a "healing journey," telling their sometimes painful, sometimes humorous stories during group-therapy sessions with great eloquence. But they distanced themselves from those elements that appeared culturally incompatible and, consequently, that did not serve to substantially inform their narratives of healing.

In fact, in the case of one Inuk resident, although he expressed an interest in the house's "Indian things" because he was part Indian himself (I took this to imply he had a non-Inuk ancestor from a southern Aboriginal group), he remained skeptical of the spiritually inclined perspectives of other residents and counsellors. In the case noted below, this resident told me of an incident where there was a persistent knocking on his door accompanied by the occasional shaking of his bed. He was certain it was another resident or likely several of them who were playing a trick on him and trying to annoy him; however, substantiating this allegation proved difficult. His counsellor suggested a more esoteric interpretation from which he distanced himself.

> LB: Yeah, someone was trying to make me believe it was some kind of spirit. At first, they said it was a bad spirit.
> GB: Who was saying it was a bad spirit?
> LB: One of the counsellors.
> GB: A counsellor?
> LB: I don't remember. And it turned it ... one of the counsellors say it was the Spirit Keeper of the West doing that. Then after a period of time, another person was saying it was my dead brother doing that. And after a period of time, that same person, she [a counsellor] told me it was – just ignore it.
> GB: So what do you think?
> LB: I don't think it was spirits.
> GB: You don't really believe in spirits?
> LB: No. (L.B., Inuk, 5 November 1997)

The resident resisted the suggested spiritual interpretations of the counsellor. Evidently, these interpretations were too elaborate for what appears, in his view, the daily exigency of life in a halfway house. His interpretation, grounded in experience within a correctional setting and familiarity with the irritating behaviour of some former inmates, points to a more banal explanation: every day one must contend with incessant acts of intimidation, ridicule, and immature pranksterism.

GREGORY M. BRASS

Conclusion

Aboriginality as a historical social construction and body of knowledge about cultural "others" has become a broad tapestry into which some residents can weave the threads of a narrated self. These acts of articulation – both to one's self (in private reflection) and before a group of residents and staff – hopefully lead to gradual transformations of personal narratives from stories centred on pain and sadness to stories about healing and renewal. Through the experience of sharing and listening to each other's stories, residents learn to reflect upon and confront forms of behaviour and ingrained attitudes that may contribute to the cycles of alcoholism and substance abuse, criminal activity, and periods of incarceration that have faced them throughout their adolescence and adulthood. At the same time, clinical staff, through their therapeutic ideology and practices, as well as through their own attitudes and personal commitments, tend to essentialize and romanticize the Aboriginal identity of residents. In some important respects, they are forced to do so. For example, the Canadian government's own bureaucratic application of Aboriginality does not fully differentiate the indigenous populations within its modern national territory; as a segment of the national population, Aboriginal peoples are mainly a legal and, in terms of incarceration and overall health disparities, a worrisome statistical category for the Canadian state. Currently, men of Aboriginal ancestry are vastly overrepresented in the incarcerated Canadian population. However, the category "Aboriginal" covers a broad range of different peoples and individuals with different backgrounds and commitments to their Aboriginal identity. Thus, on a daily basis, the staff of Medicine House must confront a significant degree of cultural, geographic, and linguistic pluralism among residents that makes the delivery of effective and culturally sensitive (or relevant and specific) therapeutic interventions and programs difficult. As part of their therapeutic approach, the staff homogenize the cultural identities of residents and construct a sense of (Aboriginal) community among residents. Residency at the house implies that one is and desires to act as a temporary member of the "medicine" community. This surrogate Aboriginal community is founded on the principles of caring, sharing, honesty, and respect. To sustain this community, clinical staff deploy a series of rhetorical devices – "the circle," "the community," "the medicines," "the medicine wheel," "the sacred fire" – that cultivate a moral imperative for the therapeutic interventions as well as invoke a common spiritual purpose among residents.

The house's therapeutic ideology and practices construct an image of Aboriginal identity that is reinforced by the sense of community and commitment to healing. This identity is for the most part a positive one that represents Aboriginality as located in a framework of spiritual awakening and renewal. At the same time, this reference to Aboriginal spirituality fits a pre-established web of social relations utilized by the Canadian state that, in turn, is rooted in the history of colonial encounter. Aboriginality subsumes the localized cultural identities of indigenous populations and is a source of identity more easily controlled, manipulated, and promoted (e.g., through the mass media) by the dominant non-Native society. The negative consequence of pan-Indianism, should it become too dominant and prevalent, is that it can seriously challenge or even thwart local expressions of cultural identity (see McIlwraith 1996). In the case of Medicine House residents, when their backgrounds and experiences diverge from the expected template, the dominant discourse of Aboriginality may even lead to a sense of confusion about one's local identity or foster a sense of cultural inferiority, especially given the increasingly hegemonic status of pan-Indian beliefs and values in recent decades.

Clinical rhetoric grounded in pan-Indianism, therefore, can be a two-sided cultural coin. For some residents, as in the case of Inuit residents, it had genuine shortcomings as a therapeutic approach. At best, these residents respectfully deferred to the interests of clinical staff and fellow residents more invested in this ideological construct. At worst, they were left confused by its generic cultural assumptions about contemporary indigenous identity. For these residents, pan-Indianism made for poor cultural currency, and accordingly, they did not invest in it. For other residents, a spirituality grounded in pan-Indianism afforded an abundance of fertile metaphors or idioms of healing and suffering through which they could articulate their experiences of pain and loss. For these individuals, pan-Indian spirituality and the rhetoric of psychological healing provided meaningful sustenance for emotional growth and personal change. And it certainly seemed that, with the help of therapists equipped with a generic cultural therapy, personal change did occur. For some, the cycle of alcohol and substance abuse was abated, and further incarceration was no longer an inevitable and inescapable reality upon leaving the halfway house. Of course, the precise role of the house and its healing practices in the subsequent course of residents cannot be determined by the type of ethnographic methods used in this study. It remains important to recognize that with – and sometimes even without – the aid of Medicine House's Aboriginal community of pan-Indian spirituality, many residents did go on to live peaceful and productive lives.

In conclusion, the findings of this study are consistent with Waldram's critically earlier work in prisons (1993, 1997), showing that there is a need to examine critically the cultural assumptions that inform a therapeutic approach and attempt to respond to the cultural needs of men of Aboriginal ancestry. Aboriginal men in prison are not a population with a single cohesive notion of social identity, although they do share a common struggle with issues of personal and collective identity. Importantly, this struggle over politically charged notions and representations of identity is not restricted to this incarcerated segment of the Aboriginal population. Rather, it is endemic to all contemporary Aboriginal peoples and their communities in the turbulent political context of the Canadian state.[14] The struggle over what constitutes an authentic Aboriginal identity – and relatedly, over what is an Aboriginal community – has various shades and can be found in a multitude of venues. Medicine House is one instance of this struggle with a particular version of the discourse of Aboriginality. Whatever the narrative decisions and impulses of residents, it was clear that the context and content of therapeutic interventions mattered greatly and that, as I have attempted to show, context and content reflected particular social structural constraints and discursive systems of their historical times.

Notes

1 Medicine House is a pseudonym. The names and initials of residents and staff as well as certain details have also been changed to protect their identities.

2 Throughout this chapter, I use the terms "Aboriginal," "Indian," "indigenous," and "Native" interchangeably. "Aboriginal" is a constitutionally recognized term (Section 35 of the Canadian Constitution) and includes status Indians (persons recognized under the Indian Act), nonstatus Indians, Métis, and Inuit.

3 By "clinical rhetoric," I mean the perspective held by Jerome Frank and Julie Frank (1991), who have argued that all forms of psychotherapeutic healing employ a ritualistic and symbolically rich form of talk therapy to empower the sufferer. Their main contention is that a healer uses rhetoric to resuscitate the morale of the sufferer.

4 Recent case studies of justice issues in localized settings identify the complexity of trying to integrate and operationalize differing legal systems (Miller 2001) and the divergence in expectations among individual community members about the role of indigenous healing practices, justice, and the court system (Denis 1997). As an illustration of the difficulties of such integration, Adam Ashforth (2005) offers a fascinating international case study on the complex relationship between medical pluralism, spiritual insecurity, and attempts to update and reform South Africa's legal system in order to address widespread fears about the apparent harm caused by witches as well as vigilantism and violent retribution against persons accused of practising witchcraft.

5 This chapter is based in part on my MA thesis (Brass 2000). The research protocol was approved by the McGill University Research Ethics Board and by the administration of Medicine House. All participants gave informed consent for my presence at group meetings and recording of their narratives in research interviews.

6 A key argument of my MA thesis (Brass 2000), which I do not address at length here, involves the interpretation of Medicine House as a kind of symbolic socializing space. Specifically, I argue that because of the house's status as a "halfway house" within the correctional system, it was located within a very liminal bureaucratic space. Because of the persistent use of narcotics and other criminalized activities among some residents, administrative and clinical staff members were forced to implement measures to discipline the residents. Consequently, the house seemed to waver between being a therapeutic community and an extension of the correctional system, as evidenced by periodic threats to limit the freedom of residents to leave the grounds of the house. Likewise, some residents saw the house as merely an extension of the system of incarceration and reverted to behaviour that was more appropriate to such an environment. Not surprisingly, this oscillation between healing and punishing within the house was an important dynamic and directly impacted the process of group therapy, the diverse meanings of therapeutic disclosure, and how residents chose to narrate their personal experiences.

7 This is an important methodological and theoretical point since my fieldwork was limited to the residential centre. Understanding the community and home experiences of residents (many of whom were able to return home on weekend visits) would have added depth to the assessment of the impact of Medicine House's therapeutic regime. The one occasion when I did escort a resident (whom I did not interview) to his community for the funeral of a family member was revealing; the experience opened up a number of questions about the potential strengths and limitations of residential therapy and the transitory nature of selfhood, especially one founded upon the narration of experiences (for discussion on the illusion of wholeness, see Ewing 1990; on the fragmentation of self, see Kirby 1991).

8   Although this definition seeks to clarify this point about what is pan-Indianism, it does not address the larger and more interesting questions about how social identity is manufactured and renegotiated within communities. Furthermore, questions about the relationships between contemporary rural and urban Aboriginal populations, especially in terms of patterns of urbanization and the effects of transmigration, require critical inquiry.

9   The Oka Crisis of 1990 was a 78-day standoff that saw militant Mohawk protesters aligned against the Sureté du Quebec (the provincial police force) and the Canadian Army. The dispute originated over the proposed expansion of a municipal golf course into a disputed area known as "the Pines" situated between the Mohawk community of Kanesatake and the town of Oka, Quebec. On 11 July 1990 a Sureté du Quebec tactical team launched an armed assault against the Mohawk protestors. In the ensuing gun battle a police tactical officer was killed. The crisis rapidly escalated when sympathizers in Kahnawake, another Mohawk community on the south shore of Montreal, blocked the Mercier bridge into the city. Eventually, the Canadian Army was called in to relieve civilian police authorities. The "Crisis" ended on 26 September 1990.

10 This flag is associated with the Oka Crisis of 1990. It is a facial profile of an Iroquois warrior within the rays of the sun set on a deep red background. The "Aboriginal Solidarity" flag is its official name, given by its creator, the late Louis Karoniaktajeh Hall, a grassroots Mohawk political activist, artist, and writer who revitalized the militant warrior society in Kahnawake Mohawk Territory, Quebec, from the 1970s through the 1990s. Its more popular name, the "Mohawk Warrior Society" flag, comes from the media. The media associated it with the open show of armed force by Mohawks who belonged to this militant group.

11 The song offers a compelling description of the sense of entrapment caused by drug addiction.

12 "The Prodigal Son" is a parable in the New Testament (Luke 15:11-32) where a man with two sons loses one to a wanton lifestyle. The "black sheep" of the family eventually mends his ways and returns to redeem the honour of his father. Basically, the parable provides the moral instruction that individuals must sometimes hit rock bottom in order to recover and find redemption. The parable has been a source of musical and lyrical inspiration for several genres, including blues, country western, classical, and contemporary rock music. One of the earliest twentieth-century renditions, "That's No Way to Get Along," by blues and folk musician Reverend Robert Wilkins (1896-1987), was later re-recorded by the Rolling Stones in 1967-68; their version was called "Prodigal Son" and can be found on the album *Beggar's Banquet,* released in 1968. The country musician Hank Williams also recorded a song called "The Prodigal Son." A number of more recent popular rock musicians, including Billy Idol, Bruce Springsteen, and Kid Rock, have either referenced the parable in song lyrics or recorded a song with that title. It appears that Neil Young has not recorded a song by that title or referenced the parable in any of his song lyrics. The parable's poetic themes of moral decay, self-destruction, and eventual spiritual redemption have obvious relevance to the suffering caused by drug and alcohol addiction and the process of recovery.

13 It is common for residents to attend self-help groups beyond the house. The staff encourage such activity.

14 Medicine House is nested within a specific historical, political, and social context and attempts to exist as an autonomous "Aboriginal" community within the hegemonic regime of the Canadian state. Through its deployment of generic symbols of pan-Indian identity, then, the microcosmic Aboriginal community of the house projects onto a larger interpretive/imagined community of Aboriginals residing within the national territory of Canada (Anderson 1991).

References

Anderson, B. 1991. *Imagined communities: Reflections on the origin and spread of nationalism*. New York: Verso.

Archer, J. 1991. Ambiguity in political ideology: Aboriginality as nationalism. *The Australian Journal of Anthropology* 2 (2): 161-70.

Ashforth, A. 2005. *Witchcraft, violence, and democracy in South Africa*. Chicago, IL: University of Chicago Press.

Beckett, J. 1988. The past in the present, the present in the past: Constructing a national Aboriginality. In J. Beckett, ed., *Past and present: The construction of Aboriginality,* 191-217. Canberra, AU: Aboriginal Studies Press.

Berkhofer, R.F., Jr. 1979. *The whiteman's Indian: Images of the American Indian from Columbus to the present.* New York: Vintage.

Brady, M. 1995. Culture in treatment, culture as treatment: A Critical appraisal of developments in addictions programs for indigenous North Americans and Australians. *Social Science and Medicine* 41 (11): 1487-98.

Brass, G.M. 2000. Respecting "the medicines": Narrating an Aboriginal identity at Nechi House. MA thesis, McGill University.

Bruner, E.M. 1986. Ethnography as narrative. In V. Turner and E. Bruner, eds., *The anthropology of experience,* 139-55. Chicago, Il.: University of Illinois Press.

Clifford, J. 1988. *The predicament of culture: Twentieth-century ethnography, literature, and art.* Cambridge, MA: Harvard University Press.

Correctional Services of Canada. 2006. *Aboriginal Initiatives Branch facts and figures: Aboriginal offender statistics.* http://www.csc-scc.gc.ca/text/prgrm/correctional/abissues/know/4e.shtml.

Csordas, T.J. 1983. The rhetoric of transformation in ritual healing. *Culture, Medicine and Psychiatry* 7 (4): 333-75.

Denis, C. 1997. *We are not you: First Nations and Canadian modernity.* Peterborough, ON: Broadview Press.

Dorais, L.J. 1999. Aboriginals: Inuit. In P.R. Magocsi, ed., *The encyclopedia of Canada's peoples,* 47-56. Toronto, ON: University of Toronto Press.

Ewing, K.P. 1990. The illusion of wholeness: Culture, self, and the experience of inconsistency. *Ethos* 18 (3): 251-78.

Frank, J., and J. Frank. 1991. *Persuasion and healing: Comparative study of psychotherapy.* 3rd ed. Baltimore, MD: Johns Hopkins University Press.

Garro, L. 2000. Cultural knowledge as resource in illness narratives: Remembering through accounts of illness. In C. Mattingly and L.C. Garro, eds., *Narrative and the cultural construction of illness and healing,* 70-87. Berkeley, CA: University of California Press.

Hollinsworth, D. 1992. Discourses on Aboriginality and the politics of Aboriginality in urban Australia. *Oceania* 63 (2): 137-55.

Kehoe, A.B. 1990. Primal gaia: Primitivists and plastic medicine men. In J.A. Clifton, ed., *The invented Indian: Cultural fictions and government policies,* 193-209. New Brunswick, NJ: Transaction.

Kirby, P. 1991. *Narrative and the self.* Bloomington, IN: Indiana University Press.

Kirmayer, L.J. 2000. Broken narratives: Clinical encounters and the poetics of illness experience. In C. Mattingly and L.C. Garro, eds., *Narrative and cultural construction of illness and healing,* 153-80. Berkeley, CA: University of California Press.

Lattas, A. 1991. Nationalism, aesthetic redemption, and Aboriginality. *The Australian Journal of Anthropology* 2 (3): 307-24.

–. 1993. Essentialism, memory, and resistance: Aboriginality and the politics of authenticity. *Oceania* 63 (3): 240-67.

Lerch, P.B., and S. Bullers. 1996. Powwows as identity markers: Traditional or pan-Indian? *Human Organization* 55 (4): 390-95.

Mattingly, C. 1998. *Healing dramas and clinical plots: The narrative structure of experience.* New York: Cambridge University Press.

McIlwraith, T. 1996. The problem of imported culture: The construction of contemporary Stó:lô identity. *American Indian Culture and Research* 20 (4): 41-70.

Miller, B.G. 2001. *The problem of justice: Tradition and law in the Coast Salish world.* Lincoln, NE: University of Nebraska Press.

Mink, L.O. 1981. Critical response: Every man his or her own annalist. *Critical Inquiry* (Summer): 777-83.

Ricoeur, P. 1984. *Time and narrative*. 3 vols. Trans. K. McLaughlin and D. Pellauer. Chicago, IL: University of Chicago Press.

Ross, R. 1992. *Dancing with a ghost: Exploring Indian reality*. Markham, ON: Octopus.

–. 1996. *Returning to the teachings: Exploring Aboriginal justice*. Toronto, ON: Penguin.

Shafer, R. 1980. Narration in the psychoanalytic dialogue. *Critical Inquiry* 7 (1): 29-54.

Snipp, C.M. 1996. Urban Indians. In F.E. Hoxie, ed., *The encyclopedia of North American Indians*, 653-55. New York: Houghton Mifflin.

Solicitor General Canada, Ministry Secretariat. 1998. *Final report: Task force on Aboriginal Peoples in Federal Corrections*. Ottawa: Supply and Services.

Tanner, A. 1979. *Bringing home animals: Religious ideology and mode of production of the Mistassini Cree hunters*. St. John's, NL: ISER Books.

Waldram, J.B. 1993. Aboriginal spirituality: Symbolic healing in Canadian prisons. *Culture, Medicine, and Psychiatry* 17 (3): 345-62.

–. 1997. *The way of the pipe: Aboriginal spirituality and symbolic healing in Canadian prisons*. Peterborough, ON: Broadview Press.

–. 2004. *Revenge of the Windigo: The construction of the mind and mental health of North American Aboriginal peoples*. Toronto, ON: University of Toronto Press.

White, H. 1980. The value of narrativity in the representation of reality. *Critical Inquiry* 7 (1): 5-28.

17

A Jurisdictional Tapestry and a Patchwork Quilt of Care: Aboriginal Health and Social Services in Montreal

MARY ELLEN MACDONALD

The mainstream image of Aboriginal people in Canada is, at best, one of trappers in remote northern communities equipped with beaver pelts and birch bark canoes and, at worst, one of blighted settlements plagued with misery. However, the reality is that 75% of this country's Aboriginal population are living off-reserve (Valentine 1992), with 50% in urban areas (Graham and Peters 2002). Just as the stereotypes of the Aboriginal population lag behind contemporary reality, so too do the needs of this growing urban population.

The goal of this chapter is three-fold. To begin, I will provide an overview of Montreal's Aboriginal population and the many "communities" contained therein. Second, I will present the jurisdictional reality faced by Aboriginal peoples seeking services in the Montreal area, focusing on the lack of attention to Aboriginal cultural issues in Montreal's current community-health model. Finally, I will discuss client, service-provider, and policymaker perspectives on the potential of an Aboriginal-specific community clinic to overcome jurisdictional barriers and respond to the needs of the local Aboriginal population. My fieldwork suggests not only that jurisdictional conundrums make it unclear who could and should have a mandate to create an Aboriginal-specific organization but further that not all Aboriginal clients are convinced that a centralized service organization would answer their needs.[1]

Montreal's Aboriginal Population

When Jacques Cartier first arrived on the island that was later to be called Montreal, he was the first European in a territory Amerindians had occupied for thousands of years. Postcontact, there was Aboriginal involvement in, as well as resistance to, European colonial development in the region. The territorial and civic organization of the growing city of Montreal mostly excluded and continues to exclude Aboriginal peoples, as will be further elaborated below.[2]

Today, despite this exclusion, thousands of Aboriginal people live in Montreal. Population counts and estimates vary dramatically: figures range from a "few thousand" to 44,645, the former quoted from various informants and the latter from the 1991 Aboriginal Peoples Survey (Statistics Canada 1991). The latter figure is often described as the number of people in the Montreal Census Metropolitan Area (CMA) who are Aboriginal, but in reality it represents those who identified as having "Aboriginal ancestry" on the census, of whom only 15.2% identified as "Aboriginal" (6,786, or 0.2%, in the CMA). In contrast, the First Nations Regional Health Survey report (FNQLHSSC 1999) states that there are 16,398 Aboriginal people in the Greater Montreal region; however, it is not clear from where this figure is drawn or whether Inuit are included in the total. Sorting through the various figures, Lévesque and colleagues (2001) conclude that the Aboriginal population in Montreal is currently between 25,000 and 30,000, mostly drawn from Quebec Aboriginal communities, but with a growing number from other provinces and the United States. Estimates of Inuit in Montreal sit between 700 and 800 (Lowi 2001; George 2000; Kishigami 1999; Mesher 2000; Statistics Canada 1991).

Although other Canadian cities have large Aboriginal populations (e.g., Winnipeg, Regina, Saskatoon, Toronto, Vancouver),[3] Montreal's Aboriginal community has a local flavour that sets it apart from other urban Aboriginal communities in Canada. A political sovereignist movement has influenced public policy in Quebec, affecting the degree of inclusion of non-Québécois cultural communities in provincial affairs.[4] Further, unlike some other Canadian cities (e.g., Vancouver and Winnipeg), Montreal has no part of town identified as an Aboriginal "ghetto"; throughout Montreal, a diversity of nations make up many Aboriginal "communities" within the larger population. For example, Montreal has an active Inuit population, something Toronto and Vancouver do not. There are two Mohawk communities (Kahnawake, Kanehsatake) and one Abenaki community (Odanak) close to the city boundaries, which can mean easier back and forth integration for some Mohawks and Abenakis and a partial option for individuals from other nations who cannot find acceptance or Aboriginal-sensitive services in the urban core. The community is enormously varied: the population is made up of members who have lived all their lives in the city as well as many who have migrated to the city from rural reserves throughout the province, country, and continent. There is no unifying service organization, no governing structure, no coherent whole or hub of the community. Although some might argue that the Native Friendship Centre of Montreal is, or at least has been at various points, the symbolic core, many self-described "community members" would dispute that claim.[5] Finally, Montreal is bilingual, providing a destination for both English- and French-speaking Aboriginal people.

There are a number of cultural and social-service organizations in Montreal attending to the heterogeneous profile and needs of the population. There are nation-specific services provided through provincial-Aboriginal agreements (e.g., the James Bay and Northern Quebec Agreement, 1975) that contribute to a "haves vs. have-nots" dynamic. These services are available only to those communities that fall within these agreements (mostly the Inuit, Cree, and Naskapi) and only for community members in good standing; members who have moved away from the northern communities and lost their active-residency claim cannot access these services. Other Aboriginal groups, such as the Mi'kmaq or

MARY ELLEN MACDONALD

Malecite, have no nation-specific assistance in the urban environment. There are "nation-blind" services in Montreal (e.g., the Native Friendship Centre, the Native Women's Shelter), but not all of these are "status-blind" as well; some, such as Health Canada's Non-Insured Health Benefits, are open only to status Indians. There are also service organizations outside the city's borders, such as Waseskun Healing Centre, a halfway house for Aboriginal offenders, and the Onen'to:Kon Treatment Centre near Kanehsatake.

Although far from comprehensive, there is a growing body of literature and policy work on the situation of urban Aboriginal peoples in Canada. In Quebec there are a number of reports that begin to paint an image of the situation of Aboriginal "communities" in the province, many of which provide comparison of the on-reserve to the off-reserve populations.[6] Little information, however, specifically addresses the urban situation or focuses on Montreal. Most of the documents that do exist on Montreal are "issue-based," providing only one facet of Aboriginal reality in Montreal.[7] There is no health or mental health assessment of the overall Aboriginal population of Montreal, nor is there a synthesis of existing reports and articles characterizing the community, its diversity, and its multiple needs. Further, there is no report that provides a comprehensive ethnographic image of the community or that looks at the success stories of healthy, well-adjusted community members.

Although the available literature falls short of providing a comprehensive overview of the urban Aboriginal situation, these reports do begin to describe general characteristics of the Montreal population. The main themes that emerge include the great heterogeneity of cultures and languages in the urban population; the cultural-identity issues that arise for members when they move off-reserve and interact with other Aboriginal and non-Aboriginal peoples; the marginality, discrimination, and poverty many Aboriginal people experience in the city; and the need for more Aboriginal-specific health and social services in the urban area, for substance-abuse treatment, and for HIV/AIDS prevention, especially for women.

Jurisdiction and Health Coverage

Notwithstanding the growing list of studies and reports, the urban Aboriginal remains "an endangered species," as an Aboriginal policy analyst put it to me, referring to the high morbidity and mortality rates in certain Aboriginal subpopulations. The Montreal Aboriginal community sits so precariously in the clash of jurisdictional and policy domains that, despite the hard work and best intentions of front-line workers and researchers, it will not become a priority of governing structures any time soon. Although there is a tapestry of jurisdictional domains that govern health-service delivery in Montreal and across the province, Aboriginal people have no clear place in this tightly woven scheme. As a result of the jurisdictional conflicts and ambiguities that beset Aboriginal peoples in Montreal, the search for adequate health care can be compared to piecing together a patchwork quilt. There is no central facility or formalized network to assist the Aboriginal person navigating the jurisdictional maze. There is no national, provincial, or local mental health policy for the urban Aboriginal person that can link the distressed client with culturally appropriate support. Finding publicly funded mental health counselling that goes beyond a conventional biomedical or psychiatric model and that acknowledges or integrates cultural or traditional approaches is a challenge for even the least distressed.

According to Quebec's Secrétariat aux affaires autochtones (SAA 1998, 11), "the growing determination of Aboriginal people to develop their identity is now an essential feature of relations with Québec." Further, it is claimed that the "Québec government intends to meet the challenges of improving relations between Aboriginal people and Quebecers as a whole, reaching development agreements, improving self-government and financial self-sufficiency of Aboriginal communities, as well as their social and economic conditions" (SAA 2001, 5). In this spirit, throughout Quebec the devolution of health and social services from governmental authorities to local First Nations and Inuit control has been steadily increasing under both the federal government (via the Health Transfer Policy, 1986) and the provincial government (via the James Bay and Northern Quebec Agreement, 1975). Services in many First Nations and Inuit communities are partially, if not entirely, locally conceived and run.

Outside Aboriginal "community" or "reserve" jurisdictions, the situation is quite different. Two recent promotional documents on Aboriginal communities in Quebec, one by the provincial government (SAA 2001) and the other by the federal government (Indian and Northern Affairs 1999) demonstrate the absence of the urban Aboriginal population from public policy: neither document includes the Montreal population in descriptions of Aboriginal communities in Quebec. A third document (SAA 1998) refers to the estimated size of the off-reserve population in the province but does not detail the Montreal community.

Interestingly, even Aboriginal groups in rural areas tend to treat "urban Natives" as invisible, owing in part to the politics of jurisdiction. Although over half of the Aboriginal population may live off-reserve, money and resources are still targeted for reserve communities, and allotments are often guarded by the on-reserve population. It is in the reserves' economic interest to keep members registered as living on the reserves so that transfer payments are maximized. For example, Health Canada will assist with the provision of health services for Aboriginal peoples within Canadian reserve jurisdictions. This assistance will follow a band member who is referred for specialist services off-reserve; it does not follow a band member who purposely moves outside this jurisdiction. Once becoming an off-reserve, or urban, Native, the individual comes under provincial and municipal jurisdiction. As one report puts it, the individual's "rights are not mobile" across jurisdictions (Quebec Native Women 2001, 42).

In some Canadian provinces, there are provincial mandates to address certain Aboriginal issues when they fall outside federal jurisdiction.[8] Further, in some Canadian cities

MARY ELLEN MACDONALD

(e.g., Winnipeg and Vancouver) the Aboriginal population is too large and visible for provincial or municipal governments to ignore. These scenarios do not apply to Montreal. Instead, the urban Aboriginal person is grouped with the mainstream culture in both provincial and municipal policy when in Montreal.[9] Although not dissimilar to scenarios in many other Canadian urban centres, the situation is further complicated in Quebec, where the francophone-anglophone linguistic and cultural tensions have been a major concern both vis-à-vis the federal government and in local politics, diverting attention from other minority issues. Quebec's concern for its own minority status in Canada casts a shadow over many local minority issues, which can create an uncomfortable place for First Nations politics. The sovereignist agenda has influenced public policy in the province throughout the past few decades. Although there are some success stories in rural communities (e.g., the James Bay and Northern Quebec Agreement), urban Aboriginal issues remain mostly invisible in the eyes of the province. Even in city politics, urban Aboriginal people are virtually nonexistent except for the mostly marginal individuals who experience problems of homelessness or present a public health concern.

Despite health-transfer agreements that shift control of services to rural Aboriginal communities and despite calls by policy analysts such as Pelletier and Laurin (1993, 41) who contend that health services in Quebec must become "more Native" and "be taken over by communities," there is no officially recognized Aboriginal "community" or band council in Montreal to which health services could be devolved. Although some people may feel that they are part of an "Aboriginal community" in Montreal, health coverage is determined primarily by the provincial government and organized by geographic sector. Although Montreal has a large Aboriginal population, it is not officially recognized as a "community," nor are there health services mandated to treat this population as Aboriginal.

Aboriginal "Community" and "Community" Health Care

The model for community health care currently in place in Quebec combines social services with health services. Quebec was the first Canadian province to create such an integrated community-service network. As political scientist Antonia Maioni contends, "the Quebec health care system is seen by many as a distinctive example of the positive role of the state in social affairs" (2001, 2). The province-wide system of community clinics, Centres locaux de service communautaire (CLSCs), provides a mix of health and social services, integrating hospitals, rehabilitation, convalescent centres, and social-service agencies in autonomous units mandated by law and ultimately co-ordinated by the provincial Ministère de la santé et des services sociaux (MSSS).[10]

The CLSC model is premised on an understanding of community that is defined by geography: one's right to attend a given clinic is based on one's postal code, which marks off urban neighbourhoods and rural regions. CLSC clinics are found throughout the province and are designed for a generic population. They are geographically accessible to all but the very remote, and they follow a liberal ethic of equality: all citizens, regardless of income or culture, who hold a valid Quebec Medicare card are welcomed at the CLSC in their region. The only services available in the CLSC that go beyond mainstream culture are linguistic-interpreter services, which are provided by regional health authorities. All CLSCs are conceived under this model, but in reality the different clinics make up a diversified set of bodies, some clinics remaining much closer to an ideal of community participation than do others. For example, some CLSCs in immigrant areas take the ethnic mix of the clientele into consideration; this may include a multilingual welcome sign on the door as well as some attention to linguistic needs and to diverse psychosocial realities. Alternative medicines or traditional healers, however, are not provided.[11]

The place for Aboriginal peoples in the CLSC community model is problematic. In leaving their communities and coming to Montreal, First Nations people enter a jurisdiction that is provincially controlled and designed. In Montreal, Aboriginal peoples are included in the provincial jurisdiction and agenda if and when they fit into the mainstream models; urban Aboriginal peoples *as Aboriginal peoples* have no distinct niche in the CLSC generally and little place in the overall Montreal health care system specifically.

Culture and community are seemingly simple concepts often used uncritically to gloss groups of people "contained" by various kinds of borders (Jewkes and Murcott 1996). Anthropology tells us, however, that neither culture nor community can be read as fixed entities but are processes given meaning and significance by the people who live them as realities (Cohen 1985). What is crucial to analysis therefore is the interpretation of the experiential aspects of everyday life. Communities are the assemblages of their members, held together by common elements that demarcate them from other groups. Communities, therefore, must be understood in relation to what stands outside the boundaries. As Cohen puts it: "Community is the entity to which one belongs, greater than kinship but more immediate than the abstraction we call 'society'" (1985, 14). A community is where one equips oneself with the knowledge needed to be social, where one acquires "culture." Awareness of a boundary is integral to having a community, and boundaries can take various forms – physical, legal, racial, linguistic – or they may exist solely in the "minds of their beholders" and thus may carry quite different meanings for people who think they belong to the same group. Community exists as symbols, as something for people "to think with," but the sharing of the symbols with other community members does not necessarily mean the sharing of all the personal meaning associated with those symbols.

This discussion of community has implications for understanding how identity and community are conceived and lived in the urban Aboriginal population in Montreal. Being Inuit in a small village in Nunavik will necessarily differ from being Inuit when navigating the urban health care system in Montreal. There are many different ways to be Aboriginal within Montreal: the expression of cultural identity may differ when at an Inuit Association gathering, compared to when working in a bank, using a local health clinic, or shopping in a unilingual French store. Cultural identity and community configurations shift as contexts shift, responding to changing reference points.

The Aboriginal community in Montreal is not a homogenous and fixed locale with clearly demarcated boundaries, either symbolic or physical. Instead, it is a dispersed, multicultural network that is spread across the Island of Montreal and that extends across the province, the country, and even the continent – a network of individuals, many of whom view themselves as a multicultural combination of Aboriginal as well as non-Aboriginal ancestries. Members of this community are often mobile, moving in and out of the city, back and forth between rural and urban communities. This movement constantly extends and reconfigures community boundaries around subunits; there is no real core but instead a number of shifting subpopulations.

Although dispersed and "invisible" without an identified hub, Aboriginal people in Montreal are not simply a "category" defined by their Aboriginal ancestry and urban address. There is a community, symbolic as it may be, with many bases of unity crosscutting the larger population. These lines of segmentation are defined by many categories, including geographical location and culture (e.g., the Inuit vs. Inuit from Nunavik vs. Inuit from Kuujjuaq, Nunavik); "the north" (e.g., Cree, Inuit) and "the south" (e.g., Mohawk, Abenaki); language (French, English, and/or Aboriginal languages); employment, poverty, and/or homelessness; and time spent in prison and/or at a residential treatment centre. Further, there are divisions internal to all categories based on such things as gender, education, class, government-defined status, religion, hangout spots, healing journeys, and sobriety. Members simultaneously belong to various segments of the larger community and seek out or claim access depending on social circumstances and need. Identity in and among these groups is formed and played out in many ways on many levels.

Aboriginal People and Montreal CLSCs

How appropriate the CLSC model is for cultural communities in the province is open to debate. My fieldwork discovered that many Aboriginal people did not find themselves included in this model and avoided the CLSC for a variety of reasons. One problem with the model is the way it geographically defines community. According to self-proclaimed community members, there is a vibrant Aboriginal community in Montreal, but it is not a geographically consolidated community. The generic definitions of community and identity that are taken for granted in the provincial health system and that underwrite the approach (and lack thereof) to culture and identity in the CLSC clash with the complex lived reality of culture and identity of some cultural communities. The end result is the creation of barriers to service delivery.

Although there is a CLSC near a downtown drop-in centre frequented by Inuit women, Inuit clients rarely use the CLSC. Most do not live in the region but simply spend their days there, so even though it may be part of their "cultural community," it is not their "postal code community," which defines access to care. Services are not available in Aboriginal languages at the CLSCs, and as a Cree social worker told me, clients avoid the CLSC because they feel that "there's nobody there that can help them, you know, especially if their English is not that good and they can't express themselves in Cree." A general practitioner at a downtown CLSC who had worked many years in a northern community tried to set up an Aboriginal practice: "I really wanted to develop a Native clientele for myself at the CLSC because I have an interest in it and I think I have some experience in it that could be useful. But I've been a bit discouraged in seeing how it would not be possible within our CLSC now. And I think in the last few years it has gone downhill."

Like any service organization, the CLSC has limits in terms of its mandate and resources. Some services (e.g., public health nursing and psychosocial services) may have leeway to be culturally responsive, but medical services do not cover alternative approaches to medicine and health, Aboriginal or otherwise. Looking for adequate and responsive care can be stressful for any client, compounding the levels of anxiety and distress they may already be experiencing. In a system facing structural and capacity limits, developing additional specific services or finely tuned responses to cultural diversity, Aboriginal or otherwise, appears to be an unattainable luxury.

If clients do not go to the CLSC, where do they go? When I asked where in Montreal he would send an Aboriginal client, a psychiatrist who works both in northern Quebec and in Montreal said: "Nothing would pop into my head. There is no resource in Montreal ... In terms of long-term psychiatric issues, there's nothing. I think communities up north would do everything possible to keep the person there rather than sending them down, no matter how sick they are ... They know that if they send them down here, they're going to get really crappy care in psychiatry."[12]

Many service providers responded to this question by saying that they might call local Cree or Inuit patient services or the Native Friendship Centre. Yet the Cree and Inuit services include only liaison assistance (e.g., interpreters and transportation) and accommodation. These organizations do not run medical services themselves, nor are their services available for non-Inuit/Cree or for those Inuit/Cree who no longer claim residency in the northern communities. Similarly, the Friendship Centre has no medical services beyond addictions counselling and some referral suggestions.

The lack of appropriate services for Aboriginal people in Montreal is underscored by the experiences of one client from a rural reserve many hours from Montreal who was in need of comprehensive care for a number of physical and mental ailments. After being in many different kinds of health services in the city, the closest fit he found was in a refugee clinic run at an inner-city CLSC. This specialized clinic has an "open-door" mandate, which overrides the policy of postal code sectorization. The clinicians at the clinic are trained to address issues of cultural dislocation, distress, and trauma. A clinic worker told me that even though this client was not a refugee, he could not find adequate, culturally sensitive services in Montreal and therefore fit their mandate exactly. Ironically, as an Aboriginal client unable to find satisfactory services either in Montreal or in his home community, this person was like a refugee in his own land.

An Aboriginal Community Clinic

A First Nations Regional Health Survey (FNQLHSSC 1999, 76) found that only 42% of the First Nations population in Montreal felt they received the same quality of services as Canadians. Zambrowsky (1986) reports that many women, despite having lived in Montreal for up to 10 years, are unable to make use of the social, educational, or legal services available to them. Another report by Quebec Native Women (2001) states that Aboriginal women in Quebec experience a lack of information about services and that their information needs are higher in urban areas. Pelletier and Laurin (1993) argue that current approaches to mental health services in Quebec are fragmented and that in place of the specialized psychological or psychiatric care and crisis intervention, a broader "global" approach to mental health intervention is needed, one that integrates such elements as self-government and economic development.

At the level of service delivery, one practical means to address the barriers and accessibility issues experienced by Aboriginal clients and to guard against fragmentation of services is to develop a centralized health and social-service clinic. The idea of a "one-stop shop" that is nation-blind and status-blind yet exclusive to the Aboriginal population is not new to Montreal; it has been discussed for years within Aboriginal organizations. Yet for many reasons, such a clinic remains only an idea despite similar models in other Canadian cities. Many different levels of bureaucracy exist for Aboriginal citizens in the urban environment, sometimes overlapping and sometimes failing to converge, leaving clients in the confusion and gaps that result from poor institutional co-ordination. The answer to the question of why there is not such a clinic already in Montreal is found partly at the level of jurisdiction and politics: who could and should design or sponsor such a clinic remains unclear. There has never been enough sustained pressure on any government body to sort this out and spearhead such a clinic.

Further, my fieldwork data suggest that not all Aboriginal clients assume that a centralized service organization would be the answer to their needs. Not only do jurisdictional conundrums make it unclear who should have the mandate to create an Aboriginal-specific organization, but neither the desire for the service nor the design of the structure is self-evident.

I received three different types of response from informants when I asked about such a clinic. The first was from policymakers and service providers who felt that services were inadequate for the majority of Canadians and therefore that any effort should first be directed at improving services generally and generically, *not* specifically at an Aboriginal clientele. A second response came from policymakers and service providers who were pessimistic about the relevance and/or possibility of this sort of clinic, their pessimism being rooted in their knowledge of governmental priorities and budgetary concerns. The aide of a Liberal member of Parliament insisted that such a culture-specific service would represent not the recognition of cultural need but a form of segregation and discrimination. Although he supported the federal multiculturalism policy, "health," he said, "is not a cultural matter." Similarly, a Health Canada administrator referred to culture as a "Pandora's box" of trouble that the government should avoid when it comes to the matter of health. The government should continue to support mainstream health services and let Aboriginal communities sort through their "cultural issues" on their own. Service providers expressed the need for culturally specific services to alleviate their frustration in trying to place Aboriginal clients in local mismatched services, but most were cautious about the potential fundability; the economic bottom line was always a deciding factor.

In contrast to these responses from professionals, the answers I received from clients were unexpected. Most clients were suspicious of and ambivalent toward Aboriginal-run services. At first, I found this strange; I had assumed that culturally specific services would be a boon for the community. I soon realized, however, that many of these clients had come to Montreal after negative experiences with services in home communities and were worried that such a model would lead to increased segregation and discrimination. It was not so much that these clients did not want a culturally sensitive health and social-service environment; it was that they did not trust that their ideals could be reached in the current social, political, and economic climate. Interestingly, no clients brought up the centralized model on their own, despite my attempts to sound out clients for potential solutions. Most seemed to find it a novel but unlikely idea when I raised it, and many claimed they had never heard of the equivalents in other cities, such as the Wabano Centre for Aboriginal Health in nearby Ottawa and the well-established Anishnaabe Health Centre in Toronto.

Contrary to service providers pointing out problems with the community-health model in Montreal, many clients were less negative about local services, telling me that mental health services in Montreal were generally adequate for their needs. Services were considered adequate, especially by those clients who were deliberately *not* seeking Aboriginal-specific services. These clients were suspicious of the culture-specific model based on their experiences in their own communities. Some were concerned that if a segregated clinic was built in Montreal, the right to go to other clinics might be removed, something clearly not acceptable. Some believed that services that were Aboriginal-run were substandard and that Aboriginal professionals were not as well-trained or as professional as non-Aboriginal providers. One woman who had negative experiences in a treatment service in her own community felt she cured her alcoholism *despite* the addictions services and said: "God forbid it's run all by Native people!" She had nothing but negative things to say about Aboriginal organizations, especially around issues of professionalism. Another client balked at the idea: "To me that sound like 'Let's have the black people sit only in the back and the white people sit only in the front!'"

Some clients said that although they were not interested in Aboriginal-specific organizations, they could understand why some Aboriginal clients would find it useful. For example, "urban Indians" who, as one client said, "get disconnected or disjointed from not being around other Natives" might find it useful. Similarly, another mentioned that having Inuktituk service providers or translators available would be helpful for rural Inuit.

So on the surface, although some clients had general concerns for the well-being of the population (e.g., "urban Indians" and those who speak Inuktituk), most did not complain about a lack of services for their personal problems. I was surprised by these responses after having heard the opposite both from service providers and in political rhetoric. The former national chief, Matthew Coon Come, speaking at a national conference on Aboriginal health,[13] had stated: "I have not even tried to address the issue of mental health and social services for First Nations, because these services are so rare as to be virtually unavailable when they are needed." Although this remark reflects the situation in many remote communities, it remained unclear whether the existing services in Montreal are really adequate for client needs. I wondered whether these clients simply have low expectations, having learned to get by in a system that has neglected them.

As I pushed further with my questioning, I uncovered another layer of opinion: many clients agreed that "in the best possible world," having an Aboriginal health and social-service centre would be a worthwhile addition for the community. "In this world," however, most were jaded and cynical on pragmatic grounds: How would it look? Who would run it? Which First Nation would be in charge? Who would be hired? What level of professionalism would be guaranteed? These sorts of questions called attention to the fragmentation of the urban community as well as to the problems in local and rural communities that have weakened the capacity of some professionals to provide true healing. Once on the topic, many clients used the clinic model as an opportunity to detail their dissatisfaction with the current system, both in Montreal and in Aboriginal communities, offering lengthy criticism, analysis, and creative ideas for improvement. Many agreed that, if it was established, they would attend such a clinic at least once, mainly out of curiosity. They also agreed that it would be useful for rural or elderly clients, those less resourceful and resilient and less apt to ask for help.

Many of the themes that emerged in my conversations with informants matched those in literature on the needs of people in the Aboriginal population and the barriers to their care (e.g., FNQLHSSC 1999; Gill et al. 1995; Lévesque et al. 2001; Quebec Native Women 2001; Petawabano et al. 1994). The following section pools ideas from interviews as well as policy documents, mapping out the "best possible world" scenario for building an Aboriginal health and social-service centre in Montreal or for improving existing services so that they are more responsive to the diversity of the Aboriginal community.

A Heterogeneous Community

An Aboriginal clinic designed for Montreal must attend to the heterogeneity in the population. There are unifying symbols ("the city") and concepts ("urban Aboriginality") that may link the Aboriginal population in Montreal, and according to Gill and colleagues: "Whether they have always lived in cities or whether they have just moved there, Aboriginal people demonstrate a will to protect and pass on their cultural identity" (1995, iii). That said, the great diversity found within the population should not be homogenized or essentialized. The heterogeneity of the population divides along individual preferences but also along group demarcations such as nation, urbanization, age, gender, education, sexuality, healing philosophy, spiritualism/religion, and class. The usefulness of any clinic would be determined more by its ability to respond to individual client identity and need than by trying to create a "one size fits all" model designed around a generic pan-Indian notion of identity or around individual health issues (e.g., HIV/AIDS, addictions).

Philosophy of Care

The clinic should be organized to meet the evolving understanding of health and wellness present in Aboriginal literature (Mental Health Working Group 2001). Approaches to health must be inclusive of a "wellness" philosophy, or "whole person care," which includes physical, mental, emotional, and spiritual health. The biomedical model that separates the mind from the body is efficacious yet limited for those who understand health as embodied in individuals and their social worlds. Although the "medicine wheel" model is supported by some community members, there are clients for whom it does not resonate. Health services that address wellness by incorporating influences such as traditional healers and Elders should be supported alongside mainstream biomedical services.

To be culturally aware, culture must not be essentialized using a rigid reading of community and tradition or a pan-Indian version of identity, nor should culture be seen simply as a marker of identity to be gathered with intake statistics. Instead, culture should be read as an emergent process that is continually invented, transformed, and recreated. Culture is embodied at both individual and community levels; clients should be approached with an openness that can tailor care to the individual client's "perspective on reality" with an awareness that individuals may negotiate between social and cultural communities and modes of belonging throughout the course of their quests for help.

Accessibility

Given the widely dispersed nature of the community, an open-door policy overriding postal code sectorization is essential. Clients should not be included or excluded based on a geographic mapping of their communities. Further, this organization should be status-blind, the identity of clients self-declared and not tied to blood quantum.[14] In addition, this organization should be sensitive to the fact that marginalized clients may have lower expectations for service delivery.

Newcomers to the city often do not know where to begin to find services. A "survival handbook" was suggested in order to help newcomers with integration. Further, advertising the clinic on Aboriginal television and in community newspapers and ensuring that

MARY ELLEN MACDONALD

front-line workers across the city were aware of such a service would increase the inclusion of the population.

Considering the meanings of space and place can provide an understanding of how a clinic could be designed to foster inclusion. The accessibility of any clinic is in part determined by its physical construction (e.g., location near a métro/subway station, disability accessible). Accessibility is also determined by a client's sense of welcome and comfort. Comfort will be experienced as a relationship between the spatial region and client identity, with identity extending beyond the corporeal self into the "space" the client chooses to take up. The clinic could become a "negative space" for some clients if it constrained their sense of self or demanded certain behaviours or profiles. The exclusion of persons based on symbolic or fixed boundaries set up around such markers as nation, status, class, sexuality, gender, or urbanization would ultimately limit the accessibility of a clinic.

Clients recounted how a particular aesthetic can increase the accessibility of a service. Having to take an elevator to the reception desk of a local CLSC acts as a barrier for some, as do the windows that jeopardize anonymity. Positive suggestions included comfortable chairs, space to hang around and "play cards," a "brown" (Aboriginal) face at the reception, and representation of the major Aboriginal languages. Further, a "family-like" style was encouraged, "where you could just sit down and relate to whoever is there or whoever you want to talk to or need to talk to."

Some clients disagreed with the model of a centralized clinic because of the stigma associated with seeking help. Instead, they felt that services should be dispersed throughout the city, attached to existing community organizations, with the service providers shifting locations instead of the clients. Others argued that many existing community organizations were already inaccessible given administrative politics; the politics that complicate the workings of many community organizations are equally present in Aboriginal organizations, along with issues that can accompany ethnic diversity. Thus many clients were concerned about the idea of linking services to existing organizations and were cynical about the politics that would develop in a new clinic. Perhaps ensuring a multicultural service staff without overrepresentation of any nation and with inclusion of as many ethnicities as possible would help to address some of this concern. Given the limited pool of trained staff to draw from in the city, however, this is an ideal rather than a practical solution. At least having some awareness of these issues is an important step.

Whereas the location was a concern when it meant a fixed affiliation with an existing organization, the actual geographic location of a clinic was not an issue for most clients. Although convenience of location is an aspect of the CLSC model, Aboriginal clients already travel all over the island, and also off the island to local First Nations communities, to get services. Clients often travel outside the city to see Elders and traditionalists, to take part in ceremonies, or to use Aboriginal-run services, relying on friends and family to help with travel arrangements. One client was continually travelling from the New Brunswick border, 8 hours away, to get services in Montreal. Having to cross town for an Aboriginal-specific clinic in order to ensure continuity of care was not an issue for most.[15] Of course, basing a clinic near a métro station is useful; basing it near other Aboriginal organizations is not necessarily a good thing given the lack of confidentiality that may result.

Unmet Needs

A number of the health and social-service needs of the urban Aboriginal population are currently being addressed by local organizations. The Association of Montreal Inuit, founded in 2000, has great potential to provide a meaningful community organization for urban Inuit, attracting community members (and Cree) to social, cultural, and sporting events, including monthly feasts with northern foods. Similarly, the Native Women's Shelter is often full. The Native Friendship Centre services 600 clients each month, has an urban-referral worker, a hospital-liaison worker, an HIV/AIDS portfolio, a diabetes program, and a tuberculosis-awareness initiative. The McGill Aboriginal Healing Clinic was developed to address sexual-abuse issues related to residential schools. Lévesque and colleagues write that 80% of employment-training programs and jobs held by the Aboriginal women in their Montreal sample were within Aboriginal organizations, a point they argue is a sign of "the emergence of an Aboriginal job market in the heart of Montreal" (2001, x-xi).

Although numerous services are available in Montreal, the list of unmet needs for the urban Aboriginal population remains extensive. Despite much praise from providers and users of the services, few would argue that these services could not be improved with more staffing, expertise, and resources. That the Native Women's Shelter often must turn away clients, that there is no equivalent for Aboriginal men, and that there are no Native shelters for clients – male or female – who are abusing substances suggest that an extension of Native services may be needed. Further, some Métis and adoptee clients feel that some services exclude clients who are not "Aboriginal enough." Clients also expressed frustration at the lack of accessible community spaces open in the evenings and on weekends.

Health and social problems continue *despite* already-existing services in the city. Many informants spoke about the lack of support for spirituality. One proposal for a centralized clinic suggested building an urban sweat lodge and establishing an Aboriginal Women's Elders Council. Three province-wide reports (Gill et al. 1995; Lévesque et al. 2001; Quebec Native Women 2001) have outlined the needs specific to Aboriginal women in urban centres, arguing that there are not enough appropriate services to attend to their realities. Many women leave rural communities in search of employment and education, and many are also escaping from violence and abuse (LaRocque 1993). Lévesque and colleagues write: "In most cases, their life in the city is characterized by isolation and a glaring lack of a broad range of resources" (2001, 2). Although the Native Women's Shelter is an essential resource, its space and mandate are limited. Women who are not actually "homeless" have needs that the shelter cannot address without the additional support of healthy individual, social, and community support networks.

MARY ELLEN MACDONALD

There also needs to be more research into the reality of Aboriginal people in the city. A clearinghouse or resource library of documents about the community would be a boon. While rumours circulate about reports, documents, or theses, finding these documents is not straightforward.

Professionalism

The professionalism required to run a health and social-service clinic is a major concern. There are clients who already believe that the quality of any Aboriginal-run service will necessarily be lower simply because it is Aboriginal. That Health Canada will fund only generic drugs for Aboriginal clients made one client suspicious following the same logic: if it is for Aboriginal clients, it must be second-rate. This client paid from his own pocket for brand-name equivalents. Confidentiality is also a problem: as one client said, "the question of confidentiality is four times as large because in the urban settings, we are the minority. There are so few of us that everybody knows everybody." Two clients with whom I spoke chose to travel off-reserve to go to more urbanized clinics for therapy because they believed their story would get "gossiped" past the boundaries of their local clinic. Gill and colleagues (1995) report that Aboriginal women experiencing family violence often have "no choice" but to leave their reserve to find "more confidential" assistance outside. Another issue is respect: a report by Quebec Native Women argues that Aboriginal women "are concerned by the lack of respect towards them once they present their status card in order to get pharmaceutical goods" (2001, 45). This phenomenon recurred in the testimony of one client who recounted a time she felt her pharmacist overstressed that she was not to drink alcohol with her medication.

Staffing and Ethnic Match

Staffing an Aboriginal clinic with Aboriginal professionals seemed obvious at first. Of course, a major problem in achieving an "ethnic match" between service providers and users is finding enough Aboriginal people to train as staff.[16] A Cree social worker said that she thought Inuit clients would be happier with Aboriginal nurses, especially if they spoke Inuktituk, but admitted: "I don't think any nurse from up north would want to come [to Montreal]." Even those Inuit nurses who do professional placements in Montreal generally choose to return to the North. Local training sites for Aboriginal social workers focus on training students to work in the North; they do not prioritize placement in urban organizations.

The notion of ethnic matching gives way when informant opinions are considered more closely. Quite simply, most clients prioritize skill over ethnicity and want someone who is well-trained, sometimes in traditional but also often in biomedical models, regardless of ethnicity. Most clients have heard stories of charlatan healers and insist that their practitioner must have skill and a solid reputation. More clients were adamant that the receptionist in a clinic be Aboriginal than the service providers. "Well-trained" includes being sensitive to cultural issues for which generic "Aboriginality" or pan-Indianism were not adequate models. Most clients also felt that both the choice of ethnic match as well as the form of healing (biomedical or traditional) should be up to the client, not a clinic policy.

Of course, some clients do prefer Aboriginal service providers and models. For some, this is an issue of language. Although for clients with French or English proficiency language is less of a concern, it can still be key, especially for issues related to mental health. One client, speaking at a health conference, made this point: "I cannot cry in English or French; I can only cry in my Native language." Further, a social worker told me that there are some communities in particular with families who, when they come to Montreal, do not want anything to do with non-Aboriginal workers. For many, however, the key question is not "Is the service provider Aboriginal?" but "Are they local?" These clients believe confidentiality will be better guaranteed if the provider is not from their own Aboriginal community.[17] This can be especially true for issues of childhood sexual abuse.

A More Practical Model?

An Aboriginal clinic in Montreal would answer the needs of some clients; however, it could never attend to the health and social-service needs of the entire population. Further, regardless of its strengths, such a clinic could never solve the problems clients confront when they leave Montreal and return home to rural communities. Such a clinic would perhaps be more successful if it was designed for the most vulnerable, such as migrants, new residents, the disabled, and the disenfranchised. Inclusion could focus on those who do not (for whatever reasons) already access specialized services, who are not comfortable in English or French, who are intimidated by the urban health care environment, and who prefer health services to also meet their cultural needs. Those who are well enough established to already have satisfying relationships with a CLSC and/or private practitioners or who are jaded by Aboriginal services should not be the target population. The clinic could also function as a consultation and training resource for mainstream services seeking to improve their delivery of care to Aboriginal clients (Kirmayer et al. 2003). Such a clinic could never be a panacea; however, although issues such as urban political representation or larger concerns such as self-government may not be best addressed from this sort of structure, the existence of such a clinic could add to the sense of community already present in Montreal and thereby help to increase capacity to tackle these other issues.

Conclusion

The Aboriginal population in Montreal is not simply a "category" defined by Aboriginal ancestry and urban address. Despite being dispersed and often invisible, there is a vibrant Aboriginal community in Montreal. Although there is a large community, there are no health services in Montreal designed to service this population as "Aboriginal." The answer to why this is the case is far from straightforward, requiring an in-depth understanding of the jurisdictional, bureaucratic, economic, and cultural context of Aboriginal reality in Montreal. This reality is shaped by systemic injustice at many different levels of governance – community, municipal, provincial, and federal. Jurisdictional conundrums make it unclear who could and should have a mandate to create an Aboriginal-specific organization.

Further, neither the desire for such a service nor the design of the structure is self-evident. Enthusiasm and support for an Aboriginal community clinic was not forthcoming from the participants in my fieldwork. The cynicism that policymakers and service providers voiced about the feasibility of such a clinic and the suspicion that clients felt toward Aboriginal-specific services both on- and off-reserve are indicative of problems endemic to the Canadian health care system generally. Although "in the best possible world" clients might prefer to have their health and social-service needs addressed in an environment that acknowledges them as deserving respect, compassion, and cultural sensitivity, "in this world" they are faced with practices rooted in a colonial history that precedes the development of the Canadian health system. That informants were generally pessimistic about the potential for such a clinic is not surprising when viewed in this historical context.

The Aboriginal community in Montreal is not easily confined, defined, or located; this reality helps to explain why it has been little researched to date. Without more research, the needs and realities of community members will continue to be little known to health care planners in the city. As this chapter has shown, the definitions of culture and identity that underwrite the approach to community in the current health system do not correspond with the complex lived reality of members of the Aboriginal community. The end result is barriers to service delivery and service accessibility. Further research on the urban experience of Aboriginal people is needed to address client marginalization and the barriers to care.

Notes

1 This chapter is drawn from an ethnographic project conducted between 1999 and 2002 designed to understand Aboriginal experiences of mental health services and policies in Montreal. This project involved participant observation with Aboriginal and non-Aboriginal policymakers, analysts, service providers, and health care clients in many local, provincial, and national locations. For more information on the methodology and scope of the project, see Macdonald (2003).

2 For a history of Aboriginal presence pre- and postcontact, see Alfred (1994), Chapdelaine (1991), Gabriel-Doxtater and Van den Hende (1995), Jenness (1955), Obomsawin (1993), Trigger (1976), and York and Pindera (1991).

3 This article focuses on Montreal, which was the site of my fieldwork.

4 This is not to say that nonsovereignist provinces or the federal state necessarily treat cultural minorities with more inclusion; the issue of inclusion/exclusion does not necessarily hang on a sovereignist mandate.

5 Friendship Centres are community-based drop-in centres for urban Aboriginal clients in urban areas throughout Canada. They may provide a wide variety of services from employment placement to tuberculosis testing.

6   Although in the literature the terms "Indian reserve," "on-reserve," and "off-reserve" are used, it is common practice in Quebec to refer to Aboriginal "communities," not "reserves," because many Aboriginal communities in the provinces are not reserves under the Indian Act (Lévesque et al. 2001, 104 n. 6).

7   There is work on substance abuse (Jacobs and Gill 2002), HIV/AIDS in street youth (Roy et al. 2000), a needs assessment for HIV/AIDS prevention (Brassard, Smeja, and Valverde 1996), a study of urban Inuit (Kishigami 1999), a report on women and the law (Zambrowsky 1986), an ethnography on Aboriginal identity at a halfway house (Brass 1999; Chapter 16), and a film on homelessness (Obomsawin 1995).

8   For example, see Ontario's Aboriginal Healing and Wellness Strategy (2000).

9   Of course, this is not the official party line of the Quebec government; see for example, Secrétariat aux affaires autochtones, which states: "Over the years, Québec has developed a position which considers Aboriginal people to be both citizens of Québec and as having their own identity" (1998, 15).

10 A new health care institution has been created in Quebec since this research was conducted. The Centres de santé et de service sociaux (CSSS) were created by merging CLSCs with residential and long-term care centres and/or with general and specialized hospital centres. This new type of institution resulted from the adoption of Bill 25 in December 2004. It is still unclear how care for Aboriginal people will be transformed under this new model, which does link remote regions of the province to urban centres and academic institutions in an effort to provide access to care. See http://www.santemontreal.qc.ca/En/portrait/csss.html (accessed 8 January 2007).

11 Although there is a clinic specifically for refugee claimants based at a Montreal CLSC, this should not be seen as an emblem of provincial concern for cultural issues. According to a clinic administrator, there is constant pressure from the MSSS to assimilate clients into the more generic model.

12 Although there are hospitals in Montreal with the mandate to provide long-term beds for northern clients, this psychiatrist did not mention them because he either was unaware of them or lumped them together with the sort of poor care that is resisted by the communities.

13 The conference, First Nations Health: Our Voice, Our Decision, Our Responsibility, was hosted by the Health Secretariat of the Assembly of First Nations and sponsored by Health Canada's First Nations and Inuit Health Branch, Ottawa, Ontario, 25-27 February 2001.

14 Although blood quantum may be used to define membership in some First Nations communities, it is inappropriate in an urban milieu where the population is culturally diverse and includes Métis, adoptees, and others of mixed descent who nevertheless self-identify as Aboriginal.

15 Interestingly, an administrator at the refugee clinic said that many clients also travel over one hour instead of attending clinics in their own neighbourhoods.

16 For a discussion of ethnic match in health care and social services, see Weinfeld (1999).

17 Similar observations are reported by itinerant clinicians who visit remote "fly-in" communities: sometimes they are entrusted with secrets or confessions that would be difficult to make to local workers because of fears about loss of confidentiality and gossip.

References

Aboriginal Healing and Wellness Strategy. 2000. *Annual report 1999/2000*. Toronto, ON: Aboriginal Healing and Wellness Strategy.

Alfred, G.R. 1994. *Heeding the voices of our ancestors: Kahnawake Mohawk politics and the rise of Native nationalism*. Toronto, ON: Oxford University Press.

Brass, G.M. 1999. Respecting "the medicines": Narrating an Aboriginal identity at Nechi House. MA thesis, McGill University.

Brassard, P., C. Smeja, and C. Valverde. 1996. Needs assessment for an urban Native HIV and AIDS prevention program. *AIDS Education and Prevention* 8 (4): 343-51.

Chapdelaine, C. 1991. Poterie, ethnicité et Laurentie Iroquoienne. *Recherches Amérindiennes au Québec* 211 (2): 44-52.

Cohen, A. 1985. *The symbolic construction of community*. London: Routledge and Kegan Paul.

First Nations of Quebec and Labrador Health and Social Service Commission (FNQLHSSC). 1999. *Report on the analysis and interpretation of the regional health survey: Quebec region*. Quebec, QC: FNQLHSSC.

Gabriel-Doxtater, B.K., and A.K. Van den Hende. 1995. *At the wood's edge: An anthology of the history of the people of Kanehsata:ke*. Kanehstà:ke, QC: Kanehstà:ke Education Center.

George, J. 21 January 2000. New organization may help Inuit of Montreal. *Nunatsiaq News*. http://www.nunatsiaq.com/archives/nunavut000131/nvt20121_09.html.

Gill, L., C. Robertson, M. Robert, and M. Ollivier. 1995. *From the reserve to the city: Amerindian women in Quebec urban centres*. Ottawa, ON: Status of Women Canada.

Graham, K.A.H., and E. Peters. 2002. *Aboriginal communities and urban sustainability*. Ottawa, ON: Canadian Policy Research Networks.

Indian and Northern Affairs. 1999. *Quebec Indian communities guide*. Ottawa, ON: Indian and Northern Affairs Canada, Quebec Region.

Jacobs, K., and K. Gill. 2002. Substance abuse in an urban Aboriginal population: Social, legal and psychological consequences. *Journal of Ethnicity and Substance Abuse* 1 (1): 7-25.

Jenness, D. 1955. *Indians of Canada*. 3rd ed. Ottawa, ON: National Museum of Canada.

Jewkes, R., and A. Murcott. 1996. Meanings of community. *Social Science and Medicine* 43 (4): 555-63.

Kirmayer, L.J., D. Groleau, J. Guzder, C. Blake, and E. Jarvis. 2003. Cultural consultation: A model of mental health service for multicultural societies. *Canadian Journal of Psychiatry* 48 (2): 145-53.

Kishigami, N. 1999. Life and problems of urban Inuit in Montreal: Report of 1997 research. *Jinbun-Ronkyu: Journal of the Society of Liberal Arts* 68 (30): 81-110.

LaRocque, E.B. 1993. Violence in Aboriginal communities. In *The path to healing: The Royal Commission on Aboriginal Peoples*, 72-89. Ottawa: Canada Communication Group, for the Royal Commission on Aboriginal Peoples.

Lévesque, C., N. Trudeau, J. Bacon, C. Montpetit, M.-A. Cheezo, M. Lamontagne, C.S. Wawanoloath. 2001. *Aboriginal women and jobs: Challenges and issues for employability programs in Quebec*. Ottawa, ON: Le Partenariat Mikimon for the Status of Women Canada.

Lowi, Emanuel. 2 November 2001. Mamaqtuq! It's Inuit feast night in Montreal. *Nunatsiaq News*. http://www.nunatsiaq.com/archives/nunavut011102/news/features/11102_2.html.

Macdonald, M.E. 2003. Hearing (unheard) voices: Aboriginal experiences of mental health policy in Montreal. PhD diss., McGill University.

Maioni, A. 2001. *"Emerging solutions": Quebec's Clair Commission report and health care reform*. Ottawa, ON: Canadian Research Policy Networks.

Mental Health Working Group. 2001. *Comprehensive culturally appropriate mental wellness framework: First Nations and Inuit health and wellness discussion document*. Ottawa, ON: Assembly of First Nations – Inuit Tapirisat of Canada.

Mesher, V. 18 February 2000. Montreal Inuit association still in its infancy. *Nunatsiaq News*. http://www.nunatsiaq.com/archives/nunavut000230/letters.html#montreal.

Obomsawin, A., writ./dir. 1993. *Kanehsatake: 270 years of resistance*. Film. Available from the National Film Board of Canada.

–, writ./dir. 1995. *No address*. Film. Available from the National Film Board of Canada.

Pelletier, C., and C. Laurin. 1993. *Assessment of violence and mental health conditions among Native peoples in Quebec*. Montreal, QC: Centre de recherche et d'analyse en sciences humaines, for Quebec Native Women.

Petawabano, B.H., E. Gourdeau, F. Jourdain, A. Palliser-Tulugak, and J. Cossette. 1994. *Mental health and Aboriginal people of Quebec*. Quebec: Gaëtan Morin, for Comité de la santé mentale du Québec.

Quebec Native Women. 2001. *Aboriginal women and health: An assessment*. Montreal, QC: Quebec Native Women.

Roy, E., N. Haley, J.F. Boivin, J.Y. Frappier, C. Claessens, and N. Lemire. 2000. HIV infection among street youth in Montreal: Aboriginal youth – a descriptive analysis. Paper presented at the Circle of Hope, Montreal.

Secrétariat aux affaires autochtones (SAA). 1998. *Partnership, development, achievement*. Quebec, QC: Gouvernement du Québec.

–. 2001. *The Amerindians and the Inuit of Québec: Eleven contemporary nations*. Quebec, QC: Gouvernement du Québec.

Statistics Canada. 1991. *Canadian census, catalog no. 11-001E*. Ottawa, ON: Ministry of Industry, Science and Technology.

Trigger, B. 1976. *The children of Aataentsic: A history of the Huron people to 1660*. Montreal, QC, and Kingston, ON: McGill-Queen's University Press.

Valentine, V.F. 1992. *Off reserve Aboriginal populations: A thumbnail sketch by numbers*. Ottawa, ON: NCC Sociodemographics Research and Analysis Project.

Weinfeld, M. 1999. The challenges of ethnic match: Minority origin professionals in health and social services. In H. Troper and M. Weinfeld, eds., *Ethnicity, politics, and public policy: Case studies in Canadian diversity,* 117-41. Toronto, ON: University of Toronto Press.

York, G., and L. Pindera. 1991. *People of the pines: The warriors and the legacy of Oka*. Toronto, ON: Little, Brown.

Zambrowsky, S.C. 1986. *Native women who are or may be in conflict with the law in the region of Montreal*. Ottawa, ON: Ministry of the Solicitor General.

18

Six Nations Mental Health Services:
A Model of Care for Aboriginal Communities

CORNELIA WIEMAN

Aboriginal peoples should be supported in the development of their own solutions, rather than having solutions imposed on or provided for them. Such a change would foster the development of more culturally appropriate, and therefore effective, services and supports.

> – THE HONOURABLE MICHAEL J.L. KIRBY, QUOTED IN *MENTAL HEALTH, MENTAL ILLNESS AND ADDICTION*

The Iroquois are in the throes of reinventing themselves yet again, a tradition that is itself seven times seven generations old. For the most part, these are wise and principled people, who understand that nothing is ever settled once and for all, and who have learned to live comfortably with uncertainty that understanding entails. Despite everything that has occurred through their long past and the uncertainty of the future, the Iroquois prepare the way for the seventh generation still to come.

> – DEAN R. SNOW, *THE IROQUOIS* (1996), 221

Six Nations Mental Health Services is a community mental health clinic that delivers a variety of psychiatric out-patient and mental health services to a rural Iroquoian community close to Brantford in southern Ontario. First opened in June 1997, it is a freestanding community mental health clinic physically located in proximity to other health and social services in Ohsweken, the central village on the reserve. The clinic currently employs 10 staff, all of whom, with the exception of the psychiatrists, are of Aboriginal ancestry, with approximately half coming from the Six Nations community and the others from other First Nations communities in Ontario and Manitoba. During the years that I worked as the general adult psychiatrist at the clinic (1997-2005), I was one of only four Aboriginal psychiatrists in Canada; it was an honour for me to work with this community.

Six Nations is a unique mental health service in a First Nations community in that it is located on a reserve, is community-run, and integrates a range of mental health services,

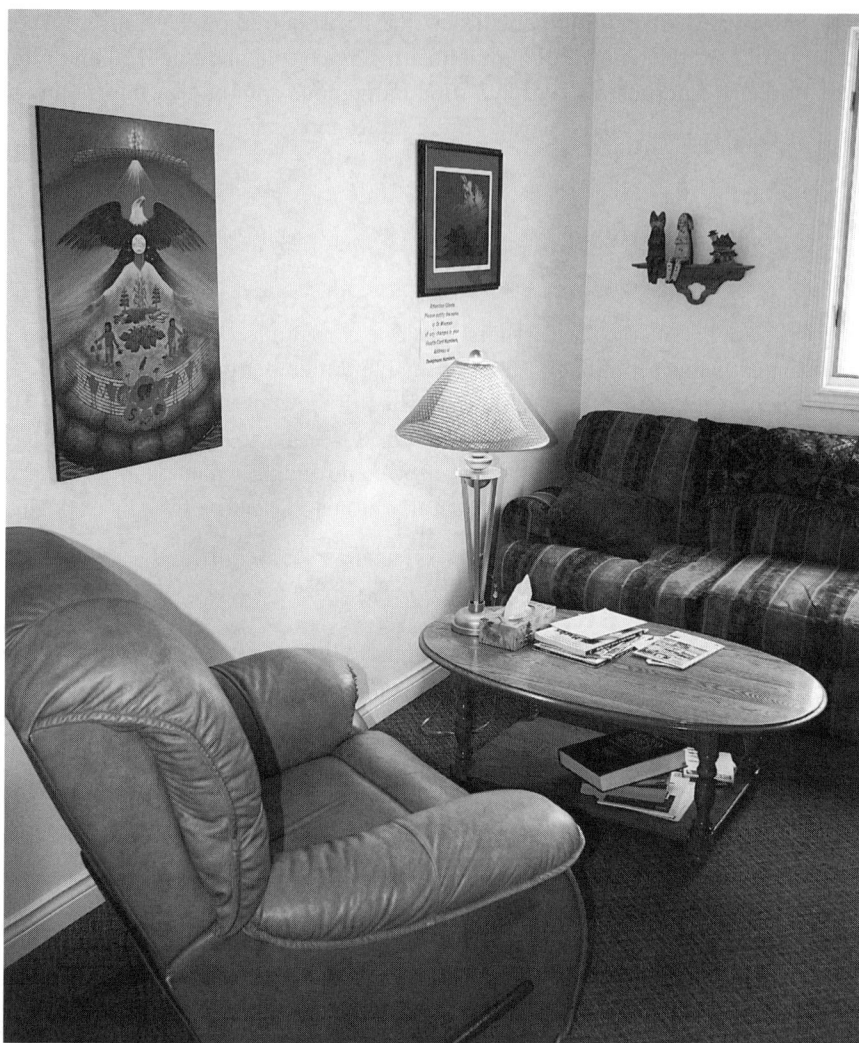

FIGURE 18.1   A deliberate effort was made by Six Nations Mental Health Services staff to have the clinical interview rooms be as comfortable as possible in order to offer a relaxing, non-intimidating environment for clinical encounters. (Photo: L.J. Kirmayer)

including psychiatry as well as access to traditional healing. To appreciate the significance of this mental health service and better understand how it originated, one needs to know something about the history of the people of Six Nations of the Grand River and their tenacity in maintaining a complex and multifaceted sense of autonomy. Importantly, I hope to show how the people of Six Nations of the Grand River have worked with a maze-like federal bureaucracy with its tangled webs of health policy. Maintaining this service has

CORNELIA WIEMAN

been a struggle against structural inequalities that has required perseverance. By providing a meaningful and much needed mental health service to a marginalized and often misunderstood client population within a rural indigenous community, this mental heath service offers a potential model for other indigenous and/or rural communities.

Six Nations of the Grand River

With a population close to 22,000, the Six Nations of the Grand River Territory, near Brantford, Ontario, is Canada's largest First Nations community. Like many First Nations communities, nearly half, or about 11,000, of the band-member population live off-reserve, and this is a significant issue for the delivery of health services in the community. The off-reserve population of Six Nations resides in neighbouring towns and cities across southern Ontario, as well as in other major urban centres throughout Canada and the United States. Six Nations gets its name from the fact that it includes all six nations of the Iroquois Confederacy – Mohawk, Cayuga, Oneida, Onondaga, Seneca, and Tuscarora.[1] The Six Nations, also referred to as the Iroquois Confederacy or Haudenosonee, is a political alliance of Iroquoian-speaking nations that formed prior to European contact and colonization of North America. Interestingly, it was the first known democratic system of government in the New World.[2]

The community of Six Nations of the Grand River was formed in the late eighteenth century, after and as a result of the American War of Independence. Under the leadership of Joseph Brant, a Mohawk who became a British officer, some Iroquoian communities in what was to become the State of New York allied themselves with the British Crown. When the American revolutionaries defeated the British and their allies, those Iroquoian communities that sided with the British under Brant were forced to move north. In 1784 the British offered these emigrant Iroquois populations a tract of land – referred to as the Haldimand Grant – that ran along the length of the Grand River in Upper Canada, or present-day south-western Ontario. The original settlement was enormous, totaling 1,150,311 hectares (Dickason 1993, 190). However, over the next 50 years, two-thirds of this original tract of land was lost, due either to revisions made by the Crown to the earlier settlement or to dubious sales and claims by squatters. By 1850 the Six Nations settlement had been reduced in size to about 19,000 hectares and changed to reserve lands. Up until 1924 Six Nations was governed under the traditional system of the Iroquois. In that year, under the Indian Act, the Dominion Government of Canada forced the community to adopt a system based on an elected band council.[3] Since that time, the Band Council has borne primary responsibility for the functioning of the community and has delivered all services, including land allotments, finalizing estates and trusts, co-ordination of emergency and police services, health and social services, elementary and postsecondary funding, and water and sewage systems. Funding for these community services comes from the Government of Canada through the Department of Indian and Northern Affairs Canada (INAC) and

Health Canada (First Nations and Inuit Health Branch) in the form of federal transfer payments. According to the information provided on an INAC website, the Six Nations of the Grand River community received $17,502,000 in the fiscal year 2005-06. This money included close to $8 million for postsecondary and elementary education, $2.3 million for community infrastructure and operations, and $785,400 for housing.

The majority of the Six Nations mental health clinic's operating funds, including salaries of administrative staff, mental health nurses, and case managers, comes from a contribution agreement that is signed annually between Six Nations Health Services and Health Canada's First Nations and Inuit Health Branch (FNIHB) through the Building Healthy Communities Program. Six Nations remains a "nontransferred" community, so these federal funding agreements are renegotiated on a yearly basis. Some of the new programs added to the clinic, such as the Crisis Intervention Worker and Intensive Case Management programs, are supported by funds from the Ontario Ministry of Health and Long-Term Care via a provincial transfer agreement. The Assertive Community Treatment Team for Brantford also has provincial funding, and this supports a worker dedicated to Six Nations clients.

Being a "Haudenosonee" Person from Six Nations

Given Six Nations of the Grand River's proximity to several surrounding municipalities, including Brantford, Hamilton, and other large towns nearby, residents have developed complex relationships, both formal and informal, with these other communities. Despite longstanding relationships with many townsfolk in these outside communities, there is a pervasive sentiment among Six Nations community members of being a distinct and separate people. Although residents in Six Nations may go into these non-Aboriginal communities to shop and to use a range of services, may send their children to school there, and may have friends and colleagues there, social and physical boundaries remain. Over the years, some of these relationships have been difficult, and this has reinforced a sense of separateness among residents of Six Nations. The recent events in Caledonia, Ontario, are a case in point: the historical loss of settlement lands and the slow pace of land claims negotiations are an ongoing source of political friction in Aboriginal and non-Aboriginal community relations. These tensions inform a collective outlook among Six Nations residents toward those surrounding communities and influence long-term patterns in social relations. Like other Iroquoian communities, due to the historical relationship to traditional lands in New York State and a tendency among young people, particularly men, to find employment in the United States (including military service and iron work),[4] collective identity may centre on being from Six Nations of the Grand River and a Haudenosonee person rather than on being defined by international or provincial borders that are relatively recent intrusions.[5] Longstanding cultural and familial ties with other Haudenosonee communities are maintained through the political and religious influences of the "long-house," which involves a traditional clan structure and system of naming. As well, competitive sports, particularly lacrosse, link Six Nations of the Grand River with other Iroquois communities and reinforce an orientation toward a wider Haudenosonee worldview. Intermarriages and peer relationships with other First Nations communities – along with shared frustrations both with the Indian Act's imposed band-council system and with participation in provincial and federal Aboriginal political forums – fortify an identity as an indigenous person. For these reasons, "being Canadian from a southern Ontario town" may not resonate as strongly as being Haudenosonee, Six Nations, or even "indigenous." Finally, for some residents, a "small-town complex" fuels apprehension of big cities like Hamilton and Toronto and contributes to the social distance between those Six Nations individuals and families who have stayed on the reserve and those who have chosen to live away from the community (Maracle 1996).

Creating and Providing Community Services in Six Nations

In recent decades, Six Nations has increasingly taken on greater responsibility for all its community services, including health. Although the Six Nations Band Council does have governance over health, unlike many other First Nations communities, it is not a "transferred community," in which responsibility for health services has been formally transferred from Health Canada to community government. In fact, there is some wariness about the health-transfer program since, from the official standpoint of the community's political leadership, health is a treaty right and transfer should not be used by the government to avoid its obligations. As in any governmental structure, health is a portfolio within the system of governance. In the case of Six Nations, an elected Band Council member supported by the bureaucratic structure holds the health portfolio and leads a community Health Committee. The Health Committee guides the delivery and planning of community health services; it is composed of 8 to 10 community stakeholders, including other elected councillors, health professionals, Elders, and community members at large. This committee has an overarching role in determining and planning for the health needs of the community. It was this committee, led by particular members, that first identified the need and worked to make Six Nations Mental Heath Services a reality. The creation of the clinic was preceded by an environmental scan of the community's health and social-service resources (Six Nations Band Council 1999). This led to a report that documented the need for improved and more timely mental health services and provided the community with a long-term mental health strategy.

Community experiences with health professionals from outside Six Nations have been mixed at best. In particular, encounters with psychiatric and other mental health services have generally been negative. Before the Six Nations Mental Health Services clinic opened, there was a psychiatrist coming to the community for a half-day of clinical consultation every 2 weeks. This arrangement was cancelled with the opening of the new clinic. Although initial use of the new mental health clinic was limited, community usage steadily increased over time as its presence became known and a level of familiarity developed with its staff, greatly facilitating the development of stronger clinical relationships and trust.

Six Nations Mental Health Services

The service includes a full complement of staff and consists of a program co-ordinator, an administrative assistant, four mental health nurses, a mental health/addictions outreach worker, two case managers, a crisis counsellor, and access to the consulting services of three part-time psychiatrists. The program co-ordinator manages the administrative and day-to-day operations of the clinic. The outreach worker, who is trained as a social worker, works mainly in the community's elementary schools, implementing mental health curriculum with youth from kindergarten to Grade 8. The outreach worker also plans and co-ordinates educational and awareness events in the community for the various health and social-service providers as well as for the general community. The mental health nurses are all registered nurses (RNs) with extensive previous experience in psychiatry and mental health. The nurses participate in the psychiatric consultation and follow-up processes and also provide intensive case management for individuals with serious mental illnesses. Each of the four mental health nurses works with a specific client population: children and youth, adults, geriatrics, and clients with concurrent substance-abuse problems. There is one case manager (RN) who handles clients through the Early Intervention in Psychosis Program. There is a psychiatry subspecialist in psychotic disorders who provides backup to the case manager one day per month. The intensive-case manager (RN) manages the clients with the most severe and complicated nonpsychotic disorders. A general adult psychiatrist provides backup to the four mental health nurses and the intensive-case manager an average of 1 to 2 days per month. There is also one psychiatrist for children and adolescents who provides psychiatric consultations only and who works with the service 1 day per month.

The primary mandate of Six Nations Mental Health Services is to serve Six Nations band members living both on- and off-reserve. However, individuals from other Aboriginal communities have been seen and treated, such as individuals from the nearby Muncie community close to London, Ontario. Clients span all age groups from children to the elderly; the youngest client seen was 4 years old, while the oldest client was 94 years old. Clients present with a wide range of symptoms that can be diagnosed according to the *Diagnostic and statistical manual* (DSM-IV) diagnostic classification on Axes I to V (American Psychiatric Association 2000). Clients followed by the clinic suffer from a variety of mental illnesses and psychosocial problems, which range from mild to severe. A 1994 needs assessment conducted in the community showed that mental health services were urgently required, being rated the third-highest priority behind only diabetes and cardiovascular care programs.

The Six Nations community has long been underserviced in terms of mental health. Community members have been somewhat reluctant to receive mental health care in the larger cities of Hamilton and Brantford, partly due to the perceived lack of cultural sensitivity of service providers. To improve accessibility, the Six Nations Mental Health Service takes referrals from a wide variety of agencies. Self-referrals consisted of 54% of all referrals in the first twelve months the clinic operated. The majority of the remainder of referrals were from family physicians (17%) and from nurses, social workers, and clinical staff of other agencies (29%). The service occasionally received referrals from an individual's family members, police and other emergency staff, and hospitals in the surrounding areas of Hamilton, Brantford, Caledonia, and Hagersville. Individuals who are referred to the clinic for psychiatric services must be under the care of a primary-care physician who is aware of and in agreement with the referral.

Services offered by the clinic include around-the-clock response to mental health crisis, psychiatric consultation, assessment, and short- and long-term follow-up as well as case management for the seriously mentally ill. Such individuals would include those who have illnesses such as schizophrenia and severe bipolar affective disorders. There are now specialized services, including access to psychosocial and vocational rehabilitation, for clients with psychotic disorders. The clinic also tries to deliver education, support, and awareness programs for clients and their families as well as for general community members. Regular clinic hours are between Monday and Friday from 8:30 a.m. to 4:30 p.m. Psychiatric services are offered on Tuesdays and Thursdays. Since 2006 the crisis-response service has operated 24 hours a day, 7 days a week. Individuals in perceived distress or crisis may call the clinic during this time. During the week, community members will be seen immediately by the crisis counsellor, who is also on-call on weekend nights. The mental health nurses rotate their on-call time slots each weekend with a partner. If called, they may speak with individuals over the phone, see them in their homes, or meet at mutually arranged places (e.g., coffee shop). The general psychiatrist provides backup to the nurses each weekend and is available 24 hours a day by phone or pager. Decisions are made about whether individuals require transportation to the nearest hospital emergency department or whether they have become settled after their visit with the nurse and can be seen in follow-up when the clinic reopens on Monday. In the first year of operation, the psychiatrist in the clinic saw a total of 126 individuals. Approximately 40% of these individuals made their initial contact with the clinic through the crisis-response service.

In the first year of service, 55% of individuals referred for psychiatric consultation and assessment were female; 84% of referred individuals were seen directly, while the remainder were either indirect consults or did not come to the clinic. Clinic staff were actively following 73% of individuals after the first 15 months that the clinic was open. The most common presenting problems were depression, suicidal ideation, and anxiety. The most common diagnoses following psychiatric assessment were mood disorders (including depression and manic depression), personality disorders, disruptive-behaviour disorders, and anxiety disorders. Although substance abuse was a comorbid condition for some individuals, the various substance-abuse treatment programs available in the community and surrounding area see the majority of those who have substance-abuse difficulties as their primary disorder. One of the mental health nurses now focuses her nursing and case-management skills on working with clients who have concurrent psychiatric and substance-abuse problems.

Clients who may be suitable for ongoing case management are discussed at the intake level by the nurses and program supervisor and are then distributed equally among the four mental health nurses, with the psychiatrist providing clinical backup. The psychiatrist may be consulted about these clients or may see them directly. In the first year of service, the average intake for case management per month was about 10 clients. Approximately 65% of the individuals seen by the clinic are followed under the case-management model; 40% of the total individuals remained in active case-management status 18 months after the clinic opened. After initial assessment, if clients meet the criteria to be followed either by the manager for early intervention in psychosis or by the manager for intensive cases, they are transferred to the appropriate nurse case manager, with backup from one of the psychiatrists. A recent option available to residents of Six Nations is to receive care from the Assertive Community Treatment Team (ACTT) operating out of Brantford. It is believed to be the first ACTT team to deliver services directly in a First Nations community in Ontario.

In addition to clinical services with clients, Six Nations also provides a wide range of educational, support, and awareness services for clients, their families, and community members. Approximately 13% of clients who were initially presented or referred requested information about mental health, mental illness, or various treatments. The clinic has compiled a large database of patient literature and pamphlets to share with clients as requested. There is a growing lending library of books and videos that are available to clients and their families. The major criticism of available materials is the lack of information directed specifically toward Aboriginal individuals and their communities. The mental health nurses also assist clients and their families in accessing other available mental health/illness resources in the surrounding communities – services that are not available within the Six Nations reserve. For example, nurses will accompany clients to their first meetings with support groups, such as groups for clients with depression and those for parents whose children have died by suicide. This support allows clients and their families to feel more comfortable in accessing these services, which they may have been reluctant to attend in the past for a variety of reasons.

Within the community, the clinic also holds biannual workshops on various themes to coincide with national-awareness weeks dedicated to mental health and mental illness. For example, issues of depression, suicide, grief, loss, and trauma are common within the community (Macmillan et al. 1996; Royal Commission on Aboriginal Peoples 1995). Clinic staff also write regular columns dealing with a variety of mental health issues for the two community newspapers; articles have included a review of the signs and symptoms of depression and information on how community members can access help if they feel they are depressed. Clinic staff participate in a phone-in health show on the community radio station every 2 to 3 months. Clinic staff also regularly take part in various community events sponsored by the other health and social-service agencies in the community in order to improve their visibility and hopefully to ease access into the mental health system. Finally, clinic staff function as facilitators in critical/traumatic-incident debriefings in the community. For example, since the clinic opened for service in 1997, there have been several traumatic events, including a shooting, several sudden deaths, and several suicides. The clinic provides support for other clinical and emergency staff, including police, emergency-response workers, and community social workers.

Challenges to Service Delivery

There are a number of service-delivery issues at the level of both the individual and the community. Aside from the local micro-level challenges associated with life in a First Nations community (e.g., occasional flare-ups in Band Council and community politics as well as in intra- and interfamilial relationships), there is a tendency for community members to mistrust "outsiders" who provide health care in the community. In part, this is because of uncertainty regarding their motivations for wanting to work in the community and their awareness of community values and perspectives. Too often there have been stories of health care providers who lack cultural sensitivity toward their Aboriginal patients. As Aboriginal individuals, clinic staff try to provide culturally sensitive care, and they achieve a greater sense of trust with their clients because they have an "insider" understanding of relevant issues within the community. Staff who are not originally from the Six Nations community have made an extra effort to meet the community, participate in various community activities, and become familiar with its members and resources. They have also been respectful of individuals' wishes to pursue traditional healing for their difficulties.[6] Clients can continue to be followed by the mental health service even if they wish to seek traditional healing. A modified version of the "shared care" approach to providing mental health services has been developed. It is common for staff to help a client of the mental health service to access traditional healing.

Initially, there was some concern from the community regarding confidentiality. For example, the clinic is located in the centre of the community, and individuals stated they did not want to be seen by others entering the building. However, one goal of the service has been to de-stigmatize mental illness and improve access to mental health services, so the decision was consciously made to locate the clinic in a central, accessible place. Initially, a lack of consumer awareness regarding mental health, mental illness, various treatments, and available services was noted. Over the long term, the plan is to improve

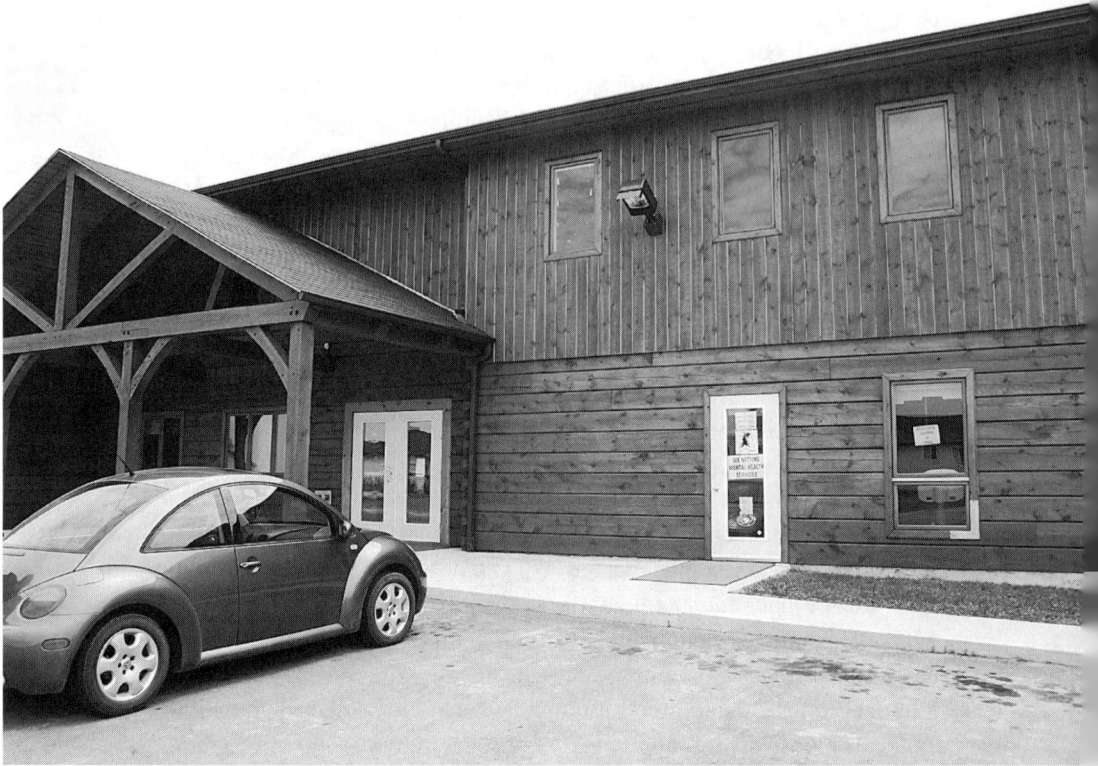

FIGURE 18.2 This is the building in which Six Nations Mental Health Services was housed for three years (2003-5). The new health building, the Whitepines Wellness Centre, which has many of the on-reserve health services under one roof, officially opened on 7 September 2007. (Photo: L.J. Kirmayer)

awareness of the availability and appropriate use of mental health services within the community by continuing education initiatives. In the future, the aim is to expand services – for example, by offering various support groups for people with similar difficulties. Recently, some of the clients of the clinic started their own peer-support group for those suffering from mood disorders, with assistance from the mental health nurses.

At the community level, there are a number of service-delivery issues. Six Nations is a community with a very complex sociopolitical context. There is a distinct delineation between more "Westernized" individuals and those with a more traditional viewpoint. It is important for any health care provider to have an understanding of this complex context in order to deliver sensitive and effective care. Prior to the clinic opening, there was a lack of psychiatric and mental health services, which resulted in the "revolving door syndrome."

CORNELIA WIEMAN

Previously, individuals with mental illnesses became acutely ill, were admitted to hospital psychiatric units in surrounding cities, and were subsequently discharged without any follow-up services being available in the community. They would then quickly deteriorate and often be re-admitted to hospital. In the year prior to the clinic opening, 17 individuals accounted for 54 separate admissions to hospital. During the first year of providing mental health services in the community, only 3 individuals were hospitalized for a total of 5 admissions. There is also a complicated administrative structure within the community, and much effort had to be put into service planning, development, and co-ordination so that the clinic's services would not overlap with those of existing agencies. Efforts were also made to improve collaboration with existing community agencies and services by promoting a "shared care" model and being available for case conferences and planning around complex cases.

There were also initial challenges involved in establishing collaborative working relationships with traditional healers in the community. Despite decades of attempts by government to suppress traditional healing and despite a previous epoch when the Western medical profession rejected and tried to discredit Aboriginal healing knowledge and practices, indigenous medical systems have not only persisted and survived but have also begun to flourish and become reinvigorated. For the most part, traditional Iroquoian health and healing systems have remained vital to community life in Six Nations.

Although some indigenous healing techniques may be largely symbolic in nature, they involve rituals with meaningful psychological and social impacts (Kirmayer 2004; Waldram 2000). It should also be kept in mind that some traditional healing methods include the use of an assortment of herbal remedies composed of organic substances with active pharmacological properties: these remedies may have significant effects on human physiology. North American indigenous pharmacological knowledge of local fauna was both extensive and empirically grounded. In the Six Nations community, some of the most obvious of these medicines are a wide variety of tobacco plants, certain species of coniferous trees (i.e., pine and cedar), and willows. Still more important, traditional healing practices have a fundamentally spiritual dimension that is central to their meaning and effectiveness for many individuals.

In the clinical work of the mental health service, there is ongoing consideration given to balancing the "medical model" with traditional, holistic approaches. Due to the efforts of authorities and others to discredit traditional healing in decades past, many traditional healers in the community work "underground" and are difficult to access. Clinic staff have worked toward establishing respectful, collaborative relationships with traditional healers for the benefit of their clients. As a group of care providers, staff have sought additional traditional teachings not only to increase their familiarity with traditional ceremonies and healing practices but also to sustain themselves in what is often very complex and challenging work.

There is a need to recognize the importance of self-care for mental health professionals. Continuing education and professional development should be an integral part of any clinical service not only to allow providers to keep abreast of new information and techniques but also to give them time away from the day-to-day strains of clinical work. Collegial support and the validation of peers, as well as opportunities to debrief, help clinicians to keep their focus and stay committed to their work. For the staff at Six Nations Mental Health Services, more traditionally aligned ways of caring for oneself and each other within the group (such as sharing meals, use of humour and storytelling, spending time as a group with Elders or traditional healers) are seen as crucial to healthy functioning at the clinic. Dealing with clients with complex health and psychosocial needs requires staff who are well from a holistic point of view themselves. It has always been the goal of Six Nations Mental Health Services to provide clinical and out-patient psychiatric services within the community that meet and even exceed the standard of care that clients would be able to access outside the community.

Finally, there remains a lack of Aboriginal health professionals across Canada and specifically in the Six Nations community. Clinic staff work in a variety of ways to try to improve access for Aboriginal students to the health professions and related programs. For example, they have provided information for school projects and student placements for young individuals in the community who show interest in a career in the health professions. They also make an effort to be visible at various career fairs, which are held several times a year in the community. Clinic staff have participated in the admissions process to the various programs of the Faculty of Health Sciences at McMaster University in Hamilton (e.g., Nursing, Medicine, Physiotherapy, and Occupational Therapy). There is an improved relationship between the postsecondary educational programs at Six Nations and the Native Students Health Sciences program at McMaster University so that more community members can receive encouragement and guidance toward a career in the health professions. In an informal way, clinic staff also function as role models to the youth in the community and have discussed establishing a more formal mentorship program for young students in the community who are interested in a health-related career.

The Impact of Health Policy

The greatest challenge to the creation and long-term sustainability of the Six Nations Mental Health Services involves the complexity of the federal and provincial bureaucratic structures and health policies that determine health-program funding for First Nations (registered or status Indian) and Inuit populations. Bureaucratic structures and policy are slow to change and often unresponsive to individual or local needs. The First Nations and Inuit Health Branch (FNIHB) is the federal department within Health Canada mandated to oversee the health-planning and program-funding requirements of Canada's First Nations and Inuit peoples. Health Canada's program funding for the Inuit and status Indian populations is delivered through the Non-Insured Health Benefits (NIHB) program, which is one of several programs delivered by the FNIHB. The NIHB program provides a range of medical services that supplement benefits provided through other private, provincial, or territorial programs. The aim of the NIHB program is to provide health services in a manner that "1) is appropriate to Inuit and status Indian's unique health needs; 2) contributes to the achievement of an overall health status for First Nations and Inuit people that is comparable to that of the Canadian population as a whole; 3) is sustainable from a fiscal and benefit management perspective; and 4) facilitates First Nations and Inuit control at a time and pace of [our] choosing" (NIHB 2000, 3). Benefits under the NIHB program include pharmacy (i.e., prescription and over-the-counter medications, medical supplies and equipment), dental care, vision care, transportation to access medical services, health care premiums (in Alberta and British Columbia only), and other health care services, such as crisis-intervention mental health counselling. The NIHB program funding is intended to "provide limited funding of last resort for professional mental health treatment for individuals and communities in at-risk, crisis situations" (NIHB 2000, 1; see also NIHB 1999). Mental health professionals from a range of disciplines, including psychology, psychiatric nursing, and social work, provide mental health services funded by the NIHB for some individuals in some communities.

As stated in the Program Directives, the mental health services provided by the NIHB are intentionally limited and primarily cover brief courses of counselling or interventions for acute crises. Indeed, a review of mental health services funding under the NIHB suggests that mental health has not been a high priority, despite the clearly documented evidence of need from community surveys and the voices of leaders who have identified better-funded and sustained mental health services in First Nations communities as a critical priority. The lack of comprehensive, adequate, and reliable funding for mental health services has wide implications for the delivery of much-needed mental health programs in First Nations communities, including Six Nations.

From the perspective of clients, there are additional challenges to consider. First Nations persons living both on- and off-reserve are confronted by many obstacles to service access; for example, if NIHB-funded counsellors practice off-reserve, there may be transportation difficulties in travelling to or attending counselling sessions. Importantly, some clients may find that the counselling they do receive lacks cultural sensitivity or cultural relevance. Youth, in particular, may feel that they are unable to relate to the counsellors available to them. NIHB-funded counsellors may vary in their competence and confidence in dealing with difficult patients, including those who are acutely suicidal. Confidentiality is an important concern for individuals considering entering into a counselling relationship and becomes even more critical in smaller communities. Individuals who have complicated histories and multiple mental health issues (e.g., relationship and family difficulties, concurrent substance abuse, domestic violence, criminal history) may be receiving services from multiple agencies, which results in care that is fragmented and inadequately co-ordinated.

The Day-to-Day Experience of Mental Health Service Delivery

The consequences of the complicated nature of the FNIHB bureaucracy and the constraints of the NIHB policy for funding mental health services are evident in the day-to-day effort to provide consistent and timely services to a range of clients. Although some clients require assistance with illness management, such as monitoring their medication, regular counselling or psychotherapy sessions, and an adequate level of social support, others may be in an acute mental health crisis. Patients with bipolar disorder (manic-depressive illness) provide a case in point. Bipolar disorder involves very distinct episodes that require intensive effort to treat. The process of stabilizing a person in the acute stage of bipolar disorder can last 6 months or longer and must be followed by regular sessions to improve functioning and prevent recurrence. But FNIHB guidelines for some regions allow funding only for up to 15 sessions in 1 fiscal year. If, by the end of those sessions, a patient who was previously stable goes into crisis again – not uncommon with bipolar disorder – either the second episode will not be covered or additional sessions will need specific FNIHB approval.

Adequate coverage for conventional psychiatric disorders is only the tip of the iceberg, however, since among the First Nations population in need of mental health services there may be other issues not generally seen among the general Canadian population. The most common set of issues concerns the intergenerational effects of the residential school experience and the "Sixties Scoop" – both of which have proven to be disastrous experiments in social engineering (Assembly of First Nations 1994, 1998; Fournier and Crey 1997; Johnston 1983). In these cases, undisclosed incidents of physical and sexual abuse may underlie a presentation of severe anxiety disorder or depression, combined with a history of alcohol and substance abuse. How reasonable is it to expect any clinician to work through this degree of complicated psychopathology in just 15 sessions? Health policymakers in the FNIHB/Health Canada need to recognize that the assessment and treatment of some forms of persistent and severe psychiatric disorders in the Aboriginal population do not fit neatly into the requirements of rigid funding schemes. The nature of some more unpredictable psychiatric disorders demands intensive interventions that more likely fit a case-management model. Aside from a clear need to substantially increase funding of mental health services overall, there is a pressing need for more flexibility in the funding model so that mental health professionals can respond in a timely and effective way to acute mental health crises and can provide intensive treatment and continuity of care that allows clients to achieve some stability. Mental health services, including psychiatry, should be available on a regular and as-needed basis in order to assist a wide range of clients.

On a final note, funding agencies and policymakers also need to understand the unique structural constraints within most First Nations communities. In particular, there is often a lack of public transportation in these places, something that directly impacts Six Nations.

Although some southern First Nations communities are literally surrounded by municipalities, even when these First Nations are situated within a shared municipal-transport grid, inexpensive and reliable public transportation is not always available to the on-reserve population because of federal, provincial, and municipal jurisdictional issues. Not everyone in these communities owns a personal automobile, nor can everyone afford to maintain one. That said, there may be a need to improve medical transportation for First Nations people with mental health problems so that they can access clinical services, keep appointments with qualified mental health professionals, and make use of appropriate social supports outside the community when these are not available locally.

Conclusion

The creation of Six Nations Mental Health Services was the result of a lengthy process based on widespread recognition of the need for action among community members. To make this service a reality, it took considerable effort and leadership among a core group of community members, long-term planning, and fierce dedication to the goal of helping those who need help the most – community members living with a severe mental illness. Once the service became a reality, even more commitment and persistence was required from the newly formed clinical team to build trust, increase recognition, and overcome barriers within the community. There is still a great deal of stigma associated with mental illness within Canadian society, and Six Nations is no exception. But these obstacles can be overcome through education and greater familiarity with mental health problems.

The experience of Six Nations Mental Health Services leads to some advice and recommendations for other First Nations communities that see a need for similar services for their community members. First, in the area of human resources, it is important to aim high in terms of professional training and to maintain high standards for ongoing educational and professional development. Clinical staff need opportunities to hone their skills as well as to stay emotionally balanced. Second, avoid a fee-for-service model and create salaried positions for clinicians. This arrangement is preferable because it is more equitable and flexible and supports all the essential work that happens outside direct patient contact, including team work, community consultation, education, mental health promotion, and program development. Third, there is a need to stay focused on evidence-based interventions and to avoid the many fads that regularly come and go in the field of mental health. In particular, there seems to be a tendency among some government funding agencies to prefer or even push for popular but unproven single-program models. History repeatedly tells us that these "one size fits all" approaches often fail because they ignore the local dynamics, diversity, and specific needs of individuals and communities. Fourth, mental health professionals should be aware of the various forms of traditional healing and develop relationships of trust and co-operation with healers in their community. This atmosphere of co-operation will make it easier for individuals to integrate traditional forms of healing in their care without denying them the best of biomedicine and psychiatry. At the same time, it is important to discuss and monitor possible side effects that the patient may experience due to interaction between a medication prescribed by a biomedical practitioner and the active ingredients contained in a traditional herbal medicine; this should be done in conjunction with a pharmacist. The services that clients are able to access at the Six Nations clinic are supported by a strong, collaborative relationship between the mental health nurse, physician, community pharmacist, and client. Finally, for the health care professional, there is a need to find opportunities for self-care and support. This issue becomes heightened in rural and remote First Nations communities where the usual stress of clinical work is amplified by limited collegial support, a demanding workload, and geographic isolation. Although continuing medical education and professional development can provide stimulation and support, there is a need to further develop networks across Canada in order to reduce the isolation of practitioners.

In summary, Six Nations Mental Health Services is a community-based mental health and psychiatric out-patient clinic, which has provided clinical support and educational services to a rural Aboriginal community since June 1997. While offering conventional medical treatment for psychiatric disorders, clinicians have strived to modify their practice in order to provide more culturally sensitive and appropriate care to community members. Six Nations has tried to establish a mutually respectful collaborative working relationship with traditional healers in the community. In this way, it aims to offer the community a "best of both worlds" approach to the prevention and management of mental disorders with the overall goal of providing culturally relevant services for the betterment of mental health at the individual, family, and community levels. The creation of this service reflects a collective effort to build a community that is fully inclusive of all its members and to make things better not just for the current generation but for future ones as well. This is a perspective that fits a forward-thinking cultural outlook well known among the Iroquois. Among traditional Iroquoian peoples, there is a firmly rooted commitment to and deference toward what is called the "Seven Generations" prophecy. The central tenet of this prophecy is a clear-minded understanding of how one's actions, attitudes, behaviours, and, in particular, decisions in this generation will affect not just the next generation but our descendants for seven generations to come. Six Nations mental health has developed with this philosophy in mind, and we look forward to its continued growth in the years to come.

Notes

1 The Tuscarora joined the Iroquois Confederacy in 1721 in response to the violent usurpation of their traditional territories by Euro-American settlers.
2 For decades historians have debated the degree to which the Iroquois Confederacy's organizational structure served as a political template in founding the democratic system of the early American colonies.

3 For more historical background, see Weaver (1978) and Shimony (1994). Although the Band Council currently provides primary leadership to the community on all official government-to-government relationships, the older traditional system remains an active and integral part of community life, as it does in many other Iroquoian communities. The long-term relationship between these two governing entities, however, has not been without political differences and ideological disagreements, especially when issues of indigenous sovereignty are perceived to be at stake.

4 Iroquois men, Mohawks in particular, have a long history of employment in the high-steel construction industry, especially in twentieth-century New York as well as in other major US and Canadian cities. This dangerous profession has been a lucrative source of income, travel opportunities, and social prestige that has powerfully shaped modern-day Mohawk and Iroquoian identity and community social relations.

5 For more on membership issues in the context of cross-border, contemporary identity, see Alfred (2005) and Simpson (2003).

6 Traditional healing refers to local knowledge and practices related to health and healing that have persisted and become reinvigorated in recent decades – despite colonization, confinement to reserves, and historical government efforts to stamp out indigenous culture (Warry 1998). Traditional healing may also include aspects of pan-Indian spirituality that have become integrated into indigenous community life and even into mainstream society – for example, "circle," "healing," smudging, sweat-lodging, and other practices generally associated with the indigenous cultures of the Great Plains (see Waldram 1997; McCormick, Chapter 15).

References

Alfred, T. 2005. *Wasáse: Indigenous pathways to action and freedom*. Peterborough, ON: Broadview Press.

American Psychiatric Association. 2000. *Diagnostic and statistical manual of mental disorders: DSM-IV-TR*. 4th ed. Washington, DC: American Psychiatric Publishing.

Assembly of First Nations. 1994. *Breaking the silence*. Ottawa, ON: Assembly of First Nations Secretariat.

–. March 1998. *Residential school update*. Ottawa, ON: Assembly of First Nations Health Secretariat.

Dickason, O.P. 1993. *Canada's First Nations: A history of founding peoples from earliest times*. Toronto, ON: McClelland and Stewart.

Fournier, S., and E. Crey. 1997. *Stolen from our embrace: The abduction of First Nations children and the restoration of Aboriginal communities*. Vancouver, BC: Douglas and McIntyre.

Johnston, P. 1983. *Native children and the child welfare system*. Toronto, ON: Canadian Council on Social Development, in association with James Lorimer.

Kirmayer, L.J. 2004. The cultural diversity of healing: Meaning, metaphor and mechanism. *British Medical Bulletin* 69 (1): 33-48.

MacMillan, H.L., A.B. MacMillan, D.R. Offord, and J.L. Dingle. 1996. Aboriginal health. *Canadian Medical Association Journal* 155 (11): 1569-78.

Maracle, B. 1996. *Back on the rez: Find the way home*. Toronto, ON: Viking.

Non-Insured Health Benefits (NIHB), First Nations and Inuit Health Branch. 1999. "Preamble." In *Interim program directive no. 7: Mental health services*, 1. Ottawa, ON: Government of Canada.

–. 2000. *1999/2000 annual report*. Ottawa, ON: Government of Canada.

Royal Commission on Aboriginal Peoples. 1995. *Choosing life*. Ottawa, ON: Royal Commission on Aboriginal Peoples.

Shimony, A.A. 1994. *Conservatism among the Iroquois at the Six Nations reserve*. Syracuse, NY: Syracuse University Press.

Simpson, A. 2003. To the reserve and back again: Kahnawake narratives of self, home, and nation. PhD diss., McGill University.

Six Nations Band Council. 1999. *Six Nations of the Grand River Territory*. Ohweken, ON: Six Nations Band Council.

Snow, D.R. 1996. *The Iroquois*. Cambridge, MA: Blackwell.

Standing Senate Committee on Social Affairs, Science and Technology. 2004. Mental illness and addiction policies and programs: The federal framework. In *Mental health, mental illness and addiction: Overview of policies and programs in Canada,* 180. Ottawa, ON: Government of Canada.

Waldram, J.B. 1997. *The way of the pipe: Aboriginal spirituality and symbolic healing in Canadian prisons*. Peterborough, ON: Broadview Press.

–. 2000. The efficacy of traditional medicine: Current theoretical and methodological issues. *Medical Anthropology Quarterly* 14 (4): 603-25.

Warry, W. 1998. *Unfinished dreams: Community healing and the reality of Aboriginal self-government*. Toronto, ON: University of Toronto Press.

Weaver, S.M. 1978. Six Nations of the Grand River, Ontario. In B.G. Trigger, ed., *Handbook of North American Indians,* vol. 15, *Northeast*, 525-36. Washington, DC: Smithsonian Institution.

19

Encountering Professional Psychology: Re-Envisioning Mental Health Services for Native North America

JOSEPH P. GONE

In the late 1870s, with the imminent closing of the western frontier, a "humanitarian" reform movement occasioned a dramatic shift in United States Indian policy. In contrast to the prevailing assumption that Western civilization must inevitably extinguish the "savage" inhabitants of the North American continent, "progressive" visionaries such as Captain Richard Henry Pratt – an Army officer initially appointed to oversee Apache prisoners at St. Augustine, Florida – sought instead to demonstrate that Native peoples could be effectively socialized into "civilized" habits under carefully controlled conditions (Adams 1995). The result of this bold experiment was the creation of a federal education policy for American Indians that dispatched Christian missionary organizations to the far reaches of the western frontier to school the wild Redman in the habits of enlightened American society (albeit principally for occupational roles judged appropriate to the Indian's station). Comparable efforts were undertaken during this same historical moment to assimilate First Nations peoples into Euro-Canadian society, with mutual influence on federal policy across the 49th parallel attested to by the report of Nicholas Flood Davin in 1879 (Miller 1996; Milloy 1999). For the next several decades, Native students who arrived at these missionary schools were stripped of any clothing and personal property, shorn of their too-long hair, dressed in Army uniforms, schooled in military drill and the industrial arts, and forbidden to speak any language but English on penalty of brutal corporal punishment. The catastrophic consequences of this policy (in which the US and Canadian federal governments openly subsidized missionary outreach by underwriting mandatory parochial education with public monies) require little elaboration for Native audiences today since the vestiges of these educational experiences – both psychological and material – still influence many of our home communities in profound ways. Certainly, the unifying slogan for these assimilative efforts, inspired by Captain Pratt himself, seemed prosaically descriptive of the enterprise at hand: "Kill the Indian, Save the Man."

Over a century later, most contemporary Tribal communities no longer fret about the Christian missionaries in their midst, as church influence is no longer wedded to the coercive power of the nation-state. Nevertheless, there are frequently instructive insights to be gleaned from cursory historical analysis. Indeed, what seems so remarkable about the missionary education complex of the late nineteenth century is that an explicit campaign of cultural eradication, coupled with coercive socialization into mainstream American and

Canadian cultural mores, was embraced and supported by *progressive humanitarians,* all in the name of *helping* the indigenous North American to *adjust* or *adapt* to quite challenging societal circumstances. In hindsight, of course, even the casual observer might readily critique the unjust colonial purposes served by the so-called progressive policies of the time, which never once interrogated the supremacist ideology that suffused the historical American and Canadian discourses of "civilization strategies" and the "Indian problem." Nonetheless, although there can be no doubt that federal policies (and the political and ideological agendas that motivate them) relative to these countries' enduring "Indian problem" have shifted dramatically in our contemporary era, as a Native person – and more specifically, as a Gros Ventre person from the United States – I remain committed to vigilant analysis and critique. Such vigilance is necessary because North America's indigenous communities still struggle for self-determination and cultural survival in an increasingly globalized world and because the US and Canadian nation-states, through their agents and agendas, still police and patrol these struggles (Jaimes 1992).

If the colonizing campaigns undertaken through church and school are no longer fashionable in America and Canada at the opening of the twenty-first century, a more recent constellation of progressive humanitarians – once again bound together in the name of helping indigenous North Americans to better adjust or adapt to challenging societal circumstances – continues to expand its influence in Native lives and communities through what might be loosely termed the "psy-fields" (Ward 2002) or the "mental health" professions. I myself am trained as a clinical psychologist and obtained my doctorate following nearly 13 years of higher education in 2001. Throughout those years, visits home to my Tribal community on the Fort Belknap reservation in Montana always presented me with a bit of a dilemma. Typically, community members inquired about my lengthy course of study in graduate school, and when I explained that I was training to become a psychologist, I immediately elicited suspicious glances and awkward jokes about "psychos" and "couches" and "mind reading." I suppose that Native North Americans are not the only people in the United States and Canada to glance askance when in the presence of a psychologist, but what does seem unique about American Indian and First Nations responses to psychology and the other psy-fields is the recognition by Native people that these endeavours are culturally alien approaches to understanding human behaviour (Gone 2003, 2006b, forthcoming b; Gone and Alcántara 2006). That is, these fields of inquiry are built on *ways of knowing* that are completely foreign to indigenous thought and practice in this hemisphere. These ways of knowing are not *our* ways of knowing – indeed, as I have already noted, many of our ancestors were forcibly taught to think in these alien ways as compulsory students in government or religious boarding schools. Nevertheless, these foreign ways of knowing now dominate the world in which many of us live, and Native people throughout the Americas have encountered psychology, psychiatry, mental health, and human services whether we wanted to or not. The anxious responses I elicited from people at home when they learned of my study of psychology suggested to me that the members of my community were still uncomfortable with the intrusion of psychology into their world.

I suspect that many Native people within the mental health professions also experience some discomfort with the intrusion of psychology and psychotherapy into our worlds, and I wish to propose that within this discomfort lies the key to envisioning a completely different kind of delivery system for mental health services. Thus I aspire to unpack here a few facets of this Native discomfort with the psy-disciplines – and especially psychology – beginning with a handful of personal and professional observations that I originally formulated during my graduate training. In so doing, I doubt that much of what I write here will be new to most Native mental health professionals. Even so, we rarely seem to openly discuss these matters, as though we are afraid that powerful outsiders, when confronted with our misgivings, might take away our hard-earned credentials. But outsiders, too – especially those in positions of authority with regard to the formulation, funding, delivery, and evaluation of mental health services – need to hear our misgivings in order to improve their efforts at effectively assisting and serving our communities. Thus the observations and recommendations I wish to summarize in this chapter have emerged from the paradoxes and contradictions that I have observed within the Native professional community – and more specifically, within the community of Native psychologists – concerned with indigenous mental health. First, I will examine why Native people bother to endure years of culturally alienating graduate education in order to become professional psychologists. Second, I will ponder why some American Indian and First Nations professionals express disdain for the scientific foundations of psychological practice while simultaneously embracing a wide variety of theoretical concepts that would seem to depend on science for their validity. Finally, I will explore how both Native and non-Native psychologists might maintain a unique role in the mental health service sector by cultivating effective alternatives to conventional therapeutic services for indigenous peoples. Note also that as an American Indian who is most familiar with the relevant professional issues in the United States, several of my examples and illustrations draw on details from the American context in particular, although political, professional, and institutional parallels in Canada will ensure, I hope, relevance for First Nations, Inuit, and Métis communities as well.

The Cultural Perils of Graduate Education for Native North America

The evident discomfort with psychology that I have observed in my own community reflects in part a Native discomfort with mainstream education more generally (Deloria 1991). The institution of formal education as we now know it in the United States and Canada is a "Western" invention and is thus understood, from the perspective of many Native people, to be adopted from our conquerors (Noriega 1992). Such formal education is clearly foreign to indigenous worldviews insofar as 30,000 years in this hemisphere produced nothing remotely resembling it. Furthermore, our experience of Western education is marked by great ambivalence. On the one hand, the colonial projects that became the United States and Canada required some form of resolution to their perennial "Indian problem," and the formal education of Native children was a primary strategy to effect civilization among the "savages" in stark assimilationist terms. On the other hand, a formal Western education is increasingly essential to finding a sustainable place within the contemporary globalized economy, and Native communities, like so many others, do not wish to be left behind. The result is a longstanding conundrum for many Native people regarding the utility and value of a Western education: under what conditions do education's vocational prospects compensate for its assimilationist transformations?

Between a Rock and a Hard Place

With regard to mainstream education, then, Native people recognize that we are caught between a rock and hard place, for learning to think like a "whiteman" forever alters the kinds of cultural experiences available to a formally educated Native person. That is, no matter how much we appreciate the concept of biculturalism (LaFromboise, Coleman, and Gerton 1993), once we learn to think certain kinds of thoughts, there is ultimately no going back to an (ab)original state of mind, as though we had never encountered such transformative ideas and perspectives. Once we learn, for example, as psychologists and other social scientists do, how to "objectify" people by studying their experiences in terms of detached and abstract concepts, there can be no complete return to experiencing social life without the occasional intrusion of such detached and abstract analysis. Perhaps a more subtle example involves the languages we speak. In the face of declining fluency in our traditional language, I have often heard my own Elders insist that our culture is in the language. By this, I take them to mean that language itself structures our thinking and knowing (and thus the "reality" that is crafted through these human activities) in nearly invisible but extraordinarily profound ways – an idea known in academic circles as the Sapir-Whorf linguistic-relativity hypothesis (Lucy 1992). Thus merely learning to speak and think in English circumscribes Native experience in ways that can never fully capture what our experience might have been if we were fluent only in our traditional languages. As professionals of any kind, then, we as Native people must acknowledge along with our Elders that formal education forever eradicates the possibility for certain kinds of cultural experiences. There is no getting around it: learning to think like a whiteman in the process of formal education necessarily implies some inability to think like our ancestors did. Thus the education of Native people in North America cannot help but invoke the colonial dynamics that originally sought the eradication of our cultures (Adams 1995; Miller 1996; Milloy 1999). And graduate training of any kind, including that in psychology, social work, counselling, or the other mental health professions is no exception.

Note here that I assume that contemporary formal education in the United States and Canada remains assimilative for contemporary Native peoples. Certainly, this is true for the underfunded public schools in the reservation bordertown of Harlem near my home reservation, in which white teachers send their own children to all-white schools in adjacent counties so they might escape the contaminating influence of the Native students they teach. But this is also true for tribally controlled educational institutions that depend on public monies and accreditation for their operation, in which curricula and pedagogy remain responsive to imposed expectations. In either case, Native students are schooled in the use of math, science, and English; socialized into prescribed modes of interpersonal interaction; channelled into certain vocational pipelines; and transformed into specific kinds of persons that even the Elders in their own communities can have difficulty recognizing. Not surprisingly, most Native people never arrive at university campuses to commence postsecondary education, and of those who do, disproportionate numbers never complete their undergraduate degrees (US Department of Education 1991). So, although I acknowledge that formal education within our respective countries has indeed evolved in many respects beyond the bald assimilationist agendas that structured it in the days of our grandparents, what remains continues to fail too many of our peoples in systematic and predictable ways.

Nonetheless, if the ideological perils of formal education burden us on the one hand, the driving need to control our own destinies as indigenous peoples in the modern world presses us on the other. For as my grandmother often reminds me in an ironically adopted idiom, there is no use in "crying over spilled milk." The history of Euro-American and Euro-Canadian subjugation of our peoples is a fait accompli (although always throughout this colonial enterprise there has been indigenous resistance). The milk is spilled, and we need sensibly to find alternative nourishment the best way that we can. Although the colonial pressures of formal education are indeed oppressive, the costs to our communities of allowing cultural outsiders to determine our collective fates are more oppressive still. And within the dominant society, the path to community control and self-determination is paved with the skills, experiences, and especially the credentials of formal education. Thus Native people are indeed between a rock and a hard place. If we truly desire to control our own destinies and preserve our cultures, formal education is nearly essential. But the requisite educational experiences transform us in permanent ways, forever altering our ability to participate in and reproduce for future generations certain cultural processes and practices that we otherwise struggle so ardently to preserve. It is this dilemma, and the discomfort produced by it, that each of us as indigenous persons must confront and negotiate.

Nowhere has this dilemma been more salient to me than at the annual conventions of American Indian psychologists and psychology graduate students convened by professor of psychology Carolyn Barcus (Blackfeet) and sponsored by Utah State University and the Indian Health Service for nearly two decades running. During my previous attendances at these conventions, I have benefited tremendously from the presence of many people who have come to be called the "Elders" of Indian psychology. Their wisdom and encouragement were invaluable to me during the formative years of my professional development and (in part) have inspired the words offered for your consideration here. Indeed, I have observed several interesting paradoxes in the words and lives of these professional pioneers, contradictions that emerge from their historical positions at the enigmatic confluence of mainstream education and cultural tradition. These contradictions are in no way unique to these Elders, for as my introductory observations suggest, all of us as Native people labouring or training in the academy or the professions must navigate the same thorny path. Nevertheless, as I look toward a professional psychology with relevance for Native communities in the twenty-first century, it stands to reason that younger indigenous psychologists must stand upon the shoulders of our forebears in order to see all the more clearly into the not-so-distant future. We can start by considering the many paradoxes that have shaped their lives and their careers as psychologists and that will surely shape ours.

The Relevance of Psychology Training?

One significant paradox that I have observed among Native psychologists at our annual conventions is a wry cynicism or even open disdain for the many years of Western education that these individuals completed in order to become practising professionals. This cynicism is not infrequently expressed in terms of the perceived irrelevance of both psychological science and psychological practice for our peoples. In fact, I remember one of our Elders of Indian psychology admonishing that if Native people want to be effective healers in our communities, we should learn at home from our own medicine people rather than embarking upon doctoral careers in psychology. This question merits further scrutiny: if graduate training in psychology is neither readily accessible nor culturally relevant for Native people, why do Tribal members pursue such training, and why do Indians and non-Indians alike in the United States (including the US Congress through its legislation of "Indians into Psychology" training programs) support efforts to recruit more Natives into the discipline?

There can be no question that doctoral education in psychology – and graduate education in general – is typically inaccessible to Indian and Aboriginal people. A host of societal factors, ranging from inadequate educational preparation to lack of adequate financial resources, conspire to ensure that most Native people could not undertake professional training in psychology even if they wanted to. In addition to these factors, however, is the perceived cultural incongruity of psychology for Native lives (Gone 2003, 2004b, 2006c, 2007, forthcoming a). I will elaborate further on this incongruity shortly, but observe here that psychological theory and practice depend on overt or covert conceptualizations of what it means to be a person living in relationship to other persons and one's milieu. I suspect it is obvious that the ways that mainstream psychology conceptualizes the person contrast markedly with the ways that our peoples have traditionally conceptualized the person (Anderson 2001; Hallowell 1955, 1976; Straus 1977; Kirmayer, Fletcher, and Watt Chapter 13). It is no wonder, then, that Western psychology seems irrelevant to the concerns of many indigenous communities.

So why is it that Native psychologists find it useful and important to complete graduate study in psychology? Speaking as a recently minted Indian psychologist, allow me to suggest that we do so primarily because doctoral training in psychology results in credentials that the dominant society recognizes. This recognition of credentials in turn allows us as Native people to assert greater control over the futures of our communities. Thus our graduate training in psychology is an important contribution to the larger project of Tribal self-determination. In pursuing these credentials, however, it is important that we never forget that they come at a price: in obtaining them, we have all "majored" in "White Studies"

(Churchill 1995), and majoring in White Studies changes us in the process. Nevertheless, especially in societies (and a world) so heavily structured by inequality, autonomy and opportunity may be the greatest antidotes to ongoing vulnerability to exploitation and oppression. Thus it may be that beyond the merely vocational and assimilationist functions of Western education lies a third alternative: the possibility for an education that *liberates* people from these vulnerabilities. This promise of a liberal education has deep roots in the West, grounded as it is in a philosophical liberalism that champions individual rights and the autonomous pursuit of happiness. Such grounding is undoubtedly assimilationist for many Native communities. However, by seeking to cultivate customary modes of critical reason and analytic engagement as a means to anchor authoritative knowing within the individual, a liberal education is likely to equip any oppressed and marginalized community with habits of mind and conduits of critique that – at least insofar as formal education can serve such purposes – hold the highest promise for enabling communities to exercise autonomy and realize a more just and meaningful world. Beyond this, of course, are more politically radical educational projects that are overtly dedicated to community building and consciousness raising, but these remain largely unavailable for Native peoples. In the end, I promote the more familiar ideals of liberal education as my own rationale/ rationalization – I leave it to individual Natives and their communities to determine whether the price of such assimilative transformations is too high to pay.

The one thing of which I am certain is that, once Native psychologists have obtained the PhD, we have an obligation to our communities to do much more and much differently than the average Euro-American or Euro-Canadian psychologist. And although I will describe my specific vision for psychologists who work with Native people in more detail later, I will assert here that, in my opinion, we cannot afford to obtain our doctorates primarily to practise individual psychotherapy in our communities. In this regard, I agree with the view expressed by an Elder of Indian psychology at one of our previous conferences: if your primary goal is to relieve individual distress and restore individual lives within indigenous communities, then become a medicine person or traditional healer – we simply need something different from our doctoral psychologists. Finally, let me conclude this discussion by confessing to some ambivalence about our efforts to recruit more Native people into doctoral-level training in psychology. In my mind, the benefits to American Indian or First Nations people of their recruitment into and retention in psychology depend on the *kind* of psychology for which they are recruited (Gone 2004a); both the mainstream discipline of psychology and future cohorts of Native students deserve a more thorough appraisal of the substantive implications of endorsing and embracing doctoral training programs for Natives in psychology.

The Utility of Psychological Science for Native North America

A second notable paradox I have encountered among Native psychologists involves the simultaneous adoption of a frank skepticism toward the scientific principles and methods of psychology on the one hand and an uncritical acceptance of a wide variety of prevailing theories and concepts from the discipline on the other. Thus it is not exceptional in our midst to dismiss even well-established research findings on the basis of our mistrust of the scientific enterprise while concurrently and routinely referencing concepts like "codependency," "addictive personality," "defence mechanisms," "chemical imbalance," "suicidality," "intergenerational trauma," "anger discharge," "assertiveness training," "communication skills," "mental health," and so forth. The irony here lies in our circulation of culturally foreign ideas and concepts in our communities, resulting in some instances in the unintentional displacement of already-disappearing indigenous concepts and understandings, together with a simultaneous rejection of the scientific basis on which such foreign concepts empirically stand or fall. I hasten to add, however, that this contradiction is not exclusive to practising Native psychologists but evident in similar form among psychological practitioners of many backgrounds and commitments (Tavris 2003). In fact, it is the dismissive attitude of many practising psychologists toward the scientific foundations of their profession that led almost two decades ago to the fracture of the disciplinary guild in the United States into the well-established American Psychological Association and the break-away American Psychological Society (now the Association for Psychological Science). Thus I posit another question for consideration: If we as Native professionals do not trust the scientific foundations of psychology as a discipline, how can we then proselytize our communities with abstract theories and concepts that otherwise emerge from a Western understanding of the "psyche"?

The Profound Implications of Divergent Ethnotheories

I mentioned earlier that psychology as an academic and professional discipline is grounded in Western ways of knowing. That is, most academic psychologists esteem a methodology of inquiry grounded in both inductive and deductive reasoning: we first propose theoretical explanations for human behaviour and then test the validity of these hypothesized explanations through careful empirical investigation (Campbell and Fiske 1959; Cronbach and Meehl 1955). For psychologists, then, the value of any given theoretical construct (e.g., "repression") supposedly depends on the kind and quality of evidence obtained in support (as opposed to refutation) of these hypothesized entities. The history of professional psychology in particular, however, demonstrates that theoretical constructs may persist in the complete absence of systematic empirical tests of their validity. For example, certain hydraulic models of the mind initially popularized by psychoanalysis continue to wield influence in modern professional psychology despite their persistent resistance to scientific study (for exceptions, see Luborsky and Barrett 2006; for critiques of Freudian theory more generally, see Crews 1996, 1998). In sum, a variety of theoretical concepts are influential in psychology that either resist scientific validation or presuppose it (pending further investigation).

These prevalent (but untested) theoretical constructs owe their un- or underwarranted professional proliferation not to any corpus of compelling scientific evidence demonstrating their explanatory power but to their resonance with the experiences, approaches, traditions, and practices of the clinicians who endorse them. Given the cultural orientations of these professionals and the cultural origins of the therapeutic traditions they embrace, it should come as no surprise that most of these concepts are typically derived from modern Western notions about mind, body, and person (which are perhaps most appropriately designated "ethnotheories" of mind and behaviour). Moreover, such Western ethnotheories not infrequently contradict Tribal ethnotheories concerning mind, body, and person. For example, one set of Western ethnotheories evident in the mental health professions tacitly posits an authentic or "true" self buried deep within each of us that is naturally inclined to unique individual expression and thus lies in wait of recognition and actualization through introspection, communication, achievement, and interpersonal validation (Ward 2002). In contrast, my own community (as but one concrete example) still tends to configure wellness (i.e., life lived "in a good way") much differently than the "mental health" of professional psychology, emphasizing respectful relationships instead of egoistic individualism and the ritual circulation of sacred power instead of the liberating enlightenment of secular humanism (Gone 1999, 2006a, 2008a, 2008b, forthcoming c; Gone, Miller, and Rappaport 1999). Such comparisons are readily apparent to most Native people familiar with the mental health professions and illuminate cultural divergences in multiple arenas in regard to "ethnopsychology": mind-body dualism versus "holistic wellness," the significance of secular versus sacred therapeutic orientations, the ascription of illness and dysfunction to endogenous rather than interpersonal causes, and so on (for additional reviews of these and other salient cultural contrasts, see LaFromboise, Trimble, and Mohatt 1990; McShane 1987; Trimble et al. 1984).

Since mainstream professional understandings would appear to contradict our complex Tribal ethnopsychologies in many significant ways, my view is that embracing and disseminating Western concepts in indigenous communities when there is no valid scientific reason to do so is counterproductive to cultural preservation and reproduction – indeed, doing so arguably represents an extension of the Euro-American and Euro-Canadian colonial enterprises. Instead, psychologists and other mental health practitioners need to collaborate more closely with the communities we serve in order to conceptualize culturally appropriate theories of the person and to employ these in designing alternative programs and services that are directly tailored to the experiences of Native peoples. Proper attention to these Tribal ethnopsychologies will guarantee that services fit the prevailing cultural norms, including those that govern communication and interpersonal interaction.

So, for example, we cannot design a culturally appropriate intervention for Native communities without first understanding in normative terms who talks with whom about what and under which circumstances (for examples of such analysis, see Basso 1990; Carbaugh 2005; Darnell and Foster 1988; Philips 1983; Sherzer and Woodbury 1987). In some important sense, then, all of us need to become "cultural" psychologists (Shweder 1991; Shweder and Sullivan 1993), attentive to the subtle but formative nuances of the predominant cultural practices and traditions within Native communities. In so doing, we will come to realize that "culture" is much more than participation in ceremony or fluency in traditional language – in fact, cultural practices comprise the almost invisible participation in shared thought and activity that need never be conscious since most people in the community are socialized into such routines. Whether psychologists learn these things as Native people living in our own communities or simply as advocates and professionals working within these settings, we are together assured that our majors in "White Studies" will not typically expose us to such matters in graduate school.

The Pressing Relevance of Scientific Epistemology

I am thus critical of the tendency for Native psychologists to adopt a host of professionally salient concepts, categories, principles, and practices – many of which persist solely because of their resonance with Western ethnopsychology as opposed to their scientific validity – without directly confronting the ideological implications of disseminating these Western cultural artifacts within Native communities. But I have also noted the reluctance of Native mental health professionals to embrace a scientific epistemology, owing to both its Western origins and its association with the colonial legacy. What, then, are we to make of the scientific enterprise itself, clearly another Western way of knowing? Before addressing this question, I must turn briefly to matters of definition. It is of course rather challenging to characterize scientific knowing with any precision given the wide range of approaches adopted by scientists of all sorts, ranging from paleontologists to particle physicists and from astronomers to evolutionary anthropologists. Nevertheless, by "scientific epistemology" I simply mean a way of knowing that privileges systematic inquiry involving the precise, investigator-independent measurement of observables that is progressively or cumulatively employed to evaluate falsifiable theoretical explications of a phenomenon. By "investigator-independent" I simply mean that such observations are dependent on the particular method used to obtain them as opposed to the particular specialist who obtains them and that any competent specialist should be able to reproduce the observations in question. Thus, for example, psychological scientists aspire to determine whether a specified clinical intervention does or does not result in the therapeutic effects claimed by the intervention's proponents using one form of scientific inquiry – the experiment – that purportedly lends itself to the establishment of reliable causal attributions (for much more detail, see Gone and Alcántara 2007).

Returning then to the question of scientific inquiry vis-à-vis the colonial legacy, there are at least two approaches that Native psychologists might adopt with regard to the scientific basis of our discipline. One is to reject a scientific epistemology as a legitimate way of knowing about human behaviour and interaction (especially in terms of causal attribution). This position could either assert that (a) scientific knowing is inherently unsuitable for assessing causal claims in the world (an assertion sufficiently contradicted, I think, by everyday technology) or that (b) human behaviour and interaction are not amenable to scientific study, particularly when it comes to causal questions (which implies, of course, that all that remains of psychology are Western ethnotheories). I reject both of these characterizations, although many Native psychologists do not. A second approach, one that I personally embrace, is that scientific knowing is *probably all that recommends psychology as a profession*

(McFall 1991, 1996, 2000; Meehl 1997). More specifically, I believe that the application of scientific methods may be the only way for human beings to establish reliable causal attribution when it comes to the evaluation of certain complex but pressing causal claims (Campbell and Stanley 1963). Thus, in contrast to the professional tendency I have observed among many Native psychologists, I am persuaded of the utility of a scientific epistemology for improving Native lives (James 2002) even as I remain skeptical of the utility of incorporating the latest clinical theories and techniques into Native service-delivery settings.

Of course, none of this is intended to assert that a scientific epistemology is the only means to know the world – indeed, an overzealous scientism would actually cripple the important work required of professional psychologists working in American Indian and First Nations communities. Instead, scientific methods are merely tools that remain available to mental health professionals for exploring certain kinds of significant questions. And despite their Western origins, these methodological tools – liberated of much of their former ideology in our postpositivist age – may have demonstrated a universal applicability for certain purposes that appears to transcend culture and time (for a discussion relevant to clinical contexts, see Meehl 1997). For my purposes here, a scientific epistemology is utterly essential to indigenous "mental health" concerns because any effective (post)colonial efforts to render psychology useful to Native communities must be methodologically equipped to establish causal claims grounded in alternative ethnopsychologies. This would seem especially important in the context of clinical intervention, where practice frequently ventures far ahead of empirical validation and where causal claims are routinely asserted yet typically remain inadequately tested – recent examples include the alleged benefits of Thought Field Therapy (Beutler 2001) and Eye-Movement Desensitization and Reprocessing (Herbert et al. 2000). As a result, the scientific foundations of psychology deserve far greater emphasis within Native-community contexts than the latest assemblage of theoretically driven concepts that routinely suffuse clinical intervention. Instead of importing and embracing Western ethnotheoretical notions and their attendant practices, mental health professionals serving Native North Americans ought to be struggling with how best to tailor a scientific epistemology to the grassroots efforts of Tribal communities that seek to more effectively combat distress and promote wellness among our peoples.

As mental health professionals, we routinely encounter a host of causal claims, including the claims of ethnotheories of all kinds – for example, scientology or neurolinguistic programming at the margins of mainstream society, but also the assertions of Native-community advocates and practitioners (Duran 2006). At least some of the more important of these can be either substantiated or not with recourse to scientific methods. Thus, in the context of mental health services for American Indian and First Nations communities specifically, I will provocatively suggest that – at least in comparison to the conventional mental health concepts, categories, principles, and practices that are so clearly grounded in Western ethnopsychology – a rigorous methodological training grounded in a scientific epistemology may be all that recommends psychology as a profession with relevance for Native communities. For even in our postpositivist era, well-trained psychologists are haunted by what Meehl (1997) has referred to as the two searching questions of positivism: "What do you mean?" and "How do you know?" Having said this, however, let me hasten to add that my endorsement here of scientific methods is not an endorsement of *scientism* – I do not think that science can speak meaningfully to many of life's questions, or even to the most important ones. Nevertheless, if scientific psychology cannot equip professionals with useful tools for the assessment of certain theoretical and causal claims – a process with evident utility for all communities, including indigenous ones – then I am not sure that it offers anything useful at all.

Creating a Niche for Professional Psychology in Native North America

A third and final paradox I have observed among Native psychologists concerns the tension between the overwhelming levels of distress in our communities and our professional monopoly in the health care service-delivery market. National epidemiological surveys of the prevalence of mental illness in America have revealed that nearly half the adult American population has suffered from a diagnosable "mental disorder" in the course of their lives (Kessler et al. 2005). Comparable state-of-the-art epidemiological studies of mental disorder within two American Indian reservation communities have identified slightly lower overall prevalence rates for a history of mental disorder in these populations (Beals et al. 2005a), but cross-cultural methodological complexities render the interpretation of these findings somewhat open to speculation (Beals et al. 2005b; Gone 2001; for an overview of the methodological limitations that plague Native mental health research in general, see Waldram 2004; Chapter 3). Nevertheless, few of us need to be persuaded that the lifetime prevalence of diagnosable psychiatric distress in many indigenous communities is much higher than in Middle America or Canada – including, for example, alcohol dependence and posttraumatic stress disorder, which Beals and colleagues (2005a) did find in higher proportions. Yet, as clinical researchers have noted for some decades, the production of psychologists (as well as psychiatrists and every other kind of mental health professional combined) is so gradual that the population of practising professionals will *never* be sufficient to meet the mental health needs of our respective national populations (Albee 1968, 1990), not to mention our indigenous ones, thereby establishing an "infinite insufficiency" of professional therapeutic resources (Gone 2003). If one believes in the efficacy of mental health services for the management of distress in Native lives, it goes without saying that the pace of preparation of mental health professionals is so discordant with the levels of distress in Native communities that it recommends despair (Nelson et al. 1992).

Thus, assuming that the delivery of some form of "mental health" services to indigenous peoples is desirable, anything that we can do to extend and multiply the natural helping resources available in our communities would seem to be the order of the day. Unfortunately, Native psychologists seem subject to the same politics of our professional guild as other psychologists. That is, the more that nonprofessionals are encouraged to provide the kind of services for which our doctoral training has supposedly prepared us, the more likely it is that we will feel insecure about the value of our many years of professional education and experience. The temptation is to preserve our status, salaries, and prestige by excluding all but the few doctoral-level initiates from the important work that we do (although "managed" health care in the United States has helped to ensure otherwise; see Cummings 1995 and McFall 2006). So I submit a final question for consideration: If the low number of mental health professionals – especially Native mental health professionals who presumably have a greater commitment to working in often isolated indigenous settings – can barely begin to meet the needs of our peoples, how might psychologists cultivate and expand the non-professional "mental health" resources available in Native communities without either re-pudiating our years of training and experience or rendering our roles obsolete?

Shifting Professional Roles

The answer to this question depends on a reformulation of what training in professional psychology must be about for future mental health service delivery in Native North America. More specifically, new generations of psychologists with aspirations of relevance for indigenous communities must be equipped not so much for direct delivery of clinical services (such as individual psychotherapy) as for innovative administration, program development, grant writing, outcome assessment, community-based research, local outreach and training, and clinical supervision (McFall 2000). That is, the effective psychologist of the future will act primarily as the steward of a locally tailored community-based service system that cultivates endogenous helping resources already existent in the community and procures additional necessary resources from outside the community. The backbone for this creative facilitation of community-accessible and culturally appropriate helping services will be partnerships with community leaders, traditional healers, and other natural helpers. These partnerships will enable professionals to learn about potentially effective therapeutic practices already employed in the community while concurrently contributing additional resources, professional legitimacy, and helpful organizational structures toward the wider availability and success of these local therapeutic efforts. Other helping interventions may need to be developed from the ground up in cultural terms and then evaluated and revised as necessary in response to measured outcomes. Still others may be locally tailored versions of more familiar professional approaches, depending on the evidence in support of their efficacy and the community's willingness to vet such activities for local relevance. These diverse skills in administration, program development, outcome evaluation, clinical supervision, and community collaboration are skills that professional psychologists should learn in the course of their graduate preparation – owing to our mandatory training in research, no other mental health professional stands as ready to develop such skills as the doctoral-level psychologist.

Additional implications of this shift in professional role are worthy of further consideration as we envision future "mental health" service systems with greater relevance for Native North America. First, professional psychologists trained at the doctoral level and bound for service in Native communities need only rarely see "clients" in individual psychotherapy during the majority of their postdoctoral careers. In fact, given the overwhelming levels of distress in Native communities and the incredible scarcity of professionals trained at the doctoral level who serve Native people, it may be time to consider whether it is actually ethical for psychologists to spend most of their time conducting individual psychotherapy in Native communities. Coincidentally, rapid shifts in health care policy are quickly rendering the practice of psychotherapy by doctorally trained clinicians less viable in the United States (Cummings 1995; McFall 2006). Thus, in America at least, psychologists in "Indian country" may now be able to assume their proper roles as creative administrators, program developers, local researchers, and clinical supervisors while reserving the therapeutic activities for compassionate and competent individuals with different skill sets and less-costly credentials. This necessarily implies that professional psychologists must obtain the necessary skills in their graduate training to be effective at program development, outcome assessment, and effective administration as a matter of course, and I therefore have recommended that such skills take precedence over training in psychotherapy within doctoral-level psychology education.

As an aside, I should note briefly that rather extensive scientific inquiry during the past few decades has examined the question of whether doctoral training and pre- and post-doctoral clinical experience lead to improved clinical outcomes for psychotherapy clients (Berman and Norton 1985; Bickman 1999; Christensen and Jacobson 1994; Durlak 1979; Hattie, Sharpley, and Rogers 1984; Landman and Dawes 1982; Smith and Glass 1977; Stein and Lambert 1984; Strupp and Hadley 1979). Interestingly, the assumption that higher levels of professional training and experience would lead to better therapeutic outcomes has not been borne out in the literature: professors, students, community members, and even computers (Selmi et al. 1990) with rather limited backgrounds in psychology or clinical practice have been proven to function as effective therapists for many people in distress. Instead of threatening our professional livelihoods, however, such scientific findings are cause for inspiration among credentialed psychologists who serve Native communities, for at the very least they promise a future with much greater availability of therapeutic resources than marginalized indigenous communities utilizing conventional service-delivery models can presently muster.

Keeping Culture in Mind

A second implication worthy of elaboration as we envision future "mental health" service systems with greater relevance for Native North America concerns the cultural appropriateness of conventional therapeutic activities for indigenous communities. I have already noted that professional psychologists within indigenous communities ought to conceptualize culturally appropriate theories of the person in an effort to ensure that local services are tailored to existing cultural norms. In this light, I have made reference to psychotherapy somewhat awkwardly, for although there is ample evidence that psychotherapy can be effective for a variety of problems that people might experience (Smith, Glass, and Miller 1980), I am less persuaded of the effectiveness and appropriateness of psychotherapy for Native communities in particular. For one thing, I am aware of no studies demonstrating the efficacy of individual psychotherapy for Native "clients" (Gone and Alcántara 2007), and for another, there seem to be many intimidating cultural barriers to providing therapy to indigenous people, regardless of whether these interventions are proven to reduce symptoms and improve functioning for non-Native people (Gone 2007, 2008a, 2008b, forthcoming c; Gone and Alcántara 2006). For example, I well remember the occasion when an older relative was referred by her physician to the Indian Health Service "behavioural health" staff for emotional support during a time of distress. She described a visit with the social worker for a single session before leaving, never to return. In recounting the incident to me, she laughed while asking, "What could that [young Euro-American] social worker possibly have to say to me?" And in a scene that might seem familiar to many Native mental health professionals, a close family member once approached me for "counselling," explaining that under no conditions would he trust someone outside our family with his difficulties and concerns.

These instances offer a glimpse into the very different worlds in which many Native people live. I have already argued that as highly educated professionals in tense (post)colonial contexts, we have the special obligation to attend very carefully to these cultural worlds prior to imposing Western psychological practices on suffering, and sometimes desperate, people. This obligation to attend to the cultural worlds of Native communities implies the aforementioned opportunity to discover already-existing therapeutic interventions as well as to develop new ones grounded adequately in the local cultural dynamics. One relevant area of inquiry, for example, with regard to the formulation of culturally tailored therapeutic interventions involves the culturally local experience and expression of emotion. The psychological study of emotion still retains a conceptual bias toward the biophysical and intrapsychic character of affect that affords little room for any primary role of social and cultural processes in the constitution of emotional experience – leading, for example, to Ekman's (1984) six universal, or "basic," human emotions. This perspective fails to recognize, however, that emotional experience is simultaneously constituted by the symbolic meanings and social interactions that render such experience intelligible in the context of human communities (Harre 1986; Kitayama and Markus 1994; Leavitt 1996; Lutz and White 1986; Shweder 1992; Shweder and Haight 1999). As a result, human emotion depends on *both* biology and culture for its realization in the lives of persons: without the requisite biology, humans would have nothing to interpret and meaningfully represent as emotion; without the requisite enculturation, humans would have only bodily sensations and perturbations with no symbolic framework of meaning to render them intelligible to self and others. The result is a fantastic diversity in emotional experience and expression around the world, and Native North America is no exception. Perhaps the best-documented instances of these divergences in the context of psychological functioning or "mental health" concerns in Native communities are Briggs' (1970) ethnography of Inuit emotion and O'Nell's (1996) exploration of Salish "loneliness" and depression.

In any case, the development of truly appropriate interventions will necessarily require that psychologists working in Native communities attain actual competency in "thinking through cultures" (Shweder 1991) – that is, in the conceptualization and exploration of cultural practice and process in social life (Gone and Kirmayer 2008). In my mind, beyond the standard variable-analytic statistical procedures that psychologists typically master in their graduate training, such competency requires professional familiarity with qualitative or interpretive methods (see, for example, Denzin and Lincoln 2005); never again should culture be considered as merely an independent variable (Valsiner 1996). Furthermore, the effective psychologist in Native North America will learn to engage and involve a variety of community leaders, cultural authorities, ritual practitioners, and natural helpers to guide our work, recognizing that the end results of our collaboration may bear little resemblance to conventional psychotherapy. And finally, we must not forget that we owe Tribal communities a systematic assessment of outcomes for these novel interventions developed in close collaboration with local community members.

Expanding Therapeutic Resources

Once we have identified or developed culturally resonant helping services for Native communities, we can then begin to expand the availability of these resources. Such expansion will necessarily require more person power. Thus a final implication worthy of elaboration as we envision future "mental health" service systems with greater relevance for Native North America concerns the cultivation and development of presently untapped human resources for the relief of distress in indigenous communities. It remains for professional psychologists to identify local people with proven track records in helping others through crisis and distress. Once such people have been identified, we might then muster our resources to support these individuals in the very efforts for which they have already demonstrated proficiency. One place to start may be within the nucleus of American Indian or First Nation life, the extended family. Extended families in Native North America have survived untold hardship over past decades (and in some cases, centuries), so it stands to reason that professional psychologists should attempt to cultivate family relationships as one important source of strength. One way to do so might be to facilitate the abilities of already-supportive members in each extended family to better assist their relatives in times of trouble. A second pool of untapped resources is the many students who matriculate at tribally controlled (or other nearby) community colleges in human-services curricula. At the University of Illinois, where I was a graduate student, the psychology department administered a Mental Health Workers Program consisting of trained undergraduates who receive academic credit for assisting members of the community in times of distress or crisis. There is no reason why similar programs could not also be developed within tribally controlled community colleges.

A third pool of untapped resources is the adolescent population in Native communities. Adolescents in Native North America clearly face great challenges in their transitions to adulthood (for a review of challenges facing American Indian adolescents, see Office of Technology Assessment 1990), and the formation of a culturally grounded peer support system does not seem out of reach for many indigenous communities. Perhaps we might even facilitate the establishment and nurturance of adolescent cultural societies (think of these as prosocial "gangs") that would create a mentored context for our youth to exercise autonomy, respect, reciprocity, and influential relationships with their Elders; such support systems might displace the antisocial gang activity that seems to be on the rise in too many of our communities. A fourth resource pool is the myriad participants in a variety of self-help groups in Native communities. These groups already thrive in many urban and reservation enclaves, providing their membership with an effective, empowering, and cost-effective "intervention" for unmanageable (or sometimes just underfulfilled) lives. Interestingly, the psychological benefits of many self-help endeavours have been empirically demonstrated (Gould and Clum 1993; Scogin et al. 1990). The list could go on and on, for the cultivation of untapped resources within Native communities is limited only by our energy and imagination. Clearly, Native communities stand to gain a great deal when professional psychologists move out of the clinic and apply our talents and expertise to the facilitation and expansion of alternative and natural helping systems that rely on nonprofessional community members for their design, availability, and efficacy (Rappaport and Seidman 1983).

Conclusion

I have summarized three paradoxes or contradictions that I have observed among Native professionals in psychology and have examined each with regard to its implications for the future of mental health services in indigenous communities. I have noted that despite the cultural incongruity of graduate education in psychology, Native professionals obtain degrees and credentials to maintain control of our own destinies (and perhaps to cultivate habits of critical and liberating inquiry). I have also asserted that we cannot reject the scientific basis of psychology and the mental health professions while simultaneously adopting and disseminating in Native communities various psychological concepts established in Western ethnopsychology. Finally, I have observed that Native professionals cannot afford to protect the privileges of our guild at the expense of greater person power in service systems of the future. Rather, the professional psychologist who aspires to future relevance in Native North America must instead act primarily as administrator, program developer, researcher, and facilitator in the discovery and expansion of culturally appropriate, demonstrably effective helping services. Progress in establishing such services for indigenous communities will require of psychologists (1) professional skills other than psychotherapy, (2) conceptual approaches that afford insight into extant cultural resources, and (3) enduring commitments to expanding the effectiveness and availability of people involved within these community-responsive helping systems. It is my concentrated wish that these words will help us to eschew the road of the so-called progressive and humanitarian assimilationist educators of the nineteenth century and thereby stimulate development of an alternative vision for mental health service delivery in Native North American communities of the twenty-first century.

Acknowledgment

This chapter was completed during the author's tenure as the Katrin H. Lamon fellow at the School for Advanced Research on the Human Experience in Santa Fe, New Mexico.

References

Adams, D.W. 1995. *Education for extinction: American Indians and the boarding school experience*. Lawrence, KS: University Press of Kansas.

Albee, G.W. 1968. Conceptual models and manpower requirements in psychology. *American Psychologist* 23: 317-20.

–. 1990. The futility of psychotherapy. *The Journal of Mind and Behavior* 11 (3): 369-84.

Anderson, J.D. 2001. *The four hills of life: Northern Arapahoe knowledge and life movement*. Lincoln, NE: University of Nebraska Press.

Basso, K.H. 1990. *Western Apache language and culture: Essays in linguistic anthropology*. Tucson, AZ: University of Arizona Press.

Beals, J., S.M. Manson, N.R. Whitesell, P. Spicer, D.K. Novins, C.M. Mitchell, for the AI-SUPERPFP Team. 2005a. Prevalence of DSM-IV disorders and attendant help-seeking in 2 American Indian reservation populations. *Archives of General Psychiatry* 62: 99-108.

–, S.M. Manson, N.R. Whitesell, C.M. Mitchell, D.K. Novins, S. Simpson, P. Spicer, and the AI-SUPERPFP Team. 2005b. Prevalence of major depressive episode in two American Indian reservation populations: Unexpected findings with a structured interview. *American Journal of Psychiatry* 162: 1713-22.

Berman, J.S., and N.C. Norton. 1985. Does professional training make a therapist more effective? *Psychological Bulletin* 98 (2): 401-7.

Beutler, L.E. 2001. Thought Field Therapy: Initial research – Editor's introduction. *Journal of Clinical Psychology* 57 (10): 1149-51.

Bickman, L. 1999. Practice makes perfect and other myths about mental health services. *American Psychologist* 54 (11): 965-78.

Briggs, J.L. 1970. *Never in anger: Portrait of an Eskimo family*. Cambridge, MA: Harvard University Press.

Campbell, D.T., and D.W. Fiske. 1959. Convergent and discriminant validation by the multitrait-multimethod matrix. *Psychological Bulletin* 56 (2): 81-105.

–, and J.C. Stanley. 1963. *Experimental and quasi-experimental designs for research*. Boston, MS: Houghton Mifflin.

Carbaugh, D. 2005. *Cultures in conversation*. Mahwah, NJ: Lawrence Earlbaum.

Christensen, A., and N.S. Jacobson. 1994. Who (or what) can do psychotherapy? The status and challenge of nonprofessional therapies. *Psychological Science* 5 (1): 8-14.

Churchill, W. 1995. White Studies: The intellectual imperialism of U.S. higher education. In S. Jackson and J. Solis, eds., *Beyond comfort zones in multiculturalism: Confronting the politics of privilege*, 17-35. Westport, CT: Bergin and Garvey.

Crews, F.C. 1996. The verdict on Freud. *Psychological Science* 7 (2): 63-68.

–, ed. 1998. *Unauthorized Freud: Doubters confront a legend*. New York: Viking.

Cronbach, L.J., and P.E. Meehl. 1955. Construct validity in psychological tests. *Psychological Bulletin* 52: 281-302.

Cummings, N.A. 1995. Impact of managed care on employment and training: A primer for survival. *Professional Psychology: Research and Practice* 26 (1): 10-15.

Darnell, R., and M.K. Foster, eds. 1988. *Native North American interaction patterns*. Ottawa, ON: National Museums of Canada.

Deloria, V., Jr. 1991. *Indian education in America*. Boulder, CO: American Indian Science and Engineering Society.

Denzin, N.K., and Y.S. Lincoln, eds. 2005. *The Sage handbook of qualitative research*. 3rd ed. Thousand Oaks, CA: Sage.

Duran, E. 2006. *Healing the soul wound: Counseling with American Indians and other Native peoples*. New York: Teacher's College.

Durlak, J. 1979. Comparative effectiveness of paraprofessional and professional helpers. *Psychological Bulletin* 86 (1): 80-92.

Ekman, P. 1984. Expression and the nature of emotion. In K. Scherer and P. Ekman, eds., *Approaches to emotion,* 319-43. Hillsdale, NJ: Erlbaum.

Gone, J.P. 1999. "We were through as Keepers of it": The "Missing Pipe Narrative" and Gros Ventre cultural identity. *Ethos* 27 (4): 415-40.

—. 2001. Affect and its disorders in a northern Plains Indian community: Issues in cross-cultural discourse and diagnosis. *Dissertation Abstracts International* 62 (6): 2957B.

—. 2003. American Indian mental health service delivery: Persistent challenges and future prospects. In J.S. Mio and G.Y. Iwamasa, eds., *Culturally diverse mental health: The challenges of research and resistance,* 211-29. New York: Brunner-Routledge.

—. 2004a. Keeping culture in mind: Transforming academic training in professional psychology for Indian country. In D.A. Mihesuah and A. Cavender Wilson, eds., *Indigenizing the academy: Transforming scholarship and empowering communities,* 124-42. Lincoln, NE: University of Nebraska Press.

—. 2004b. Mental health services for Native Americans in the 21st century United States. *Professional Psychology: Research and Practice* 35 (1): 10-18.

—. 2006a. "As if reviewing his life": Bull Lodge's narrative and the mediation of self-representation. *American Indian Culture and Research Journal* 30 (1): 67-86.

—. 2006b. Mental health, wellness, and the quest for an authentic American Indian identity. In T. Witko, ed., *Mental health care for urban Indians: Clinical insights from Native practitioners,* 55-80. Washington, DC: American Psychological Association.

—. 2006c. Research reservations: Response and responsibility in an American Indian community. *American Journal of Community Psychology* 37 (3-4): 333-40.

—. 2007. "We never was happy living like a Whiteman": Mental health disparities and the postcolonial predicament in American Indian communities. *American Journal of Community Psychology* 40 (3-4): 290-300.

—. 2008a. "I came to tell you of my life": Narrative expositions of "mental health" in an American Indian community. Manuscript submitted for publication.

—. 2008b. Psychotherapy and traditional healing in American Indian cultural contexts: Exploring the prospects for therapeutic integration. Manuscript submitted for publication.

—. Forthcoming a. Introduction: Mental health discourse as Western cultural proselytization. *Ethos,* 36 (3).

—. Forthcoming b. The Pisimweyapiy Counselling Centre: Paving the red road to wellness in northern Manitoba. In J.B. Waldram, ed., *Aboriginal healing in Canada: Studies of therapeutic meaning and practice*. Ottawa, ON: Aboriginal Healing Foundation.

—. Forthcoming c. "So I can be like a Whiteman": The cultural psychology of space and place in American Indian mental health. *Culture and Psychology* 14 (3): 369-99.

—, P.J. Miller, and J. Rappaport. 1999. Conceptual self as normatively oriented: The suitability of past personal narrative for the study of cultural identity. *Culture and Psychology* 5 (4): 371-98.

—, and C. Alcántara. 2006. Traditional healing and suicide prevention in Native American communities: Research and policy considerations. Unpublished report contracted by the Office of Behavioral and Social Sciences Research, National Institutes of Health.

—, and C. Alcántara. 2007. Identifying effective mental health interventions for American Indians and Alaska Natives: A review of the literature. *Cultural Diversity and Ethnic Minority Psychology* 13 (4): 356-63.

—, and L.J. Kirmayer. 2008. On the wisdom of considering culture and context in psychopathology. Manuscript submitted for publication.

Gould, R.A., and G.A. Clum. 1993. A meta-analysis of self-help treatment approaches. *Clinical Psychology Review* 13: 169-86.

Hallowell, A.I. 1955. *Culture and experience*. Philadelphia: University of Pennsylvania Press.

–. 1976. *Contributions to anthropology: Selected papers of A. Irving Hallowell*. Chicago, IL: University of Chicago Press.

Harre, R. 1986. An outline of the social constructionist viewpoint. In R. Harre, ed., *The social construction of emotions*, 2-14. Oxford: Basil Blackwell.

Hattie, J.A., C.F. Sharpley, and H.J. Rogers. 1984. Comparative effectiveness of professional and paraprofessional helpers. *Psychological Bulletin* 95 (33): 534-41.

Herbert, J.D., S.O. Lilienfeld, J.M. Lohr, et al. 2000. Science and pseudoscience in the development of Eye-Movement Desensitization and Reprocessing: Implications for clinical psychology. *Clinical Psychology Review* 20 (8): 945-71.

Jaimes, M.A. 1992. *The state of Native America: Genocide, colonization, and resistance*. Boston, MS: South End.

James, K., ed. 2002. *Science and Native American communities: Legacies of pain, visions of promise*. Lincoln, NE: University of Nebraska Press.

Kessler, R.C., P. Berglund, O. Demler, R. Jin, K.R. Merikangas, and E.E. Walters. 2005. Lifetime prevalence and age-of-onset distributions of DSM-IV disorders in the National Comorbidity Survey Replication. *Archives of General Psychiatry* 62: 593-602.

Kitayama, S., and H.R. Markus. 1994. *Emotion and culture: Empirical studies of mutual influence*. Washington, DC: American Psychological Association.

LaFromboise, T., H.L.K. Coleman, and J. Gerton. 1993. Psychological impact of biculturalism: Evidence and theory. *Psychological Bulletin* 114 (3): 395-412.

–, J.E. Trimble, and G.V. Mohatt. 1990. Counseling intervention and American Indian tradition: An integrative approach. *Counseling Psychologist* 18 (4): 628-54.

Landman, J.T., and R.M. Dawes. 1982. Psychotherapy outcome: Smith and Glass' conclusions stand up to scrutiny. *American Psychologist* 37: 504-16.

Leavitt, J. 1996. Meaning and feeling in the anthropology of emotions. *American Ethnologist* 23 (3): 514-39.

Luborsky, L., and M.S. Barrett. 2006. The history and empirical status of key psychoanalytic concepts. *Annual Review of Clinical Psychology* 2: 1-19.

Lucy, J.A. 1992. *Language diversity and thought: A reformulation of the linguistic relativity hypothesis*. Cambridge: Cambridge University Press.

Lutz, C., and G.M. White. 1986. The anthropology of the emotions. *Annual Review of Anthropology* 15: 405-36.

McFall, R.M. 1991. Manifesto for a science of clinical psychology. *Clinical Psychologist* 44: 75-88.

–. 1996. Making psychology incorruptible. *Applied and Preventive Psychology* 5: 9-15.

–. 2000. Elaborate reflections on a simple manifesto. *Applied and Preventive Psychology* 9: 5-21.

–. 2006. Doctoral training in clinical psychology. *Annual Review of Clinical Psychology* 2: 21-49.

McShane, D. 1987. Mental health and North American Indian/Native communities: Cultural transactions, education, and regulation. *American Journal of Community Psychology* 15 (1): 95-116.

Meehl, P.E. 1997. Credentialed persons, credentialed knowledge. *Clinical Psychology: Science and Practice* 4 (2): 91-98.

Miller, J.R. 1996. *Shingwauk's vision: A history of Native residential schools*. Toronto, ON: University of Toronto Press.

Milloy, J.S. 1999. *"A national crime": The Canadian government and the residential school system, 1879-1986*. Winnipeg, MB: University of Manitoba Press.

Nelson, S.H., G.F. McCoy, M. Stetter, and W.C. Vanderwagen. 1992. An overview of mental health services for American Indians and Alaska Natives in the 1990s. *Hospital and Community Psychiatry* 43 (3): 257-61.

Noriega, J. 1992. American Indian education in the United States: Indoctrination for subordination to colonialism. In M.A. Jaimes, ed., *The state of Native America: Genocide, colonization, and resistance*, 371-402. Boston, MS: South End.

Office of Technology Assessment, US Congress. 1990. *Indian adolescent mental health*. Washington, DC: US Government Printing Office.

JOSEPH P. GONE

O'Nell, T.D. 1996. *Disciplined hearts: History, identity, and depression in an American Indian community*. Berkeley, CA: University of California Press.

Philips, S.U. 1983. *The invisible culture: Communication in classroom and community on the Warm Springs Indian reservation*. New York: Longman.

Rappaport, J., and E. Seidman. 1983. Social and community interventions. In E. Walker, ed., *The handbook of clinical psychology*, 1089-1122. New York: McGraw-Hill.

Scogin, F., J. Bynum, G. Stephens, and S. Calhoon. 1990. Efficacy of self-administered treatment programs: Meta-analytic review. *Professional Psychology: Research and Practice* 21 (1): 42-47.

Selmi, P.M., M.H. Klein, J.H. Greist, S.P. Sorrell, and H.P. Erdman. 1990. Computer-administered cognitive-behavioral therapy for depression. *American Journal of Psychiatry* 147 (1): 51-56.

Sherzer, J., and A.C. Woodbury, eds. 1987. *Native American discourse: Poetics and rhetoric*. Cambridge: Cambridge University Press.

Shweder, R.A. 1991. *Thinking through cultures: Expeditions in cultural psychology*. Cambridge, MA: Harvard University Press.

–. 1992. "You're not sick, you're just in love": Emotion as an interpretive system. In P. Ekman and R.J. Davidson, eds., *The nature of emotion: Fundamental questions,* 32-44. New York: Oxford University Press.

–, and M.A. Sullivan. 1993. Cultural psychology: Who needs it? *Annual Review of Psychology* 44: 497-523.

–, and J. Haight. 1999. The cultural psychology of the emotions: Ancient and new. In M. Lewis and J.M. Haviland-Jones, eds., *Handbook of emotions*, 2nd ed., 397-414. New York: Guilford.

Smith, M.L., and G.V. Glass. 1977. Meta-analysis of psychotherapy outcome studies. *American Psychologist* 32: 752-60.

–, G.V. Glass, and T.I. Miller. 1980. *The benefits of psychotherapy*. Baltimore, MD: Johns Hopkins University Press.

Stein, D.M., and M.J. Lambert. 1984. On the relationship between therapist experience and psychotherapy outcome. *Clinical Psychology Review* 4: 127-42.

Strauss, A.S. 1977. Northern Cheyenne ethnopsychology. *Ethos* 5 (3): 326-57.

Strupp, H.H., and S.W. Hadley. 1979. Specific versus nonspecific factors in psychotherapy. *Archives of General Psychiatry* 36 (10): 1125-36.

Tavris, C. 2003. The widening scientist-practitioner gap: A view from the bridge. In S.O. Lilienfeld, S.J. Lynn, and J.M. Lohr, eds., *Science and pseudoscience in clinical psychology,* ix-xviii. New York: Guilford.

Trimble, J.E., S.M. Manson, N.G. Dinges, and B. Medicine. 1984. American Indian concepts of mental health: Reflections and directions. In P.B. Pedersen, N. Sartorius, and A.J. Marsella, eds., *Mental health services: The cross-cultural context,* 199-220. Thousand Oaks, CA: Sage.

US Department of Education. 1991. *Indian nations at risk: An educational strategy for action*. Washington, DC: US Department of Education.

Valsiner, J. 1996. Editorial: After the first year. *Culture and Psychology* 2 (1): 5-8.

Waldram, J.B. 2004. *Revenge of the Windigo: The construction of the mind and mental health of North American Aboriginal peoples*. Toronto, ON: University of Toronto Press.

Ward, S.C. 2002. *Modernizing the mind: Psychological knowledge and the remaking of society*. Westport, CT: Praeger.

20
Conclusion: Healing / Invention / Tradition

LAURENCE J. KIRMAYER, GREGORY M. BRASS, AND GAIL GUTHRIE VALASKAKIS

As the contributions to this volume make clear, notions of tradition and healing are central to contemporary efforts by Aboriginal peoples to confront the legacy of injustices and suffering brought on by the history of colonization. Through individual and community-based initiatives as well as larger political and cultural processes, Aboriginal peoples in Canada are involved in healing their traditions, repairing the ruptures and discontinuities in the transmission of traditional knowledge and values, and asserting their collective identity and power.

Any approach to mental health services and promotion with Aboriginal peoples must consider these ongoing uses of tradition to assert cultural identity. However, it is important to recognize that tradition itself is both received and invented: built in equal measure of wisdom transmitted across the generations and of creative visions of how the many strands of knowledge available today from diverse cultures of the world can be woven together in new patterns. Even though oral tradition works to maintain an unbroken chain of teachings, collective history is retold in new ways in each generation, using contemporary images and vocabulary. Living traditions are always works in progress.

Academics and scholars also belong to communities, professional associations, and social networks that embody traditions – shared value systems, intellectual interests, and philosophical questions that have been collectively debated and discussed for decades, centuries, or even millennia. The clinical disciplines of psychology, psychiatry, and other mental health professions are more recent traditions that consist of not only accumulated scientific knowledge or technical skills but also systems of cultural values and practices. Recognizing that mental health professionals belong to communities and that their practices are part of a "tradition" provides a way to think about the conflict and complementarity between different healing practices. Differences may reflect superficial choices of models, metaphors, or materials, but they also may point toward deeper conflicts in values. Making these different values explicit is a necessary step toward respectful co-existence or developing a meaningful integration of Aboriginal and academic psychological perspectives on mental health and healing. In this concluding chapter, we consider some of the models of healing in current circulation and discuss their implications for Aboriginal mental health policy, services, and interventions.

Universal Aspects of Healing

In his account of the universal dimensions of symbolic or interpersonal healing, Jerome Frank (1973) argued that all systems of healing involve theories of illness that characterize different types of affliction, defined roles for the healer and the afflicted person, a designated place and time for healing rituals, and expectations for recovery. Within this cognitive and social framework, the specifics of a healing ritual unfold. Frank later revised his argument in light of the elaborate nosology of contemporary psychology, which split "mental illness" into many discrete diagnostic entities with specific treatments; but at the level of general morale and malaise, and in terms of the "nonspecific effects" of expectation and placebo, this basic structure of healing remains (Frank and Frank 1991; Young 1988).

In his famous essay "The effectiveness of symbols," Claude Lévi-Strauss (1967) used the example of the Kuna healers of Panama to outline a structural theory of healing. The sick person's condition is mapped symbolically onto a mythic story or landscape. Movement along the narrative trajectory or across the symbolic landscape then corresponds to changes in the individual's condition, from sickness to health. For Lévi-Strauss, it is the structural parallels between the myth and the individual's illness that account for the effectiveness of the ritual, but this leaves unclear the actual processes of transformation and their material substrate.[1]

James Dow (1986) elaborated Lévi-Strauss' account, suggesting that personal experiences of suffering were attached to affect-laden cultural symbols. The transformation achieved through the ritual or narrative thus modifies the individual's emotional state. This emotional transformation could account for changes in the way the person thinks about and experiences body, self, and others. Through psychophysiological mechanisms, such healing could also result in actual changes in bodily functioning (Kirmayer 2003b).

In an account close to that of Dow, Kirmayer (1993) suggested that the process of transformation in healing can be understood in terms of the social, cognitive, and physiological effects of metaphor. Healing rituals redescribe individual and collective experiences of suffering in new terms. These metaphorical redescriptions can then be transformed according to the cognitive dynamics of the metaphor. There is a rich literature on the cognitive processes that underlie the production and understanding of metaphors that offers ways to further develop a cognitive account of the psychological effects of symbolic healing (Kirmayer 2003b, 2004).

Metaphor theory suggests that we can understand the cognitive transformations of symbolic healing with reference to our ability to think in terms of different images, frames, and stories. Even though metaphorical thinking allows great fluidity and creativity, strong and moving metaphors are grounded in both bodily experience and core social symbols and institutions. This cognitive process has analogues at many levels of experience, so we can recognize a hierarchy of healing processes involving transformations of

experience at multiple levels: bodily, emotional, cognitive, self-reflexive, family inter-
actional, communal, social, and political (Kirmayer 2004). As we move up this hierarchy,
we also move outward, so what heals the individual necessarily has impact on wider social and political spheres.

Spirit Matters: Myth, Metaphor, and Archetype

Metaphors work in an intermediate representational space between the archetypal and
the mythic. The archetypal level refers to the universal or given in experience, which is
present either because it is hardwired into our brains or because it emerges, more or less
inevitably, from basic facts of human existence. These existential universals may be related
to our bodily, emotional, and social experience or to our own awareness of basic experiential facts like the presence of other minds and wills as well as our own and others'
mortality.

Myth refers to the overarching narratives or stories that make sense of the human
condition by weaving together all its disparate strands. Myths are "maps of meaning"
(Peterson 1999) but are especially those maps or narratives located at the centre of a
community's identity.[2] Here, the term "myth" connotes not an absence of truth but a displacement of the literal by the metaphorical through the seamlessness, immediacy, and
facticity of collective stories. The value of myth and storytelling can be easily appreciated
in terms of psychological processes of making meaning and coherence from often quixot-
ic life experience (King 2003). Traditional stories and myths are also emblems of identity
that circulate among Aboriginal peoples, providing opportunities for mutual understanding and participation in a shared world.

Although this account of healing emphasizes personal and social meaning, it is rooted
in the materialistic ontology and epistemology of science; it deals with what can be seen
and felt, and it assumes that healing processes can be explained in terms of material
forces, influences, and mechanisms. Whether healing is grounded in the body or in psychological and interpersonal processes, its mediators, mechanisms, and outcomes can, in
principle, be reliably observed and measured. But many forms of Aboriginal healing are
based on a different ontology, one that acknowledges the presence of a spirit world. In
this view, affliction involves not only the bodies, psyches, and social relations of individuals but also their relations to a world in which nonhuman persons play an active role in
the lives and fate of human beings, either through their visible actions or in an invisible
spirit realm. Traditionally, shamanistic healing was based on an animistic ontology in which
everything in the universe is recognized as a living being, including not only the animals
and plants but also the landscape and forces of nature (Ingold 2004). In the contemporary
world, healing is no longer so closely associated with this animistic ontology but invokes
a broad notion of spirituality.

Spirituality refers to the sense that there is another realm of value and meaning, larger than the individual psyche or the social world, to which the person can feel connected. This connectedness has esthetic, psychological, and ethical consequences, providing a sense of calmness, clarity, and guidance in one's life. Spirituality is attractive for many because it sidesteps the politics, doctrines, and dogmas of religious institutions to emphasize the individual quest for meaning and experience of the sacred (Torrance 1994). The focus on spirituality puts Aboriginal traditions and newer hybrid forms of healing and spiritual practice on an equal footing with established, institutionalized religions in terms of truth, efficacy, and moral value.

Another way to approach spirituality is in terms of the interpretive strategies used to understand experience. Biomedical explanation uses materialist explanations: everything can be understood in terms of physical mechanisms, laid bare by technical means that allow systematic observation and precise measurement. Psychology adds another level of explanation in terms of the importance of the meanings of events to individuals. We need to know how someone understands an event to appreciate what impact it will have for them. And personal meaning derives from larger cultural meanings that give events their evocative power through developmental experiences and social reinforcement. The interaction of individual and cultural meaning opens onto a third level of interpretation of experience that has been termed the "mythopoetic" (Rowley 2002). This recognizes that the meanings conveyed by myth are not only personal but also concern larger webs of connection that draw in culture, history, the social world, and the environment. Learning from a myth, participating in a ritual, seeking spiritual wisdom are all ways of getting access to larger patterns of meaning not subsumed by material or psychological levels of explanation. Myth cannot be reduced to a psychological explanation because "the mythic narrative is an articulation of an experience with transcendence" (Rowley 2002, 494). The esthetic and psychological response to the ritual retelling of a myth is an identification not with a character but with the whole mythic structure.[3] The Haida term *qqaygaanq*, often translated as *story, myth,* or *tale,* comes from the root *qqay,* meaning *full, old,* or *round,* and from the suffix *–gaang,* meaning *enduring* or *continuing to be* (Bringhurst 1999, 27). This expresses very well the notion of myth as a story in which we apprehend the beginning, middle, and end all at once in a circle or cycle that draws us into the fullness of the timeless moment of transcendence.

Myth, dream, and ritual offer the participant a glimpse of visionary experience in which deeper connections among phenomena are felt or understood. For many Aboriginal peoples, this sense of transcendence is tied to place and landscape as much as to any specific cultural content or context. "Ontologically speaking, the mythopoetic experience articulates that creation or landscape precedes existence, which precedes essence. The preexisting state of landscape provides continuity and eventually community. As one engages the landscape and its extension, culture, individuals can engage other people" (Rowley 2002, 498-99).

The Way of Animal Powers

If men would ... seek what is best to do in order to make themselves worthy of that toward which they are so attracted, they might have dreams which would purify their lives. Let a man decide upon his favorite animal and make a study of it, learning its innocent ways. Let him learn to understand its sounds and motions. The animals want to communicate with man.

– BRAVE BUFFALO, TETON SIOUX, QUOTED IN F. DENSMORE,
TETON SIOUX MUSIC (1981), 172

Cross-cultural comparative research on healing has often used the shamanistic traditions found among some indigenous peoples as a model of the most basic system of medicine (Fabrega 1979; Waldram 2004). Shamanism was practised in small-scale hunter-gatherer societies without highly differentiated roles. Many authors have assumed that shamanism therefore resembles the forms of healing that emerged early in human prehistory, and the images found in archaeological sites have been interpreted in terms of the symbolism of contemporary shamanistic traditions (Clottes and Lewis-Williams 1996; Vitebsky 2001). This view has been criticized, however, for conflating and confounding quite different traditions and as an obstacle to understanding the specificity of Aboriginal traditions (Kehoe 1996). Nevertheless, at the level of symbolic structure and process, there are important similarities across even quite disparate forms of healing (Kirmayer 2004).

Traditionally, Aboriginal peoples had their entire religion, economy, and sense of well-being built up around arduous hunts and transactions with animals, birds, fish, and mammals as well as with other creatures and supernatural beings (Tanner 1979). Although ways of life have changed, something of this sensibility persists for many people, sustained in part by retellings of mythic stories that anchor and enliven Aboriginal identity.

The anthropologist Marie-Françoise Guedon (1984) described Tshimsian shamanism as a technology of image or metaphor. Each shaman has spirit helpers who take the form of animals or objects. In healing rituals, the patient's illness is explored and worked on through these symbols. Some of these symbols are unique to a specific tradition with its authorizing myths, arts, and ritual practices, but they may also have a level of meaning that is universally intelligible. For example, animals are natural symbols that stand for ways of being that are potentialities not only because of our mimetic capacities, or enactment of culturally acquired meanings, but because of the physical substance and organization of our being. Understanding how these images work to convey a bodily habitus and moral meaning is important for our theories of healing.

Shamanistic practice can be understood in terms of the cognitive theory of metaphor. The movement through an extended metaphor transforms the representation of experience; to the extent that the representation shapes experience, this transformation will change the way that participants think and feel. Indeed, the ordering of a series of meta-phors itself supplies an implicit metaphoric structure that may be spatial or temporal. Thinking about illness in these metaphoric terms provides the shaman a picture with which he can work. It anchors hidden and complex phenomena in something more familiar. It thus provides a readily mastered scenario in which symbolic actions make sense and can move the individual's representation of bodily suffering toward images of health and wholeness.

In many shamanistic traditions, the healer's knowledge and power come from his or her own encounter with illness. An acute illness (or self-inflicted crises through fasting and other privations during a vision quest) confirms one's calling to become a healer and begins a process of initiation through which the shaman gains spirit helpers and acquires the ability to see or travel in the spirit realm, where afflictions can be diagnosed and treated. The shaman, then, is an example of the archetype of the wounded healer, who draws his or her authority from a personal initiatory illness and survival (Kirmayer 2003a).

In recent decades, shamanistic practices have undergone a popularization in North America both in New Age spirituality and in academic circles interested in myth and heal-ing (Atkinson 1992). Neo-shamanism has become the subject of weekend workshops for middle-class Americans. These activities offer a pastiche of ideas and practices borrowed from diverse traditions, often with a strong undercurrent of the values of individualism and self-development that mirror the dominant society. They appeal to non-indigenous people from diverse backgrounds and also provide those who claim Aboriginal knowledge or background (whether or not it is bona fide) with a marketable product in the form of their spiritual and ritual expertise. Even though the questionable authenticity and mar-keting of these practices raise concerns about cultural appropriation (Aldred 2000), the ongoing exchange between Aboriginal healing practices and New Age spirituality is part of a response to real problems in the dominant value systems of the West. Behind this interest in Aboriginal healing traditions lies a broader search for meaning driven by the lack of connectedness to others in the community and the limitations of the materialism that characterize North American society (Kasser 2002).

Ecocentrism and Aboriginal Identity

As many of the contributions to this volume show, connection to the land has played an important role in Aboriginal conceptions of personhood and wellness. Disruption of this link has been a major contributor to the social suffering endured by Aboriginal commun-ities. Indigenous peoples can be defined through the historical fact that they have a com-mon experience of displacement, marked by the dispossession of their lands and way of life, due to interactions with settlers and colonial regimes. They can also be defined in terms of their relationship to the land and to place (although many indigenous peoples were nomadic, this way of life has its own strong sense of place, associated with seasonal cycles of social and subsistence activities). The traditional relationship to the land was not ownership but something more intimate; in Chapter 2 Durie and colleagues call it "custodianship," or "looking after the land for the sustainable benefit of the environment and humankind alike, 'Mother Earth' taking on a literal meaning, the sacred inscribed in a totemic landscape." At a conference on Aboriginal mental health research in Perth in 2005, Kimberley Smith described this relationship in striking terms that evoked the qualities of emotional attachment and moral concern: "The land is our mother. We must care for it. We need to be needed by the land."

The effects of colonization, then, have not simply been displacement or appropriation of land but an undermining of the cultural meanings of land in the sense of self and personhood:

> The meaning of land emerges in the historical specificity and cultural practice of Native North American lifeworlds. It is enacted and acted upon every time Native people hunt or fish, plant gardens, visit the graves of ancestors, offer tobacco to spirit rocks, or acknowledge the interrelatedness of these experiences of everyday life. But the meaning of land is also expressed in the stories people tell about heritage and ceremony, people and places, travel, conflict and loss. Not only the ownership of land but also the meaning of land was erased and devalued on the policies that emerged to exterminate or acculturate Indians. (Valaskakis 2005, 94)

The devaluing and disruption of the communal connection to land is a pivotal historical loss in the lives of Aboriginal peoples, but it has an echo in the experience of non-Aboriginal people. Suffering from fragmentation of identity and alienation from the world around us, many individuals are attracted by a myth of Edenic harmony and more specifically by the imagery and promise of a life lived with greater simplicity and enjoyment of the natural world (Brody 2000; Merchant 2003). First Nations peoples and Inuit of Canada and Native Americans in the United States are held up as the bearers of a spiritual tradition of living in harmony with the earth. Although this should not be taken to mean that every action by every individual or community was always an expression of some ecological wisdom or equipoise (Krech 1999), it does mean that living on the land encourages a sensory and sensual connection to the physical environment, a view of the natural world as having power and presence, and a respect for the lives of nonhuman beings (Abram 1996). These connections are what have been strained, severed, or displaced by the insistence of an urban way of life that sees the environment as raw material for consumption in the ravenous hunger of commerce and industrialization. This suggests that what Aboriginal healing traditions that are rooted in the land have to offer non-Aboriginal society resides in certain attitudes that reaffirm the sensual appreciation of nature, an acknowledgment of the human dependence on the environment, and a recognition of the place of nonhuman persons in imagination and reality.

In Aboriginal understandings, "human beings are themselves powerless individuals and collectivities whose control over their lives comes from interactions with empowered spirits, from a negotiation with non-human and other-than-human forces of nature. The hierarchies of spiritual relations that sustain and empower Indians are located in the range of living beings that are embodied in the natural world, in the environment, animal, other-than-human persons, which like the land itself, specify the significance of place and extend the presence of time" (Valaskakis 2005, 100).

Among Stó:lô communities in the Fraser River Valley near Vancouver, British Columbia, for example, the focus of present-day efforts to protect sacred sites is not limited to burial mounds and other locations where ancestral activities were known to have occurred (and can be proven archaeologically) but also includes anomalous rock formations, parts of the local river, specific forested areas, and even entire mountains where mythic events are remembered to have occurred long ago and that are still regarded as containing "power" accessible to some (Carlson, McHalsie, and Blomfield 2001; Mohs 1994; Pokotylo and Brass 1997). These sacred sites are integral to contemporary community life and vital to the continuation of traditional healing and spiritual activities (Jilek 1982; Nabokov 2006) but are in direct collision with the economic interests and value system of a capitalistic industrial society intent on continued resource extraction, greater urban development, and the creation of publicly accessible spaces.

Clearly, what an Aboriginal person experiences while growing up on and continuing to live close to the land will be quite different from the experience of a Euro-Canadian born and raised in a city. The experiential and social realities of Aboriginal culture should not be confused with the imaginative projections of city folk who long for simpler times – although for many urban Aboriginal people dispossessed of land and tradition, the predicament and the longing may be similar. Defining authentic Aboriginal identity in terms of commitment to ecocentric values, however, would constitute another form of essentialism and oppression (Sissons 2005). The urban environment allows for a relocation and reinvention of Aboriginal identity in ways that can, in turn, reshape the nation-state (as has happened with the recognition of New Zealand as a bicultural state) and that can exert still wider influence through emerging notions of indigeneity that link rural and urban environments with bonds of affinity and affection.

Pan-Indianism, Hybridity, and Healing

Much work on symbolic healing emphasizes the individual level of transformations, but in reality, all healing practices have fundamental social dimensions. The greatest power and efficacy of a healing ritual may be felt not in terms of its direct impact on the afflicted person but in the ways it transforms interactions with others, changing the perception of the sick person, his or her family, or the social life of a whole community.

Notions of health, illness, and healing play a central role in the discourse of Aboriginal identity in many communities (Johnston 2002). In her ethnographic work, Naomi Adelson has shown how the Cree notion of "being alive well" *(miyupimaatisiiun)* serves both to organize social life and to create a sense of collective identity (Adelson 1998, 2000a). As described by Tanner and Adelson in Chapters 11 and 12, respectively, contemporary Cree communities have available a variety of healing practices drawn from Christianity, Cree traditions, pan-Indianism, and popular psychology that provide settings and symbols to articulate social suffering and narrate personal and collective transformations (Adelson 2000b; Tanner 2004). In some cases, there are divergences and disagreements between adherents of different traditions, but many share a concern with achieving wellness through living a morally upright life, defined not only in religious or spiritual terms but also in relation to the community and the land.

In recent years, pan-Amerindian healing movements have enjoyed increasing popularity in Aboriginal-run treatment centres (Waldram 1997; Brass, Chapter 16). Participants in Aboriginal spirituality and healing come from diverse cultural, socioeconomic, and personal backgrounds; pan-Indianism offers them membership in a larger spiritual diaspora. Often this identity is acquired through participation in healing ceremonies. To take part, one must learn the symbolic system and mythic underpinning to which the healing process is attached. This positions the healer not only as the ritual expert but also as the bearer of "tradition." Faced with a group of people who do not belong to one community with a long history of shared experience and tacit knowledge, the healer must find or develop commonalties among participants' experiences and weave them together to make a coherent story, with links to cultural identity and tradition that can foster the interpersonal and spiritual dimensions of the healing process.

The sharing, intermixing, hybridization, and marketing of healing traditions evoke two polarized positions. On the one hand are those who protest when an Aboriginal healing tradition is treated as a commodity – not only because they are angry about the appropriation and selling of indigenous cultural capital but also because they believe that to be properly understood, effective, and ethical, a healing practice must be embedded in the larger system of meanings and practices of a community, with its history and ongoing ways of life. On the other hand are those who argue that certain healing traditions are obviously of universal relevance because they tap into pan-human spiritual truths.

In traditional societies, by definition, individuals share a common background of knowledge and experience. This ensures that they have some exposure to a common core of symbols and conventional ways of understanding the world and so bring specific assumptions to the healing process. It also makes it more likely that particular symbolic actions will be powerfully and predictably evocative for them, resonating with long experience, calling forth rich memories and associations, and activating strong emotions that are shared with, or at least intelligible to, others in their family, entourage, or community.

How, then, do symbols work when they are not drawn from a shared worldview or ethos that is grounded in bodily experiences through early childhood learning? Unfamiliar symbols must be given new meaning, be accompanied by more or less explicit instructions on how to interpret or understand them, or be decoded in terms of some more universal "archetypal" understanding. In some instances, individuals first exposed to a new healing practice may be left "cold" and unmoved. Only with further preparation and repeated exposures over time do they find that the ritual or ceremony speaks to them. In other instances, individuals may have a profound and compelling experience from the start. This may reflect their own preparedness based on previous learning and expectations as well as a level of personal identification with the setting, participants, or the ceremony as a whole. Of course, throughout their participation they are reflecting on the fact that this form of healing comes from a shared heritage. It thus has emotional resonance as an emblem of identity that can be a source of collective pride and belonging. All that is needed to benefit from this aspect of the healing ritual is a sense of the seriousness of the occasion, respect for the practice, and a desire to feel connected to the other participants or to a shared history and tradition.[4]

This is illustrated in Joseph Couture's story of his pilgrimage from Alberta to visit the healer Raymond Whitehair in Wyoming:[5]

> In the spring of 1971, about eight of us with our families and girlfriends, parents, whoever, drove fourteen hours – we were only given time off from our jobs for the weekend, but we drove nonstop all Friday night to get there. And we saw things happen, so we had to stay three weeks. And during that time all of us fasted for the first time ... and saw extraordinary things I had no idea were possible. I had no inkling at all that there were such real life people called "medicine people," healers. I had no idea; that was just something Indians didn't talk about. But I thought all these years that every treaty for sure learned about these people because they were there ...
>
> The churches were down on these kind of people, but they knew about it because the families were extended families, and every extended family had a medicine person or two in there somewhere – had or still have. And so Harold and I did a lot of travelling together and went to ceremonies nonstop for the next two years, all over Alberta. There weren't many places at that time; there weren't many sweat lodges and certain ceremonies, so you travelled a long way to see the ceremony.[6]

Couture's journey – his experience of fasting and subsequent participation in the sweat lodge and other ceremonies – has all the elements of a rite of initiation identified by van Gennep (1960): separation from everyday life (the long night's journey to Wyoming); entry into a liminal state (through fasting and other ceremonial activities); and the assumption of a new identity – in this case, expressed through a continued quest to seek out and participate in ceremonies. However, when it occurs in a situation where individuals are uprooted from tradition and community, the last phase becomes less stable and demands from participants an active effort to reconstruct communities of shared experience that can validate their new insights and stabilize their new knowledge in a way of life. This turns the heightened feeling of communion achieved during the ritual experience into a sustained and solid sense of belonging to a community – which can be a specific local community or a wider pan-Indian community of shared ceremonial experience (Valaskakis 2005). Later in his account, Couture describes how he and others worked to build new social contexts for living out one's identity as a Native, including Native study programs, counselling work in prisons with offenders, and healing practices offered as an Elder to others making journeys to visit him. He also drew from the writings of transpersonal psychology and philosophy to find perspectives consistent with his experiences in Aboriginal spirituality.

Symbol and Ceremony

Even without a strong identification with the healing ritual as part of one's cultural heritage or without formal preparation for understanding and participation, there are many levels of symbolic meaning built into healing practices that are immediately accessible to any participant. These include the basic sensory and affective meanings of natural symbols conveyed through their physical properties. Beyond this, the order or structure of a healing symbol or ceremony also conveys specific knowledge. To illustrate this natural symbolism of healing practices, consider two examples drawn from pan-Indian spirituality: the medicine wheel and the talking circle.

The medicine wheel, a circle divided into four quadrants, representing the mental, physical, emotional, and spiritual dimensions of the person, embodies the notion of wholeness and harmony in human experience (Mussell 2005; McCormick, Chapter 15). Through its roundness and symmetry, the medicine wheel is a natural symbol for balance, inclusiveness, and completeness.[7] The medicine wheel provides a model of the person that gives equal weight to the spiritual dimension of experience, which must be balanced with thinking (rationality), feeling (emotional appraisal), and the physical understanding that comes through engagement of the bodily senses. The quadrants of the circle may also be mapped onto other symbolic systems, including features of the environment and the social world. Indeed, the medicine wheel may be used to depict and diagnose imbalances in larger spheres of life (see Figure 20.1).

The circle with four quadrants is a common representation of wholeness and plenitude in many traditions, notably in Buddhism, where the mandala has a similar structure (Jung 1972). The Buddhist mandala is used as an objective of meditation to guide the person toward an understanding of wholeness, harmony, and balance (Leidy and Thurman 1997).

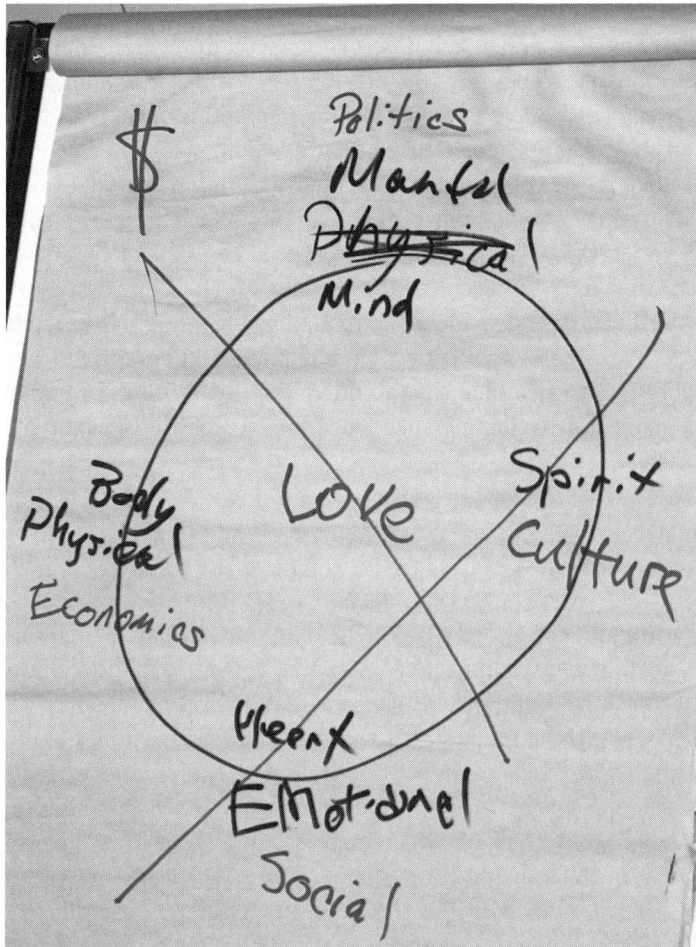

FIGURE 20.1   From a workshop on "Integrative health and healing: Co-learning our way to expanding wholeness through restoration of relationships with the land," Eskasoni, Quebec, 2003. (Photo: L.J.

Like the mandala, the medicine wheel may be elaborated with many levels of correspondence. The four elements of the medicine wheel – mental, physical, emotional, and spiritual – correspond roughly to Jung's distinction in the theory of psychological types between the personality dimensions, or functions, of thinking, sensation, feeling, and intuition (Jung 1976). This convergence developed before Jung had much knowledge of or contact with Native Americans (something he did pursue later), which suggests that these distinctions reflect some general insights into human experience.[8]

A talking circle sets up an order in which each person takes a turn speaking while others listen respectfully and attentively. The speaker takes as much time as needed, and then the next person speaks. The protocol of the circle, with its turn-taking and attention given to the speaker, has multiple effects: it honours the voice of the individual, treating each person's speech as a gift to the group or community and offering in return the gift of attentiveness. The spaciousness of having enough time to speak and waiting one's turn (knowing with calm certainty that it will come) prevents a competition for the floor in which those who speak more loudly and forcefully dominate while others are silenced. The circle is inherently egalitarian insofar as each person gets a turn and all are accorded time according to the desire of each to speak. In this way, the circle honours the individual voice and gives each person's experience and perspective equal weight. The protocol of the circle is a corrective to situations where individuals have been silenced by oppressive circumstances, whether within the family, community, or larger political spheres. Of course, each circle also has its own dynamics that sometimes may re-enact situations of oppression and abuse, but hopefully these become opportunities for reflection and a corrective response from participants (Picou 2000).

Healing circles differ from talking circles in the protocol and expectations. Participants are encouraged to tell specific types of stories centred on themes of suffering, trauma, loss, grief, and healing, and there is increased tolerance for and expectation of intense affect as these stories are recounted. The healing circle thus serves cathartic functions (Scheff 1979) and allows a group to bear witness to the suffering of each individual. In telling their stories, individuals are able to narrate their experiences in ways that give them new meaning and coherence and to receive social validation. Of course, the intensity and experience are regulated by a group process that provides a narrative structure with which to make sense of an individual's experience, either by explicit example or by the group's response to specific narrative turns or modes of explanation. Thus the stories tend to fit a narrative that is structured like a journey, with specific stages or way stations marked off (Lane et al. 2002). This structure has parallels at both individual and collective, or community, levels.

Both the talking circle and the medicine wheel embody notions of balance, harmony, and wholeness. Both provide maps or models of the nature of affliction and its potential transformation. In use, both serve as vehicles to establish and affirm respect for the individual that are compensatory to the violations of these same values whether at the level of the family or at a larger political level. Indeed, part of the current healing efficacy of these protocols and symbols for Aboriginal people resides in the fact that they can work simultaneously at multiple levels to address the compounded insults and injuries that constitute historical trauma.

Historical Trauma

Healing is always predicated on some notion of the nature of affliction. In recent years, the metaphor of trauma has gained currency as a way to talk about personal and collective injuries suffered by Aboriginal peoples (Manson et al. 1996). The suffering of current generations is understood in terms of the transgenerational transmission of collective and historical trauma (Brave Heart 1993, 1999; Duran and Duran 1995; Serbin and Karp 2004). Wider recognition of the pervasive effects of this history of violence and oppression is relatively recent, following on the oral testimony and reports of the Royal Commission on Aboriginal Peoples. One important consequence of this was the establishment of the Aboriginal Healing Foundation, which was mandated to support healing projects that would address the transgenerational effects of the residential schools. Along with the increase in attention to trauma in mainstream psychology and the experiences of American Indian veterans in the United States and Canada, this has encouraged a view of the current mental health problems of Aboriginal peoples as stemming from large-scale traumatic events that followed colonization and forced assimilation. Individuals recounting their personal stories of domestic violence or other traumatic events may situate this account as related to larger historical events affecting their community or Aboriginal peoples as a whole. Historical trauma is linked to a collective discourse of a sometimes-assumed experience of grief and loss and to an awareness of cycles of abuse in Aboriginal communities.

Notions of historical trauma have borrowed from studies of the transgenerational impact of the Holocaust, which show both enduring effects and resilience (Kellerman 2001; Sigal 1998). But the situation of Jews during and after the genocidal regime of Nazi Germany and that of indigenous peoples suffering invasion and colonization differ in many potentially significant ways, including the following: (1) colonization and its oppressive institutions took place over hundreds of years; (2) for Aboriginal peoples extermination was usually not so direct, systematic, and complete; in many instances, the aim of the colonizers was cultural assimilation or marginalization rather than murder; (3) in addition to enduring violent attacks and systematic oppression, Aboriginal peoples experienced nonviolent but profound transformations in ways of life that made it difficult for them to maintain their cultures, traditions, and social structures; and (4) there was no end to the war and no liberation, only a gradual and uneven recognition of injustices, limited restitution, and small changes in policies. As a result of these differences, Aboriginal people have many ongoing reminders of historical trauma that are coupled with current stresses that range from discrimination to ambiguous social status; their losses are multiple and intertwined; and the potential communal sources of resilience, coping, and rebuilding have been undermined. Given these differences, the transgenerational effects of the history of "historical trauma" among Aboriginal peoples requires its own study.

Whitbeck and colleagues (2004) discuss the notion of historical trauma among American Indian people as developed especially in the writing of Brave Heart (1993, 1999; Brave Heart and Le Bruyn 1998). Despite the historical reality and aptness of the metaphor of historical trauma, there are two basic unresolved empirical questions: (1) Is there, in fact, a distinctive pattern of distress (what would, in medical terminology, be called a "syndrome") that characterizes the outcome of historical trauma? Or do the effects of colonization, sedentarization, violence, loss, and grief overlap completely with the same mental health problems defined by psychiatry, differing not at the level of the individual but only in the frequency of the problem in the population and in the likelihood of multiple co-existing problems (comorbidity), especially alcohol and substance abuse? And (2) Is there a distinct, direct, and specific causality? That is: "Are we dealing with actual historical issues or more proximate grief and trauma from the daily lives of often economically disadvantaged people who live with constant overt and institutionalized discrimination, severe health issues, and high mortality rates? The current conditions may be related to historical causes, however, the origins of the symptoms may be contemporary experien-ces?" (Whitbeck et al. 2004, 119). This second question raises the problem of understand-ing the mediation of historical effects, which may be at the level of the individual through conscious memory or unconscious psychological processes or at the level of society through family, community, and larger political processes that determine the circumstances of opportunity and adversity in individuals' lives.

To address these questions, Whitbeck and colleagues (2004) examined the notion of historical trauma as a mental health problem empirically, first with focus groups of Elders and then with a survey of adults who were not directly affected by the residential schools or by the "worst atrocities of ethnic cleansing." They conducted two focus groups with Elders on two reservations in the upper midwestern United States. The Elders identified a range of losses associated with historical traumas. Foremost among the cultural losses was loss of language; this was followed in frequency by erosion of traditional family and community ties, loss of land, and broken treaty promises. The Elders described the feel-ings commonly associated with these losses as primarily anger and depression.

Based on the focus groups, Whitbeck and colleagues (2004) developed two scales: (1) the Historical Loss Scale, which assessed frequency of thinking about perceived losses by asking the respondent how often 12 specific types of loss come to mind; and (2) the His-torical Loss Associated Symptoms Scale, which asked for specific symptoms related to anger, depression, anxiety, and posttraumatic stress disorder (PTSD). They administered these scales to a sample of 143 adult parents of children aged 10 to 12 years on two reserves in Ontario and two reservations in the upper midwestern United States.[9] They found that many participants reported thinking daily or more often about the whole range of historical losses, especially loss from the effects of alcoholism on our people (45.9%), loss of respect for Elders by our children and grandchildren (37.5%), loss of our language (36.3%), loss of respect by our children for traditional ways (35.2%), loss of our culture (33.7%), and loss of our traditional spiritual ways (33.2%). In terms of associated symptoms, the most common (reported often or always in association with thinking about these losses) were anger (23.8%), feeling uncomfortable around white people when you think of these losses (21.4%), and fearful or distrust the intentions of white people (15.7%). Structural-equation modelling found that perceived historical loss was significantly related to symptomatology. The relationship was stronger for anger and interpersonal symptoms, which included fear and mistrust of white people, shame, and avoiding reminders of his-torical losses.

These results are from a small study that needs replication and extension. They suggest, however, that thinking about historical loss is a common experience for people in these communities and that it is associated with distress. Nonetheless, the symptoms do not fit postraumatic stress disorder but are more closely associated with feelings of anger, fear, and mistrust. This accords with the findings from other studies of individuals exposed to massive and pervasive trauma: the symptoms of anxiety and avoidance characteristic of PTSD are only one dimension of distress that covers many other domains related to sense of trust, justice, and meaningfulness in the world (Silove 1999). Indeed, anger and mistrust are crucial elements in this situation because, like avoidance, they may become obstacles to the re-establishment of safety and solidarity both within the traumatized community and in relations with others.

Grief and the Dynamics of Community Healing

The analysis of healing projects funded by the Aboriginal Healing Foundation suggests that recognizing the historical legacy of the residential schools – one major aspect of historical trauma for Aboriginal peoples in Canada – is an important step in the process of individual healing (Archibald 2006a; Brant Castellano 2006; Kishk Anaquot Health Research 2006; Stout 2003). As an externalizing attribution that locates the origins of suffering in social and political events, the focus on historical trauma has several important effects: it diminishes individuals' tendency to blame themselves and others close to them for their misfortune by encouraging an understanding of their behaviour as an outcome of forces beyond their control; it valorizes their suffering as a way to bear witness to historical injustices; and it points the way to social and political action aimed at redressing past wrongs and righting the structural violence that persists (Wesley-Esqimaux and Smolewski 2004).

Recounting one's own story of trauma safely and with some healing benefit requires a receptive audience that bears witness (Kirmayer 1996). The quality of this bearing witness depends on the relationship of Aboriginal people to the larger society where their stories can be validated, honoured, and commemorated. Encountering wilful ignorance and disbelief from others can be as great a violence as the original event. Wider recognition of the role that historical trauma has played in shaping the lives of Aboriginal people provides a social context that allows individuals and communities to tell their stories in ways that can begin the process of personal and collective transformation from helpless victim, through courageous survivor, to creative thriver.

The trauma-centric perspective has rhetorical power but raises complex issues for identity and healing. Not all suffering stems from overt violence or traumatic events. The emphasis on narrating personal trauma in contemporary psychotherapy is problematic because many forms of violence against Aboriginal people are structural or implicit and thus may remain hidden in individual stories. Creating a prototypical narrative of historical trauma gives authority and credibility to some accounts while marginalizing and casting doubt on others. Having the right sort of story of suffering, then, can be a source of social status within the community and a politically powerful instrument.

It is tempting to focus only on the stories that can be told about explicitly traumatic events and use these to explain the persistent inequities, but these individual events are part of larger historical formations that have profound effects for both individuals and communities that are harder to describe. The impact of these damaging events is not encoded as declarative knowledge but "inscribed" on the body in the form of one's habitual responses and stance toward the world or else built into ongoing social relations, roles, practices, and institutions (Kirmayer, Lemelson, and Barad 2007). Social analysis is necessary to delineate these structural forms of violence and oppression.

At the same time, focusing on large-scale historical events as the primary sources of collective trauma and individual psychological suffering may eclipse other more discrete but equally devastating losses and stressors that occur in the life of a family or community, such as the slow deterioration of a parent from dementia or the sudden and untimely loss of a child. Individuals have their own stories and predicaments. Although "the personal is political," it is not *only* political. Addressing individual suffering requires psychological understanding, attention to the dynamics of specific families, and consideration of the individual's cultural and spiritual values and aspirations. Conflating the personal and political may not allow the clarity and specificity needed to respond to the unique aspects of problems that beset individuals or communities.

Beyond the focus on trauma, the notion of collective historical grief has been used to acknowledge the profound sense of loss of continuity and tradition as a people. Loss evokes a range of responses: grief but also anger, fear, insecurity, depression, hopelessness. Each of these emotions has social and moral consequences: anger calls others to account to demand redress; fear motivates withdrawal, avoidance, and acquiescence. Grief is the most open of these responses and thus contains possibilities for healing and transformation (Boss 1999). Grief can be a "washing with tears" that opens us to both past and future. Through mourning what was lost, we commemorate the past, contributing to historical memory, identity, and tradition. By acknowledging the pain and vulnerability of loss, we remain open to others and, ultimately, to the possibility of renewal and reconstruction. The inability to grieve may be an unwillingness to acknowledge loss and therefore an inability to recognize what is valued, which must be regained in other ways.

These dynamics of anger, fear, and grief occur not only in individuals' inner psychic space but also in the give and take of family and community relationships as well as in larger political arenas involving people who may see themselves or be labelled as perpetrators, victims, and bystanders. Demanding justice and accountability, bearing witness, acknowledging responsibility, sorrow, and regret, and offering forgiveness are all part of a moral economy that works to build a society in which Aboriginal individuals, nations, and peoples can achieve health and healing.

The Politics of Healing

There is a basic tension between the authority of tradition and the autonomy of individuals in a pluralistic society. This presents a complex social and political conundrum for contemporary nation-states.[10] For example, Denis (1997) discusses the legal controversy over the case of "Joseph Peters" (the name is fictitious but the case is real) and his Coast Salish community. In 1988 Peters was compelled to undergo an initiation *(syewen)* organized by the Elders in response to his wife's request to help him with his alcohol abuse and marital problems. Subsequently, he successfully sued the Elders for "assault, battery and false imprisonment." This case illustrates basic conflicts between protecting and upholding individual human rights, on the one hand, and respecting the collective healing and religious practices of an indigenous community, on the other. There is a difference between spirituality as private source of meaning and as a socially sanctioned and regulated domain of tradition, serving collective identity. Although framed in terms of the survival of specific traditions, identities, and ways of life, communal engagement with spiritual practice reflects inevitable tensions between individual and community found everywhere: community offers belonging, support, and collective wisdom at the cost of individual freedom (Bauman 2001).

The many forms of traditional healing that are currently undergoing a renaissance across diverse cultures and communities must be considered from this larger perspective. The resurgence of interest in traditional practices like the sweat lodge (Bucko 1998) and their adoption by Aboriginal communities that never had such traditions are part of a more global movement of regenerating Aboriginal identity and exploring the significance of an evolving tradition in the contemporary world (Washburn 1996). Sharing traditions and participating in healing traditions identified as Native or Aboriginal are basic ways to affirm a collective identity and to connect historical knowledge and wisdom to one's lived experience and everyday life. The compelling experiences, personal transformations, and new insights that come from participation in healing can give emotional immediacy, intensity, and conviction to Aboriginal identity.

Of course, in some hands, Aboriginal spirituality becomes a product, open to commercialization. The relationship between this commercialization and the healing power of "authentic" tradition needs careful study. Claims to authenticity may be efforts to protect a "pure" tradition, regulate the political use of social power, and prevent the distortion or loss of spiritual truth. Such claims may also be ways to police identity that function as a form of cultural or political oppression in which new versions of indigenous identity are undermined and invalidated (Sissons 2005). Authenticity may be a cultural construction, but it has ethical, political, psychological, and pragmatic consequences.

To a large extent, traditional healing draws its authority from its rootedness in a local community with a shared social life. The traditional healer lives in the community, and his or her efficacy and moral conduct are open to scrutiny. Traditional healing practices involve local contexts of power that should not be immune from critical examination. Removed from this local moral economy, commodified, and placed in circulation on a global market, the ethics of healing undergo a radical transformation, and the risks of inauthenticity, bad faith, and exploitation grow. Many Aboriginal communities today are exposed to a great many different sorts of healers and practices, each claiming to be especially effective, and one marketing tool is the appeal to cultural authenticity.

One option is to bring Aboriginal healing practices under the umbrella of the institutions that regulate conventional mental health institutions. For example, in Manitoba, the Eyaa-Keen Centre, directed by Mel and Shirley Chartrand, has received accreditation in behavioural-health services from the Commission on Accreditation of Rehabilitation Facilities International, a nongovernmental organization that provides independent reviews.[11] Eyaa-Keen provides individual counselling programs that address issues related to PTSD and to the transmission of historical trauma. A key intervention is a type of breath work through which participants are trained to be more "aware of the present moment." "This awareness allows individuals to safely become increasingly cognizant of what is, and is not, working in their lives and ... to focus on life aspects that require further work."[12] The treatment provided by Eyaa-Keen combines Aboriginal values and notions of spirituality and healing with contemporary approaches to counselling. This integration made accreditation more feasible than it would be for traditional forms of healing that do not incorporate the protocols and perspectives of mainstream counselling and psychotherapy.

The risk of accepting external accreditation is that the core cultural values and human connection that characterize indigenous healing may be displaced by bureaucratic institutions and technical standards. Another alternative is providing people with the knowledge needed to judge the quality and relative merits of different treatment options. This would include both a sense of the range of options and some criteria for assessing whether a healer or program is credible and likely to be helpful. With or without such information, the human qualities and ethical conduct of the healer must be given the greatest weight. Credibility, authenticity, and safety may be found, then, not in asserting some privileged access to spiritual wisdom or tradition but in basic human qualities of empathy and compassion, self-criticism and humility, openness and willingness to engage in dialogue, respect for others, and commitment to stay available and engaged over the long term.

Healing the Body Politic

Political and social activism can be a path toward healing. Activism shifts the focus from "blame the victim" to recognition of oppressive systemic structures. Engagement with the aspirations of a community or a people offers an immediate sense of purpose and direction. It requires building functional ties to community to develop solidarity and both individual and collective efficacy. If successful, such activism brings great rewards not only in terms of social recognition, power, and economic resources but also in terms of a renewed sense of both individual and collective agency.

Developing this political power and presence, however, is not straightforward. Most current Aboriginal communities were created by or in response to colonizing powers. In the case of some hunter-gatherer peoples, current communities have brought together extended families that had no tradition of living together and that may have had previous conflicts. Aboriginal communities represent new forms of social life with their own uncharted and complex dynamics. Communities vary in their level of integration, support, and social capital. The old forms of power that grew out of a local community and way of life have been supplanted by the massive and impersonal bureaucratic apparatus of the state.

Each community has its own history, political issues, and aspirations. These local dynamics inform negotiations for health services with government-funding bodies or outside agencies. For example, as Wieman (Chapter 18) describes, the Six Nations' decision to create and deliver mental health services for its community members reflects a desire to maintain its autonomy and sense of self-reliance; at the same time, the community is currently embroiled in a complex land claims dispute that is rooted in the American Revolutionary War over 200 years ago. What effect does this have on community well-being as well as on individual mental health and the delivery of services and access to other needed services in neighbouring non-Native municipalities? This historical and political situation contrasts markedly with that of First Nations bands on the Canadian Prairies, whose demands for funding of health services may be linked to the provisioning of a "medicine chest" promised in the treaties their ancestors signed with the Queen's representatives in the 1870s (Lux 2001) – demands that are now tied to fiduciary responsibilities protected under the Canadian Constitution. This, in turn, contrasts with the precisely worded legal language of the regional agreement signed between the James Bay Cree and the Governments of Canada and Quebec in the 1970s, where health services and broader notions of a collective Cree identity have evolved in parallel (Salisbury 1986). In sum, every First Nations community has its own history and political platform that influence its approach to health services and that shape the ways political engagement itself can be healing or divisive.

There are complex political issues within communities as well. Small communities may exert powerful forces on individuals to silence dissent. Challenging violence and abuse within families, extended networks of kin, and communities threatens existing structures of power and privilege. It takes great courage to confront this abuse, whether at the level of domestic violence or in the machinations of local politics. Fox and Long write that "an important and quite painful step in the healing process involves naming the people, circumstances, and social structures that cultivate violence and perpetuate individual and collective unwellness" (2000, 271). Notwithstanding the importance of local control and self-determination, outside support from extended social networks, other communities, organizations, and professionals may be crucial to enabling vulnerable or disempowered individuals to speak out against oppression and to work for change within their communities.

All these issues take on a different cast in the urban contexts where the majority of Aboriginal people now live. Urban Aboriginal populations consist of people from diverse backgrounds with varying levels of cultural identification and are usually not as closely knit as rural or reserve communities. In the urban setting, there may be a shift from Aboriginal identity centred on "tribal" belonging toward Aboriginality as ethnicity (Sissons 2005). This views Aboriginal people as just another ethnocultural group within the multicultural mosaic of Canada. The consequence is a lack of recognition of their unique history and priority as First Peoples and a fragmented or "artificial" community with little to hold it together beyond the stereotypes and discrimination of the dominant society. Against these divisive forces, the growing number of urban Aboriginal organizations and institutions – along with pan-Indian ceremonialism, mass media like the Aboriginal Peoples Television Network, the Aboriginal Achievement Awards, and other regional and national cultural events – are contributing to increased cohesion across diverse cultures and traditions. Ultimately, Aboriginal identity will be sustained both by increasing cultural and historical awareness and by the circulation of people between rural and remote communities and the urban environment.

Youth, Gender, and Empowerment

The Aboriginal population is a young population, and efforts to address the mental health issues of Aboriginal communities must actively engage youth and consider their unique dilemmas. The cumulative effects of internal colonialism on cultural identity and continuing tensions between the values of Aboriginal peoples and mainstream society complicate the efforts of Aboriginal youth to forge their identities and find their ways in the world. The forces of globalization have introduced diverse cultures to even the most remote Aboriginal communities. The identity of youth is inscribed in a world culture – indeed, through mass media and Internet exchanges, many Aboriginal youth may feel they share more with distant peers than with other generations within their own communities. For most, however, this sort of virtual community cannot replace the intimacy, material support, or practical resources through which local relationships prepare one to navigate a future. Nor do the images of youth-oriented consumer culture propagated by mass media fit with the realities of poverty, unemployment, and other obstacles faced by youth in many Aboriginal communities.

Despite important social and cultural differences across Aboriginal peoples, young people played a vital role in traditional community life. The notion of a prolonged period of adolescence as a distinct phase in the lifecycle between childhood and adulthood was not sharply drawn; by their mid- to late teen years, young people were functioning as adults in the community with responsibilities for subsistence activities and raising families. The community context for the socialization of youth has changed dramatically with colonialism. Adolescence and young adulthood have become prolonged periods with ambiguous demarcation and social status. Marking a departure from traditional times, where "everyone was important and everyone had a role" (Carpenter 1999), colonialism and sedentarization resulted in impoverished roles and opportunities within many communities, leaving youth without clearly defined direction.

In many societies, the transition from youth to adulthood was marked by rites of passage that subjected youth to arduous trials and then conferred a new and valued social status, whether as a warrior, hunter, and potential head of a family or through other adult roles appropriate to one's gender, lineage, and experience (van Gennep 1960; Turner 1967). The challenge of these rites engaged youth and guided them along a socially prescribed path. This was particularly important for young males at the peak of their energy and impulsivity. The loss of these traditions has left youth without comparable structures to foster identity and consolidate their engagement with and commitment to the community. In the absence of formal rites of passage, young men have improvised their own trials and ways of belonging, but these tend to reflect the ethos of the peer group rather than of the whole community.

There are important gender differences in the ways that culture change has affected traditional roles. For young women, there has been more continuity in social roles, and many are involved in childrearing as well as in work and school (McElroy 1975). They may suffer from role strain as they try to fulfil multiple tasks (Kirmayer et al. 2003). Young men, in contrast, have experienced a profound disjuncture between traditional roles and the limited opportunities available to them in many Aboriginal communities. The high suicide rates among Aboriginal young men can be related to this loss of valued status and direction (Kirmayer 1994). The discontinuity in roles and the emergence of adolescence as a prolonged life stage requires adaptations within communities to provide meaningful opportunities and constructive roles for young people to develop their potential.

Some years ago, Margaret Mead (1970) distinguished between traditional societies, in which this hierarchy and order worked well and were sufficient to prepare young people for their social roles, and *posttraditional* societies, in which the rapidity of change cast youth adrift to find their own way with limited guidance from the patterns and protocols that worked for the previous generation. The acceleration in culture change threatens to up-end the natural sequence of cultural transmission across the generations. Everyday life in these communities necessarily takes new forms, not seen in traditional times, and individuals face new problems unanticipated in the thousands of years of precontact existence, or indeed, even in the earlier years of colonization, prior to the advent of the telecommunications and transportation technologies, networks, and institutions that have accelerated globalization. When change happens too rapidly and when old ways seem irrelevant to new predicaments, young people try to become their own leaders. This is one way to understand the dynamics of urban gangs and the new peer groups that have emerged in Aboriginal communities with sedentarization.

Recognition of the development predicament of youth points to the need to re-establish forms of initiation that lead toward viable identities in the contemporary world. Rites of passage that reconnect youth with Elders and with traditional understandings of the land can strengthen identity, self-esteem, and sense of belonging in ways that improve their ability to go forward with a sense of personal and collective continuity and purpose (Lertzman 2002).

Programs to promote mental health that are oriented toward empowerment aim to restore positive mental health and a strong sense of cultural identity by giving youth an active role in designing and implementing programs that meet their needs. Health promotion, with its emphasis on empowerment, may represent a contemporary alternative to traditional practices that accorded meaningful roles to youth as vital contributors to the community (Cargo et al. 2003). The language of empowerment is problematic for some both because of the emphasis on "power," rather than on other values like relatedness, and because of the tacit assumption that members of the dominant group and its institutions have power that they can bestow on others – a dynamic that would seem to re-enact the domination and paternalism of colonization even at the moment it claims to be sharing or transferring power. Empowerment works as a root metaphor, however, if we understand power as a placeholder for many different forms of presence and commitment and if we recognize that in acts of empowerment, power is not bestowed by one group on another but stems from within the individual and the group and that the function of the powerful other is recognition and acknowledgment rather than tutelage and legitimation.

Rethinking Mental Health Services

Rapid change has challenged Aboriginal identity and resulted in dramatic generation gaps between youth, adults, and Elders. These changes affect the whole population; therefore, mental health services and health promotion must be directed at both individual and community levels. The social origins of prevailing mental health problems require social solutions. However, conventional models of service and approaches to health promotion require rethinking if they are to be consonant with Aboriginal realities, values, and aspirations.

In most urban areas, mental health services have not been adapted to the needs of Aboriginal clients, and this is reflected in low rates of utilization. Although conventional psychiatric practice tends to focus on the isolated individual, the treatment of mental health problems as well as prevention and health promotion among Aboriginal peoples must focus on the family and community as the primary locus of historical trauma and the source of restoration and renewal.

There are distinctive features of Aboriginal communities that make it difficult to deliver conventional mental health care and prevention programs. Compared to the urban centres where most models of care have been developed, Aboriginal communities are small, and many are geographically distant from major cities. This results both in fewer material resources for medical and social services and in multiple roles being played by a few individuals. These practical constraints have been exacerbated by government policies that lead to insufficient support for mental health services for Aboriginal communities.

As a result of the size and scale of Aboriginal communities, there is little opportunity for the sort of anonymity that protects the practitioner's professional role in large cities. This anonymity has both ethical and practical uses: it provides privacy and safety for clients who wish to talk about embarrassing matters, and it allows the helper to have some respite from being constantly "on-call." In small communities, helpers are often related to the people they are helping and have no way to step back from their role; this can rapidly lead to "burnout." Since 1999 many more Aboriginal people have been involved in training and healing projects funded by the Aboriginal Healing Foundation, but, as of yet, few Aboriginal people have pursued advanced professional training in mental health.

Language is a basic conveyor of culture, and most people are connected to their emotions and intimate thoughts most readily in their first language or language of everyday life. Few health professionals working in Aboriginal communities have made the effort to learn local languages, and little mental health information has been translated. Culture, however, is a much broader issue than language and includes notions of personhood, interiority, and experience (ethnopsychology), patterns of family and social interaction, and basic values that must be central to any mental health program. A new generation of people able to put together local knowledge about health and healing with the most useful aspects of psychiatry and psychology is emerging. Aboriginal heritage is no guarantee that a professional will be culturally sensitive, however, both because of the diversity of traditions, which may differ from one's own, and because of the implicit cultural values and assumptions of psychiatry itself. A cultural critique of psychiatry is necessary to open up the space where creative reformulations of theory and practice can take place.

Psychotherapy and other mental health interventions assume a particular cultural concept of the person with associated values of individualism and self-efficacy (Bellah 1985; Gaines 1992; Kirmayer 2007). These approaches may not fit well either with traditional Aboriginal cultural values or with contemporary realities of reserve or settlement life. There is a need to rethink the applicability of different modes of intervention from the perspective of local community values and aspirations. Because the healing projects that the Aboriginal Healing Foundation has funded are initiated and carried out largely by Aboriginal people themselves, some of this rethinking is occurring through the implementation of healing centres and other interventions (Archibald 2006b). Family and social-network approaches that emphasize the relational self may be more consonant with Aboriginal culture, particularly if they are extended to incorporate some notion of the interconnectedness of person and environment (Lafromboise, Trimble, and Mohatt 1990; Speck and Attneave 1973; Trimble et al. 1984).

Individual identity and self-esteem, which are central to health and well-being, may draw strength and depth from collective identity. Where the collective is devalued, individuals may suffer corresponding wounds to their esteem and to their social "capital," power, and mobility. Collective identity, however, is not simply intrinsic or internal to a specific ethnocultural group or community. It is created out of interactions with a larger cultural surround, which may impose disvalued identities and marginalized status. Accordingly, improving Aboriginal mental health demands attention to the values, attitudes, and actions of the dominant society as well. In the contemporary world, identities are often multiple, mixed, or hybrid. Individuals who are bilingual, bicultural, and "bispiritual" are increasingly the norm. The mental health implications of such complex identities are only beginning to receive careful study (e.g., LaFromboise, Coleman, and Gerton 1993; Moran et al. 1999).

Mental health services and health promotion with Aboriginal peoples must go beyond the focus on individuals to engage and empower communities. Aboriginal identity itself can be a unique resource for mental health promotion and intervention. Knowledge of living on the land, community, connectedness, and historical consciousness all provide sources of resilience. At the same time, the knowledge and values held by Aboriginal peoples can contribute a vital strand to the efforts of other peoples to find their way in a world threatened by environmental depredation from the ravages of consumer capitalism.

Government and professional responses to social pathologies that aim to provide more health care services or to support traditional forms of healing, although essential, do not address the most fundamental causes of suffering. Community development and local control of health care systems are needed – not only to make services responsive to local needs but also to promote a sense of individual and collective efficacy and pride that contributes to positive mental health. Ultimately, political efforts to restore Aboriginal rights, settle land claims, and redistribute power through various forms of self-government hold the keys to healthy communities (Warry 1998).

Research on the social problems that Aboriginal populations face has important implications for health-service delivery and mental health promotion, as well as for social and community psychiatric theory and practice more generally. However, research and program development must be fully collaborative through broad-based partnerships with Aboriginal communities (Macauley et al. 1999). To work productively with indigenous communities and peoples, researchers must understand the philosophical grounding of indigenous political perspectives and indigenous intellectual and ethical traditions (Biolsi and Zimmerman 1997; Deloria 1969; Smith 1999; Turner 2006).

Trickster (Re)Makes the World

Contemporary anthropology understands culture as an abstraction of a fluid, shifting, and complex mix of different streams of knowledge and practice that have their own contradictions, conflicts, and dynamics. Individuals use these resources to interpret their experiences, construct their identities, and find social positions that afford them a sense of meaning and purpose in their lives. Persons, institutions, and communities that position themselves as the arbiters of tradition try to maintain and defend values and institutions that are necessarily under constant challenge and renegotiation.

Yet this too is a half-truth since the preservation and persistence of values is crucial for well-being. Culture represents a measure of stability in our lives, a platform or foundation on which to build. Compared to other animals, our brains continue to develop and remain malleable for a long time, precisely so that we can acquire a culture (Wexler 2006). Hence it is the responsibility of Elders to hold and pass on the accumulated learning of family, community, people, and, indeed, humanity as a whole. Tradition itself is a cultural invention: a way to preserve, honour, and protect collective histories and to reinvest in stories, dreams, and visions that define the ethical and esthetic terms of personal virtue and a good life.

Reflecting on the historical oppression of the Crow people, Lear (2006) provides an account of cultural transformation centred on the problem of how to continue to define a good life – and oneself as a virtuous person within that way of life – when all the social structural features of that life are shattered, its practices prohibited or drained of meaning through an array of direct attacks and indirect forms of subversion. A vibrant culture has clear social roles, standards of excellence associated with those roles, and the possibility of one's becoming a person who embodies those ideals (Lear 2006, 42). Radical social change under conditions of violent suppression of a way of life and its traditions undermines the cultural resources for self-fashioning, rendering them not only inaccessible but also progressively antiquated, "primitive," and unintelligible. Lear suggests that to be able to find meaning in the radically altered circumstances that have rendered a traditional way of life senseless and impossible to perform requires the "imaginative excellence" of a poet who can take up the past and refigure it in ways that both create new fields of meaning and open up new forms of social space.

Even without the active efforts of others to destroy a culture, the world changes, and, as traditions become hidebound, it is the function of the artist at the margins of society to play with conventions, pointing out their absurdities, pushing imagination past the self-made limits that confine it. The artist as iconoclast, a modern invention, is a transfiguration of an older mythic figure, the trickster (Hyde 1998). The trickster is the most sophisticated animal power, the one who does humans one better, not by brute force but through sharp wit and the fearless will (or cosmic clumsiness) to turn everything upside down. In North American indigenous mythology, the trickster is portrayed as a solitary animal (coyote, raven, hare, spider) driven by boundless hungers for food and sex (Carroll 1984). The trickster is simultaneously the buffoon, clown, and wildcard – whose actions are destructive of order and restraint – and the culture hero who brings the foundational gifts of civilization: fire, language, and the knowledge and powers that create culture in all its symbolic wealth and variety. The trickster is like the artist, exploring the extremes of human imagination and bringing new ideas and possibilities from the margins back to the centre. The trickster pushes past the norms and bounds of culture not to teach us caution but to discover ways to remake the world.

The dramatic growth of indigenous literary and scholarly traditions over the past three decades is testimony to the strength and resilience of indigenous communities and peoples both in North America and in other colonized regions of the world (Vizenor 1999). The acerbic style and devastating wit of the late Vine Deloria Jr. (1969), a formidable Lakota intellectual, showed that an American Indian scholar could not only pick a fight and handily win his own verbal battles but could also enjoy wide social influence. His writing has inspired two generations of indigenous scholars and scholarship with the unapologetic message, directed at "settler societies," that Onkwehonwe (Mohawk for "original people") will once again live free (see Alfred 2005). Along with others, Vine Deloria Jr.'s writing represents an Aboriginal intellectual movement in North America that has much to contribute to understanding and finding remedies for the issues of cultural creativity and survival that face both Aboriginal peoples and the larger society.

The spirit of the trickster is evident in the work of many contemporary Aboriginal artists like Carl Beam, Lawrence Paul Yuxweluptun, or Brian Jungen (Augaitis 2005; Ryan 2000). The trickster reveals the process of cultural stereotyping by subverting conventional forms, as seen for example in James Luna's performance of 1987, *The Artifact Piece,* in which he put himself on display in a museum glass case, lying motionless for hours, surrounded by plaques with bits of information about his social identity (Luna, Lowe, and Smith 2005). This "piece" forces us to think about the way that Aboriginal and non-Aboriginal segments of society reciprocally construct each other's identity. Aboriginal identity cannot be understood or transformed without corresponding transformations of the collective identity of the dominant society, which builds the museums that put Aboriginal artefacts and histories on display. Identities circulate throughout society, and everyone contributes to their meaning and value through their responses, whether deliberate or unwitting. Aboriginal and non-Aboriginal peoples carry each other's "shadow" – Jung's term for those aspects of identity and experience forced out of awareness to preserve an idealized version of the self. Along with the structural violence that maintains health disparities (Farmer 2004), these psychological dynamics contribute to the stereotyping and discrimination that keep the forces of colonial oppression alive.

Concern for the well-being of Aboriginal peoples, therefore, is not only a matter of basic empathy, humanitarian values, historical justice, and human rights – although this would be more than enough to bring it front and centre. Our capacity to develop and maintain a pluralistic society that respects and nurtures creative difference depends crucially on ongoing dialogue with indigenous peoples. Indeed, the issues go far beyond the future of Canadian society, for they engage the globe both as a single superordinate world system and as an ecological environment of which we are a troublesome part. Profound climatic changes, brought on by the explosive growth of urban industrial society and the insatiable appetites of consumer capitalism, make the problem of living in balance with nature vital to the future of all of humanity. Consistent with indigenous perspectives rooted in the experience of living close to the land, the division between the humanly constructed world and the natural environment has broken down; we need new metaphors for our habitation of the earth, metaphors that allow us to fuse our sense of human community with serious commitment to wise stewardship of the planet.

There are two broad meanings of "indigenous": as a political predicament of colonized peoples in settler societies who became isolated minorities in their own lands; and as people living close to the land in a particular place. In the former sense, indigenous experience is contrasted with that of immigrants and settlers; in the latter sense, the contrast is with cosmopolitan or diasporic peoples. However, these two aspects of indigeneity are related. What distinguishes many indigenous traditions is a strong sense of place, of recognizing the spiritual, historical, ethical, and esthetic dimensions of connection to land. But there are inevitable tensions between such indigenous constructions of the self and the global or planetary networks in which we all are increasingly enmeshed. Both of these poles of identity are important, and as Anthony Appiah (2006) has argued, some version of "rooted cosmopolitanism" is urgently needed on our fractious and fragile planet. Without romanticizing or distorting the complexity of the cultural traditions and current lives of indigenous people, it remains likely that value systems emphasizing connectedness, community, and living in harmony with the land hold keys to both Aboriginal resilience and our collective survival.

Acknowledgments
Portions of this chapter are adapted with permission from L.J. Kirmayer, C. Simpson, and M. Cargo, Healing traditions: Culture, community and mental health promotion with Canadian Aboriginal peoples. *Australasian Psychiatry* 11 (suppl.) (2003): 15-23, http://www.tandf.co.uk/journals.

Notes
1 That the Kuna healers use an esoteric vocabulary that is mostly unintelligible to their patients further limits Lévi-Strauss' account (Sherzer 1983).
2 Of course, there is an archetypal level to myth and a mythic level to archetype, so these terms mark off segments in the cyclical process of making meaning.
3 Indeed, as Lévi-Strauss (1969) showed, myths embody larger cognitive structures that think through us.
4 Of course, this does not preclude a more playful, humorous, and ironic stance as embodied in the mythological figure of the trickster.
5 Dr. Joseph Couture, a Cree/Métis Elder, educator, psychologist, and healer, received the 2006 Aboriginal Achievement Award for his work in health. The citation notes: "As the first Aboriginal person to receive a

PhD in psychology, Dr. Joe as he is affectionately known, has not only built bridges of understanding between two cultures but has systematically affected generations of educators and students with his straightforward and profound traditional healing methods." See http://www.naaf.ca/html/dr_j_couture_e.html (accessed 3 June 2008).

6 From an interview by LJK with Joseph Couture, Montreal, May 2000.

7 There is a Māori analogue to the medicine wheel in the notion of *Te Whare Tapa Wha,* described by Durie and colleagues in Chapter 2, in which health is conceived of as a four-sided house in which each wall represents one aspect: *taha wairua* (spirituality), which includes a healthy relationship to the environment as well as to Māori cultural identity; *taha hinengaro* (mind), which includes thinking and feeling; *taha tinana* (physical health); and *taha whānau* (relationships).

8 There has been a circulation of ideas between Jungian psychology and Aboriginal healing traditions (e.g., Gustafson 1997; Sandner 1979). To some extent, this reflects that Jung borrowed directly from indigenous traditions – studying Innu tradition through the work of Frank Speck (1977) and meeting with Elders in the American Southwest. However, the generality of these models suggests that many traditions have used similar natural symbols to depict basic intuitions about universal features of human experience (Abramovitch and Kirmayer 2003; Petchkovsky, San Rocque, and Beskow 2003). Aboriginal people have found resonances between traditional wisdom and the ideas of Jungian psychology (Stephenson 2003).

9 Although Aboriginal peoples in the United States and Canada share common ancestry, there are important differences in their historical experiences. For example, there have been considerable differences between the two countries in the funding, administration, years of operation, curriculum, and activities of Indian residential schools. There are 72 Indian residential schools still operating in the United States, most under Tribal directorship.

10 For example, a major concern in post-Apartheid South Africa has been how to exercise appropriate legal and judicial authority in such a diverse, medically pluralistic, and ontologically rich context (Ashforth 2005).

11 They note on their website that "Eyaa-Keen Centre, Inc. is the only Aboriginal organization in Canada and most likely in North America accredited as an Aboriginal Traditionally based Traumas Treatment program." See http://www.eyaa-keen.org/whatnew.htm (accessed 9 February 2007).

12 Eyaa-Keen Centre brochure, http://www.eyaa-keen.org (accessed 4 June 2008).

References

Abram, D. 1996. *The spell of the sensuous: Perception and language in a more-than-human world*. New York: Vintage.

Abramovitch, H., and L.J. Kirmayer. 2003. The relevance of Jungian psychology for cultural psychiatry. *Transcultural Psychiatry* 40 (2): 155-63.

Adelson, N. 1998. Health beliefs and the politics of Cree well-being. *Health* 2 (1): 5-22.

–. 2000a. *"Being alive well": Health and the politics of Cree well-being*. Toronto, ON: University of Toronto Press.

–. 2000b. Re-imagining Aboriginality: An indigenous peoples' response to social suffering. *Transcultural Psychiatry* 37 (1): 11-34.

Aldred, L. 2000. Plastic shamans and Astroturf Sun Dances: New Age commercialization of Native American spirituality. *American Indian Quarterly* 24 (3): 329-52.

Alfred, T. 2005. *Wasáse: Indigenous pathways of action and freedom*. Peterborough, ON: Broadview Press.

Appiah, A. 2006. *Cosmopolitanism: Ethics in a world of strangers*. 1st ed. New York: W.W. Norton.

Archibald, L. 2006a. *Decolonization and healing: Indigenous experiences in the United States, New Zealand, Australia and Greenland*. Ottawa, ON: Aboriginal Healing Foundation.

–. 2006b. *Final report of the Aboriginal Healing Foundation, vol. 3, Promising practices in Aboriginal communities*. Ottawa, ON: Aboriginal Healing Foundation.

Ashforth, A. 2005. *Witchcraft, violence, and democracy in South Africa*. Chicago, IL: University of Chicago Press.

Atkinson, J.M. 1992. Shamanisms today. *Annual Review of Anthropology* 21: 307-30.

Augaitis, D., ed. 2005. *Brian Jungen*. Vancouver, BC: Vancouver Art Gallery and Douglas and McIntyre.

Bauman, Z. 2001. *Community: Seeking safety in an insecure world*. Cambridge, UK: Polity Press.

Bellah, R.N. 1985. *Habits of the heart: Individualism and commitment in American life*. Berkeley, CA: University of California Press.

Biolsi, T., and L.J. Zimmerman, eds. 1997. *Indians and anthropologists: Vine Deloria, Jr., and the critique of anthropology*. Tucson: University of Arizona Press.

Boss, P. 1999. *Ambiguous loss: Learning to live with unresolved grief*. Cambridge, MA: Harvard University Press.

Brant Castellano, M. 2006. *Final report of the Aboriginal Healing Foundation,* vol. 1, *A healing journey: Reclaiming wellness*. Ottawa, ON: Aboriginal Healing Foundation.

Brave Heart, M.Y.H. 1993. The historical trauma response among Natives and its relationship with substance abuse: A Lakota illustration. *Journal of Psychoactive Drugs* 35 (1): 7-13.

–. 1999. *Oyate ptayela*: Rebuilding the Lakota Nation through addressing historical trauma among Lakota parents. *Journal of Human Behavior and Social Environment* 2: 109-26.

–, and L.M. Le Bruyn. 1998. The American Indian Holocaust: Healing historical unresolved grief. *American Indian and Alaska Native Mental Health Research* 8 (2): 56-78.

Bringhurst, R. 1999. *A story as sharp as a knife: The classical Haida mythtellers and their world*. Vancouver, BC: Douglas and McIntyre.

Brody, H. 2000. *The other side of Eden: Hunters, farmers and the shaping of the world*. Vancouver, BC: Douglas and McIntyre.

Bucko, R.A. 1998. *The Lakota ritual of the sweat lodge: History and contemporary practice*. Lincoln, NE: University of Nebraska Press.

Cargo, M., G. Grams, J.M. Ottoson, P. Ward, and L.W. Green. 2003. Empowerment as fostering positive youth development and citizenship. *American Journal of Health Behavior* 27 (suppl. 1): 566-79.

Carlson, K.T., A.J. McHalsie, and K. Blomfield. 2001. *A Stó:lô-Coast Salish historical atlas*. Vancouver, BC: Douglas and McIntyre; Seattle: University of Washington Press.

Carpenter, J. 1999. The Elders have waited for young people to ask such things. In P. Kulchyski, D. McCaskill, and D. Newhouse, eds., *In the words of Elders: Aboriginal cultures in transition,* 217-54. Toronto, ON: University of Toronto Press.

Carroll, M.P. 1984. The trickster as selfish-buffoon and culture hero. *Ethos* 12 (2): 105-31.

Clottes, J., and D. Lewis-Williams. 1996. *The shamans of prehistory: Trance and magic in the painted caves*. New York: Harry N. Abrams.

Deloria, V., Jr. 1969. Anthropologists and other friends. In *Custer died for your sins: An Indian manifesto,* 78-100. London, UK: Macmillan.

Denis, C. 1997. *We are not you: First Nations and Canadian modernity*. Orchard Park, NY: Broadview Press.

Densmore, F. 1981. *Teton Sioux music*. Bulletin of the Bureau of American Ethnology, no. 61. Washington, DC: Government Printing Office.

Dow, J. 1986. Universal aspects of symbolic healing: A theoretical synthesis. *American Anthropologist* 88: 56-69.

Duran, E., and B. Duran. 1995. *Native American postcolonial psychology*. Albany: State University of New York Press.

Fabrega, H.J. 1979. Elementary systems of medicine. *Culture, Medicine and Psychiatry* 3: 167-98.

Farmer, Paul. 2004. *Pathologies of power: Health, human rights, and the new war on the poor*. Berkeley, CA: University of California Press.

Fox, T., and D. Long. 2000. Struggles within the circle: Violence, healing and health on a First Nations reserve. In D. Long and O.P. Dickason, eds., *Visions of the heart: Canadian Aboriginal issues,* 2nd ed., 271-301. Toronto, ON: Harcourt Canada.

Frank, J.D. 1973. *Persuasion and healing: A comparative study of psychotherapy.* Rev. ed. Baltimore, MD: Johns Hopkins University Press.

–, and J.B. Frank. 1991. *Persuasion and healing: A comparative study of psychotherapy.* Baltimore, MD: Johns Hopkins University Press.

Gaines, A.D. 1992. From DSM-I to III-R: Voices of self, mastery and the other: A cultural constructivist reading of U.S. psychiatric classification. *Social Science and Medicine* 35 (1): 3-24.

Guedon, M.F. 1984. Tsimshian shamanic images. In M. Seguin, ed., *The Tsimshian: Images of the past, Views for the present,* 174-211. Vancouver, BC: UBC Press.

Gustafson, F. 1997. *Dancing between two worlds: Jung and the Native American soul.* New York: Paulist Press.

Hyde, L. 1998. *Trickster makes this world: Mischief, myth, and art.* New York: Farrar, Strauss and Giroux.

Ingold, T. 2004. A circumpolar night's dream. In J. Clammer, S. Poirier, and E. Schwimmer, eds., *Figured worlds: Ontological obstacles in intercultural relations,* 25-57. Toronto, ON: University of Toronto Press.

Jilek, W.G. 1982. *Indian healing: Shamanic ceremonialism in the Pacific Northwest today.* Surrey, BC: Hancock House.

Johnston, S.L. 2002. Native American traditional and alternative medicine. *Annals of the American Academy* 583: 195-213.

Jung, C.G. 1972. *Mandala symbolism.* Princeton, NJ: Princeton University Press.

–. 1976. *Psychological types.* Princeton, NJ: Princeton University Press.

Kasser, T. 2002. *The high price of materialism.* Cambridge, MA: MIT Press.

Kehoe, A.B. 1996. Eliade and Hultkrantz: The European primitivism tradition. *American Indian Quarterly* 20 (2): 377-92.

Kellermann, N.P. 2001. Transmission of Holocaust trauma: An integrative view. *Psychiatry* 64 (3): 256-67.

King, T. 2003. *The truth about stories: A Native narrative.* Toronto, ON: House of Anansi Press.

Kirmayer, L.J. 1993. Healing and the invention of metaphor: The effectiveness of symbols revisited. *Culture, Medicine and Psychiatry* 17 (2): 161-95.

–. 1994. Suicide among Canadian Aboriginal peoples. *Transcultural Psychiatric Research Review* 31 (1): 3-58.

–. 1996. Landscapes of memory: Trauma, narrative and dissociation. In P. Antze and M. Lambek, eds., *Tense past: Cultural essays on memory and trauma,* 173-98. London, UK: Routledge.

–. 2003a. Asklepian dreams: The ethos of the wounded-healer in the clinical encounter. *Transcultural Psychiatry* 40 (2): 248-77.

–. 2003b. Reflections on embodiment. In J. Wilce, ed., *Social and cultural lives of immune systems,* 282-302. New York: Routledge.

–. 2004. The cultural diversity of healing: Meaning, metaphor and mechanism. *British Medical Bulletin* 69 (1): 33-48.

–. 2007. Psychotherapy and the cultural concept of the person. *Transcultural Psychiatry* 44 (2): 232-57.

–, L.J. Boothroyd, A. Tanner, N. Adelson, E. Robinson, and C. Oblin. 2003. Psychological distress among the Cree of James Bay. In P. Boss, ed., *Family stress: Classic and contemporary readings,* 249-64. Thousand Oaks, CA: Sage.

–, R. Lemelson, and M. Barad. 2007. Introduction: Inscribing trauma in culture, brain, and body. In L.J. Kirmayer, R. Lemelson, and M. Barad, eds., *Understanding trauma: Biological, psychological and cultural perspectives,* 1-20. New York: Cambridge University Press.

Kishk Anaquot Health Research. 2006. *Final report of the Aboriginal Healing Foundation,* vol. 2, *Measuring progress: Program evaluation.* Ottawa, ON: Aboriginal Healing Foundation.

Krech, S. 1999. *The ecological Indian: Myth and history.* New York: W.W. Norton.

LaFromboise, T., H.L. Coleman, and J. Gerton. 1993. Psychological impact of biculturalism: Evidence and theory. *Psychological Bulletin* 114 (3): 395-412.

–, J.E. Trimble, and G.V. Mohatt. 1990. Counselling intervention and American Indian tradition: An integrative approach. *Counseling Psychologist* 18 (4): 628-54.

Lane, P., Jr., M. Bopp, J. Bopp, and J. Norris. 2002. *Mapping the healing journey: The final report of a First Nation research project on healing in Canadian Aboriginal communities*. Ottawa, ON: Solicitor General Canada.

Lear, J. 2006. *Radical hope: Ethics in the face of cultural devastation*. Cambridge, MA: Harvard University Press.

Leidy, D.P., and R.F. Thurman. 1997. *Mandala: The architecture of enlightenment*. New York: Asia Society Galleries and Tibet House.

Lertzman, D.A. 2002. Rediscovering rites of passage: Education, transformation, and the transition to sustainability. *Conservation Ecology* 5: http://www.consecol.org/vol5/iss2/art30.

Lévi-Strauss, C. 1967. *Structural anthropology*. New York: Basic Books.

–. 1969. *The raw and the cooked*. New York: Harper and Row.

Luna, J., T. Lowe, and P.C. Smith. 2005. *James Luna: Emendatio*. Washington, DC: National Museum of the American Indian, Smithsonian Institution.

Lux, M.K. 2001. *Medicine that walks: Disease, medicine and Canadian Plains Native people, 1880-1940*. Toronto, ON: University of Toronto Press.

Macauley, A.C., L.E. Commanda, N. Gibson, M.L. McCabe, C.M. Robbins, and P.L. Twohig. 1999. Participatory research maximises community and lay involvement. *British Medical Journal* 319: 774-78.

Manson, S., S. Beals, T.D. O'Nell, J. Piasecki, and D. Novins. 1996. Wounded spirits, ailing hearts: PTSD and related disorders among American Indians. In A.J. Marsella, M.J. Friedman, E.T. Gerrity, and R.M. Scurfield, eds., *Ethnocultural aspects of post-traumatic stress disorders: Issues, research and clinical applications,* 255-84. Washington, DC: American Psychological Association.

McElroy, A. 1975. Canadian Arctic modernization and change in female Inuit role identification. *American Ethnologist* 24: 662-86.

Mead, M. 1970. *Culture and commitment: A study of the generation gap*. Garden City, NY: Natural History Press.

Merchant, C. 2003. *Reinventing Eden: The fate of nature in Western culture*. New York: Routledge.

Mohs, G. 1994. Stó:lô sacred ground. In David Carmichael et al., eds., *Sacred sites, Sacred places,* 184-208. London, UK: Routledge.

Moran, J.R., C.M. Fleming, P. Somervell, and S.M. Manson. 1999. Measuring bicultural ethnic identity among American Indian adolescents: A factor analytic study. *Journal of Adolescent Research* 14 (4): 405-26.

Mussell, W.J. 2005. *Warrior-caregivers: Understanding the challenges and healing of First Nations men*. Ottawa, ON: Aboriginal Healing Foundation.

Nabokov, P. 2006. *Where the lightning strikes: The lives of American Indian sacred places*. New York: Viking.

Petchkovsky, L., C. San Roque, and M. Beskow. 2003. Jung and the dreaming: Analytical psychology's encounters with Aboriginal culture. *Transcultural Psychiatry* 40 (2): 208-38.

Peterson, J.B. 1999. *Maps of meaning: The architecture of belief*. New York: Routledge.

Picou, J.S. 2000. The "Talking Circle" as sociological practice: Cultural transformation of chronic disaster impacts. *Sociological Practice: A Journal of Clinical and Applied Sociology* 2 (2): 77-97.

Pokotylo, D., and G.M. Brass. 1997. Interpreting cultural resources: Hatzic site. In J.H. Jameson Jr., ed., *Presenting archaeology to the public: Digging for truths,* 156-65. Lantham, MD: Altamira Press.

Rowley, K.E. 2002. Re-inscribing mythopoetic vision in Native American studies. *American Indian Quarterly* 26 (3): 491-500.

Ryan, A.F. 2000. *The trickster shift: Humour and irony in contemporary Native art*. Vancouver, BC: UBC Press.

Salisbury, R.F. 1986. *A homeland for the Cree: Regional development in James Bay, 1971-1981*. Montreal, QC, and Kingston, ON: McGill-Queen's University Press.

Sandner, D. 1979. *Navaho symbols of healing: A Jungian exploration of ritual, image and medicine*. Rochester, VT: Healing Arts Press.

Scheff, T.J. 1979. *Catharsis in healing, ritual, and drama*. Berkeley, CA: University of California Press.

Serbin, L.A., and J. Karp. 2004. The intergenerational transfer of psychosocial risk: Mediators of vulnerability and resilience. *Annual Review of Psychology* 55: 333-63.

Sherzer, J. 1983. *Kuna ways of speaking: An ethnographic perspective*. Austin, TX: University of Texas Press.

Sigal, J.J. 1998. Long-term effects of the Holocaust: Empirical evidence for resilience in the first, second, and third generation. *Psychoanalytic Review* 85 (4): 579-85.

Silove, D. 1999. The psychosocial effects of torture, massive human rights violations, and refugee trauma. *Journal of Nervous and Mental Disease* 187 (4): 200-7.

Sissons, J. 2005. *First peoples: Indigenous cultures and their futures*. London, UK: Reaktion Books.

Smith, L.T. 1999. *Decolonizing methodologies: Research and Indigenous peoples*. London, UK: Zed Books.

Speck, F.G. 1977 [1935]. *Naskapi: The savage hunters of the Labrador Peninsula*. Norman, OK: University of Oklahoma Press.

Speck, R.V., and C.L. Attneave. 1973. *Family networks: Retribalization and healing*. New York: Pantheon.

Stephenson, C. 2003. A Cree woman reads Jung. *Transcultural Psychiatry* 40 (2): 181-93.

Stout, M.D. 2003. *Aboriginal people, resilience and the residential school legacy*. Ottawa, ON: Aboriginal Healing Foundation.

Tanner, Adrian. 1979. *Bringing home animals: Religious ideology and mode of production of the Mistassini Cree hunters*. St. John's, NF: ISER Books.

–. 2004. The cosmology of nature, cultural divergence, and the metaphysics of community healing. In C.J.S. Poirier and E. Schwimmer, eds., *Figured worlds: Ontological obstacles in intercultural relations*, 189-222. Toronto, ON: University of Toronto Press.

Torrance, R.M. 1994. *The spiritual quest: Transcendence in myth, religion, and science*. Berkeley, CA: University of California Press.

Trimble, J.E., S.E. Manson, D.G. Dinges, and B. Medicine. 1984. American Indian concepts of mental health: Reflections and directions. In P. Pederson, N. Sartorius, and A.J. Marsella, eds., *Mental health services: The cross-cultural context*, 199-220. Beverly Hills, CA: Sage.

Turner, D.A. 2006. *This is not a peace pipe: Towards a critical indigenous philosophy*. Toronto, ON: University of Toronto Press.

Turner, V. 1967. *The forest of symbols: Aspects of Ndembu ritual*. Ithaca, NY: Cornell University Press.

Valaskakis, G.G. 2005. *Indian country: Essays on contemporary Native culture*. Waterloo, ON: Wilfred Laurier University Press.

van Gennep, A. 1960. *The rites of passage*. Chicago, IL: University of Chicago Press.

Vizenor, G. 1999. *Manifest manners: Narratives on postindian survivance*. Lincoln, NE: University of Nebraska Press.

Vitebsky, P. 2001. *Shamanism*. Norman, OK: University of Oklahoma Press.

Waldram, J.B. 1997. *The way of the pipe: Aboriginal spirituality and symbolic healing in Canadian prisons*. Peterborough, ON: Broadview Press.

–. 2004. *Revenge of the Windigo: The construction of the mind and mental health of North American Aboriginal Peoples*. Toronto, ON: University of Toronto Press.

Warry, W. 1998. *Unfinished dreams: Community healing and the reality of Aboriginal self-government*. Toronto, ON: University of Toronto Press.

Washburn, W.E. 1996. The Native American renaissance, 1960 to 1995. In B.G. Trigger and W.E. Washburn, eds., *The Cambridge history of the Native peoples of the Americas*, vol. 1, *North America Part 2*, 401-74. New York: Cambridge University Press.

Wesley-Esquimaux, C.C., and M. Smolewski. 2004. *Historic trauma and Aboriginal healing*. Ottawa, ON: Aboriginal Healing Foundation.

Wexler, B.E. 2006. *Brain and culture: Neurobiology, ideology, and social change*. Cambridge, MA: MIT Press.

Whitbeck, L.B., G.W. Adams, D.R. Hoyt, and X. Chen. 2004. Conceptualizing and measuring historical trauma among American Indian people. *American Journal of Community Psychology* 33 (3-4): 119-30.

Young, A. 1988. Unpacking the demoralization thesis. *Medical Anthropology Quarterly* 2 (1): 3-16.

Contributors

Naomi Adelson, PhD, associate professor, Department of Anthropology, York University, Toronto, is a medical anthropologist specializing in Aboriginal health issues. Her book *"Being alive well": Health and the politics of Cree well-being* (2000) documents the social, cultural, and political factors that both impinge upon and define health for the Cree of Great Whale River in northern Quebec. More recently, she has conducted research on a series of related subjects that include the growth of traditional therapies in relation to community cultural-renewal projects, social suffering, and expressions of stress among the women in this community.

Gregory M. Brass, MA, is Anishnawbe (Saulteaux) and currently a doctoral candidate in anthropology at McGill University. After completing his master's degree at McGill in 2000, he worked as a federal public servant on the National Homelessness Initiative, focusing on Aboriginal and youth homelessness issues. He has also worked in museums and in the area of cultural heritage across Canada and the United States. He has conducted ethnographic research in a correctional setting and a hospital emergency ward and co-ordinated the Aboriginal Mental Health Research Team. His current research interest is in cancers and medical pluralism among the Aboriginal population.

Jacob (Jake) A. Burack, PhD, is professor of school/applied developmental psychology in the Department of Educational and Counselling Psychology at McGill University and a researcher in the Clinique spécialisée de l'autisme at Hôpital Rivière-des-Prairies. As director of the McGill Youth Study Team, he and his students conduct research on issues of social, emotional, behavioural, and academic risk and well-being among Aboriginal adolescents from remote regions in northern Quebec.

Michael J. Chandler, PhD, is a developmental psychologist working at the University of British Columbia. The focus of his ongoing program of research is to explore the role that culture plays in constructing the course of identity development by shaping young people's emerging sense of ownership of their personal and cultural past and their commitment to their own and their community's future well-being. These efforts have earned Dr. Chandler the Izaak Walton Killam Memorial Senior Research Prize and the Izaak Walton Killam Teaching Prize and have resulted in his being named a Peter Wall Institute for Advanced Studies Distinguished Scholar in Residence. His research and scholarly efforts have also led to his being named Canada's only Distinguished Investigator of both the Canadian Institutes of Health Research and the Michael Smith Foundation for Health Research. Most recently, Professor Chandler's program of research dealing with identity development and suicide in Aboriginal and non-Aboriginal youth was singled out for publication as an invited monograph of the Society for Research in Child Development. He is currently engaged in studies of adolescent identity formation in Aboriginal communities.

Dara Culhane, PhD, is an associate professor of anthropology at Simon Fraser University who has worked in the field of Aboriginal health since 1974. From 1992 to 1994 she served as deputy director of Social and Cultural Research for the Royal Commission on Aboriginal Peoples (RCAP). In this capacity, she co-ordinated the RCAP Life History Projects and the Residential School Research Project. She is author of *An error in judgment: The politics of medical care in an Indian-white community* (1987) and *The pleasure of the Crown: Anthropology, law and First Nations* (1998), and she is co-editor (with Leslie Robertson) of *In plain sight: Reflections on everyday life in Downtown Eastside Vancouver* (2005), winner of the 2006 George Ryga Award for Social Awareness in Literature. Her current research interests focus on experimental ethnographic methodologies, marginalization, and urban studies. In 2006 she co-ordinated "People Like You," an ethnographic performance created collaboratively with women suffering HIV+/AIDS and hepatitis C, and in 2007 she directed "Stories and Plays," an ethnographic theatre project in collaboration with the Postive Outlook Program, Vancouver Native Health Society.

Mason Durie, MB ChB, is professor and deputy vice chancellor (Mäori) of Massey University. He is from Rangitane, Ngäti Kauwhata, and Ngäti Raukawa. He attended Te Aute College and studied medicine at the University of Otago. He trained in psychiatry at McGill University, Montreal. At McGill he developed an interest in both community and transcultural psychiatry. When he was appointed director of Psychiatry at the Palmerston North Hospital, he took a lead in applying the community psychiatric model to the New Zealand context. From 1986 to 1988 he was a commissioner on the Royal Commission on Social Policy and subsequently the chair in Mäori Studies at Massey University in 1988. His continuing interest in health, mental health, and social policy is reflected in an extensive range of publications and research involvements. He has also contributed to the broader field of Mäori development and has published widely on contemporary Mäori realities and the significance of identity to social and economic growth. In recognition of his research and publications, he was made a Fellow of the Royal Society of New Zealand in 1995. In 2001 he was appointed a Companion of the New Zealand Order of Merit.

Georges Henry Erasmus was born at Fort Rae, Northwest Territories, in 1948. He is a past president of both the Indian Brotherhood of Northwest Territories (later the Dene Nation) and the Denendeh Development Corporation, former two-term national chief of the Assembly of First Nations, and former co-chair of the Royal Commission on Aboriginal Peoples. Since 1998 he has been president and chair of the Aboriginal Healing Foundation and currently is also the chief negotiator for the Dehcho First Nations. Mr. Erasmus was appointed a Member of the Order of Canada in 1987, and in 1999 he was promoted to Officer. He has been awarded honorary doctorates by several Canadian universities, including the University of Toronto, Queen's University, the University of Manitoba, and the University of Western Ontario.

Jo-Anne Fiske, PhD, is professor of women's studies and anthropology at the University of Lethbridge, where she is currently dean of Graduate Studies. Her work is grounded in feminist legal anthropology and political economy. She has worked on questions of Aboriginal women's health, customary law, and colonialism. She has published widely, most recently in *Atlantis, Journal of Legal Pluralism, Western Journal of Nursing Research,* and *BC Studies*. She is co-author (with Betty Patrick, chief, Lake Babine Nation) of *Cis dideen kat – When the plumes rise: The way of the Lake Babine Nation* (2000). She is currently working on a manuscript, *The im/moral frontier: Contested histories of the residential school*.

Christopher Fletcher, PhD, is an associate professor in the Department of Anthropology at the University of Alberta. He has diverse research interests in medical and ecological anthropology. He has worked collaboratively with First Nations and Inuit peoples for over a decade in the Northwest Territories, Nunavik, Nunavut, and Nitassinan (Labrador). His research and publications have focused on Aboriginal health and healing, cultural concepts and practices in social and mental health, cultural landscape, kinship, and cross-cultural dissemination of research results. He also maintains an active interest in video and new media applications in research processes, cultural preservation, and knowledge translation.

Joseph P. Gone, PhD, is assistant professor in the Department of Psychology (Clinical Area) and the Program in American Culture (Native American Studies) at the University of Michigan in Ann Arbor. An enrolled member of the Gros Ventre tribe of Montana, he obtained his BA in psychology at Harvard University in 1992 and his PhD in clinical and community psychology at the University of Illinois at Urbana-Champaign in 2001. As a cultural psychologist, Gone addresses in his research the key dilemma confronting mental health professionals who serve Native American communities, namely how to provide culturally appropriate helping services that avoid the neo-colonial subversion of local thought and practice. He has published articles and chapters concerning the ethnopsychological investigation of self, identity, personhood, and social relations in American Indian cultural contexts vis-à-vis the mental health professions.

Ernest Hunter, MD, is an Australian psychiatrist trained in adult, child, and cross-cultural psychiatry in the United States who has been working in remote indigenous communities across northern Australia for two decades. He is currently regional psychiatrist with Queensland Health, servicing communities in Cape York, and adjunct professor at the University of Queensland.

Grace Iarocci, PhD, is an associate professor of clinical psychology and Michael Smith Foundation for Health Research Scholar in the Department of Psychology, Simon Fraser University, and an adjunct professor in the Faculty of Health Sciences. Her research has focused on risk and protective factors associated with educational outcomes among Aboriginal adolescents living in remote communities across Canada. In British Columbia she is involved in investigating educational policy initiatives designed to promote educational achievement among Aboriginal youth.

Lori Idlout is executive director of Isaksimagit Inuusirmi Katujjiqatigiit (Embrace Life Council) in Iqaluit. As a young mother of four, Ms. Idlout started her career with the Government of the Northwest Territories in 1997 in the Department of Health and Social Services. The passion and commitment her mentor taught her have grounded her in her career in the health and social-service fields. Ms. Idlout has worked for the Office of the Interim Commissioner as a policy analyst. Once the Government of Nunavut came into being on 1 April 1999, she maintained her position within the Department of Health and Social Services. Later that year, Ms. Idlout made a career move that also benefited her outlook on supporting Inuit self-reliance. Ms. Idlout joined the team of highly skilled staff and board members of the Nunavut Social Development Council. After beginning her term there as a policy analyst, she went on to become the acting executive director until staff of the mother organization, Nunavut Tunngavik Inc., became the new council members. She then returned to the Department of Health and Social Services to become the director for Policy and Planning. She is now on secondment to the Isaksimagit Inuusirmi Katujjiqatigiit, where she has led development of the mandate and office of the council, which aims to support Nunavummiut and encourage them to value life.

Laurence J. Kirmayer, MD, is James McGill Professor of Psychiatry, director of the Division of Social and Transcultural Psychiatry, McGill University, and director of the Culture and Mental Health Research Unit, Institute of Community and Family Psychiatry, Sir Mortimer B. Davis – Jewish General Hospital. He is also editor-in-chief of *Transcultural Psychiatry*, a quarterly scientific journal. From 1987 to 1993, he was a psychiatric consultant for Inuulitsivik Health Centre in Nunavik. He has conducted research on Inuit concepts of mental health and illness and risk factors for suicide among Inuit youth as well as on determinants of distress among the Cree of northern Quebec. He is co-director of the National Network for Aboriginal Mental Health Research, funded by the Institute of Aboriginal Peoples' Health of the Canadian Institutes of Health Research. His most recent co-edited book is *Understanding trauma: Integrating biological, clinical and cultural perspectives* (2007).

Michael J. Kral, PhD, CPsych, is an assistant professor in the Departments of Psychology and Anthropology, University of Illinois at Urbana-Champaign, and an assistant professor in the Department of Psychiatry, University of Toronto. Since 1994, he has been working on suicide-prevention and community wellness research with Inuit in Nunavut, and is involved in a new circumpolar study of Indigenous youth resilience across Siberia, Alaska, Nunavut, Greenland,

and northern Norway. In his work, he continues to exlore the community-based participatory action research process. His current research documents and tries to understand how indigenous communities develop their own successful suicide-prevention and wellness programs/activities, particularly by and for youth. He co-edited the book *Suicide in Canada* (1998).

Christopher E. Lalonde, PhD, is an associate professor of psychology at the University of Victoria. He is also director of the Network Environment for Aboriginal Health Research (Vancouver Island and Coastal Region). His research interests include identity development and social development in childhood and adolescence. He is currently collaborating with First Nations in British Columbia and Manitoba on a research program that aims to better understand why the promotion of Aboriginal culture and self-determination is associated with decreased suicide rates.

Mary Ellen Macdonald, PhD, is a medical anthropologist with postdoctoral training in pediatric palliative care. She is currently a new investigator with the New Emerging Team: Family Caregiving in Palliative and End-of-Life Care, a project of the Canadian Institutes of Health Research (CIHR). She holds academic appointments in Oncology and the School of Nursing at McGill University as well as an adjunct appointment in Anthropology at the University of Victoria. The study she reports in this volume comes from her doctoral work on Aboriginal mental health policy in Montreal (McGill University, 2003). In addition to her interests in palliative care and bereavement research, her current research continues to involve urban Aboriginal health issues in Montreal. Currently, she is co-investigator on a CIHR grant partnered with the Montreal Native Friendship Centre examining tuberculosis in the urban Aboriginal community.

Rod McCormick, PhD, is a member of the Mohawk Nation and works as an associate professor in the Department of Education and Counselling Psychology at the University of British Columbia. For seven years Dr. McCormick was director of the Native Indian Teacher Education Program at the same university. He also works as a mental health consultant for various Aboriginal healing organizations and governments. His research focus is on effective Aboriginal healing practices as well as on Aboriginal counsellor education.

Helen Milroy, MBBS, FRANZCP, is a descendant of the Palyku people of the Pilbara region in Western Australia. Currently, she works as a consultant child-and-adolescent psychiatrist with the Bentley Health Service. She is an associate professor with the Faculty of Medicine and director for the Centre for Aboriginal Medical and Dental Health at the University of Western Australia. Her research interests include the impact of childhood trauma, grief and mortality, and indigenous therapies.

Ronald Niezen, PhD, is Canada Research Chair in the Comparative Study of Indigenous Rights and Identity and a professor of anthropology at McGill University. He is an anthropologist with wide-ranging research experience: with the Songhay of Mali, with the Cree communities of Quebec, Ontario, and Manitoba, and with the Sami of Finland. He taught for nine years at Harvard University and held visiting positions at the University of Winnipeg and at Åbo Akademi University in Finland. His current research elaborates on the findings of his book *The origins of indigenism* (2003), with a variety of new perspectives on the transnational lobbying of indigenous peoples and nongovernmental organizations, including the implications of new uses of media for identity construction. He has also published *A world beyond difference* (2004), which considers the relationship between cultural difference and globalization. His current work continues to explore the challenges to prosperity and mental health faced by particular indigenous communities and applies this knowledge more broadly to global struggles for recognition and self-determination.

Rhoda Root, PhD, is director of Adult Services at the West Montreal Readaptation Centre. She has extensive experience working with people with disabilities and with Aboriginal children and families. Her research focus is on risk, resilience, wellness, and educational outcomes among Aboriginal adolescents in a northern community.

Colin Samson, PhD, is a sociologist and director of the Humanities Program at the University of Essex, England. He has been working with the Innu peoples of the Labrador-Quebec peninsula since 1994. Much of his research has sought to understand the health impacts and human rights implications of forced changes to the Innu way of life. His book *A way of life that does not exist: Canada and the extinguishment of the Innu* (2003) won the International Council for Canadian Studies' Pierre Savard Award in 2006. In 2004 he was invited to testify at the UN Working Group on Indigenous Populations on the connections between Canada's land confiscation practices and Innu mental health. He is currently writing a book on the health, psychological, and environmental benefits of cultural continuity for indigenous peoples around the world. In 2009 he will embark upon a film project with the Innu of Natuashish.

Cori Simpson has a Master's degree from the Frost Centre for Canadian and Native Studies at Trent University in Peterborough, Ontario. Her master's research project was entitled "In the eyes of the state: Indian Agents, agency and resistance in Kahnawake." Her research interests include social history, Indian policy, relations between Kahnawake and the state, and interdisciplinary methodologies. Simpson is a Mohawk of Kahnawake.

Caroline L. Tait, PhD, is an assistant professor at the University of Saskatchewan. She received her doctorate in anthropology from McGill University and has a bachelor of arts degree from McGill University in anthropology and a master's degree from the University of California at Berkeley. Dr. Tait was a Fulbright Scholar and Visiting Fellow at Harvard University in the Departments of Anthropology and Social Medicine during the 1995-96 academic year. Her research spans North America, contrasting Canadian and American public health responses to substance abuse by pregnant women.

Adrian Tanner, PhD, is Honorary Research Professor, Department of Anthropology, Memorial University, Newfoundland. He has conducted fieldwork among the James Bay Cree since the 1970s and is the author of a classic monograph on Cree spirituality. His expertise is in the interaction of notions of religion, land use, and politics in Aboriginal identity and communal life. From 1996 to the present, he has been involved in research on the healing movement among the Cree of Quebec, a study of a number of local spiritual-based initiatives being taken to address social and mental health problems in the Cree communities of Mistissini, Waswanipi, and Nemeska, Quebec.

Gail Guthrie Valaskakis, PhD, was director of Research, Aboriginal Healing Foundation, until her death in July 2007. She was Distinguished Professor Emeritus of Concordia University in Montreal, where she served as professor and as vice dean and dean of the Faculty of Arts and Sciences, for eleven years. She researched and wrote extensively on the social and cultural changes in Aboriginal identity. She was a founding member of the boards of Waseskun Native Half-Way House (1989), the Montreal Native Friendship Centre (1974-82), on which she served as president, and the Native North American Studies Institute and Manitou Community College (1970-75). She served on the Advisory Boards of the Institute of Aboriginal People's Health and the National Collaborating Centre for Aboriginal Health. Dr. Valaskakis received a National Aboriginal Achievement Award in 2002 for her contributions to the development of Aboriginal media in Canada.

James B. Waldram, PhD, is a professor in the Department of Psychology at the University of Saskatchewan. A medical anthropologist, he has researched and written extensively about Aboriginal health for twenty-five years. He is currently working on indigenous health issues in both Canada and Belize. His most recent books include *The way of the pipe: Aboriginal spirituality and symbolic healing in Canadian prisons* (1997), *Revenge of the Windigo: The construction of the mind and mental health of North American Aboriginal peoples* (2004), and (with D. Ann Herring and T. Kue Young) *Aboriginal health in Canada: Historical, cultural and epidemiological perspectives,* 2nd ed. (2006).

Robert Watt, BSc, is presently working as the communication officer/specialist for the Nunavik Regional Board of Health and Social Services. As the past director for the National Aboriginal Health Organization's Ajunnginiq Centre, Mr. Watt has had the opportunity to travel within all the Canadian Inuit regions, conducting workshops in order to identify national priorities relating to health and wellness (2001-3). Prior to this, Watt was involved in Nunavik cultural affairs for several years as an elected official within the Avataq Cultural Institute, promoting, protecting, and preserving Inuit language and culture in northern Quebec (1998-2001).

Cornelia Wieman, MSc, MD, FRCPC, is Canada's first female Aboriginal psychiatrist. She is a member of the Ojibway Nation and originally from the Little Grand Rapids reserve in northern Manitoba. From 1997 to 2005, she practised psychiatry at a community mental health clinic based on the Six Nations of the Grand River Territory. She is co-director of the Indigenous Health

Research Development Program and an assistant professor in the Department of Public Health Sciences, Faculty of Medicine, University of Toronto. She is a co-investigator on several research initiatives funded through the Canadian Institutes of Health Research – Institute of Aboriginal Peoples Health, including the National Network of Aboriginal Mental Health Research and the New Emerging Team on Understanding and Acting on Aboriginal Suicide.

Index

Aase, J., 206-7
Aatami, Pita, 312n7
Abel, E., 203-4, 209
Abenaki, 382, 387
Aboriginal Achievement Awards, 460, 467-68n5
Aboriginal Career-Life Planning Model, 346
Aboriginal counselling. *See* counselling psychology
Aboriginal Healing Foundation (AHF), xii, 25-26, 275, 453, 455, 463
Aboriginal health. *See* health
Aboriginal Health Studies, 162-63
Aboriginal intellectual movement, 466
Aboriginal Peoples Survey, 13, 206
Aboriginal Peoples Television Network, 460
Aboriginal rights, 24, 46, 51, 398n9, 464
"Aboriginal Solidarity" flag, 366, 378n10
Aboriginal women. *See* women
Aboriginality, 56-74; blood quantum, 57-60, 66, 392, 398n14; cultural orientation, 5(f), 57, 62-73; definition, 73, 356, 358, 362-64, 460; ethnic identity, xiii, 20-24, 396, 442-47, 464; ethnographic research, 18-20, 362-64; legislative and self-identification, 60-62; self-narratives, 355, 361, 365-74; social construction, 375
Aborigine, 3-28; culture areas, 5(f), 62-64, 71, 73n5, 73n6; definition, 5-6, 243, 377n2, 468n9; demographics, 3-7, 4(f), 28n1, 28n3, 43-44, 87; history, 7-14; life expectancy, 6, 254; mortality rates, 6, 46-47; as the Other, 21, 243, 357, 362, 375; political system, 113-14; reconciliation and reparations, 25-26; social justice goals, 51-52; worldviews, 38-39, 47-49, 338, 352
abuse: child, 14, 82, 165, 211, 306, 318-19; contributing factors, 302, 312n9; domestic, 143-46, 156, 156n2, 302-3; physical, 310; residential

schools, xii, 26, 152-53, 157n8, 302-3, 345-46, 394. *See also* alcohol/substance abuse; sexual abuse
acculturation: acculturative stress, 69, 193-94n13, 194n14; cross-national studies, 74n8; measurement of, 64-69, 74n9; search for identity, 85; social engineering, 250. *See also* assimilation; cultural continuity
adaptation: adolescence, 96, 461; forced, 129-30; resilience, xvi, 89-90; sociocultural, 62, 82-83, 316, 348-49; urbanization, 12
addictions, 112-13, 170-71, 174, 369, 378n11
Adelson, N., 117, 272-86, 448
adolescence: adaptation, 96, 461; development, 86-95, 225, 460-62; drug surveys, 93-94; personal persistence, 222-25; puberty rituals, 94. *See also* youth
adoptions, 9, 204, 351
adversity and resilience, 88-90, 214
affective disorders, 17
agency: collective, xix, 267, 315-30, 459-60; personal, 28, 36, 326-27
Ahia, C.E., 346
AIDS, 318, 383, 392, 394, 398n7
Akaneshau, 129-30, 135
Alarcón, R.D., 72-73
Alaska, 65, 73n1, 325
Alberta, 73-74n7, 357, 449
alcohol/substance abuse: alcohol dependency, 15-18, 44, 66, 205-6; ARBE-related, 208, 215n4; binge drinking, 190, 205-6, 252-53; conception of, 310, 348-50; controlled drinking communities, 319; epidemiology, 15-18, 61, 66, 205-6, 221, 228-42; gas sniffing, 125(f), 127-28, 171; genetic predisposition, 44; glue sniffing, 17; Innu, 110-11,

Canadian Medical Association, 207

capitalism, xv, 467

career and vocational counselling, 150(f), 337, 346, 352, 407, 422-23, 425

Cargo, M., 134

Carpenter, J., 461

Carstens, P., 251

Cartier, Jacques, 381

catharsis, 451

Catholic Church, 23, 276, 359

Cayuga, 403

cedar, 360, 364

Center for Epidemiological Studies Depression Scale (CES-D), 63

Centres de santé et de service sociaux (CSSS), 398n10

Centres locaux de service communautaire (CLSCs), 385, 398n10. *See also* CLSC model

ceremonies: cleansing, 339, 345, 360; Cree mourning, 367-68; drug use, 94; gatherings, 261-63, 267-68, 306; healing, 267, 340, 345, 347, 350, 359, 365; hunting groups, 256-58; initiation, 457; pan-Indian, 261-62; peace pipe/pipe ceremony, 261, 274-75, 340; Pow-Wows, 26, 66, 172, 261, 263-64, 350; puberty rituals, 94; relationship to land, 451(f); sacred fire, 365, 375; shaking tent ceremony, 281-82, 285n3, 286n7; smudging, 359-60, 364, 417n6; spirit dances, 340; Sun Dance, 9, 11, 66; symbols, 450-52; Vision Quest, 339-40, 343

Chance, N.A., 65

Chandler, M.J., 19, 68, 83-84, 134, 188-89, 192n5, 221-46, 328

Chartrand, Mel and Shirley, 458

child development. *See* development

children: adoptions, 9, 204; child abuse and neglect, 10, 14, 82, 165, 211, 306, 318-19; child care services, 239-40; child-welfare policies, 10-11, 41; domestic roles, 147, 149; forced removal, 9-11, 45-46, 128, 237, 351; gas sniffing, 125(f), 127-28; gatherings/hunting groups, 254-58, 262-63; infant mortality, 46, 110, 254; Mäori, 45; mental health data, 16-17; society's children, 198. *See also* development; fetal alcohol syndrome (FAS); residential schools

Choudhuri, A., 60-61

Christianity: authority from, 151; conversion, 187, 272-78, 374; demonic possession, 305; East

Cree, 257, 264-65, 267, 448; evangelical, 23, 305; Whapmagoostui community, 276-85; wilderness concepts, 147. *See also* missionaries; residential schools

Christopher, J., 72

Chumash, 94

Churchill Falls, 118, 136n6

Cicchetti, D., 89

circles/circle ceremonies: healing, 26, 98, 163, 275, 364-65, 417n6, 452; sentencing, 26; sharing, 26, 98; spiritual, 26, 370; talking, 26, 450-52

citizenship, 46, 398n9

civilization, 9-10, 147, 155-56, 245, 273, 420, 422

Clarkson, M., 17

cleansing ceremony, 339, 345, 360

Clifford, J., 362

CLSC model, 385-96; accessibility, 387-89, 392-94; background, 389-91; confidentiality, 395-96, 398n17; cultural sensitivity, 388-89; effectiveness, 396; heterogeneity, 391-92; location, 393-94, 398n15; philosophy of care, 392; professionalism, 390, 395; staffing and ethnic match, 395-96; unmet needs, 394-95. *See also* Six Nations Mental Health Services

cluster suicides, xvii, 179, 183-85, 189, 190. *See also* suicide

Clyde River, 293

cocaine/crack cocaine, 17, 170-72, 369

cognitive theory, 68, 342, 441-45

Cohen, A., 386

cohort, 90, 209, 425

collective identity/collectivism: Aboriginality, 6, 19-21, 311, 442; agency, xix, 267, 315-30, 404-5, 459; family interdependence, 327; globalization, 14; healing, 267, 327, 464; historical grief, 452-56, 459; incarceration, 376; knowledge systems, 39, 457; self-determination, 328; and suicide, 180-81, 189-92; survival, 467

College of Psychiatrists' mental health guidelines, 36

Collignon, B., 312n3

colonial legacy: Australia/New Zealand, 36, 38; double-bind theory, 128-33; health/health care, 27-28, 45-46, 397; historical trauma, xii, 187-88, 452-56, 463; intergenerational, 208; sociocultural impact, 7-28, 133-35, 165, 327-28, 440, 446; suicide, 185-86, 190. *See also* residential schools; spiritual colonization

crowding, 123, 237

Csordas, T.J., 359

Culhane, D., 160-75

cultural continuity, 221-46; acculturation/ discontinuity, 68, 84, 186-87, 249; implications for policy, 243-46; importance of, 133-34; languages, 39; recuperation, 274-76, 280-81, 284-85; theory, 19-20, 222-28; transformation, 7, 305-11, 460-62, 465-67. *See also* suicide

cultural genocide, 154-55, 350

cultural sensitivity: education, 90-91; health services, xix, 48-49, 57-52, 341-43, 376, 390, 431-35, 463-64; resource distribution, 165

culture: cohesion, 460; concept of, 24, 57, 68, 291, 465; cultural gaze, 362-63; culture areas, 5(f), 62-64, 71, 73n5, 73n6; deculturation, 40-41, 70, 129-34, 136n10; ethnographic research, 50, 64-71, 464-67; loss of, 212-13, 249, 454; persistence of, 22, 222-28, 465-67; reaffirmation/ renewal, 24-27, 242, 340-41; revitalization, 14, 263, 359; suppression/oppression, 7-9, 14, 28, 272-78, 281, 284, 286n8, 327-28; as therapy, 193-94n13, 376; and well-being, xi. *See also* Aboriginality; healing movement

culture-bound syndrome, 312n4

culture camps, 306-07, 325

Das, V., 165-66

Davin, N.D./Davin Report, 9, 419

Davis, J., 52

Davis Inlet, 109, 115-16, 119, 122, 123(f), 127, 135n2, 190

Day, A., 90

de Rios, M.D., 94

deculturation, 129-34, 136n10

deep listening, 50

Degnen, C., 321

Delgamuukw case, 156n5

Dell, D., 134

Deloria, Vine, Jr., 466

demographics: cultural-ecological regions, 5(f); geographic distribution, 4(f); health indicators, 37(t); Inuit, 4-5, 289; Labrador, 4; language groups, 5(f), 22; Montreal, 381-83; mortality rates, 6, 43, 46-47, 110-11, 135nn1-2, 152, 157n11; Northwest Territories, 4; population trends (Australia/New Zealand), 43-44, 46; population trends (Canada), 3-7, 28n1, 87;

pre-Columbian population, 28n3; psychiatric disorders, 15-18; suicide risk factors, 224-28; worldwide indigenous groups, 38

demon possession, 300(f), 304-5, 312n10

Denedeh/Dene First Nation, 318

Denis, C., 457

Department of Indian and Northern Affairs Canada (INAC), 403-4

Department of Northern Affairs and Natural Resources, 316

depression: Beck Depression Scale, 227; Canadian Community Health Survey, 17; cultural linkage, 49, 63, 84, 293-94; diagnostic methods, 16, 63; ecocentric connection, 300-1, 300(f), 310; elementary students, 88; rates of, 47, 408; risk factors, 117, 179; Sixties Scoop, 414; symptoms, 16, 17

Desautels, D., 122

detachment, 344-45

development, 80-100; adolescence, 86-95, 225-28; cultural contexts, 81-83, 225; family contexts, 95; moral, 303, 305, 308-10, 365, 375, 378n12; peer contexts, 93-95; risk and resilience, 83-86, 88-91; school contexts, 90-93; self, 84-86, 445; sociocultural factors, 86-95; variation/deviation dynamic, 82-83

developmental psychology, 99-100

Devereux, G., 57

Devlin, A., 192n4

devolution, 239

diabetes, 6, 8, 44, 46

diagnosis: communication styles, 49, 51; cultural orientation, 64-69; *Diagnostic and statistical manual* (DSM), 49; diagnostic frameworks, 14-17, 48-49, 63, 69, 406-7. *See also* DSM-III-R disorder; DSM-IV; DSM-IV-TR

Dick, L., 312n8

diet, xix, 8, 254, 295

Dilco Ojibway Child and Family Services, 192n4

disabilities, 6, 46, 211-13

discipline, 307-8

discourse: Aboriginality, 21-24, 356, 362-64, 376-77, 448; alcohol abuse/FAS, 196-97, 205-6, 214; colonial/neocolonial, 142, 154, 157n12, 245, 420; healing and health concepts, 42-43, 164, 199-200, 321; historical trauma, 453; political rights, 58-59; race, 205, 214; spatial, 143-44, 151-55; victimization, 140-41

behaviour, 17, 408; domestic violence, 16; emotional distress, 7-15; FAS, 204-8, 210-11; health surveys, 14-18; posttraumatic stress disorder (PTSD), 16-17, 454-55; psychiatry, 14-18, 430; service utilization studies, 15; suicide, 17, 221, 228-42; transition, 52n3

epilepsy, 298

epistemic violence, 245

epistemology, xx, 47-49, 338, 428-30, 435, 442

Erasmus, Georges, xi-xii

Erikson, E., 191-92

Escobar, A., 329

Eskimos, 65

ethics, 167-68, 448, 458, 463

ethnicity, 20-24, 39-41, 51, 395-96. *See also* Aboriginality; identity

ethnographic research: Aboriginality, 18-20, 362-64; alcohol/substance abuse, 398n7; Australia, 50, 74n8, 363; child development, 94; counselling, 341, 344-45; cultural practices, 50, 64-71, 464-67; depression, 433; drug use, 93-94; emotions, 433; ethnotheories, 426-29; FAS-related, 209; healing, 444-45; Nunavik, 291-92; race, 58-59, 209; residential schools, 19; social suffering, 166-67. *See also* narratives/narrative research

ethnopolitics, 152

ethnopsychology, 291, 299-300, 427-28, 435, 463

etiology, 86, 185-88

evidence-based medicine, 415-16

existential concepts, 349-50

extinguishment, 127

Eyaa-Keen Centre, 458, 468n11

eye contact, 49

Eye-Movement Desensitization and Reprocessing, 429

FAE. *See* fetal alcohol effects

faith, community healing, 272-86

family/family cohesion: destabilization, 119, 298, 307; family therapy, 95, 98-99, 342-43, 345, 350-51, 434-35; and healing, 99, 338-39; mental health, 302-3, 306-7

family structure: clan system, 405; hunting groups, 253-58; single-parent, 95. *See also* kinship systems

family violence, 6, 395

Fanon, F., 131, 246

FAS. *See* fetal alcohol syndrome

FASD. *See* fetal alcohol spectrum disorder

father's rights, 144-45, 156n2

feasts, 256(f), 262

Fekete, J., 146

Ferron, J., 141

fetal alcohol effects (FAE), 196, 204, 208, 215n4

fetal alcohol spectrum disorder (FASD), 204, 205, 208, 212-13, 215n4

fetal alcohol syndrome (FAS), 196-216; background, xviii, 196-200, 204-8, 215n4; creating an epidemic, 208-11; FAS/FAE children, 196; the "G" case, 200-2, 215n2; impact, 196, 211, 213-14, 318; learning disabilities, 136n12; pathology, 202-4; prevalence rates, 204, 210, 212, 215n5, 215nn9-10; prevention activities, 206, 211, 320; rates, 207, 210, 212-13, 215nn8-10; screening, 215n5; secondary disabilities, 211-13; society's children, 198

field work. *See* methodology

film program, 323-25

Fine, M., 173

First Nations: demographics, 3-4; foster-care rates, 10; Governance Act (FNGA), 12; Governance Initiative, 246n1; health indicators, 37(t); infant mortality, 46, 110, 254; Information Governance Committee, 17-18; Inherent Right to Self-Government Policy, 326; living conditions, 13; membership, 59-62; mental health resources, 434-35; nonstatus Indians, 4, 10-12, 60, 357, 377n2; Regional Health Survey, 17, 29n7, 382, 389; status Indians, 4, 10-12, 110, 180, 357, 377n2, 383, 412-13. *See also* bands; colonial legacy; Indian Act; Iroquois/Iroquois Confederacy; Métis

First Nations and Inuit Health Branch (FNIHB), 12, 201-2, 398n13, 404, 412-14

Fisher, P.A., 98

fishing, xiii, 295

Fiske, J.-A., 140-57

Flanagan, T., 94-95

Fletcher, C., 289-312

Flower of Two Soils Re-Interview Study, 17

food: country food, 23, 262, 290, 292-95, 309; dog meat, 66; as medicine, 293-94; reliance on store food, 8, 254, 261; and well-being, 170, 293-95

forgiveness, 303, 345

Fort Belknap, 420

Fort George, 278

Foster, D.A., 65

foster care, 10, 351

Lassiter, C., 117
Lattas, A., 363
Laurin, C., 385, 389
Lawrence, Caleb, 278, 286n6
Leacock, E.B., 136n5
Leader, A., 199-200
Lear, J., 465
Lejac residential school, 148(f), 149, 157n10
Lemoine, P.H., 215n3
Lévesque, C.N., 382, 394
Lévi-Strauss, C., 441, 467n1, 467n3
Levy, J.E., 194n14
liberalism, 11, 157n12, 326, 363, 386, 425
life expectancy, 6, 254
life projects, 329
life stories, 97, 152. *See also* narratives/narrative research; storytelling
lifestyle, 8, 342
local control: Australia, 325-26; child care services, 239-40; formal education, 423-24; Hamlet Councils, 319, 322; health care, 19, 241-42, 329-30, 464; Health Transfer Agreements, 326, 384; Iroquois Band Council, 403-6, 417n3; Nunavut, 319-21; political autonomy, 45, 84, 116, 132, 213, 240-42; and suicide rates, 68, 241-42, 244-46, 318. *See also* self-government
Lock, M., 165-66, 198
loneliness, 16, 149, 179, 433
Long, D., 459
longhouse, 405
longitudinal studies, 91, 96
Luna, James, 466

Macdonald, M.E., 329, 381-98
Macrae, J.A., 154
mainstream health services: alcohol/substance abuse, 347-49; approaches to healing, 68, 341-43, 441-45, 458; clinical rhetoric, 377n3; cognitive theory, 68, 342, 441-45; counselling, 341-43, 458; psychology, 365; treatment programs, 347-49, 390, 396, 458
Maioni, A., 385
Makivik Corporation, 312n7
Malecite, 383
Mancinelli, J.A., 190
mandala, 450-51
mania, 14

Manitoba: Cross Lake crisis, 178-89, 192n2, 193n10; Eyaa-Keen Centre, 458, 468n11; FAS survey, 208; hydroelectric development, 178; incarceration data, 357; murder rates, 211; substance abuse survey, 18. *See also* Iroquois/Iroquois Confederacy
Mäori, 36-52; cultural identity, 39-41, 43, 468n7; demographics, 43, 46-47; healing methods, 39, 47-49; health and well-being, 42-43, 46-49; history, 38, 40; *Hua oranga* concept, 49; identity transitions, 39-41; language, 39; origins, 37-38; political representation, 45; sovereignty (*mana*), 328; suicides, 47, 183; *tangata whenua* concept, 38; *Te taura tieke*, 50; *Te Whare Tapa Wha* concept, 42-43, 468n7; workforce development, 47, 49-50; worldviews, 38-39
marginalization: cultural/socioeconomic, 40, 69-70; health care service, 397; health conditions, 199-200, 309; inner-city women, 165; medical treatment, 136n8; social distress, 7, 13-14, 21, 27; stereotypes, 363-64; suicide, 185, 187-88
Marmot, M., 36
marriage, 143, 253, 257, 262, 304-5
mass media: Aborigine stereotypes, 21, 180, 208, 274; access to, 284-85, 290, 308-9, 460; "G" case (FAS), 200-2; impact, 13-14, 85; suicide, 180, 191, 192n2
materialism, xv, 13, 64-65, 68, 74n9, 120, 127, 445
Mattingly, C., 365-66
Mauss, M., 183, 291
McCormick, R.M., 98, 193n12, 337-52
McEachern, Allan, 156n5
McGill Aboriginal Healing Clinic, 394
McGillivray, Jane, 112-14
McMaster University, 412
McMichael, P., 329
McNicoll, P., 310
McShane, D.A., 64
Mead, M., 461
medical evangelism, 128-29, 136n8
medical pluralism, 377n4
Medicine Community Circle, 360-62
Medicine House, 355-62, 364-65, 372, 375-76, 377n1, 377nn6-7, 378n14
medicine people, 449
medicine wheel, 26, 338, 365, 370, 375, 392, 450-52, 468n7
medicine woman, 371

medicines: bad medicine, 74n10, 371; medicinal plants, 26, 112, 339, 350, 360, 364, 411, 416; respect for, 136n8, 360-62, 370-71, 373, 375; words as, 355, 360

Meehl, P.E., 430

memory/memoryscape, 26, 117, 152, 154, 188, 292, 454, 456

mental disorders. *See* mental illness

mental health: Aboriginal experience, xv, 14-18, 46-49, 193-94n13; concepts, xiv-xv, 14, 17, 49, 297-302, 310, 318; determinants, xix, 44-46, 207-8, 452-55; Elders' views, 298-309; indicators, 37(t); mind-body dualism, 427; *ngarlu* concept, 49; oppression, xix, 45-46, 207-8, 452-55; promotion of, 18, 96-100, 440, 462; residential instability, 13; socioeconomic factors, 44-45, 70, 86-99, 236-42, 303. *See also* community wellness; ecocentrism; mental illness; well-being

mental health profession: Aboriginal professionals, 47, 49-50, 401, 406, 411-12, 463; diagnostic frameworks, 14-17, 48-49, 63, 69, 406-7; mental health guidelines, 36, 317; misunderstandings, 111-21; narrative therapy, 97-98, 365-66; neurolinguistics, 429; shifting roles, 431-32, 434; therapist/healers, 337, 345. *See also* counselling psychology; psychiatry; psychology; training

mental health services, 419-35; Aboriginal community clinics, 178-79, 395-96; access, 387-89, 392-94, 397, 407, 409-12, 413-15; approaches, xx, 51, 80-81, 97-98, 291-92, 320-21; barriers, 347-48; bicultural, 47-48, 291-92, 330, 337, 343-44, 352, 409-10; Brighter Futures, 320-21; community/local control, 19, 68, 241-42, 327-28; culture-related, 48-49, 57-52, 341-43, 390, 392, 409; facilitators survey, 344-47; funding, 414-15; health coverage, 12, 383-85, 389, 397, 412-15; health research teams, 50; language used, 388, 393, 396, 463; Mäori *Hua oranga* concept, 49; rethinking, 47-49, 51, 329-30, 441-42, 462-64; shared care, 407, 411, 415-16; Western clinical approach, 47-49, 329; youth as resource, 87, 434-35. *See also* CLSC model; Six Nations Mental Health Services; treatment programs

mental illness: ARBE-related, 208; contemporary views, 14, 441; cultural linkage, 49, 51, 348-49; demographics, 6-7, 47; ecocentric views, 298-309; historical trauma, xii, 187-88, 452-56, 463;

negative identities, 40-41, 191-92; organic mental disorders, 60; physical/organic causes, 298-99, 309; prevalence rates, 15, 430; psychological causes, 299-303; spirit possession, 304-5, 312n10; stigmatization, 415. *See also* suicide

mental retardation, 196, 298

Mesoamericans, 7

metaphor, 442-45

methadone, 172

methodology: ethics, 167-68; field work, 17, 50, 311n2, 358-59, 377n7, 433; identity narratives, 358-59, 365-66, 377n7; indigenous research, 50; interview protocols, 227-29; qualitative research, 19; scientific epistemology, xx, 47-49, 338, 428-30, 435, 442. *See also* epidemiology; ethnographic research; surveys

Métis: demographics, 4; education, 28n4; foster care, 10; health care, 12; hospital admissions, 60-61; identity, 398n14; legacy of colonization, 6-7; in Montreal, 394; school dropout rates, 92; status, 12, 21; suicide rate, 17

Métis National Council, 6

Middlebrook, D.L., 318

migration, 7, 12-13, 28-29n5, 40, 316-17, 357-58, 378n8, 396

Mi'kmaq/Mi'qmaq, 253, 276, 382-83

Millennium Development Goals, 51

Miller, J.R., 157n11

Milloy, J., 151-52, 157n11

Milroy, H., 36-52

Minas, H., 72-73

mineral claims, 118

mining, 118-20, 136n7, 186-87

Ministère de la santé et des services sociaux (MSSS), 385, 398n11

Minnesota Multiphasic Personality Inventory (MMPI), 59, 66

minority groups, xvi, 71, 94, 96, 146

missionaries: conversion, 272-78, 316; cultural engineering, 187, 245; cultural suppression, 273, 278, 281, 284, 286n8; history, xix, 7-8, 109, 114; Indian education, 147, 419-20; perceived role, 245, 273. *See also* residential schools

Mistissini, 255(f), 256(f), 258-59, 259(f), 262-63

MMPI. *See* Minnesota Multiphasic Personality Inventory

Mohatt, G., 67, 338

Mohawk, 361, 372-73, 382, 403, 417n4. *See also* Iroquois/Iroquois Confederacy; Oka Crisis
Mohawk Warrior Society, 366
Montana, 420
Montreal, 381-98; Aboriginal population, 381-83, 396-97; Association of Montreal Inuit, 394; "community" health care, 385-87; jurisdiction and health coverage, 383-85, 389-90, 397. *See also* CLSC model; Oka Crisis
morality: alcohol/substance abuse, 201-2, 205, 299; double-bind theory, 132; Durkheim theory, 121; hunting groups, 23, 254, 256-57; moral development, 303, 305, 308-10, 365, 375, 378n12; moral geography, 140-42, 144, 147, 149, 151-56, 157n6; moral order, 10, 12, 27-28; moral philosophy, xx, 14, 183, 263, 266, 443-44, 446, 448; moral responsibility, 41, 199, 213, 223, 456-58; moral worth, xviii, 172, 198, 212
Morphy, F., 37
mortality rates, 6, 43, 46-47, 110-11, 135nn1-2, 152, 157n11
motor vehicle accidents, 6, 17
mourning ceremony, 367-68
MSSS. *See* Ministère de la santé et des services sociaux
multiculturalism, 24, 86, 133, 393
murder, 211
Muscogee (Creek) Indians, 349
Mushuau Innu, 114-16, 121-29
Musqueam Reserve, 344
myth, 442-45, 465-67, 467nn2-3

Napoleon (Yup'ik peoples). *See* Yup'ik
narratives/narrative research: Aboriginal identity reconstructions, 355-77, 377n7; narrative therapy, 97-98, 365-66; Saulteaux, 355, 360-62, 367-68; school memories, 152; storytelling, 50, 325, 341, 412, 443-44, 452; Vancouver narratives, 166-73
Naskapi, 368-72
National Aboriginal Community Controlled Health Organization (NACCHO), 325-26
National Aboriginal Day, 285n2
National Aboriginal Health Organization, 6, 25
National Aboriginal Health Strategy, 42
National Aboriginal Youth Strategy, 87
National Health and Medical Research Council, 50
National Health Survey (Australia), 45

National Native Alcohol and Drug Abuse Program (NNADAP), 320-21
National Post, 154
National School Based Youth Risk Survey, 87
Native Friendship Centres, xx, 13, 382-83, 388, 394, 397n5
Native Students Health Sciences, 412
Native Women's Association of Canada, 6
Native Women's Shelter, 383, 394
Natuashish, 121-27
nature, 22, 340, 343, 364, 445-47, 467
Navajo, 117, 359
Nechi Institute, 112, 127
negative identities, 40-41, 191-92
Neider, J., 66
Nelms-Matzke, J., 210
Nemeska, 262
neo-colonialism, 153-54, 157n12, 198, 363
neo-conservatism, 141
neo-liberalism, 51, 157n12, 166
neo-Shamanism, 445
networks, 97, 464
New Age, 23, 112, 445
New France, 316
New Testament, 378n12
New York State, 403-4, 417n4
New Zealand, 36-52; Aotearoa, 37, 38; biculturalism, 45, 447; counselling models, 41-43; demographics, 43-44; disability rates, 46; health indicators, 37(t), 44-46; indigenous workforce, 47, 49-50; mental health guidelines, 36; mortality rates, 46-47; Pākehā middle class, 40. *See also* Māori
Newfoundland, 111, 115. *See also* Innu
Newfoundland Child Welfare Protection Act, 128
Nguyen, V.K., 163-64
Niezen, R., 134, 178-94
Nishnawbe, 188
non-human persons, 22, 295-96, 442, 446
Non-Insured Health Benefits (NIHB), 12, 383, 412-13
nonstatus Indians, 4, 10-12, 60, 357, 377n2
Northern Flood Agreement, 178
Northern Plains Indians, 66
Northwest Passage, 316
Northwest Territories, 4, 22, 317-30
Northwest Territories Health Promotion Survey, 18

Northwest Territories Mental Health Framework, 317

Norway House, 180

Nunatsiavut, 4

Nunavik, 4, 8, 18, 289, 291-92, 315

Nunavut, 315-30; background, xix, 22, 45, 315-17; Bathurst Mandate, 317; Brighter Futures, 320-21; community wellness, 317-19; demographics, 4, 315-16; Embrace Life Council, 328; film/video project, 323-25; Hamlet Councils, 319, 322; settlements, 316-17

Nunavut Arctic College, 298, 319

Nunavut Wildlife Act, 320

nurses, 179, 192n1, 395-96, 406

Nutak, 115

NWT Housing Corporation, 319

obesity, 8, 46

Odanak, 382

Odawa, 63, 85-86

Ohsweken, ON, 401

oil drilling, 119-20

Ojibwa, 22, 63, 85-86, 253

Oka Crisis, 24, 366, 378nn9-10

Okanagan region, 251

Okwí:Rase, 80

Oneida, 403

O'Neil, J., 199-200, 329

O'Nell, T.D., 433

Onen'to:Kon Treatment Centre, 383

Onondaga, 403

Ontario, 4, 180. *See also* Iroquois/Iroquois Confederacy; Sioux Lookout

Ontario Native Women's Association, 156n4

ontology, 267, 442-43

oppression, xix, 7, 28, 45-46, 207-8, 327-28, 363-64, 452-55

oral traditions, 97, 440. *See also* narratives/narrative research; storytelling

ownership scale, 64-65, 68, 74n9

pan-Indianism: background, xix-xx, 378n8; ceremonies, 261-62; healing, 129, 396, 417n6, 447-50; identity, 20-24, 378n14, 392; religion, 23, 263-65, 267; spiritual healing, 358-60, 362, 365, 368, 370-71, 374-75; spirituality, 26, 284-85, 356, 364, 417n6, 450-52

Panama, 441

parenting: childrearing practices, 305-9, 320; hunting groups, 254-58; quality, 10, 45, 82, 187; styles, 19, 95, 302, 305-9, 310

pass system, 11

paternalism, 200, 462

Patterson, T.C., 146

Paul, K.W., 17

peace pipe/pipe ceremony, 261, 274-75, 340

Peary, Robert, 312n4

Peavy, R.V., 342

Peck, Edmund, 278

peer counselling, 320

peer groups, 93-95, 410, 434-35, 461-62

Peers, M., 154, 272

Pelletier, C., 385, 389

Pelletier, W., xi

Penashue, Elizabeth, 132

Penashue, Hank, 119

Penashue, Peter, 327

Pentecostal Church, xviii, 23, 261-62, 264-65, 267, 276, 283

personhood: cultural concept, 291; individual competence, 83-86; life projects, 329; loss of, 117-21, 134-35, 446; notions of, 22-23, 291; personal agency, 326-27; self-concept, 91; self-continuity, 222-28. *See also* identity

Peschard, K., 163-64

Peters, E., 164

Peters, Joseph, 457

physical abuse, 10, 310, 345-46

pibloktoq, 312n8

Pietacho, J.-C., 121

Pimicikamak Cree Nation Health Services, 178-79

place: colonial, 146-55; concepts, 141-43; domestic, 143-46; expressive, 141, 143; sense of and identity, 311, 312n3, 445-46; social contexts, 140-41, 155

Plains Indians, 63, 71, 73-74n7, 112-13, 127, 263-65, 359

plant medicines, 26, 112, 339, 350, 360, 364, 411, 416

Plateau Indians, 63

pluralism, 365, 375

Poehnell, G., 346

poisonings, 6, 209

Pokue, Dominic, 115

policy: best practices, 243-46; community wellness, 317; Comprehensive Land Claims Policy,

race research/eugenics, 58

racism: East Cree, 258, 269n6; legislation, 41-42, 46; marginalizing, 22, 213; Oka Crisis, 24, 366, 378nn9-10. *See also* assimilation; stereotypes

Ramsay, Jack, 145

Rankin Inlet, 319

rape, 6

Rastafarianism, 40

RCMP. *See* Royal Canadian Mounted Police

Reading, J., 199-200

reconciliation, xi, 25, 154, 157n7, 275, 285nn1-2, 303

Red Road, 365

regional autonomy, 45

religion: dualism, 257, 264; and healing, xviii, 359; organized, 23, 276; traditional forms, 257, 263, 266, 276, 282-83. *See also* spiritual colonization

relocation, 8, 114-18, 121-27, 249, 298, 316-17

renal disease, 44

The Report Newsmagazine, 153-54, 157n8

research. *See* epidemiology; ethnographic research; methodology

reserve system: background, 7-8, 13, 28-29n5, 93, 250-53; British Columbia, 68, 344; critiques of, 250-51; demographics, 193n6; East Cree, 258-61; FAS research, 208-11; Indian Act, 250-53; Musqueam, 344; Quebec, 398n6; reserve culture, 251

residential schools, 146-55; abuses, xii, 26, 152-53, 157n8, 302-3, 345-46, 394; apology for, 285n1; Fort Resolution, 148(f); Inuit, 317; legacy, 18-19, 140, 157n7, 165, 186-87, 191, 199, 207, 249, 275, 455; Lejac residential school, 148(f), 149, 157n10; mortality rates, 152, 157n11; Northwest Territories, 317; Saint Mary Residential School at Mission, 157n9; St. Joseph Christian School, 186; system of, xii, 8-10, 25, 28, 142, 147-51, 168, 351, 419-20, 468n9; vocational education, 148(f), 150(f)

Residential Schools Settlement Agreement, 25

resilience, 88-90, 214, 464, 466

resistance, 143-44, 152, 155

restorative justice, 356-57

retraditionalization, 341

Rich, G., 122

Rich, Judith, 119

Richardson, E.H., 66

Richardson, R., 66

rights: Aboriginal, 24, 46, 51, 398n9, 464; human, 27, 46, 115, 135

risk factors, 83-90, 211, 224-28

risky behaviour, 87-88, 93-94, 109-11

rites of passage, 41, 94, 461

ritual: stages of, 344. *See also* ceremonies

Roberts, D., 211

Robinson, G.C., 200, 210

Rochette, L., 17

Rock, Allan, 127-28, 246n1

Rockwood, W., 115-16, 134

Rolling Stones, 378n12

Root, R., 80-100

Ross, R., 357

Round Lake Treatment Center, 350-51

Rowles, G., 145

Roy, C., 60-61

Royal Australian and New Zealand College of Psychiatrists, 36

Royal Canadian Mounted Police (RCMP), 145, 182, 298, 312n7, 316

Royal Commission on Aboriginal Peoples (RCAP): Aboriginal counselling, 342, 351; Aboriginal health reports, 24-25, 87, 193n11, 201, 214, 453; assimilation/relocation, 8, 14; mission of, 275; suicide reports, 25, 117, 121

rural communities, 12, 28-29n5, 237, 385, 391, 394, 396, 403

Ruskin, J., 143

Sack, W.H., 67, 88

Sacred Assembly, 275, 285n2

sage, 360, 364

Sahlins, M., 126

Said, E., 243

Salish, 160-61, 433, 457

Salluit, 293, 295, 308

Sampson, E.E., 327

Samson, C., 109-36, 190

Sapir-Whorf hypothesis, 422

Saskatchewan, 60-61, 73-74n7, 357, 359

Saulteaux, 60-61, 355, 360-62, 367-68

savages, 7, 19, 419-20, 422

Schedule for Affective Disorders and Schizophrenia-Lifetime Version (SADS-L), 63

Scheper-Hughes, N., 136n8

schizophrenia, 14, 44, 49, 60, 132, 300(f)

school, 90-93, 152, 263, 306-7, 309, 316-17. *See also* education; residential schools

Schwarz, M.T., 117

scientific epistemology, xx, 47-49, 338, 428-30, 435, 442

scientific psychology, 425-30, 435

scientism, 429-30

scientology, 429

Scott, J.C., 251

Scott, K., 166

seals/seal industry, 317

Secrétariat aux affaires autochtones (SAA), 384, 398n9

sedentarization: impact, xv, 114-18, 128, 453-54, 461-62; Innu, 136n4; policy and theory, 8, 249-54. *See also* settlements

self-continuity, 83, 222-28

self-definition, 42, 60-62, 71-72, 74n12

self-destruction, 109-11. *See also* suicide

self-determination, 42, 317, 329-30, 423, 424

self-esteem: collective, 19-20; cultural identity, 85, 133, 296; personal, 36, 121, 207, 327, 464

self-government: East Cree, 269n5; Inherent Right to Self-Government Policy, 326; Iroquois Band Council, 403-4, 405-6, 417n3; political autonomy, 84, 116, 239-42, 396, 464; suicide rates, 244-46. *See also* local control

self-help groups, 163, 435

self-identity, 83, 87, 91, 146, 398n14

self-reliance, 459

Seneca, 403

sentencing circles, 26

settlements: arbitrary communities, 8; Cree, 252-53, 258-61; Inuit, 23; Iroquois Confederacy, 403; legacy, 263; Nunavut, 316-17; social theory, 250-53. *See also* reserve system

settler societies, 466

sex industry, 161

sexual abuse: children, 9, 10, 19, 128, 396; counselling victims, 345-46; cycles, 302-3; rates, 6, 16; treatment programs, 394. *See also* residential schools

Shafer, R., 366

shaking tent ceremony, 281-82, 285n3, 286n7

shamans, 257, 281, 296(f), 297, 304, 316, 442, 444-45

Shangana-Tsonga, 94

sharing circles, 26, 98

Sheshatshiu, 109-15, 119, 127-34, 190, 196

Shore, B., 72

Shore, J.H., 62-63

Shushep Mark, 114

Simpson, C., 3-28, 134

Sioux, 59, 66-67, 444

Sioux Lookout, 180, 188, 192n4

Six Nations Band Council, 403-6, 417n3

Six Nations Mental Health Services, 401-17; access, 409-12, 413-15; background/description, xx, 401-9, 415-16; bureaucracy, 412-15; challenges to, 409-12; community relations, 404-6, 459; demographics, 406-7; Early Intervention in Psychosis Program, 406; facility, 402(f), 410(f); impact of health policy, 412-13; operating funds, 404; services offered, 407-8; staffing, 406, 411-12, 415-16

Six Nations of the Grand River. *See* Iroquois/ Iroquois Confederacy

Sixties Scoop, 10, 239, 414

sleep paralysis, 304

Sluyler, Andrew, 157n6

smallpox, 43

Smith, Adam, 126

Smith, D.W., 203

Smith, K., 446

smudging, 359, 360, 364, 417n6

Snow, D.R., 401

social activism, 458-60

social capital, 326

social class/status, 164-65, 453

social cohesion, 120-21, 311

social competence, 81-86

social Darwinism, 58

social definition, 165, 273-74

social engineering, 117, 250-51

social justice, 51-52, 163

social networks, 97, 464

social pathology, 249-53

social psychiatry, 311

social suffering, 3, 166-67, 207, 212-13, 249-53, 311. *See also* spiritual colonization

social workers, xx, 10, 128, 164, 204, 395, 407, 409

socioeconomic health factors, 44-46, 70, 236-42, 303

socioeconomic status (SES), 237

Sokol, B., 83, 84

Tait, C.L., 3-28, 72-73, 196-216
talk therapy, 325, 355, 377n3
talking circles, 26, 450-52
Tanner, A., 249-69, 370, 448
Tanzania, 251
Te Hoe Nuku Roa, 40
Te taura tieke, 50
teasing, 308
technologies of power, 245
Tester, F.J., 310
theft, 308
therapy: addiction-oriented, 112-13, 170-71, 174,
    369, 378n11; behaviour, 342; bilingual, 47-48,
    382, 388, 464; cognitive, 342; culture as, 193-
    94n13, 376; family, 95, 98-99, 342-43, 345, 350-
    51, 434-35; group, 43, 98-99, 342-43, 350-51,
    356, 360-65; logotherapy, 349; mainstream
    approaches, 68, 341-43, 441-45, 458; Mäori
    Hua oranga concept, 49; multiple family group
    therapy (MFGT), 98-99; narrative, 97-98, 365-66;
    resistance to, 362, 372-73; talk therapy, 325,
    355, 377n3; Thought Field Therapy, 429. *See
    also* counselling psychology; psychotherapy;
    treatment programs
Thule people, 315
time, experience of, 39
tobacco, 26, 360
Tobin, Brian, 136n6
Toronto, 109, 405
Torres Strait Islanders: children, 46; demographics,
    44; health determinants, 44-46; language
    diversity, 39; mental health guidelines, 36;
    mortality rates, 46-47; origins, 38; Tree of Life
    concept, 43; workforce development, 49-50
tort claims, 25
trade alliances, 7
trading posts, 253, 257-58, 262, 278
tradition: commodification, 21, 448, 458; gather-
    ings, 261-63, 267-68, 306; as health determin-
    ant, 318; knowledge systems, 39, 43, 68, 191,
    243-44, 263, 297, 320, 440; loss of, 454; re-
    articulation, xiv, xxi, 14, 24-27, 193-94n13,
    263, 340-41, 359; rites of passage, 41, 94,
    461; traditionality scales, 67
traditional healing: access, 409, 411, 415-16;
    methods, 39, 47-49, 193-94n13, 417n6; renais-
    sance, xiii-xiv, 457-60; traditional healers, 386,
    411, 425, 449, 457-58

training: Aboriginal professionals, 47, 49-50, 395-
    96, 401, 406, 411-12, 415-16, 463; community
    wellness, 319-21; employment training pro-
    grams, 193n10, 394; graduate education, 420-
    25, 430-31, 434-35; professional, xx, 162-63,
    394, 415, 424, 432, 440, 463; psychology,
    422-24; relevance, 420, 424-25; suicide inter-
    vention, 178-79, 193n10; top-down, 319-21
trappers/trapping, xiii
trauma: collective/individual, 26, 190; historical
    trauma, xii, 16, 27, 187-88, 452-56, 463; nor-
    malization of self-destruction, 190-91; post-
    traumatic stress disorder (PTSD), 16-17,
    454-55; transgenerational effects, 452-55;
    trauma theory, 26-27, 455-56
treaties and agreements: Health Transfer, 326,
    384, 405; history, xi, 45, 449, 454, 459; Innu
    land claims, 113, 118, 135n3; James Bay and
    Northern Quebec, 254, 260-61, 286n5, 312n7,
    382, 384, 385, 459; military treaties, 7; North-
    ern Flood Agreement, 178; residential schools,
    25; treaty Indians, 60, 74n12, 197-98
treatment programs: alcohol/substance abuse,
    252, 328-29, 340-41, 347-51, 362, 408; Associa-
    tion of BC First Nations Treatment Programs,
    345-46; best practices, 243-46; biculturalism,
    47-49, 337, 343-44; British Columbia, 340-46,
    350-51; community-based, 350-51, 365, 448;
    cultural sensitivity, 47-50, 274, 337, 340-44,
    359, 390, 416, 463; evidence-based, 415-16;
    Eyaa-Keen Centre, 458, 468n11; family support,
    95, 98-99, 342-43, 345, 350-51, 434-35; main-
    stream health services, 174, 347-49, 390, 396,
    458; McGill Aboriginal Healing Clinic, 394;
    Medicine House, 355-62, 364-65, 372, 375-76,
    377n1, 377nn6-7, 378n14; outpatient, 163, 171;
    physical and sexual abuse, 345-46; posttraumat-
    ic stress disorder (PTSD), 458; psychosis, 406,
    408; residential, 163, 171, 355-78, 377n7; St.
    John's children's treatment program, 128-29;
    suicide intervention, 178-79, 193n10, 347;
    12-step programs, 359. *See also* Medicine
    House; Six Nations Mental Health Services
tribes, 40, 221, 229, 427, 460. *See also* bands; First
    Nations
trickster myth, 465-67, 467n3
Trimble, J., 71, 338
truancy, 95

Truth and Reconciliation Commission, 25
Tshakapesh, Simeon, 127-28
Tshikapisk Foundation, 136n11
Tshiskutamashun, 129, 133
tuberculosis, 6, 8, 316
Tulugardjuk, , Lucy, 323
Turnbull, C.M., 269n2
Tuscarora, 403
Tutchone, 269n3

unemployment, 6, 208
United Nations Permanent Forum on Indigenous
    Issues, 51
United States Congress, 424
United States Indian policy, 419-20
University of Illinois, 434
urbanization: adaptation, 12-13, 460; cosmopol-
    itanism, 467; health and social services, xx,
    390-91, 394; industrial development, xv, 118-21,
    186-87, 249, 447; Mäori, 40; morality, 12, 27-28;
    urban migration, 13, 28-29n5; urban networks,
    161
Utah State University, 423
Utshimassits, 109-10, 119, 120

Valaskakis, G.G., xxii, 440-68
Vallee, F., 297-98, 312n6, 312n10
values, shared, 68, 440, 452, 467
van Gennep, A., 344
Vancouver, BC, 160-75; Aboriginal health, 162-63;
    demographics, 160-62; Health and Home Pro-
    ject, 163-74, 174-75nn1-3; Musqueam Reserve,
    344; narratives, 166-73; poverty and health,
    163-65
Vancouver Island, 344
Vancouver/Richmond Health Board, 161
vandalism, 122
victims, and blame, 458-60
vigilantism, 377n4
villages, Innu, 116-17
villagization, 251
violation, sense of, 42
violence: colonial, 152-53; cultural discontinuity,
    84; domestic, 143-46, 155; history of, 452-55;
    interpersonal, 14, 116-17, 174, 252, 273, 303,
    318; mental health symptoms, 300(f)
Vision Quest, 339-40, 343
visions/dreams, 443

vocational counselling, 337, 346, 352, 407, 422-
    23, 425
vocational education, 148(f), 150(f), 407, 422-23,
    425
Voisey's Bay, 119-20
voting rights, 24

Wabano Centre for Aboriginal Health, 390
Wachowich, N., 317
Waldram, J.B., 56-74, 134, 205-6, 359, 365, 376
"walking out" ceremony, 262-63
Walter, E.V., 141-43, 151
Walton, W.G., 278
Ward, J.A., 180
Ward, S.C., 420
warriors, 91, 365-66, 378n10, 461
Warry, W., 325
Waseskun Healing Centre, 383
Waswanipi, 262, 263
Watkins, Edwin, 278
Watt-Cloutier, Sheila, 292
Watt, R., 289-312
Ways Forward, 42
Weisner, T.S., 59
Weiss, L., 173
welfare, 114, 197-98
well-being: collective, 116; connectedness, 311;
    country food, 293-95, 309; Cree notion of, 448;
    and culture, xi-xii; family-centered, 320; holistic
    perspective, 42, 162-63, 295, 338, 392, 427,
    443; hunting and camping, 293, 295-96; well-
    ness philosophy, 392, 427, 466-67. *See also*
    community wellness; mental health
Wemigwans, J., 213
Wente, M., 196, 204
Werner, H., 99-100
Westermeyer, J.J., 66
Western Australian Aboriginal Child Health
    Survey, 45
Western education, 421-22
Western ethnotheories, 427
Western Identification Scale, 65
whaling, 286n5, 293-94, 316
Whapmagoostui community, 117, 276-85,
    286nn5-6
Whitbeck, L.B., 453-55
White, R., 136n4
White Paper on Indian Act, 11-12

Printed and bound in Canada by Friesens
Set in Amerigo and Antique Olive by Artegraphica Design Co. Ltd.
Copy editor: Robert Lewis
Proofreader: Lesley Erickson
Indexer: Lillian Ashworth